Atlas of PET/CT in Oncology - Volume 1

Zhiming Yao • Sijin Li
Editors

Atlas of PET/CT in Oncology - Volume 1

Brain, Head and Neck Cancers

PEOPLE'S MEDICAL PUBLISHING HOUSE
PMPH

Springer

Editors
Zhiming Yao
Nuclear Medicine
Beijing Hospital, National Center of Gerontology, Institute of Geriatric Medicine, Chinese Academy of Medical Sciences
Beijing, China

Sijin Li
Nuclear Medicine
First Hospital of Shanxi Medical University
Taiyuan, Shanxi, China

ISBN 978-981-99-1171-4 ISBN 978-981-99-1172-1 (eBook)
https://doi.org/10.1007/978-981-99-1172-1

Jointly published with People's Medical Publishing House, PR of China

This Springer imprint is published by the registered company Springer Nature Singapore Pte Ltd.
The registered company address is: 152 Beach Road, #21-01/04 Gateway East, Singapore 189721, Singapore

Foreword

As an important part of medical imaging, PET/CT plays an increasingly significant role in molecular imaging in precision medicine. Its advantages and clinical value have been gradually recognized, and it has been widely used in clinical practice. Every year, millions of patients around the world (nearly 900,000 cases/year in China) receive early, accurate diagnosis and precise treatment after PET/CT examination, this benefits patients, their families, and society.

The medical technology is advancing and the knowledge is changing with each passing day. Doctors, technicians, and graduate students of nuclear medicine, clinicians urgently need to further comprehensively and systematically master PET/CT-related knowledge and its clinical application value.

In order to adapt to the rapid development of nuclear medicine in China and meet the needs of medical staff, we organized 171 first-line outstanding nuclear medicine experts and scholars from 27 university hospitals and 16 first-class hospitals at Grade 3 in China, and we carefully selected the best and most complete cases from our respective units to compile this *Atlas of PET/CT in Oncology* composed of four volumes, which lasted 2 years. *Atlas of PET/CT in Oncology* consists of four volumes, which are Volume of Nerve and Head and Neck Tumors, Volume of Thoracic Tumors, Volume of Abdominal and Pelvic Tumors, and Volume of Lymph and Blood and Bone Soft Tissue Tumors. Each volume has its own chapters with different tumors, with imaging analysis of typical cases as the main line, integrating PET/CT expertise, clinical, imaging, and pathology-related content. The specific contents include: clinical overview, PET/CT diagnostic points, typical and atypical imaging manifestations, and PET/CT manifestations of diseases that are easily confused. This book is mainly FDG PET images, with some PET images of multiple imaging agents; mainly common tumors, with some rare tumors. Each volume is relatively independent and interrelated, with rich content and clear images.

The purpose of this book is to focus on clinical practice, meet clinical needs, and improve the ability of image analysis. In the process of writing, we kept emphasizing the novelty, practicability, readability, and comprehensiveness and systematicness of knowledge. Our original intention is to offer you a comprehensive, systematic, and exquisite desk book. After the publication of the Chinese version of this Atlas, we were invited by Springer Publishing House to publish the English version. We are very happy to share this Atlas with more readers. We believe it will bring pleasant surprises to our readers!

Thanks to the experts for their precious time, valuable experience, and intelligence for the writing of the book. We would like to pay tribute to their meticulous work style and academic attitude!

Beijing, China — Zhiming Yao
Taiyuan, Shanxi, China — Sijin Li

Preface I

With the continuous development and promotion of PET/CT technology, more and more attention has been paid to its clinical application. To correctly interpret the molecular imaging of PET/CT examination, nuclear medicine physicians should have solid clinical knowledge and other skills, including the professional diagnostic ability of nuclear medicine and radiology imaging. PET/CT perfectly combines metabolic imaging with anatomical structure imaging, which is of great value in the diagnosis, staging, and curative effect monitoring of tumors. Therefore, tumor imaging has become the most important application of PET/CT. Due to the variety of tumors and complicated imaging manifestations, qualified PET/CT interpreter is required to have extensive experience and vision for PET/CT signs and diagnosis of all kinds of tumors. The series of Atlas of PET/CT in Oncology compiled by Professor Zhiming Yao and Professor Sijin Li include detailed tumor PET/CT images provided by PET/CT diagnostic experts from 33 hospitals in China. It systematically displays and summarizes PET/CT examination mode, imaging characteristics of PET and CT in various tumors, as well as key points of differential diagnosis of tumors. This atlas will become an excellent reference book for clinicians such as tumor PET/CT diagnostic experts, oncologists, radiologists to inquire systematically, quickly grasp the imaging characteristics and apply PET/CT for tumor diagnosis. It is my great honor to recommend this series of books, and sincerely hope that it will be helpful to your clinical work.

Xi'an, China | Jing Wang

Preface II

PET/CT is currently the most mature equipment in molecular imaging. The world's commercial PET/CT came out in May 2001, and then the first PET/CT was introduced in Chinese mainland in 2002. According to the data of *National Nuclear Medicine Survey Results Briefing in 2020* released by the Chinese Society of Nuclear Medicine, the number of positron imaging equipment has reached 427 sets, including 404 sets of PET/CT, 23 sets of PET/MR, and 71 sets of domestic equipment, and they are distributed in 391 medical institutions in 31 provinces, municipalities directly under the Central Government and autonomous regions in Chinese mainland, 68.8% of which belong to nuclear medicine departments, and the rest in medical imaging departments, independent PET/CT centers, and radiology departments. The total number of annual PET/CT examinations is nearly 850,000 cases, of which more than 800,000 cases are tumor imaging, accounting for 94.5%.

One-time whole-body PET/CT imaging determines the holistic and interdisciplinary diagnostic model of PET/CT. Therefore, the doctors engaged in PET/CT diagnosis are interdisciplinary talents, who should not only have extensive medical clinical and imaging expertise, but also have profound diagnostic skills in various specialties. Since PET/CT is mainly used for tumor imaging, it is very important for PET/CT doctors to be familiar with the characteristics, diagnosis, and differential diagnosis of PET/CT tumor imaging.

The atlas approach is particularly suitable for imaging medicine, where diagnosis is based on images. The series of *Atlas of PET/CT in Oncology* (four volumes), compiled by Professor Zhiming Yao, Professor Sijin Li, and other PET/CT experts with clinical experience in China mainland, are the first systematic PET/CT atlas in the field of oncology in China, with a total of 902 cases. Each case contains not only a brief medical history and relevant imaging and pathology data collected as much as possible, but also a brief analysis of the case with reference to monographs and historical documents, which highlights the PET/CT sign of tumors of each system, the key points of diagnosis and the characteristics of the lesions that need to be identified.

The authors hope this systematic Atlas of PET/CT in Oncology compiled in Chinese become a desk book of PET/CT diagnosticians, a PET/CT tool for clinicians for a quick reference, a reference book for clinical oncology and radiotherapy physicians to systematically understand the application of PET/CT in tumor diagnosis and treatment. Now, at the invitation of Springer Publishing House, the English version of *PET/CT Atlas of Tumor* will be published, making it available to readers around the world. I hope and believe that it will help scholars from the East and the West to exchange experiences, learn from each other's strengths, so as to improve the clinical application level of PET/CT, promote the training of professional talents, and promote the development of imaging medicine.

Beijing, China — Wanying Qu

Preface III

PET/CT is an advanced technology. It is a molecular imaging that combines pathology, morphology, and functional metabolism. It has been greatly developed in recent years. Although China's PET/CT is not the first to start, with the development of science and technology, China already has 23 PET/MR sets and 404 PET/CT sets as of December 31, 2019. PET examinations are well received by clinicians and they have accumulated a certain experience.

The series of *Atlas of PET/CT in Oncology* compiled by Professor Zhiming Yao, Professor Sijin Li, and experts from 33 hospitals in China is the first systematic PET/CT Atlas in the field of oncology in China. With a practical and realistic professional attitude, they have systematically summarized the PET/CT image characteristics of various tumors, which has good use value and academic value. It is really commendable.

Beijing, China Xiujie Liu

Acknowledgments

We would like to thank all the contributors to the book, who are identified by their contributions. We wish to acknowledge the staff of the Departments of Nuclear Medicine at Beijing Hospital and The First Hospital of Shanxi Medical University, and Royal Philips for their assistance during the preparation of this book.

Contents

Editors and Contributors

About the Editors

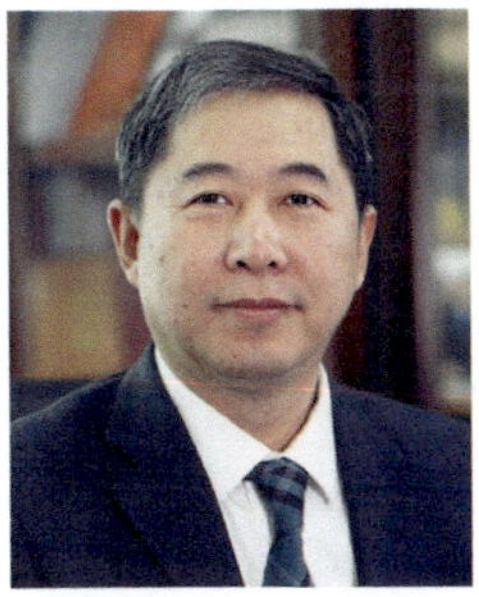

Sijin Li, MD, PhD, served as the Former President of the Chinese Society of Nuclear Medicine. Currently, he holds the position of Director, Professor in the Department of Nuclear Medicine at the First Hospital of Shanxi Medical University. He serves as the Chief Editor of *Chinese Journal of Nuclear Medicine and Molecular Imaging*.

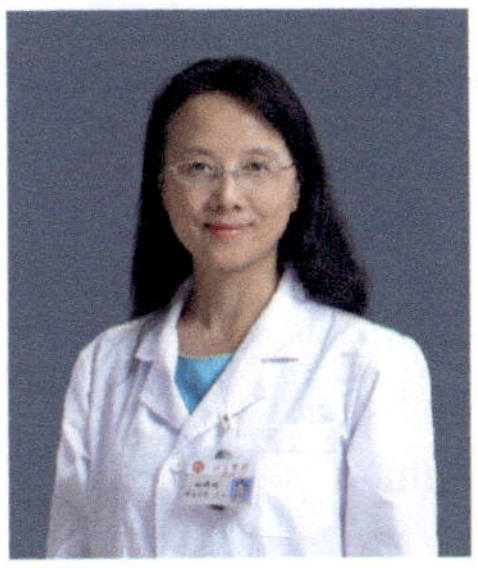

Zhiming Yao, MD, PhD, is the Chief expert, Professor in the Department of Nuclear Medicine at Beijing Hospital, National Center of Gerontology, Institute of Geriatric Medicine, Chinese Academy of Medical Sciences.

She is a member of the Standing Committee in the Chinese Society of Nuclear Medicine. She holds the position of Vice President within the Committee of Nuclear Medicine Equipment and Professional Technology, China Association of Medical Equipment. She is an Executive Editorial Board Member of the *Chinese Journal of Nuclear Medicine and Molecular Imaging*.

Chief Editor

Zhiming Yao, MD, PhD Beijing Hospital, National Center of Gerontology, Institute of Geriatric Medicine, Chinese Academy of Medical Sciences, Beijing, China

Sijin Li, MD, PhD Shanxi Medical University, Molecular Imaging Precision Diagnosis and Treatment Collaborative Innovation Center, Taiyuan, Shanxi, China

Consultant

Yaming Li, MD, PhD The First Hospital of China Medical University, Shenyang, Liaoning, China

Associate Editor

Hao Xu, MD, PhD The First Affiliated Hospital of Jinan University, Guangzhou, Guangdong, China

Wei Fan, MD, PhD Sun Yat-sen University Cancer Center, Guangzhou, Guangdong, China

Guoren Yang, MD Shandong Cancer Hospital, Jinan, Shandong, China

Yuetao Wang, MD, PhD The First People's Hospital of Changzhou, The Third Affiliated Hospital of Soochow University, Changzhou Key Laboratory of Molecular Imaging, Changzhou, Jiangsu, China

Editorial Board Member

Lin Ai, MD Beijing Tiantan Hospital, Capital Medical University, Beijing, China

Weibing Miao, MD, PhD The First Affiliated Hospital of Fujian Medical University, Fuzhou, Fujian, China

Xiaoli Lan, MD, PhD Union Hospital, Tongji Medical College, Huazhong University of Science and Technology, Wuhan, Hubei, China

Zhenguang Wang, MD, PhD The Affiliated Hospital of Qingdao University, Qingdao, Shandong, China

Linfa Li, MD, PhD Cancer Hospital of the University of Chinese Academy of Sciences, Hangzhou, Zhejiang, China

Contributors

Lin Ai Beijing Tiantan Hospital, Capital Medical University, Beijing, China

Congxia Chen Beijing Hospital, National Center of Gerontology, Institute of Geriatric Medicine, Chinese Academy of Medical Sciences, Beijing, China

Shaoming Chen The First Affiliated Hospital of Fujian Medical University, Fuzhou, Fujian, China

Wei Fan Sun Yat-sen University Cancer Center, Guangzhou, Guangdong, China

Shui Jin Zhejiang Cancer Hospital, Hangzhou, Zhejiang, China

Xiaoli Lan Union Hospital, Tongji Medical College, Huazhong University of Science and Technology, Wuhan, Hubei, China

Dacheng Li The Affiliated Hospital of Qingdao University, Qingdao, Shandong, China

Linfa Li Cancer Hospital of the University of Chinese Academy of Sciences, Hangzhou, Zhejiang, China

Xueying Ling The First Affiliated Hospital of Jinan University, Guangzhou, Guangdong, China

Xiaoping Lin Sun Yat-sen University Cancer Center, Guangzhou, Guangdong, China

Bin Long Zhejiang Cancer Hospital, Hangzhou, Zhejiang, China

Tingting Lu Shandong Cancer Hospital, Jinan, Shandong, China

Yaping Luo Department of Nuclear Medicine, Peking Union Medical College Hospital, Chinese Academy of Medical Sciences, Beijing, China

Weibing Miao The First Affiliated Hospital of Fujian Medical University, Fuzhou, Fujian, China

Rong Niu The First People's Hospital of Changzhou, Changzhou, Jiangsu, China

Weiqiang Pang Zhejiang Cancer Hospital, Hangzhou, Zhejiang, China

Chun Qiu The First People's Hospital of Changzhou, Changzhou, Jiangsu, China

Xiaoliang Shao The First People's Hospital of Changzhou, Changzhou, Jiangsu, China

Yuetao Wang Changzhou Key Laboratory of Molecular Imaging, The First People's Hospital of Changzhou, The Third Affiliated Hospital of Soochow University, Changzhou, Jiangsu, China

Yun Wang Zhejiang Cancer Hospital, Hangzhou, Zhejiang, China

Zhenguang Wang The Affiliated Hospital of Qingdao University, Qingdao, Shandong, China

Hao Xu The First Affiliated Hospital of Jinan University, Guangzhou, Guangdong, China

Guoren Yang Shandong Cancer Hospital, Jinan, Shandong, China

Xuemei Ye Zhejiang Cancer Hospital, Hangzhou, Zhejiang, China

Feifei Zhang The First People's Hospital of Changzhou, Changzhou, Jiangsu, China

Jie Zhang Union Hospital Affiliated to Tongji Medical College of Huazhong University of Science and Technology, Wuhan, Hubei, China

Shan Zheng The First Affiliated Hospital of Fujian Medical University, Fuzhou, Fujian, China

Zhiming Yao Department of Nuclear Medicine, Beijing Hospital, National Center of Gerontology, Institute of Geriatric Medicine, Chinese Academy of Medical Sciences, Beijing, China

Academic Secretary

Wen Chen Beijing Hospital, National Center of Gerontology, Institute of Geriatric Medicine, Chinese Academy of Medical Sciences, Beijing, China

Xinzhong Hao The First Hospital of Shanxi Medical University, Shanxi, China

Wenchan Li Beijing Hospital, National Center of Gerontology, Institute of Geriatric Medicine, Chinese Academy of Medical Sciences, Beijing, China

Ping Wu The First Hospital of Shanxi Medical University, Shanxi, China

Hui Zhu Beijing Hospital, National Center of Gerontology, Institute of Geriatric Medicine, Chinese Academy of Medical Sciences, Beijing, China

Part I

PET/CT of Central Nervous System Neoplasms

General Introduction

1

Hao Xu

1 Clinicopathological Overview

1.1 Intracranial Tumors

Intracranial tumors are generally classified into either primary or secondary tumors, accounting for 1–2% of all adult malignancies. Primary tumors may originate from brain tissue, meninges, cranial nerves, blood vessels, pituitary gland, embryonic remnant tissue, etc. Secondary tumors develop when malignant tumors metastasize or invade into the brain from other organs. Intracranial tumors can occur at any age, mainly at the age of 20–50 years. In children and adolescents, tumors are more common in the midline of the posterior fossa, such as medulloblastoma, craniopharyngioma, and pineal area tumors. Glioma is commonly seen in adult patients, followed by meningioma, pituitary tumor, schwannoma, primary central nervous system lymphoma, etc. In elderly patients, glioma and brain metastases are common. There was no significant gender difference in the incidence of primary intracranial tumors. Intracranial tumors have a poor prognosis, hence being the second cause of death in adult neurological diseases. The morbidity and mortality of children's brain tumors are the second most common systemic tumors in children.

The etiology of intracranial tumors has not been fully elucidated, and the possible precipitating factors include genetic, physical, chemical, and biological factors. Clinical manifestations of most brain tumors are symptoms caused by intracranial hypertension; tumor infiltration and destruction of the brain; brain localization symptoms caused by cerebral nerves, including mild hemiplegia, aphasia, and convulsions; as well as mental symptoms such as personality and behavior changes, visual or auditory hallucinations, and aculalia. The incidence and duration of neurological symptoms and signs caused by brain tumors vary with the type and location of the tumor.

The pathological classification of intracranial tumors is mainly based on the histological features of the tumors. In 2007, tumors of the central nervous system (CNS) were classified into seven types, viz., tumors of neuroepithelial tissue, tumors of cranial and paraspinal nerves, tumors of the meninges, lymphomas and hematopoietic neoplasms, germ cell tumors, tumors of the sellar region, and metastatic tumors. In 2016, the World Health Organization (WHO) issued a new classification of CNS tumors, which for the first time used molecular features in addition to histology to define CNS tumor entities. In comparison with the 2007 CNS WHO classifications, major changes of the 2016 update concluded the following: (1) formulating concept of how CNS tumor diagnoses are structured in the molecular era; (2) major restructuring of diffuse gliomas, with incorporation of genetically defined entities; (3) major restructuring of medulloblastomas, with incorporation of genetically defined entities; and (4) major restructuring of other embryonal tumors, with incorporation of genetically defined entities and removal of the term "primitive neuroectodermal tumor."

1.2 Intraspinal Tumors

Intraspinal tumors account for 10–20% of the CNS tumors and are classified into primary and secondary types. Primary intraspinal tumors are those that originate in the spine, including spinal cord, nerves, blood vessels, maters, adipose tissues, and bony structure. They are important components of the CNS tumors. Secondary intraspinal tumors mainly refer to systemic malignant tumors that spread into the spinal canal via blood or brain tumors that metastasize into the spinal canal via cerebrospinal fluid.

Based on the location of the tumor in relation to the spinal cord, intraspinal tumors are classified into three groups: extradural tumors, intradural extramedullary tumors, and intramedullary tumors. Most of the intraspinal tumors are

H. Xu (✉)
The First Affiliated Hospital of Jinan University, Guangzhou, Guangdong, China
e-mail: txh@jnu.edu.cn

Z. Yao, S. Li (eds.), *Atlas of PET/CT in Oncology - Volume 1*, https://doi.org/10.1007/978-981-99-1172-1_1

benign and gross total resection is the preferred treatment approach. Although the prognosis for most of postoperative patients is good, surgical outcomes will still be affected by many factors. For patients receiving incomplete tumor resection during the operation, there is still no consensus on the postoperative adjuvant therapy.

2 Clinical Application of PET/CT

2.1 Intracranial Tumors

Imaging findings of ^{18}F-FDG PET/CT in intracranial tumors mainly show the CT feature of lesions and the uptake level of ^{18}F-FDG which is related to the metabolic activity of glucose in tumor cells. For example, high-grade gliomas have a high degree of malignancy and abnormally high metabolic activity of glucose. ^{18}F-FDG PET imaging shows markedly high uptake in lesions, viz., hypermetabolic lesions. The uptake of ^{18}F-FDG in the lesions is higher than that in the white matter and close to or higher than that in the gray matter. On the other hand, low-grade gliomas have a low degree of malignancy, grow slowly, and have low metabolic activity of glucose, i.e., on ^{18}F-FDG PET imaging, they show low FDG uptake, and the uptake of ^{18}F-FDG in the lesions is lower than or close to that in the white matter. Nevertheless, some benign gliomas, such as pilocytic astrocytoma and ganglioglioma, may also show high uptake of ^{18}F-FDG. Hence, in patients with intracranial space-occupying lesions suspected to be glioma, if ^{18}F-FDG PET imaging shows markedly high uptake in lesion, with peritumoral edema and space-occupying effect on CT scan, high-grade gliomas can be considered. On the contrary, in patients with low-grade gliomas, ^{18}F-FDG PET imaging shows unremarkable uptake in lesion, no or mild peritumoral edema, and usually unremarkable space-occupying effect on CT scan. Gliomas should be differentiated from metastatic brain tumors and intracranial lymphomas. In the metastatic brain tumors, multiple lesions are commonly seen, which may be small ones, but the peritumoral edema is remarkable, some of which have a ring-shaped zone of radioactivity. Most of the primary tumor lesions in patients with metastatic brain tumors can be detected by PET/CT imaging. The lesions of intracranial lymphoma frequently arise in the midline of the brain, have intense uptake of ^{18}F-FDG and mild peritumoral edema, and commonly present as multiple lesions.

Different types of intracranial tumors have various imaging appearance. The imaging assessment of the tumors includes determining their properties, possible grades or margins, and follow-up of therapeutic effects. Currently, the imaging methods mainly include CT, MRI, PET/CT, PET/MRI, etc. ^{18}F-FDG PET/CT can be used to differentiate the recurrence and radiation necrosis after the treatment of malignant gliomas, assess the treatment response, predict the prognosis, make a diagnosis of low-grade gliomas or their malignant transformation, make a differential diagnosis of their recurrence, select the location of tumor biopsy, and delineate the radiation field.

Principles of CNS tumor imaging recommended by the National Comprehensive Cancer Network (NCCN) Guidelines (CNS tumor part) are as follows: (1) MRI is a gold standard for diagnosing brain tumors. (2) CT is recommended when MRI is contraindicated (e.g., patients with claustrophobia and in vivo implant). (3) MR spectroscopy (MRS) assesses metabolites within tumors and normal tissue. MRS may be useful in differentiating tumor from radiation necrosis or tumor recurrence. MRS may be helpful in grading tumors or assessing response. The area most abnormal in MRS would be the best place to target for a biopsy. (4) MRI perfusion measures cerebral blood volume in tumors. It may be useful in differentiating grade of tumor or tumor versus radiation necrosis and area of highest perfusion would be the best place. (5) ^{18}F-FDG PET scanning assesses metabolism within tumor and normal tissue by using radiolabeled tracers. It may be useful in differentiating tumor from radiation necrosis or tumor recurrence. It may also correlate with tumor grade or provide the optimal area for biopsy.

2.2 Intraspinal Tumors

^{18}F-FDG PET/CT is not commonly used for the diagnosis of intraspinal tumors due to its non-special performance, whereas MRI is the main technique for detecting the tumors. MRI without and with contrast is the most valuable technique for diagnosing intraspinal tumors in clinical practice. Basically, MRI is used to determine the location of tumors, such as extramedullary, intramedullary, epidural, or extramedullary subdural tumors. Also, it can be used to distinguish bone-to-soft tissue interfaces, compressive or invasive bone destruction, and the degree of nerve or paravertebral tissue involvement. As for MRI sequences, T_2WI and contrast-enhanced T_1WI are the most valuable for diagnosing intraspinal tumors, both of which can well demonstrate the external and internal features of the tumors. CT imaging can be used to show the degree of bone destruction in detail. For those who are contraindicated to MRI studies, CT with contrast can be used to better diagnose the tumors. The traditional posteroanterior, lateral, and flexion-extension radiographs of the spine still have unique diagnostic advantages in determining the presence/absence of spinal instability or spinal deformity. As the recently introduced techniques for multimodal molecular imaging in clinical practice, PET/MRI and PET/CT-MRI may have more clinical value for preoperatively evaluating the intraspinal tumors.

2 PET/CT of Gliomas

Lin Ai

Primary tumors of the brain parenchyma are thought to be derived from pluripotent neural stem cells. Gliomas are tumors originating from glial cells. Currently, the 2016 WHO classification of CNS tumors has been widely accepted. Currently, ^{18}F-FDG is a frequently used tracer. In general, the metabolic activity of low-grade gliomas is lower than that of normal gray matter, while the metabolic activity of high-grade gliomas is close to or higher than that of normal gray matter. Nevertheless, the ^{18}F-FDG metabolic activities in gliomas of different grades overlap greatly. Tumor imaging with amino acid tracers provides good lesion-to-background contrast and is superior to that with ^{18}F-FDG in assessing the grade of gliomas. Still, there are certain overlaps of amino acid metabolic activities in these gliomas.

1 Low-Grade Diffuse Astrocytomas

Low-grade astrocytomas are well differentiated but grow invasively, with poorly defined margins and relatively slow growth. Astrocyte-derived tumors are predisposed to become malignant. About two-thirds of low-grade astrocytomas occur in the supratentorial region of the brain, most of which are in the frontotemporal lobe. About 20% of the tumors involve deep gray matter nuclei, especially the thalamus. About a third of the tumors are located in the infratentorial region. Low-grade astrocytomas account for 50% of pediatric brainstem tumors, most of which are located in the pons and less in the medulla oblongata. The astrocytomas sometimes have cystic changes and calcification and generally rare bleeding. Microscopically, the tumors are diffusely infiltrated and densely packed and have mild to moderate nuclear atypia but little or no mitosis. ^{18}F-FDG PET shows the degree of radioactive tracer uptake in low-grade gliomas is close to that in normal white matter, while ^{11}C-MET brain imaging shows mildly to moderately increased metabolism in the tumors (Figs. 2.1, 2.2, and 2.3). The differential diagnosis mainly includes anaplastic astrocytoma, oligodendroglioma, cerebral ischemia, and encephalitis.

L. Ai (✉)
Beijing Tiantan Hospital, Capital Medical University,
Beijing, China

Z. Yao, S. Li (eds.), *Atlas of PET/CT in Oncology - Volume 1*, https://doi.org/10.1007/978-981-99-1172-1_2

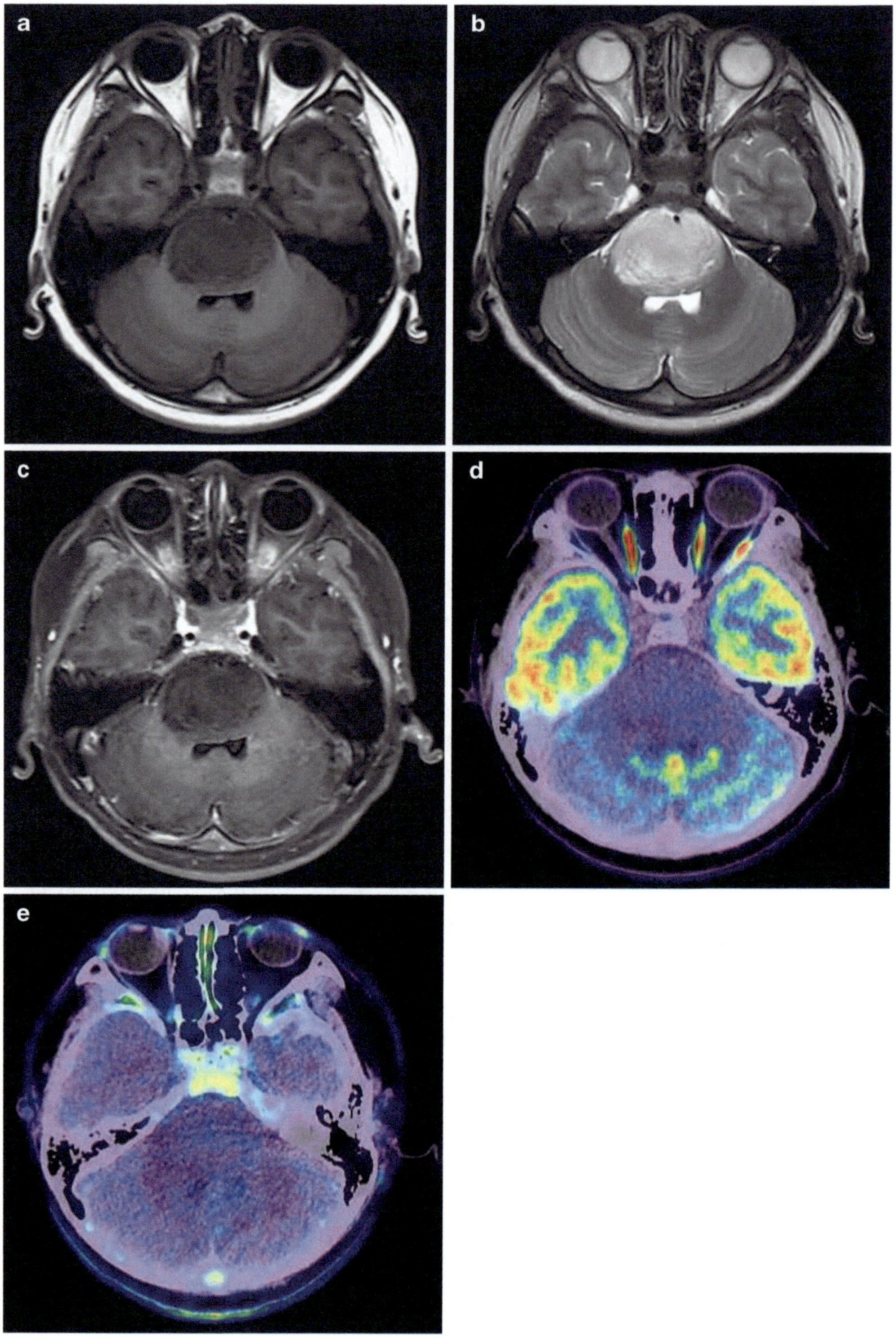

Fig. 2.1 Low-grade diffuse astrocytomas of the brainstem (Grade I). (**a–c**) T_1WI, T_2WI, and contrast-enhanced T_1WI sequences of MRI. The pons are remarkably swollen and the compressed fourth ventricle becomes smaller and the mass is not enhanced by contrast-enhanced imaging. (**d**) ^{18}F-FDG PET imaging. Only mild uptake of the radioactive tracer in lesion of the pons. (**e**) ^{11}C-MET PET. Unremarkable uptake of the radioactive tracer in lesion of the pons

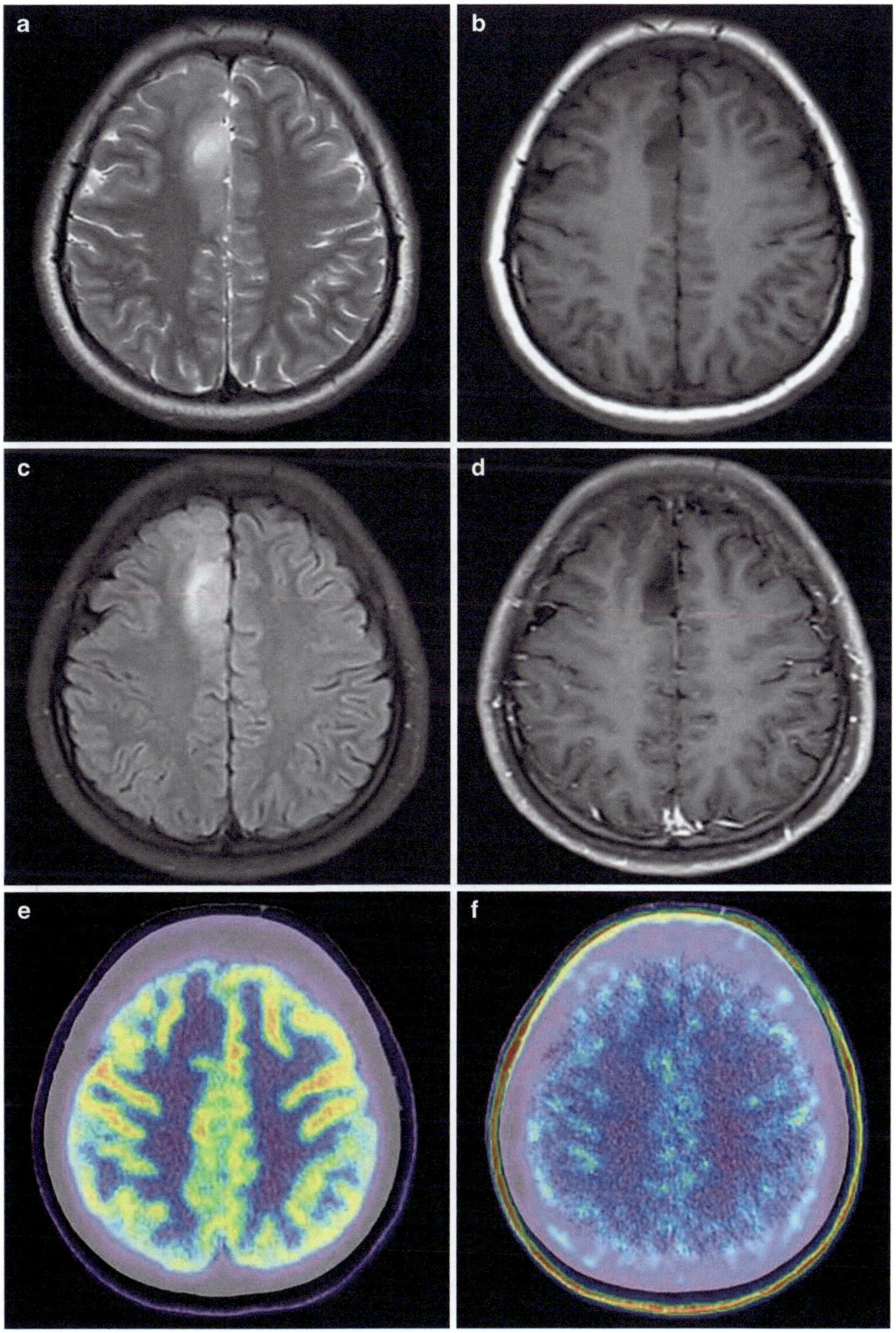

Fig. 2.2 Low-grade diffuse astrocytomas (Grade I). (**a–d**) T_2WI, T_1WI, FLAIR, and contrast-enhanced T_1WI sequences of MRI. Poorly defined margins of the mass in the right frontal cortex, focal gyral swelling, disappearance of the sulcus, and no enhancement on the MRI. (**e**, **f**) ^{18}F-FDG PET and ^{11}C-MET PET. The metabolic activity of both glucose and methionine is significantly lower in the lesions than that in the cortical

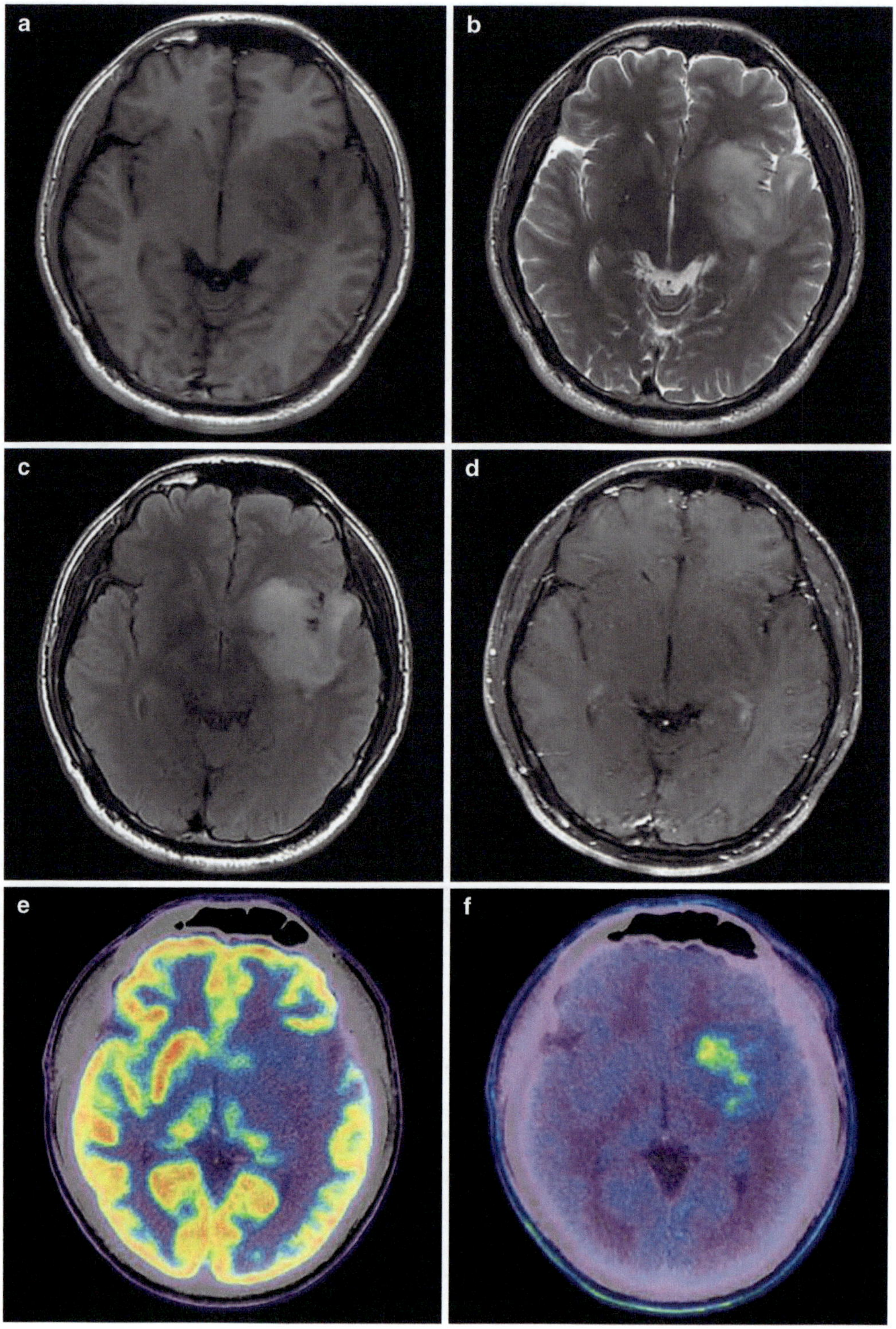

Fig. 2.3 Low-grade diffuse astrocytomas (Grade II). (**a–d**) T_1WI, T_2WI, FLAIR, and contrast-enhanced T_1WI sequences of MRI show diffuse masses in left frontal, temporal, and insular lobes, with poorly defined margins and no remarkable enhancement by contrast-enhanced imaging. (**e**, **f**) ^{18}F-FDG PET and ^{11}C-MET PET: a mildly increased metabolic activity of glucose in the lesion and a significantly increased metabolic activity of methionine in the insular lobe part of lesion

2 Oligodendrogliomas

Most oligodendrogliomas occur in the cortex and subcortex. They are well-differentiated, slow-growing, but diffusely infiltrating tumors. Of these tumors, 85–90% are located in the supratentorial region, most common (50–65%) in the frontal lobe, followed by the parietal lobe, temporal lobe, and occipital lobe, while rare in the posterior cranial fossa and spinal cord. Tumor calcification is frequently noted. In the brain imaging, the ^{18}F-FDG uptake of the tumor is close to that of the white matter, while the ^{11}C-MET uptake of the tumor is significantly increased (Figs. 2.4, 2.5, and 2.6). The differential diagnosis mainly includes low-grade diffuse astrocytomas, ganglioglioma, encephalitis, and cerebral ischemia.

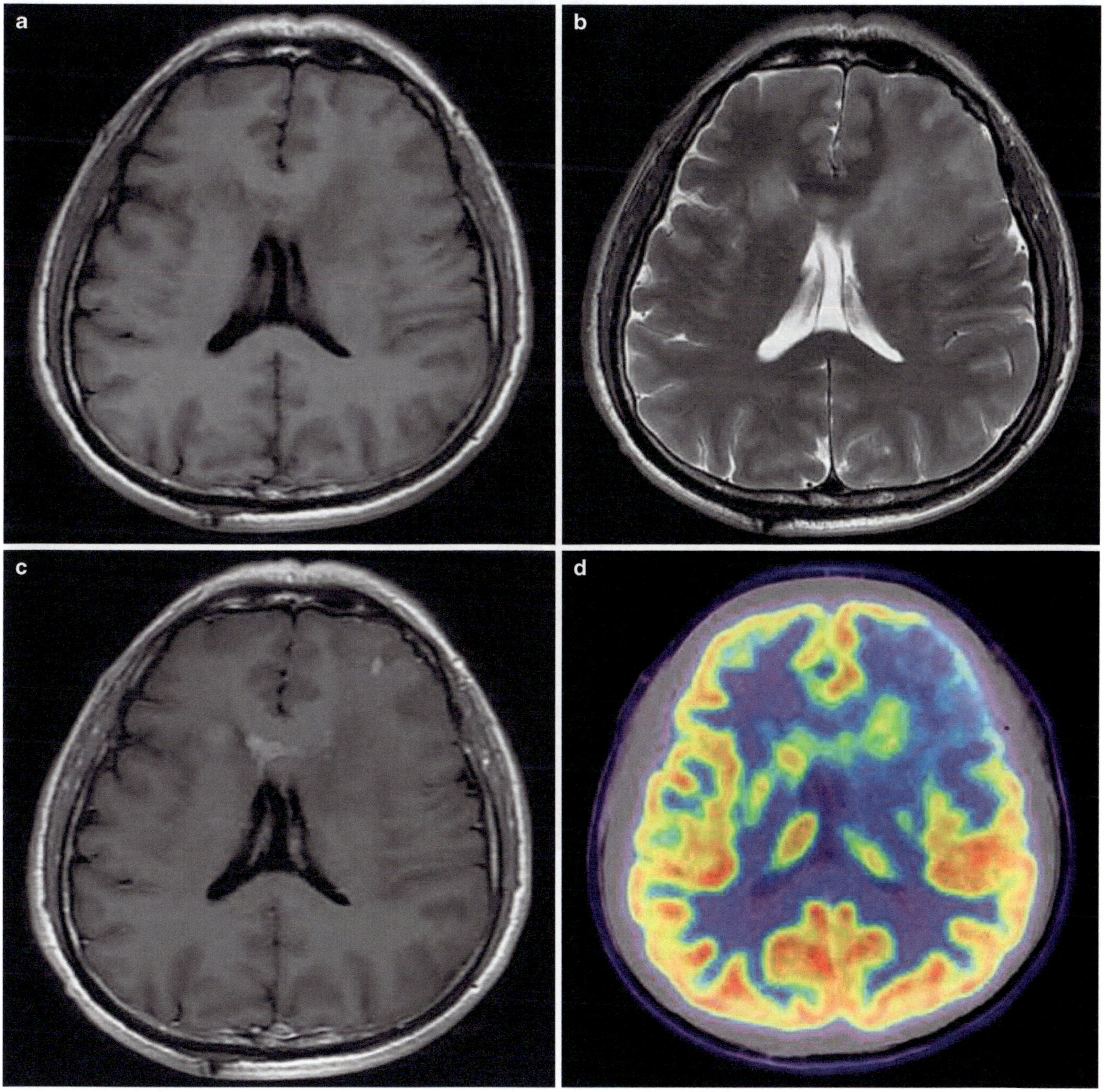

Fig. 2.4 Oligodendrogliomas (Grade III). (**a–c**) MRI T_1WI, T_2WI, and contrast-enhanced T_1WI MR sequences. Diffuse long T_1 and T_2 signals noted in the mass of bilateral foreheads (predominant left side) and the knee of the corpus callosum, with heterogeneous signals, poorly defined margins, and patchy enhancement within the lesion by contrast-enhanced imaging. (**d**) ^{18}F-FDG PET. Compared with the white matter, the lesion shows generally increased metabolic activity of glucose and more significantly in partial regions

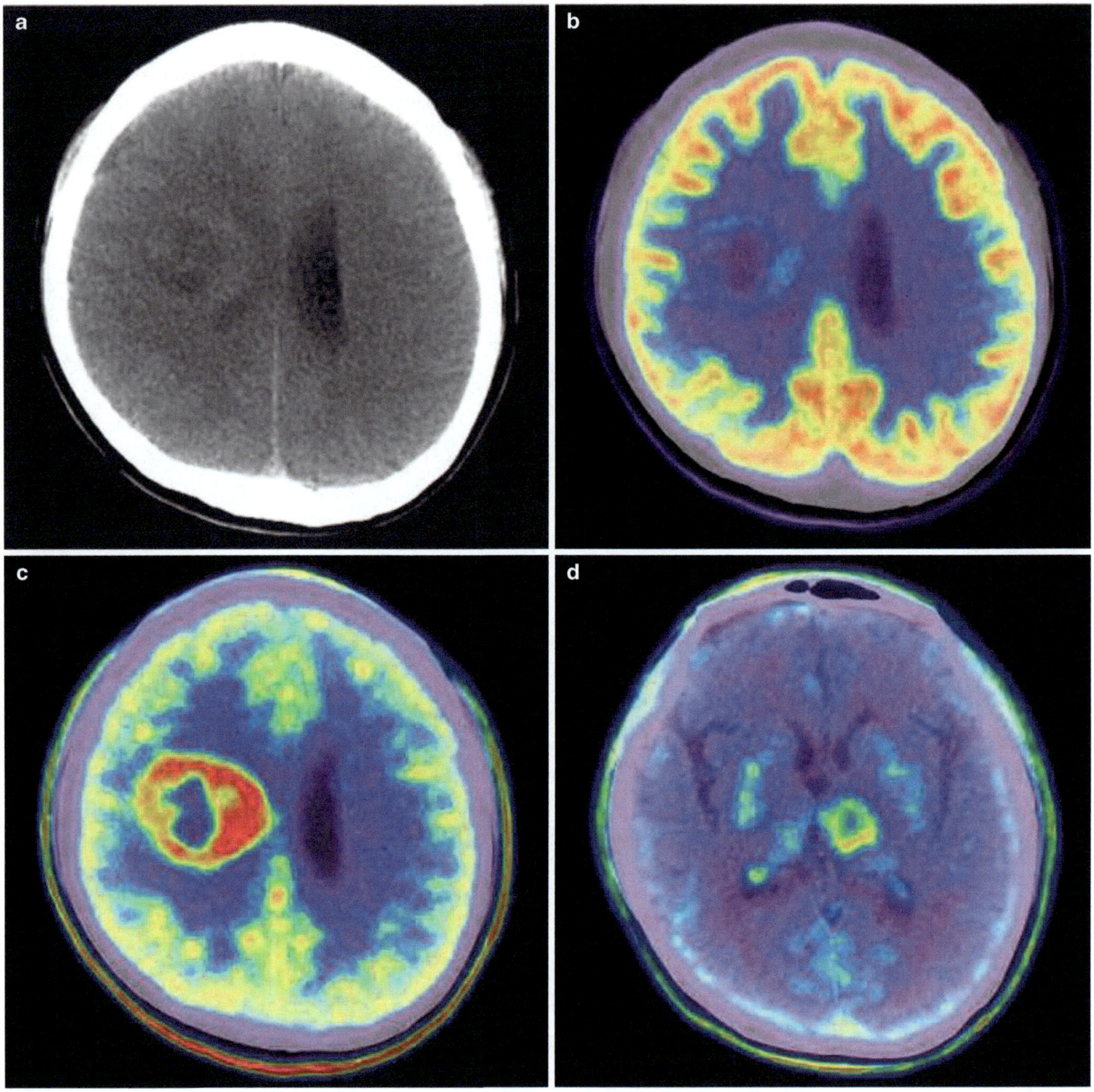

Fig. 2.5 Oligodendrogliomas (Grade III). (**a**) CT scan without contrast. A heterogeneous intensity mass is noted adjacent to the right lateral ventricle with poorly defined margins, moderate edema around it, and the compressed right lateral ventricle. (**b**) ^{18}F-FDG PET. The metabolic activity of glucose in the mass increases in an irregular ring shape. (**c**) ^{11}C-MET PET. The uptake of methionine at the margins of the lesion significantly increased in an irregular ring shape. (**d**) ^{11}C-MET PET at follow-up 1 year after surgery. Increased metabolic activity in a ring shape in lesion in the lateral thalamus, indicating spread metastasis

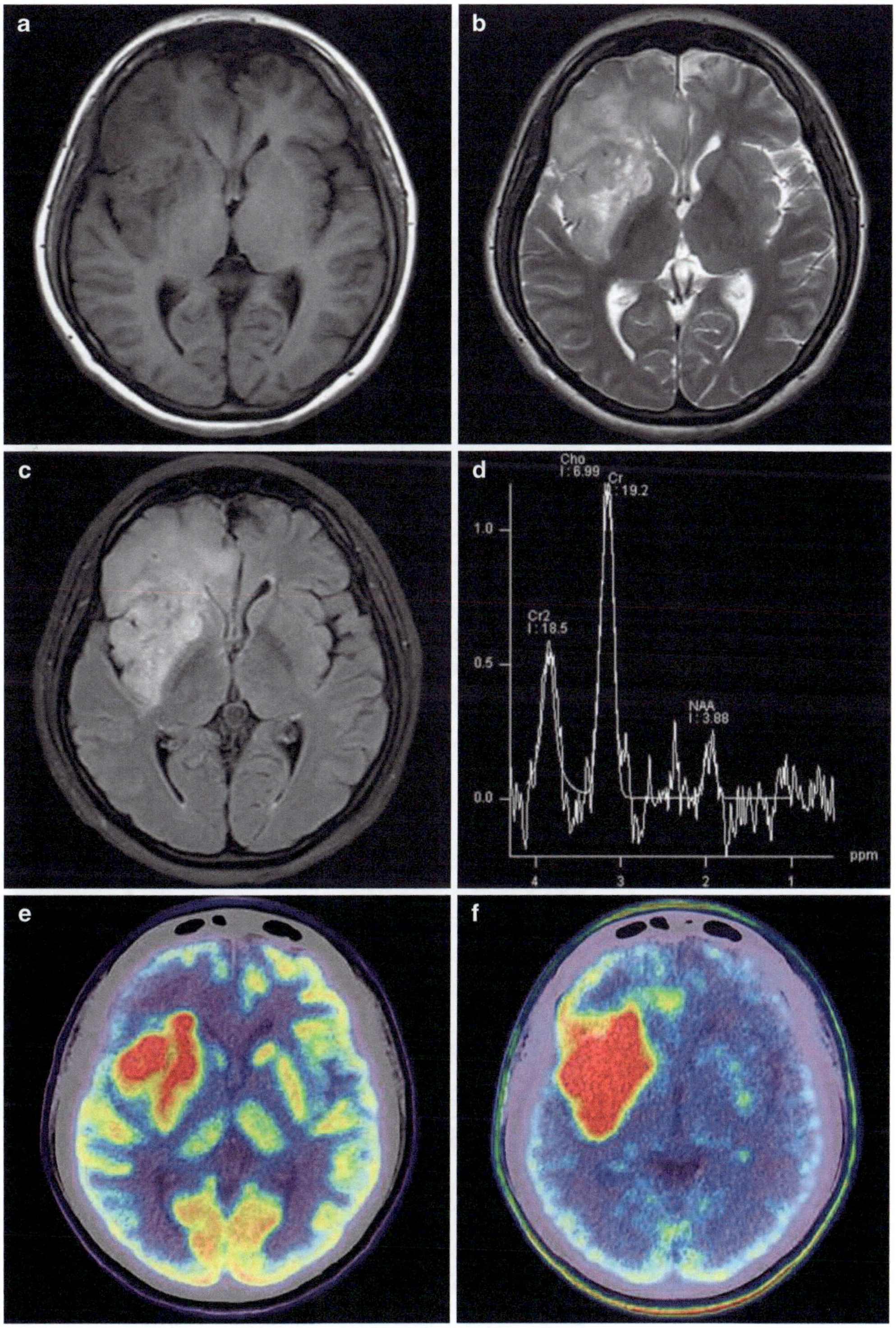

Fig. 2.6 Oligodendrogliomas (Grade III). (**a–d**) MRI T_1WI, T_2WI, FLAIR, and MRS sequences. Heterogeneous signals noted in the diffuse mass of the right frontal and insular lobe and basal ganglia, with poorly defined margins as well as significantly decreased NAA peak and significantly increased Cho peak in the MRS sequence. (**e**, **f**) ^{18}F-FDG PET and ^{11}C-MET PET. A significantly increased metabolic activity of both glucose and methionine in the mass; the latter is more severe

3 Glioblastomas

Glioblastomas are the most common primary intracranial tumors with rapid growth, space-occupying effect, and remarkable peritumoral edema. The tumor blood supply is abundant, and intratumoral bleeding is frequently noted. The tumors occur most frequently in the cerebral hemisphere, which easily involve subcortical white matter and deep periventricular white matter, and invade along the corpus callosum and corticospinal tract. Basal nuclei and thalamus are also commonly involved. Glioblastomas rarely occur in the cerebellar hemisphere and spinal cord. The tumor volume varies greatly. Primary glioblastomas are generally large and accompanied by necrosis, whereas secondary glioblastomas usually develop from small tumor tissues of low-grade astrocytomas. Glioblastoma has a high proliferation index (MIB-1), generally exceeding 10%. ^{18}F-FDG PET imaging of glioblastomas indicates that the glucose uptake varies greatly, but most of them show a high uptake. ^{11}C-MET brain imaging shows an increased uptake of the radioactive tracer in solid components of the glioblastomas as well as the absence of metabolism in the regions with cystic necrosis (Figs. 2.7 and 2.8). The differential diagnosis includes brain abscess, brain metastases, primary central nervous system lymphoma, and demyelination.

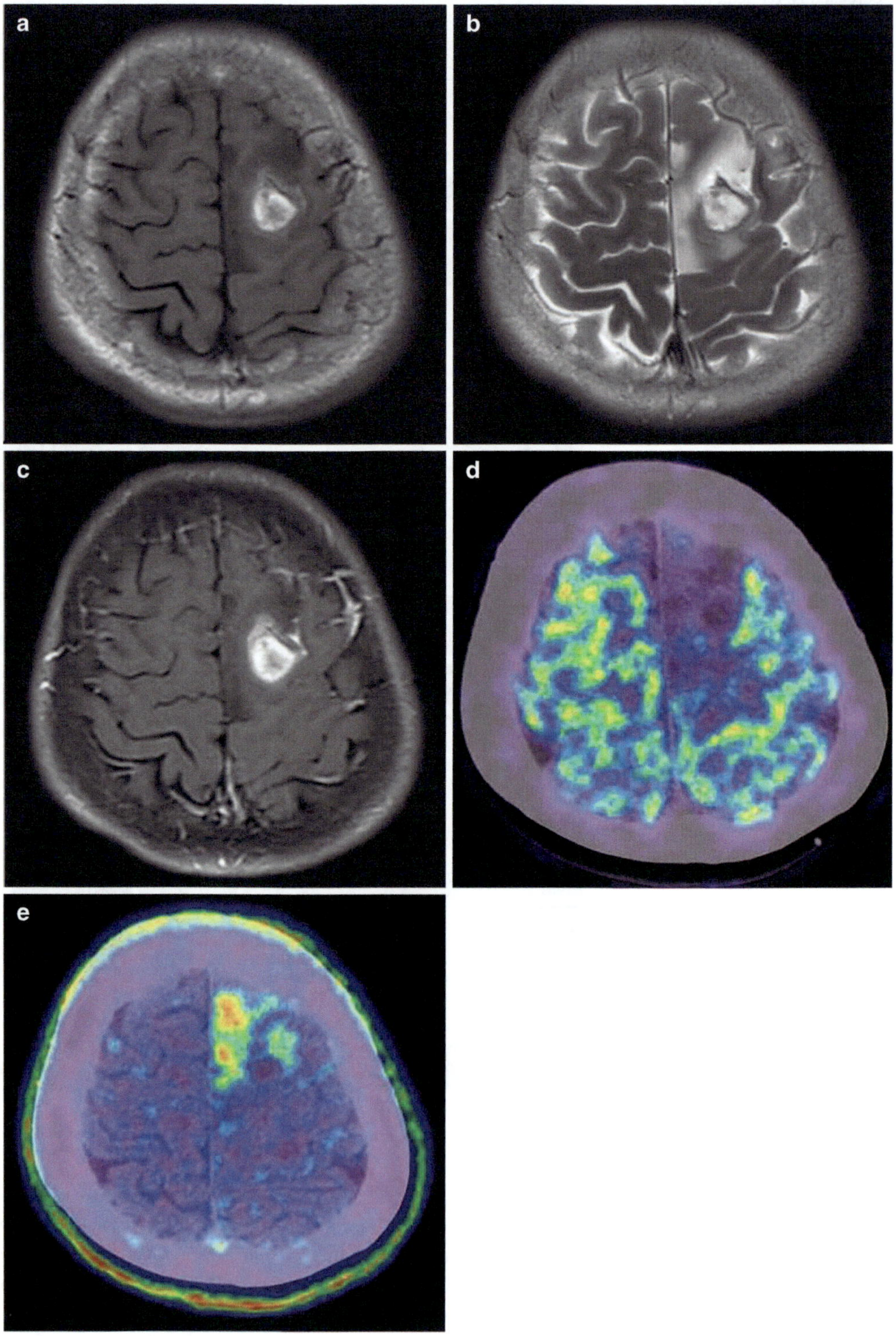

Fig. 2.7 Glioblastomas (Grade IV). (**a–c**) MRI T_1WI, T_2WI, and contrast-enhanced T_1WI MR sequences. Short T_1 and long T_2 heterogeneous signals noted in the left frontal lesion, indicating a hemorrhagic lesion, with mild-to-moderate enhancement at the margins of the hemorrhage signal by contrast-enhanced imaging. (**d, e**) ^{18}F-FDG PET and ^{11}C-MET PET. Glucose metabolism in the mass was significantly lower than the cortex, and only focal metabolism is slightly increased, while the metabolic activity of methionine around the hemorrhage signal is significantly increased, suggesting a complex hemorrhagic lesion

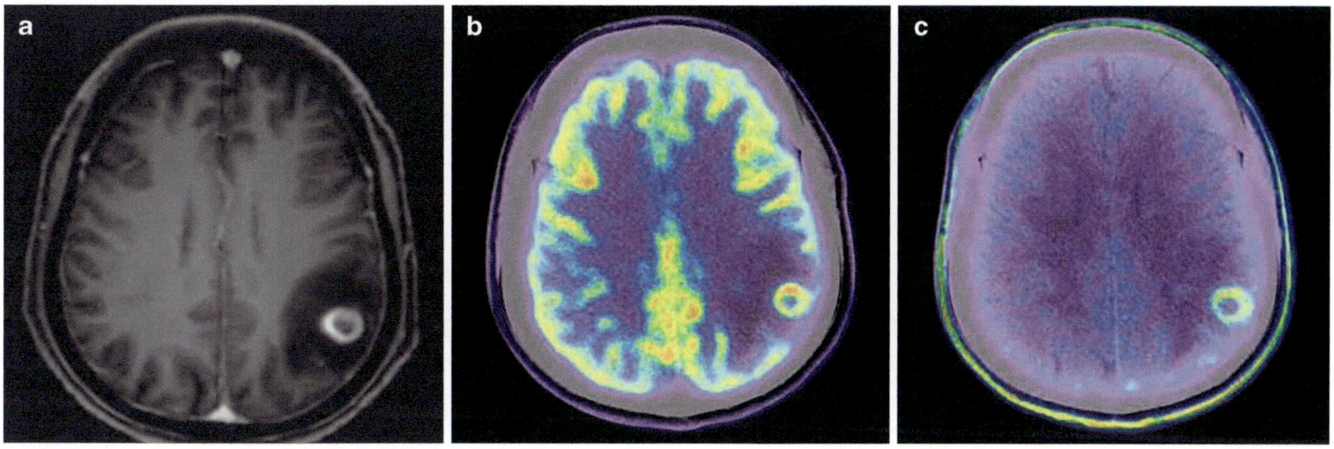

Fig. 2.8 Glioblastomas (Grade IV). (**a**) Contrast-enhanced T_1WI. A contrast-enhanced annular lesion in the left parietal cortex, with remarkable perifocal edema. (**b**, **c**) ^{18}F-FDG PET and ^{11}C-MET PET. Ring-increased metabolic activity of both glucose and methionine in the annular lesion shown on MRI

PET/CT of Meningiomas

3

Xueying Ling and Hao Xu

1 Clinical Overview

1. Epidemiology: Meningiomas are the most common intracranial benign tumors, accounting for 20% of intracranial tumors, and increase with age. The mean age of onset is 58 ± 15 years. Benign meningiomas have a male-to-female ratio of approximately 2:3, and anaplastic and malignant meningiomas are slightly more common in males.
2. Pathology: Gross appearance: spherical, flat (carpet-like), saddle-shaped (dumbbell-shaped) tumors.

   Spherical tumors are often located at the convexity or the cerebral ventricle; flat tumors are usually located at the base of the brain and extensively attached to the dura mater; saddle-shaped tumors are commonly located at the bony ridge at the base of the skull or the free margin of the cerebral dura mater.

   Most meningiomas have a capsule, while few meningiomas have no capsule and grow invasively.

   Meningiomas are firm or rubbery in consistency and may have calcification or ossification, with infrequent cystic changes as well as tortuous blood vessels on the surface.

   Most meningiomas are grayish white in color, while due to hemorrhage and necrosis, few are soft in consistency, dark red in color, and fleshy in shape.

   Meningiomas can invade the skull and lead to its reactive hyperostosis or bone destruction. In severe cases, they can even invade beyond the skull and into the scalp.

   Its blood supply mostly comes from the external carotid artery system, and a few come from the cortical branches of the internal carotid or vertebrobasilar arteries. Venous return is usually through the dural attachment.

   The adjacent brain tissue may have varying degrees of edema.
3. Prognosis: Meningiomas grow slowly and have a long course of disease.

   The course of both atypical and malignant meningiomas is relatively short.
4. Clinical management: There are no specific symptoms or signs. The symptoms are associated with the site of the tumor, including headache, visual impairment, and paralysis of limbs, or the first symptom is epilepsy. Some patients are diagnosed by chance.

   The diagnosis mainly depends on imaging studies, such as CT and MRI.

   The main treatment is surgical excision. For patients with abundant blood supply, postoperative recurrence, or unresectable meningiomas, radiotherapy is an appropriate and effective treatment modality.

2 PET/CT Diagnostic Points

1. ^{18}F-FDG PET/CT: Different degrees of FDG uptake, mostly mild increased FDG uptake in the lesion. Round, flat, or lobulated space-occupying lesion with slight hyperdensity; the broad base connected with bone lamellae and meninges; moderate homogeneous enhancement and dural tail sign; cystic changes; calcification noted in about a quarter of cases; peritumoral edema of different sizes; reactive hyperostosis osteosclerosis commonly noted in local skull and also bone destruction.
2. MRI appearance: Of meningiomas, 85–90% occur in the supratentorial region, half of which are located in the floor of the anterior and middle cranial fossae. The most common site is the cerebral convexity, followed by parasagittal regions, parafalcine regions, and base of skull including sphenoid ridge, olfactory sulcus, and cerebellopontine angle. The lesions display intermediate T_1-

X. Ling · H. Xu (✉)
The First Affiliated Hospital of Jinan University, Guangzhou, Guangdong, China
e-mail: txh@jnu.edu.cn

Z. Yao, S. Li (eds.), *Atlas of PET/CT in Oncology - Volume 1*, https://doi.org/10.1007/978-981-99-1172-1_3

weighted and intermediate T_2-weighted signal intensities, part of which show slightly longer T_1-weighted and slightly longer T_2-weighted signals and homogeneous signals. Peritumoral edema has T_1-weighted and T_2-weighted long signal intensities.

3 Typical Cases

A 43-year-old female presented with recurrent headache for 2 years. Chordoid meningioma (WHO grade II) was found at surgery (Fig. 3.1).

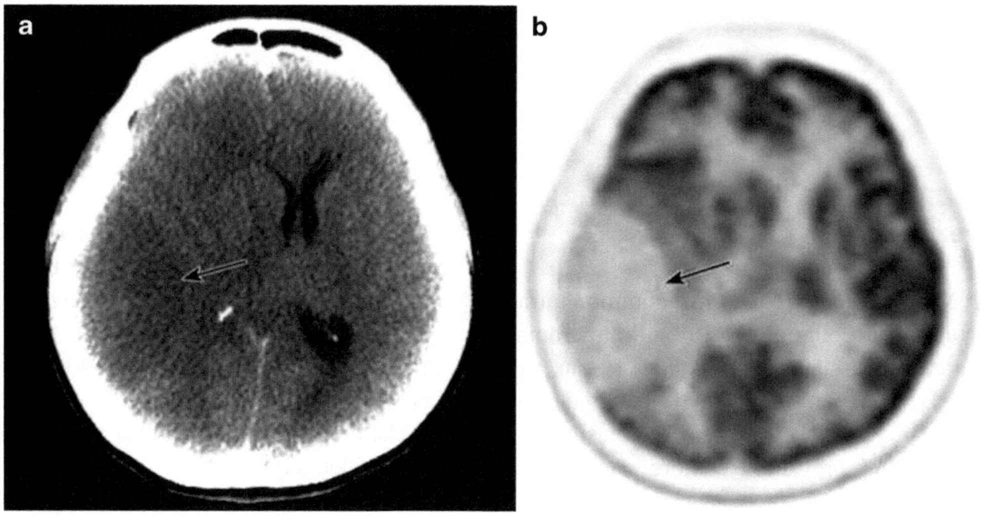

Fig. 3.1 ^{18}F-FDG PET/CT images of meningiomas. (**a**) Axial CT. (**b**) Axial PET. (**c**) Axial PET/CT. (**d**) Axial CT (bone window). (**e**) Axial T_1WI. (**f**) Axial T_2WI. (**g**) Contrast-enhanced axial T_1WI. (**h**) Contrast-enhanced coronal T_1WI. Figures **a–d**: PET/CT shows a hypodensity lesion with low uptake of FDG (comparable uptake in white matter) and reactive hyperostosis osteosclerosis in local skull (black arrow). Figures **e–h**: MRI without contrast shows long T_1-weighted and long T_2-weighted signals, remarkable and homogeneous enhancement, as well as dural tail sign in the coronal plane (white arrow)

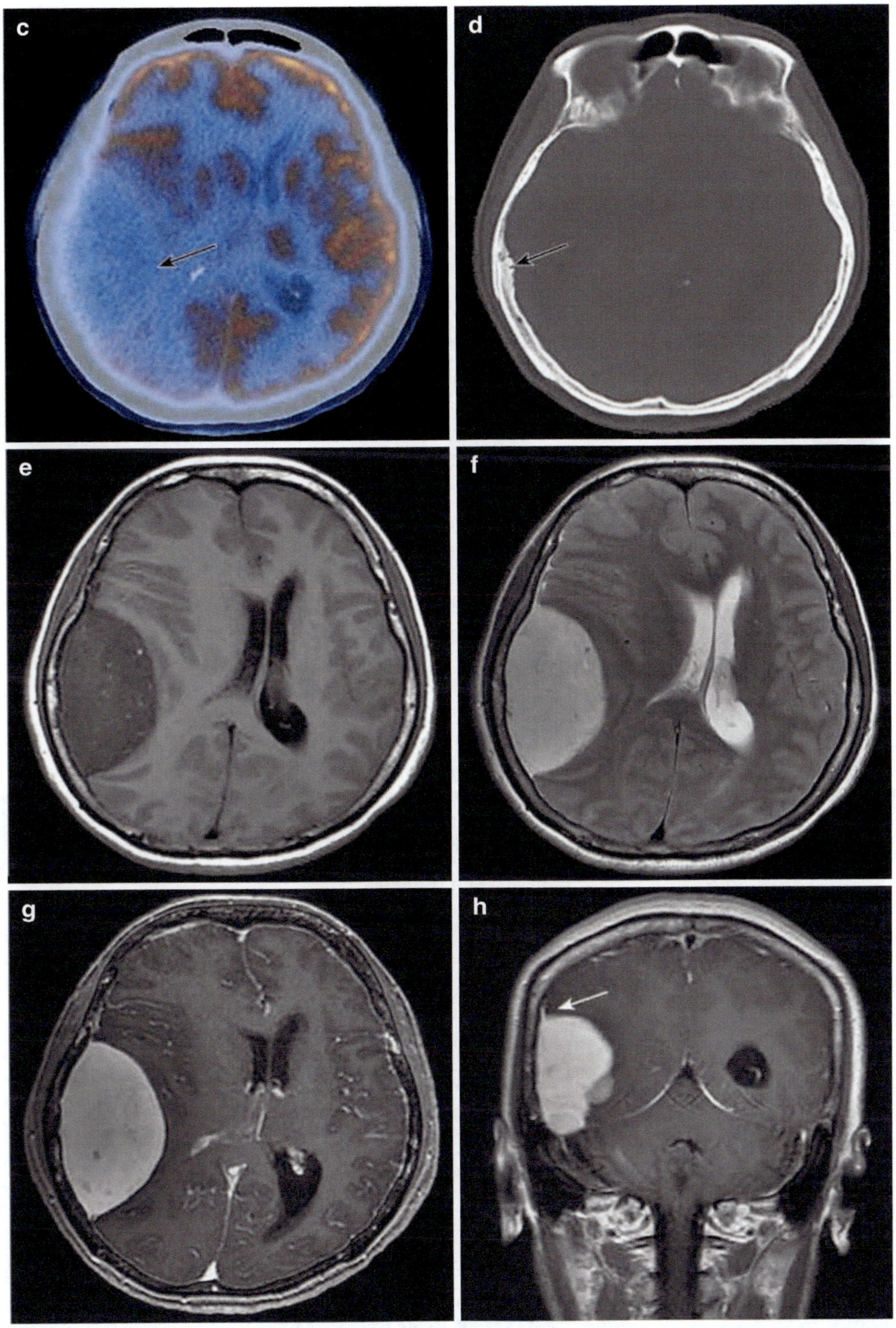

Fig. 3.1 (continued)

4 Rare Cases

Case 1: A 9-year-old male presented with progressive loss of bilateral vision caused by the meningioma in the saddle region (Fig. 3.2).

Case 2: A 64-year-old male complained of left limb weakness with headache and dizziness. Final diagnosis was the postoperative recurrence of parietal atypical meningioma (WHO grade II) (Fig. 3.3).

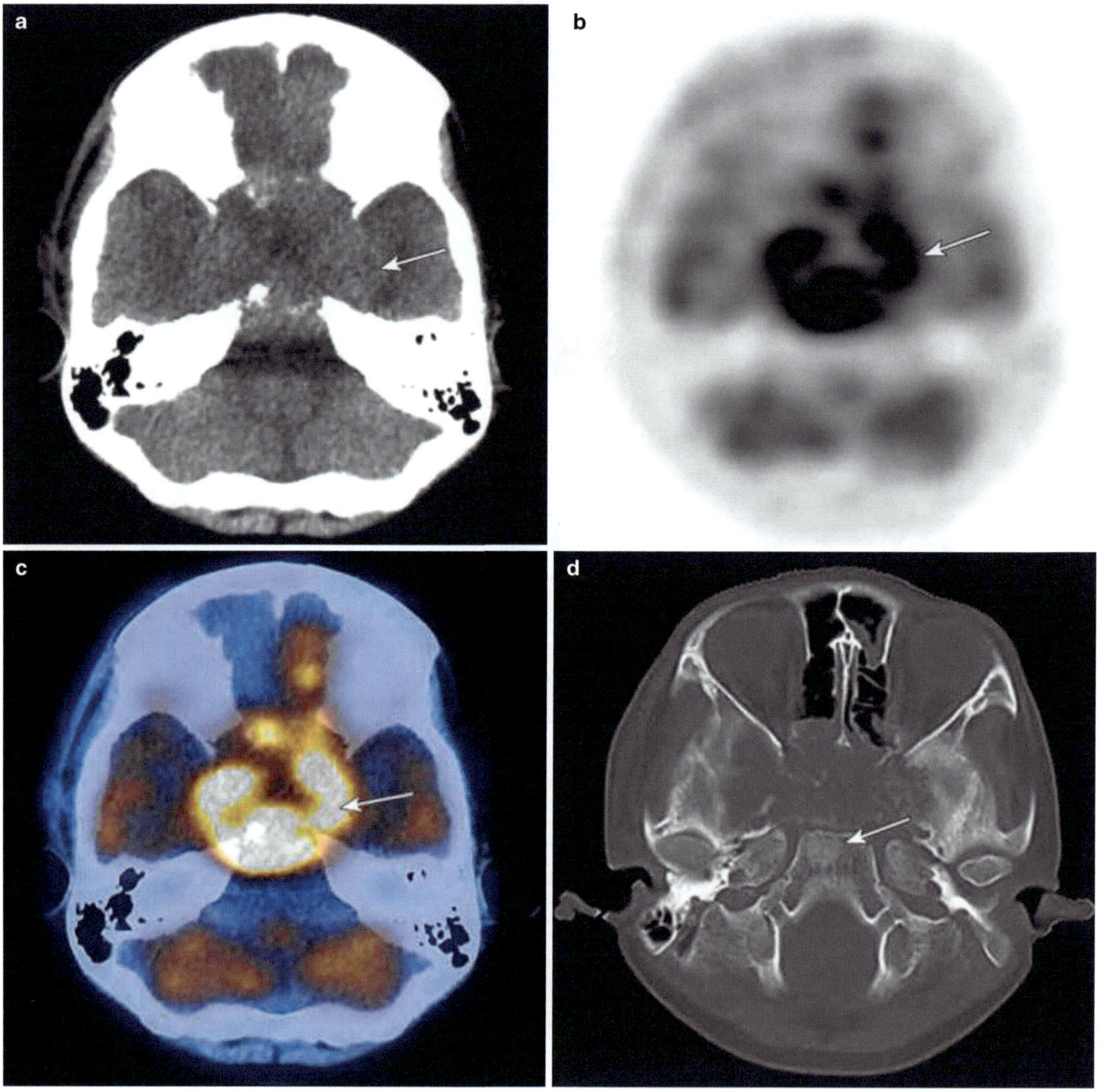

Fig. 3.2 ^{18}F-FDG PET/CT images of meningiomas. (**a**) Axial CT. (**b**) Axial PET. (**c**) Axial PET/CT. (**d**) Axial CT (bone window). PET/CT shows a slight hyperdensity lesion with hypodensity necrosis in the center, high uptake of FDG (significantly higher than the cortical uptake), extensive osteolytic bone destruction in the saddle region, and occipital osteoblastic bone destruction (white arrow). Postsurgery pathology was atypical meningioma with rhabdoid features (WHO grades II–III)

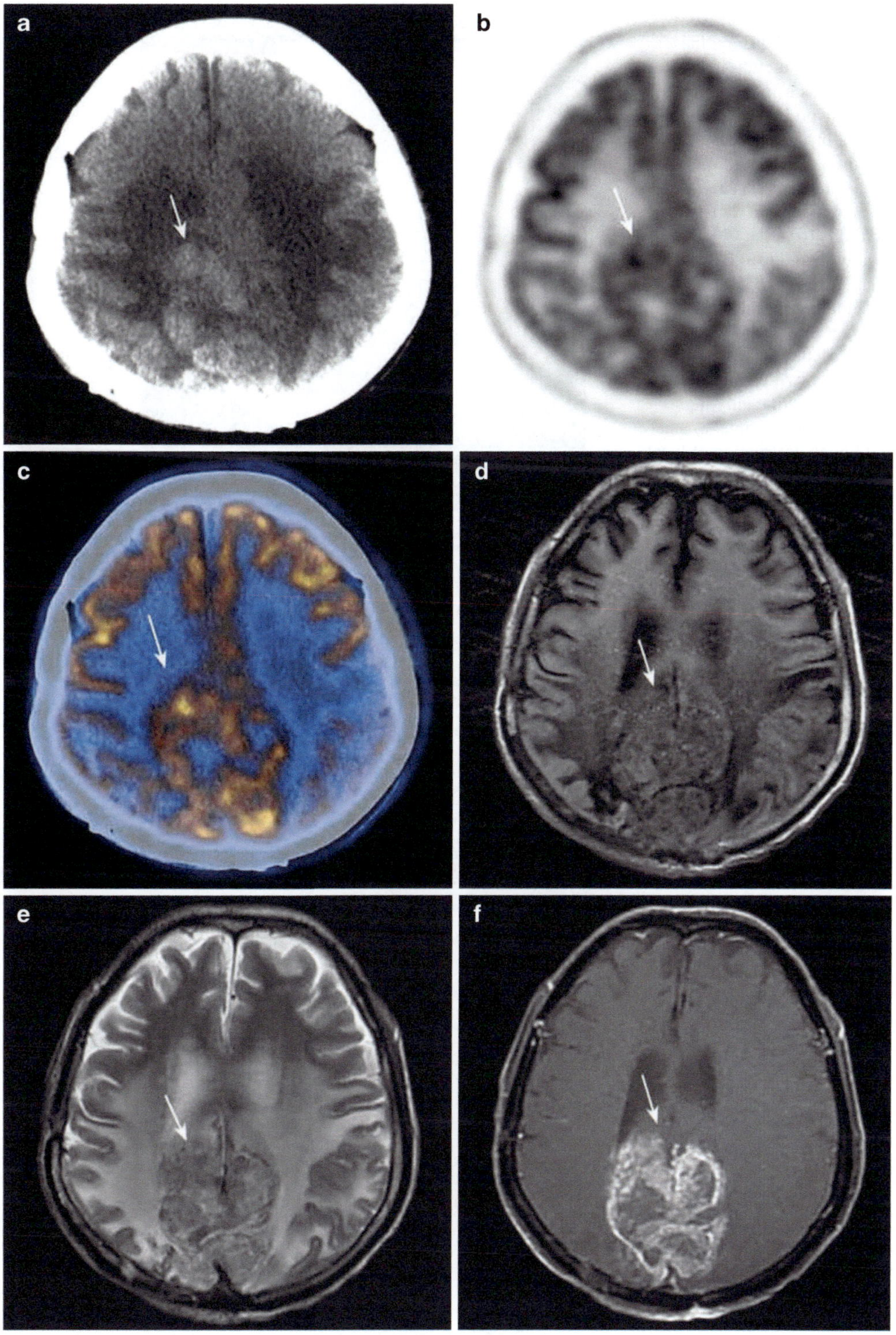

Fig. 3.3 ^{18}F-FDG PET/CT images of meningiomas. (**a**) CT. (**b**) PET. (**c**) PET/CT. (**d**) MRI T_1WI. (**e**) MRI T_2WI. (**f**) Contrast-enhanced MRI T_1WI. On PET/CT, the meningioma (arrow) shows slight hyperdensity and increased uptake of FDG (close to the cortical uptake); hypointensity on T_1WI, hyperintensity on T_2WI, and heterogeneous enhancement, accompanied by massive cerebral edema

5 Differential Diagnosis

Meningiomas with an increased uptake of FDG should be differentiated from malignant tumors, such as metastatic tumors and lymphomas.

1. **Metastatic tumors**: There are primary tumors found elsewhere in the body or having history of malignant tumors (Fig. 3.4).
2. **Primary central nervous system lymphoma**: Blood perfusion is not high in lymphomas, whereas it is significantly high in meningiomas.

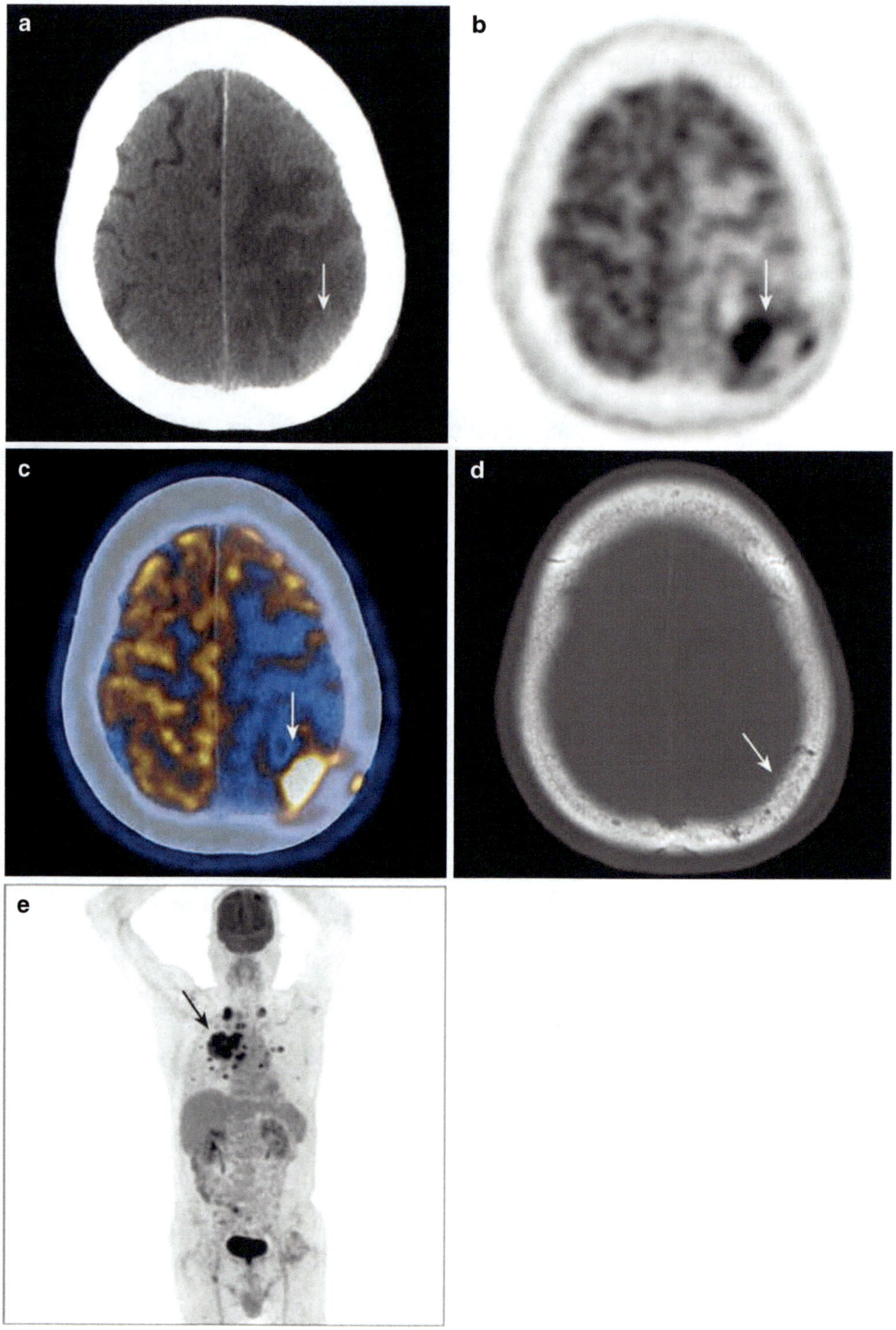

Fig. 3.4 ^{18}F-FDG PET/CT images for the differential diagnosis of meningiomas from metastasis. A 71-year-old male presented with right central bronchogenic carcinoma with multiple metastatic tumors: (**a**) Axial CT; (**b**) axial PET; (**c**) axial PET/CT; (**d**) axial CT (bone window); and (**e**) PET MIP image. On PET/CT, the left parietal meningeal metastasis shows a semi-circular space-occupying lesion of isodensity, with a high uptake of FDG (significantly higher than the cortical uptake) and mild bone destruction of local skull (white arrow), accompanied by massive cerebral edema in the left frontal and parietal lobes. PET MIP image shows primary lesions of the right lung cancer (black arrow)

6 Summary

PET/CT is not the main imaging technique for the diagnosis of meningiomas but can be used for the differential diagnosis of meningiomas from metastatic tumors.

PET/CT of Lymphomas

4

Xueying Ling and Hao Xu

1 Clinical Overview

1.1 Epidemiology

Primary central nervous system lymphoma (PCNSL) accounts for 1–5% of intracranial tumors. More than 90% of PCNSL belongs to diffuse large B-cell lymphoma (DLBCL) and accounts for less than 1–4% of all non-Hodgkin's lymphomas, and only about 2% of the PCNSL originates from T-lymphocytes. PCNSL occurs at any age, most commonly at ages of 60–70 years in patients with normal immune function and at ages 37–43 years in those with acquired immunodeficiency syndrome (AIDS). PCNSL rarely occurs in children, at an average age of 10 years. The incidence of PCNSL is higher in men than in women.

1.2 Pathology

1. Lesions are soft in consistency and various in color, without a clear interface with brain tissue and neither a capsule.
2. Multifocal or solitary growth. Intracranial hemorrhage, cystic changes, or necrosis is rare.
3. Microscopically, tumor tissues are interlaced with brain tissues, patchy in distribution, arranged in clusters, or distributed diffusely. Tumor cells are characterized by centering on blood vessels and showing flower-like growth, arranging in layers, and forming a sheath of cells surrounding the vascular tissue.
4. Lesions have remarkable space-occupying effect, whereas those without space-occupying effect in local regions are rare and show extensive tissue infiltration.

1.3 Prognosis

Pathologic types of lymphoma have no effect on prognosis, and among these types, there is no statistically significant difference in survival.

Favorable prognostic factors include an age of no more than 60 years and a good general condition.

About 1/4 patients are curable.

1.4 Clinical Management

Clinical manifestations of PCNSLs vary according to their locations.

PCNSL can be indicated by imaging studies but should be confirmed by histopathological evidence.

A comprehensive treatment mode combining systemic chemotherapy with intrathecal chemotherapy plus whole brain radiotherapy is most commonly used.

X. Ling · H. Xu (✉)
The First Affiliated Hospital of Jinan University, Guangzhou, Guangdong, China
e-mail: txh@jnu.edu.cn

Z. Yao, S. Li (eds.), *Atlas of PET/CT in Oncology - Volume 1*, https://doi.org/10.1007/978-981-99-1172-1_4

2 PET/CT Diagnostic Points

1. ^{18}F-FDG PET/CT: The uptake of ^{18}F-FDG in lesions is usually higher than that in gray matter. The lesion is solitary or multiple, round or oval, and irregular mass, and it shows slight hyperdensity, fewer with calcification, hemorrhage, or cystic changes.
2. Contrast-enhanced CT: A mild to moderate enhancement is noted in the lesions, and the delayed enhancement is more remarkable. Vascular enhancement is noted in some lesions. Peritumoral edema is generally mild to moderate, and the space-occupying effect varies from mild to severe.
3. MRI: Lymphomas usually occur in the periventricular white matter, basal nuclei, and corpus callosum, more commonly in the supratentorial region than in the subtentorial one. The lesion shows homogeneous signals (slightly longer T_1 and slightly longer T_2 signals, homogeneous signals, and DWI hyperintensity). On contrast MRI, the lesion is significantly enhanced and appears as a mass or clenched fist. Peritumoral edema of lymphomas is less severe than that of high-grade gliomas.

3 Typical Cases

Case 1: A 74-year-old male was admitted to the hospital due to headache, with lymphomas in the left basal ganglia and at the trigone of the left temporal, parietal, and occipital lobe (Fig. 4.1).

Case 2: A 73-year-old male complained of left limb weakness with headache and dizziness. The lymphomas (confirmed by stereotactic biopsy) adjacent to the right lateral ventricle (right basal ganglia and thalamus) were found on PET/CT (Fig. 4.2).

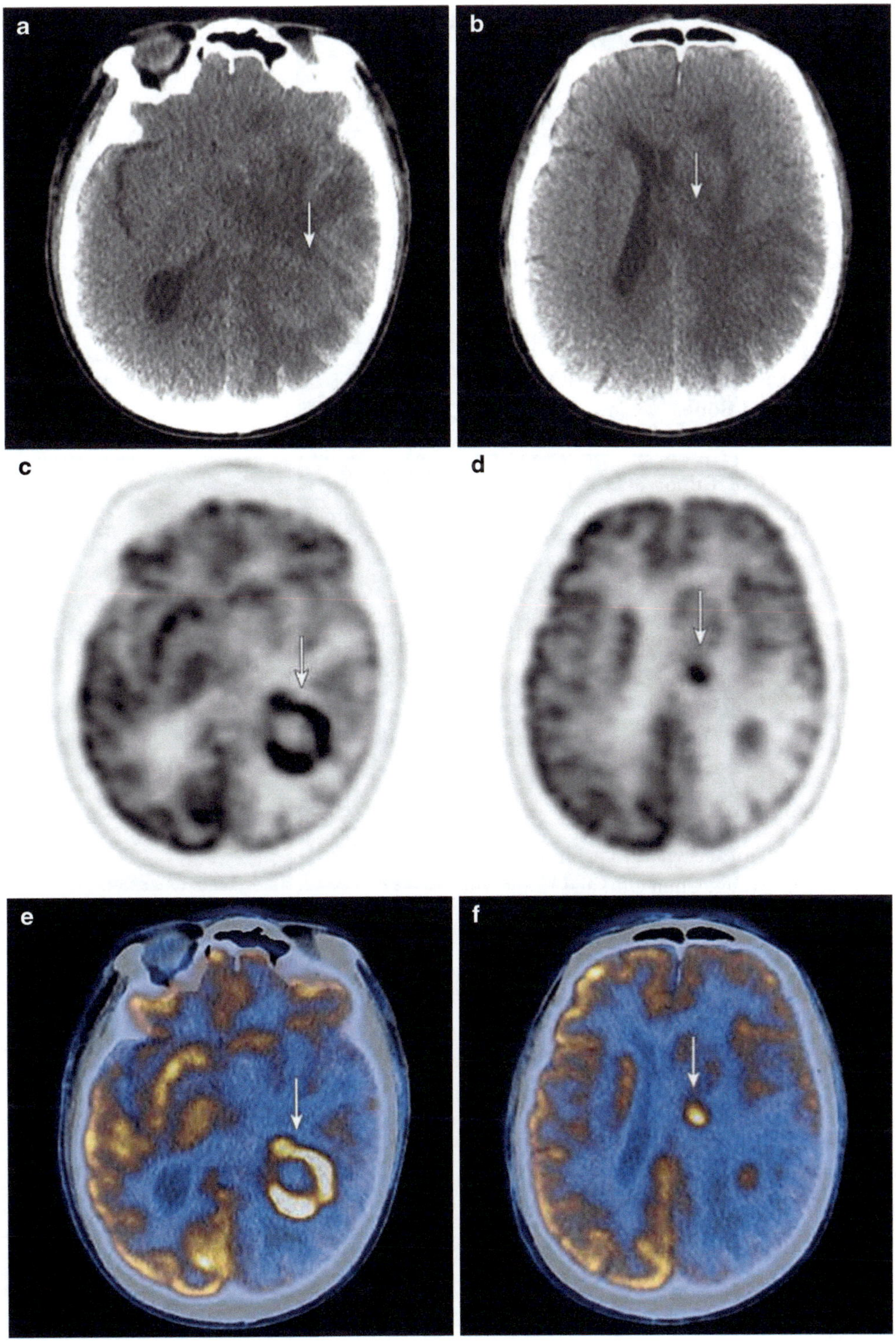

Fig. 4.1 ^{18}F-FDG PET/CT images of lymphomas. (**a**, **b**) Axial CT. (**c**, **d**) Axial PET. (**e**, **f**) Axial PET/CT. PET/CT shows slight hyperdensity (white arrow) and a nodular, irregular, ring-like, and high uptake of FDG (higher than the cortical uptake), with massive surrounding edema. Pathology from stereotactic biopsy was lymphoma

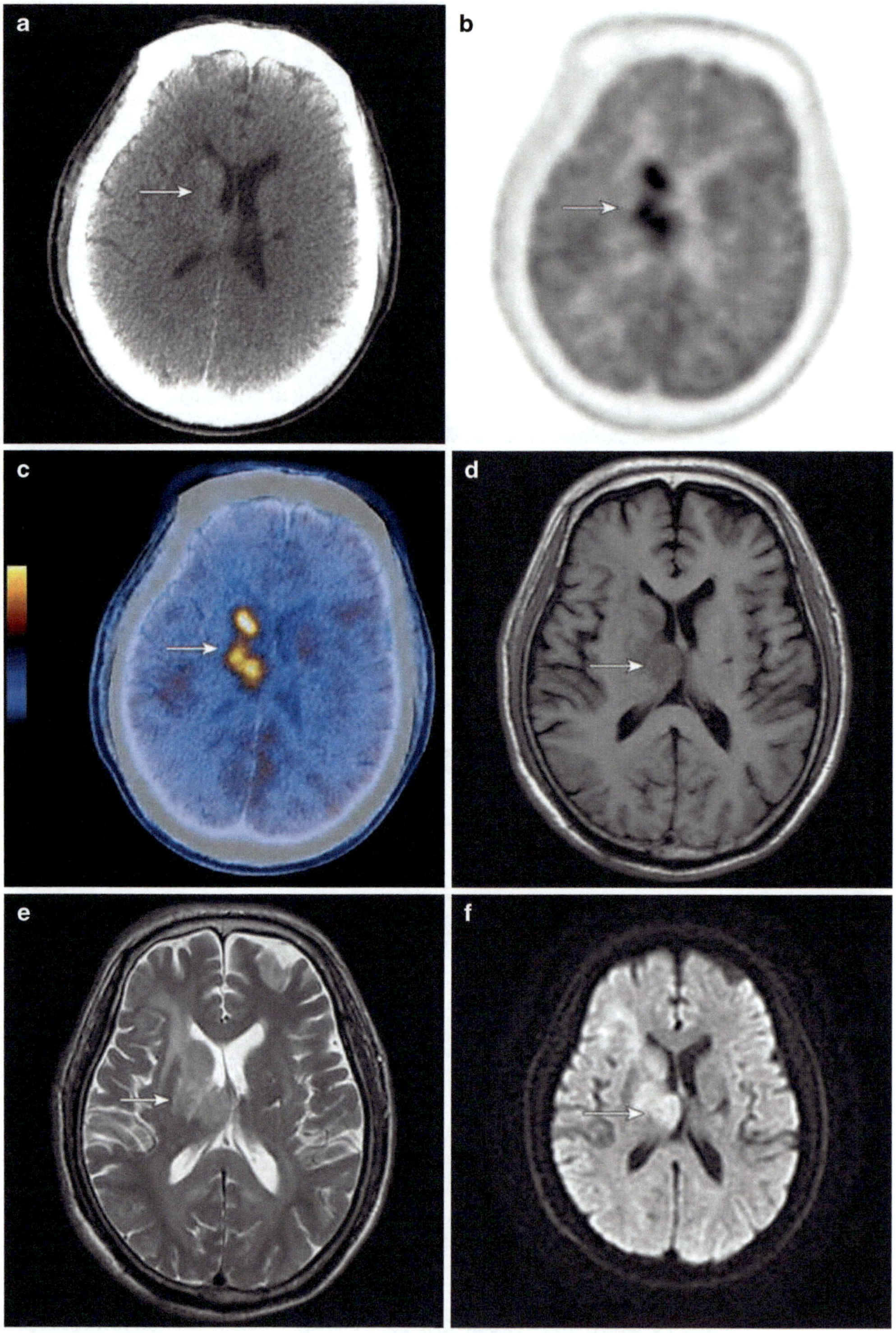

Fig. 4.2 ^{18}F-FDG PET/CT images of lymphomas. (**a**) Axial CT. (**b**) Axial PET. (**c**) Axial PET/CT. (**d**) Axial T_1WI. (**e**) Axial T_2WI. (**f**) Axial DWI. (**g**) Contrast-enhanced axial T_1WI. PET/CT shows slight hyperdensity (white arrow) and multiple nodular increased uptake of FDG (significantly higher than the cortical uptake) lesions with mild surrounding edema. Slight hypointensity on T_1WI, slight hyperintensity on T_2WI, slight hyperintensity on DWI, and mild to moderate enhancement after contrast agent administration

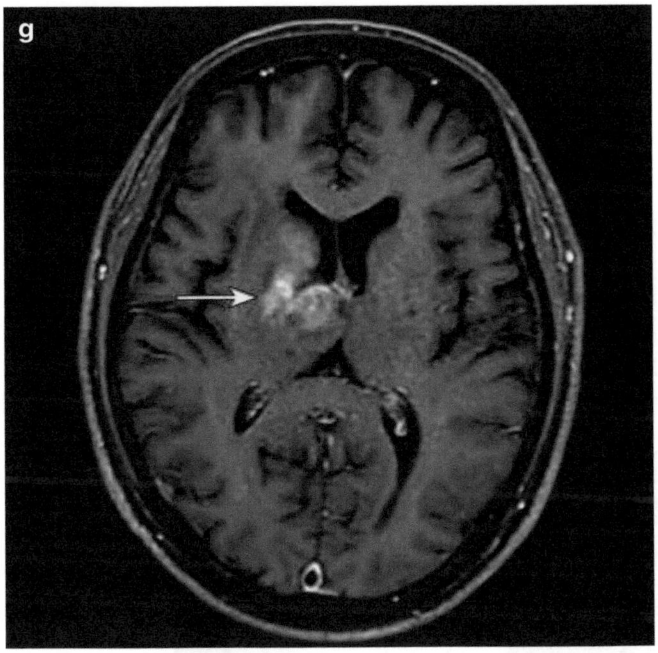

Fig. 4.2 (continued)

4 Rare Cases

A 64-year-old male presented with fever for more than 1 month (Fig. 4.3).

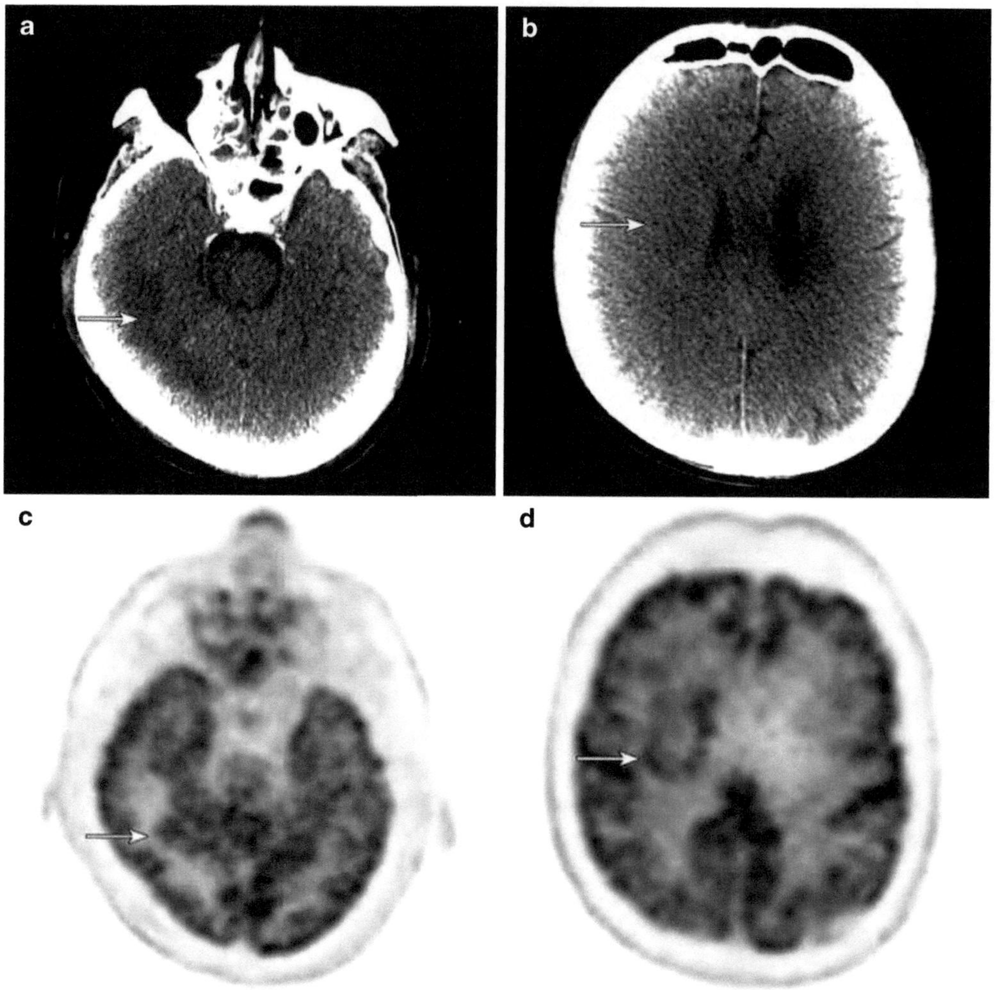

Fig. 4.3 ^{18}F-FDG PET/CT images of lymphomas. (**a, b**) Axial CT. (**c, d**) Axial PET. (**e, f**) Axial PET/CT. (**g**) Axial T_1WI. (**h**) Axial T_2WI. (**i, j**) Axial DWI. (**k, l**) Contrast-enhanced axial T_1WI. Lymphomas in the right periventricular region and the corona radiata (white arrow); PET/CT shows isodensity, nodular, and tiny patchy FDG uptake (close to the cortical uptake) lesions with mild to moderate edema in the surrounding area; slight hypointensity on T_1WI, slight hyperintensity on T_2WI, slight hyperintensity on DWI, and remarkable nodular and spotty enhancement after contrast agent administration

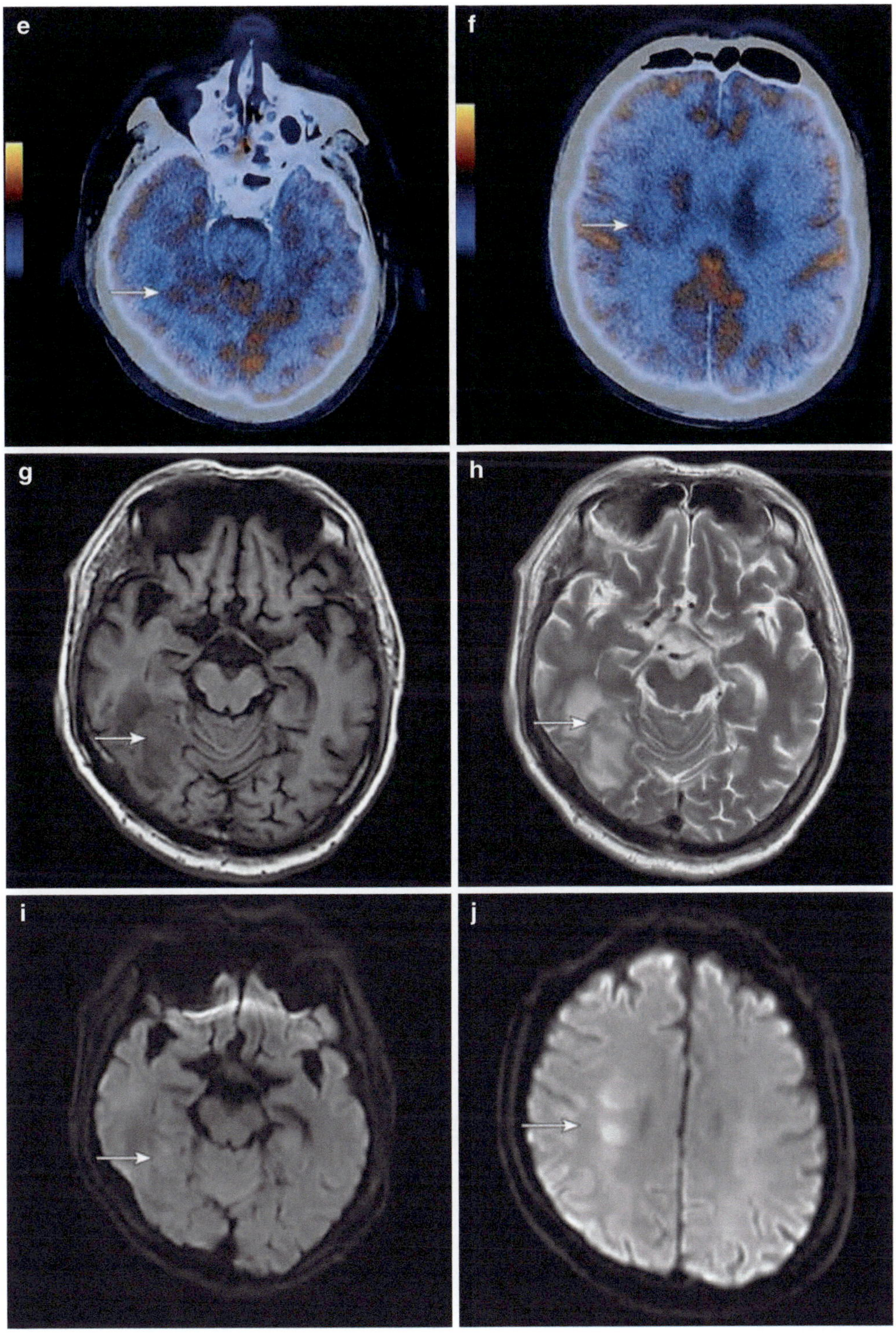

Fig. 4.3 (continued)

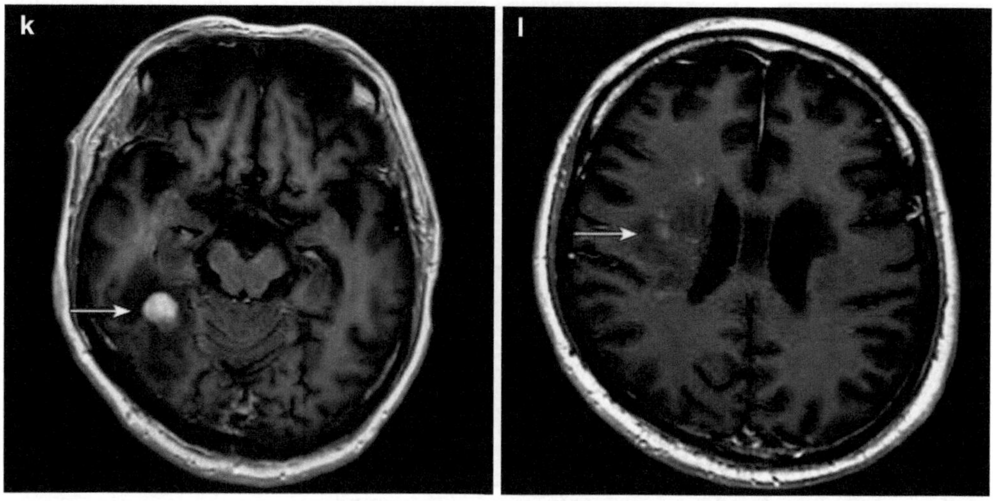

Fig. 4.3 (continued)

5 Differential Diagnosis

PCNSL with increased uptake of ^{18}F-FDG should be differentiated from high-grade gliomas, metastatic tumors, etc.

1. High-grade gliomas: Cystic changes and necrosis are commonly seen in high-grade gliomas, with significantly heterogeneous enhancement and high blood perfusion. Mass space-occupying effect and peritumoral edema of lymphomas are more severe in the gliomas than in PCNSL (Fig. 4.4).
2. Metastatic tumors: The metastases usually occur at the corticomedullary junction and have severe peritumoral edema, with primary tumor history or primary lesions identified in other parts of the body (Fig. 4.5).
3. PCNSL with low uptake of ^{18}F-FDG should be differentiated from low-grade gliomas, inflammatory granuloma (Fig. 4.6), demyelinating disease, etc.

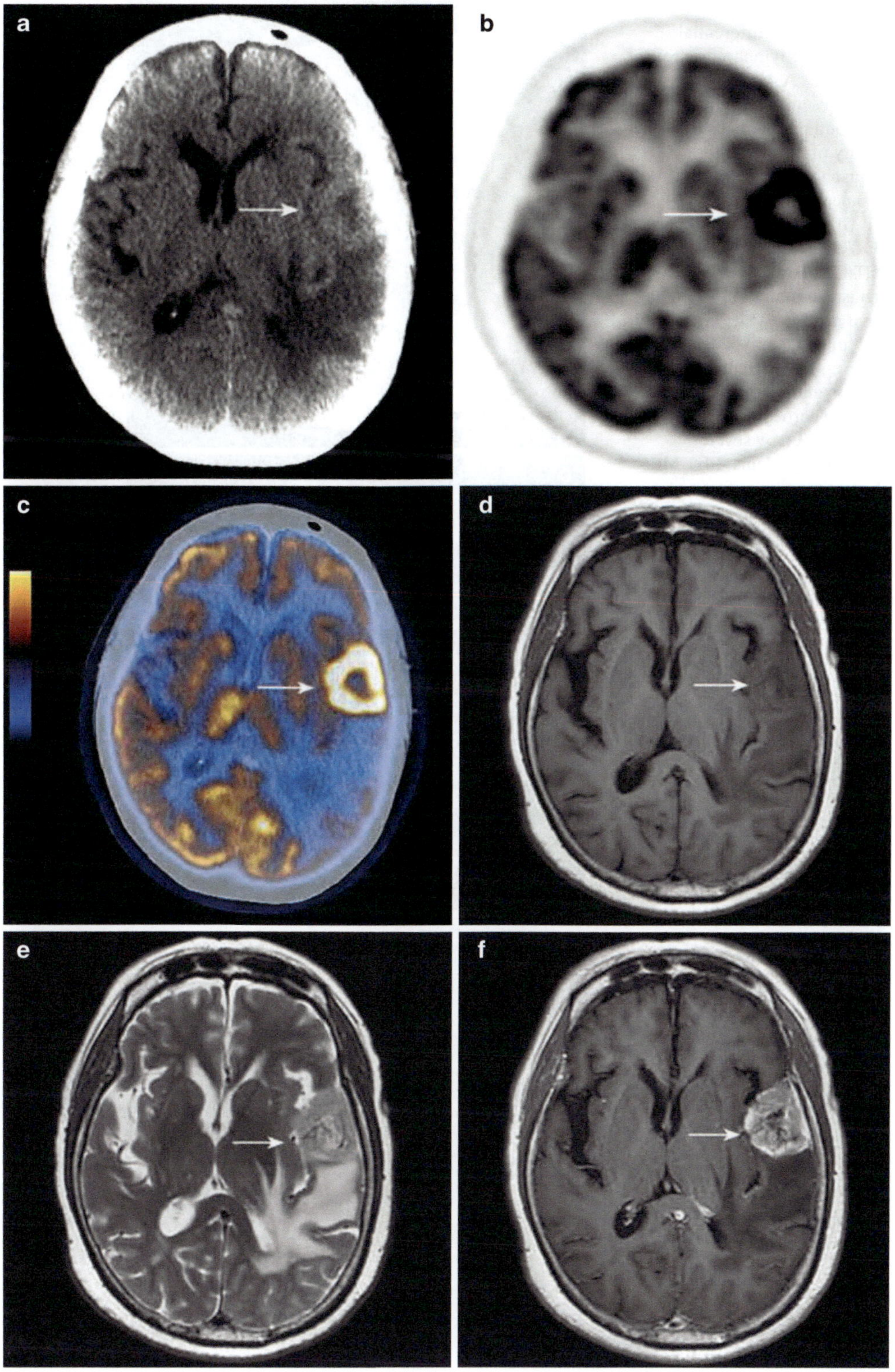

Fig. 4.4 ^{18}F-FDG PET/CT images for the differential diagnosis of lymphomas from glioblastoma. A 72-year-old female complained of headache for more than 3 months, with slurred speech for 2 weeks. (**a**) Axial CT. (**b**) Axial PET. (**c**) Axial PET/CT. (**d**) Axial T_1WI. (**e**) Axial T_2WI. (**f**) Contrast-enhanced axial T_1WI. PET/CT shows left temporal mass (white arrow) with mixed density (low-density necrosis in the center) and irregular ring-like high uptake of FDG (significantly higher than the cortical uptake), accompanied by severe surrounding edema; hypointensity on T_1WI, hyperintensity on T_2WI, and irregular ring-like enhancement after contrast agent administration. Postsurgery pathology was glioblastoma

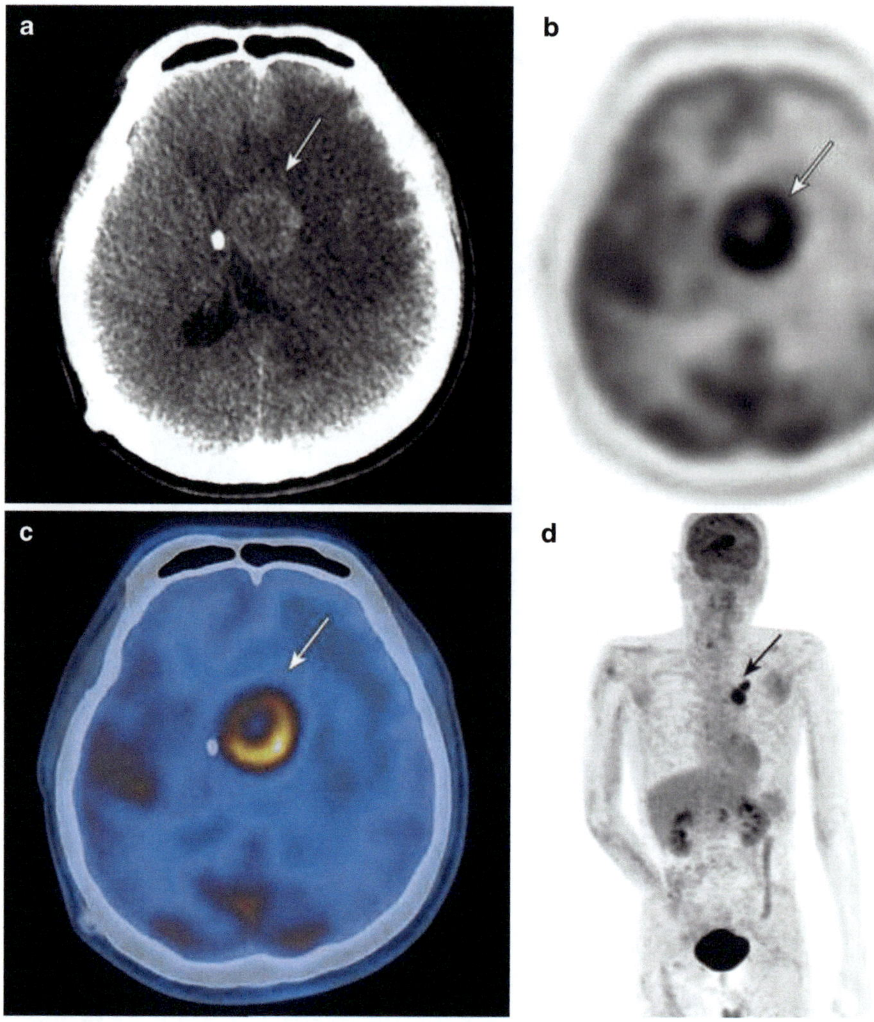

Fig. 4.5 ^{18}F-FDG PET/CT images for the differential diagnosis of lymphomas from metastasis. A 44-year-old male presented with headache and vomiting, with a surgical history of cerebellar hemispheric tumor (metastatic adenocarcinoma). (**a**) Axial CT. (**b**) Axial PET. (**c**) Axial PET/CT. (**d**) PET MIP image. PET/CT shows a new metastatic tumor in the left basal ganglia (white arrow) with mixed iso-hypodensity and ring-like high uptake of FDG (significantly higher than the cortical uptake), accompanied by severe surrounding edema. PET MIP shows the primary focus of the left upper lung cancer (black arrow)

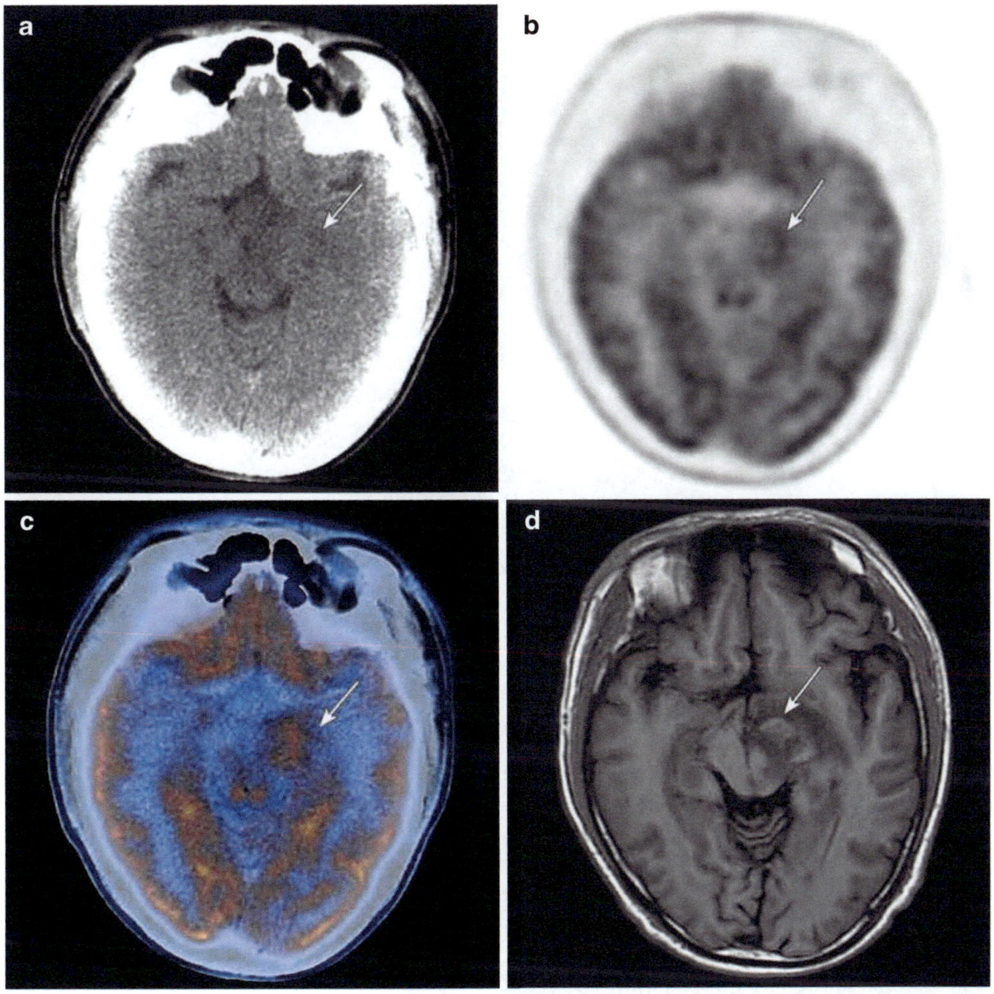

Fig. 4.6 ^{18}F-FDG PET/CT images for the differential diagnosis of lymphomas from inflammatory granuloma. A 40-year-old patient presented with recurrent headaches for more than 1 year. (**a**) Axial CT. (**b**) Axial PET. (**c**) Axial PET/CT. (**d**) Axial T_1WI. (**e**) Axial T_2WI. (**f**) Axial DWI. (**g**) Contrast-enhanced axial T_1WI. PET/CT shows isodensity lesions (white arrow) with increased FDG uptake (close to the cortical uptake), surrounded by edema. Isointensity on T_1WI, slight hypointensity on T_2WI, slight hyperintensity on DWI, as well as tiny, ring-like, and spotty enhancement after contrast agent administration. Inflammatory granuloma in the left cerebral peduncle was found at surgery

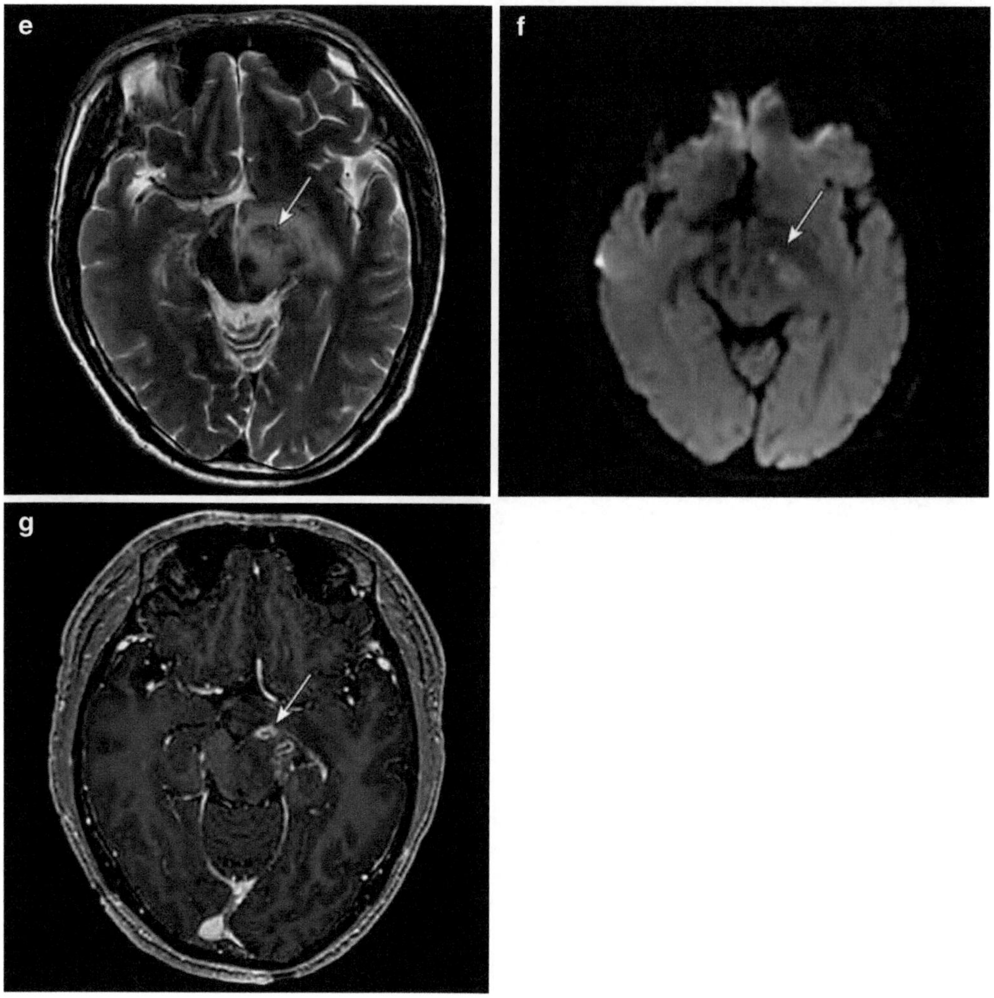

Fig. 4.6 (continued)

6 Summary

^{18}F-FDG PET/CT has an important value in the diagnosis and efficacy evaluation of PCNSL. By virtue of a high FDG uptake in the cerebral cortex, combining with MRI, we can make a more accurate diagnosis of PCNSL.

Further Reading

Albano D, Bosio G, Bertoli M, et al. ^{18}F-FDG PET/CT in primary brain lymphoma. J Neuro Oncol, 2018, 136(3):577-583.

Huang Sui-Qiao, Huang Li. Diagnostic imaging of CNS difficult cases. Beijing: People's Medical Publishing House, 2010

5 PET/CT of Germinomas

Lin Ai

1 Clinical Overview

Intracranial germinomas are mostly located adjacent to the midline structure, 80–90% in the midline, 1/2–2/3 in the pineal region, 1/4–1/3 in the suprasellar region, and 5–10% in the basal ganglia region. The size of germinomas varies depending on their location. The germinoma in the pituitary stalk can cause symptoms when it is very small, while that in the pineal region can grow to a large size if not causing hydrocephalus by invading the tectum and the central canal. About 20% of intracranial germinomas are multifocal and usually occur simultaneously in the pineal region and the suprasellar region. Germinomas are generally solid tumors and brittle in consistency and can infiltrate adjacent tissues. Intratumoral cystic changes, small focal hemorrhage, and cerebrospinal fluid spread are commonly seen. Mitosis is common in germinomas, but necrosis is rare.

2 PET/CT Diagnostic Points

The imaging diagnosis of germinomas mainly depends on CT and MRI. ^{18}F-FDG PET usually shows a mild to moderate increased uptake of FDG, and ^{11}C-MET PET shows a remarkable increased uptake of ^{11}C-MET in germinomas (Figs. 5.1, 5.2, and 5.3). Germinomas should be differentiated from other tumors in the pineal region, such as pineocytoma, other types of germ cell tumors, Langerhans cell histiocytosis, etc.

L. Ai (✉)
Beijing Tiantan Hospital, Capital Medical University, Beijing, China

Z. Yao, S. Li (eds.), *Atlas of PET/CT in Oncology - Volume 1*, https://doi.org/10.1007/978-981-99-1172-1_5

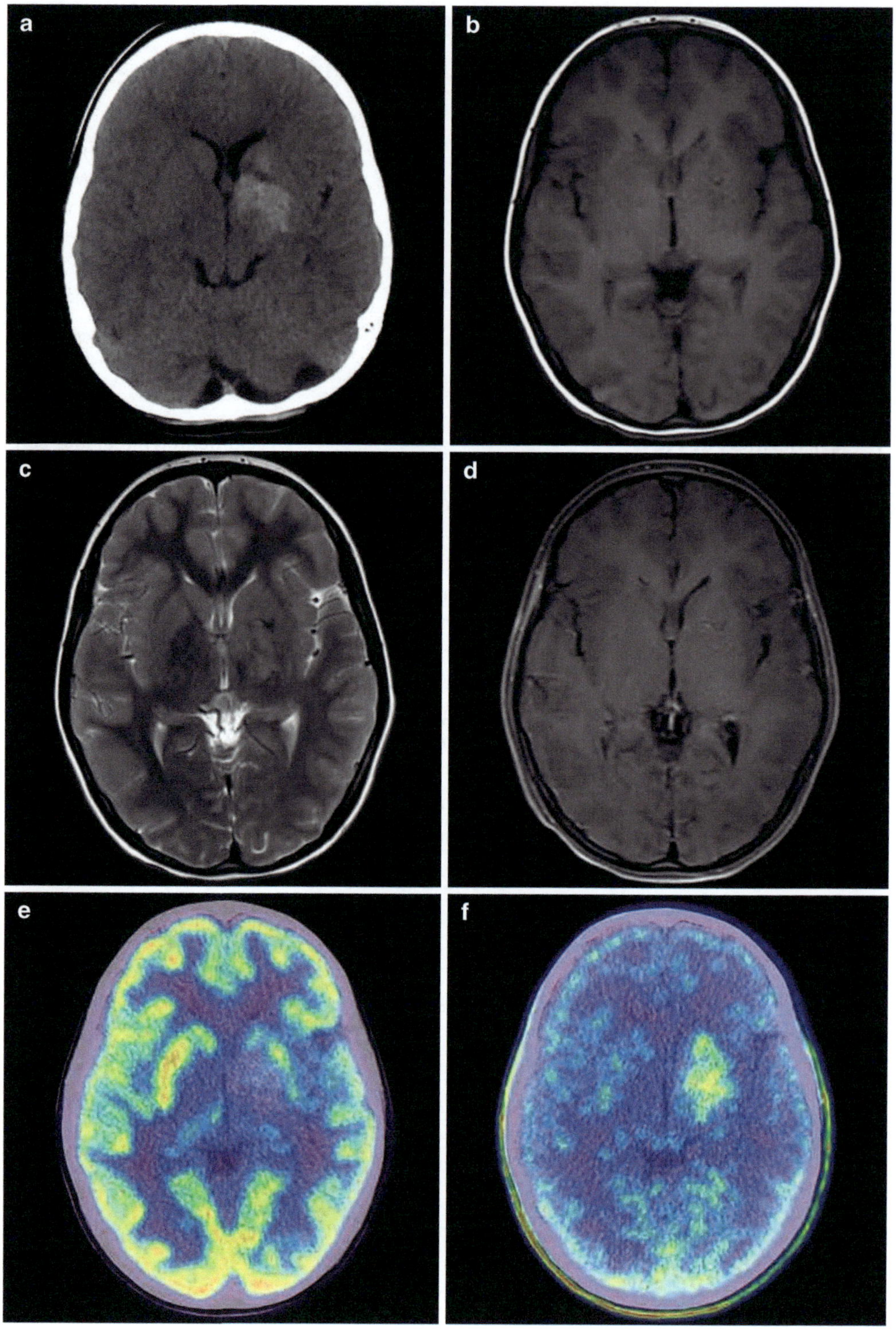

Fig. 5.1 Germinomas. (**a**) CT. A hyperintensity mass noted in the left basal ganglia, without remarkable space-occupying effect. (**b**). Mildly abnormal hypointensity on T_1WI. (**c**) Slight hyperintensity on T_2WI, with poorly defined margins. (**d**) No remarkable enhancement on contrast-enhanced T_1WI sequence. (**e**) ^{18}F-FDG PET showing a significantly decreased metabolic activity of glucose in the lesion than in the contralateral basal ganglia. (**f**) ^{11}C-MET PET showing a significantly increased metabolic activity of methionine in the lesion than in the contralateral side. The findings of both CT and MRI suggest a germinoma

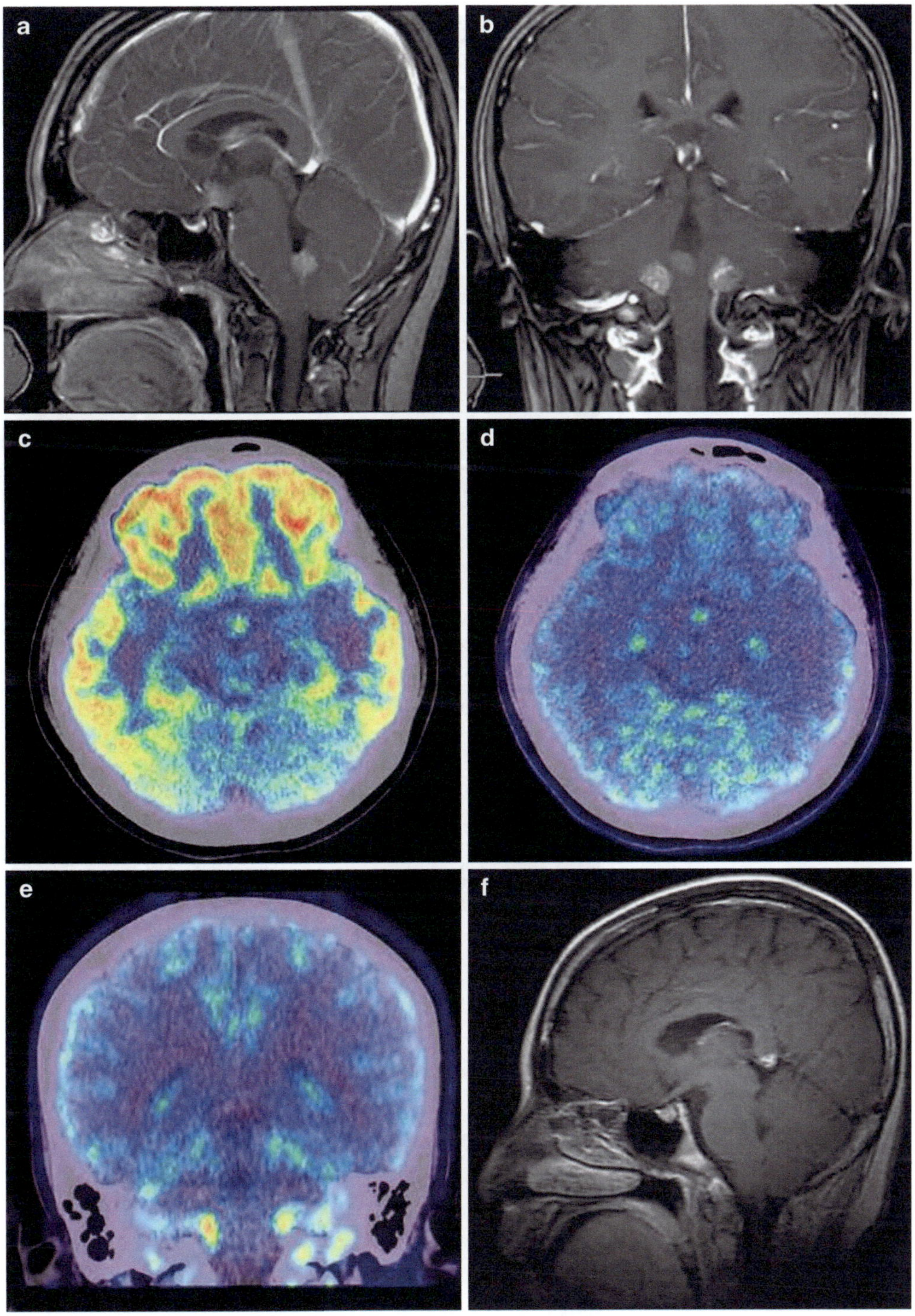

Fig. 5.2 Germinoma metastases. (**a, b**) Sagittal and coronal contrast-enhanced MRI indicates multiple enhanced nodules in the hypothalamus, lower part of the fourth ventricle, and lateral region to the fourth ventricle. (**c**) ^{18}F-FDG PET shows a high uptake of glucose in the sellar nodules. (**d, e**) ^{11}C-MET PET shows a moderately increased MET uptake in the sellar nodules and a slightly increased MET uptake in the nodules lateral to the fourth ventricle. (**f**) Two months after radiotherapy, a re-examination of MRI with contrast shows a disappearance of the enhanced nodules in the suprasellar region and the fourth ventricle

Fig. 5.3 Germinomas. (**a**) MRI with contrast shows two enhanced nodules in the pineal region and the suprasellar/hypothalamic region. (**b**) ^{18}F-FDG PET shows a mild uptake in the pineal region. (**c, d**) ^{11}C-MET PET shows significantly increased MET uptake in the pineal lesion and in the sellar lesion

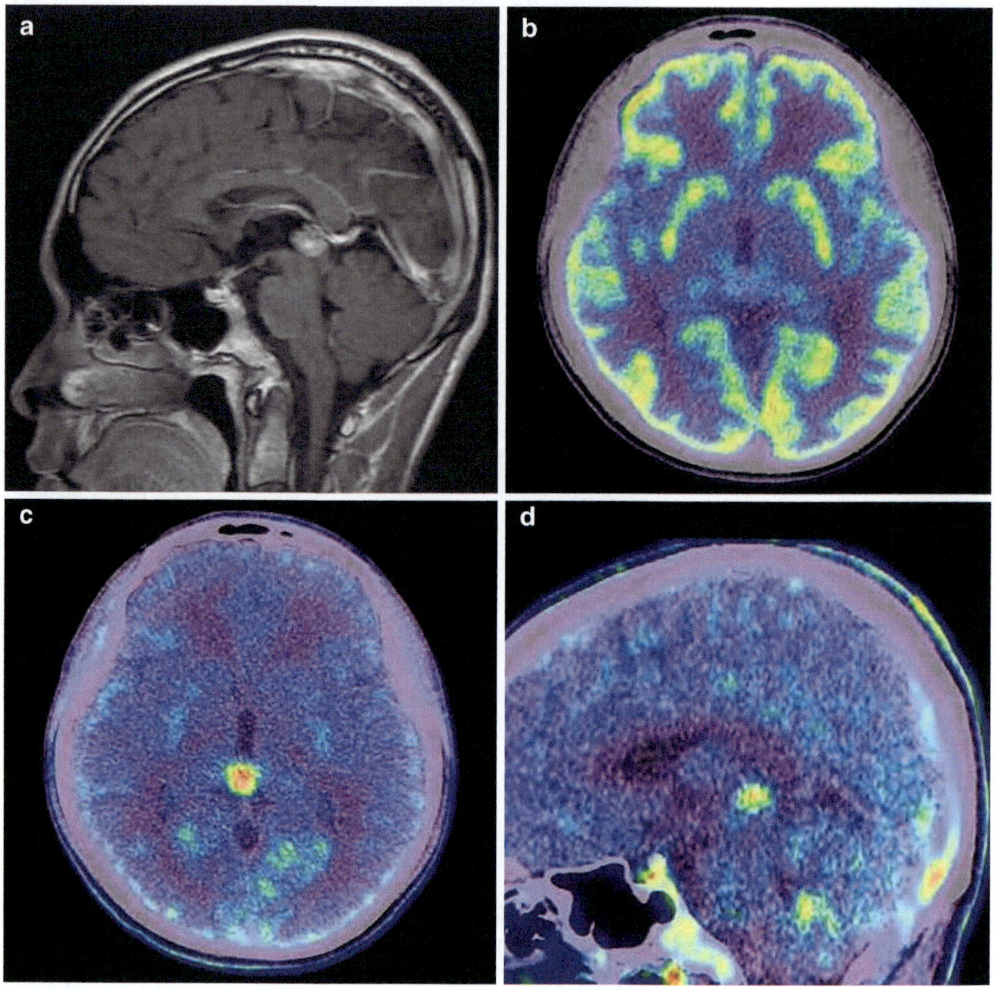

PET/CT of Metastatic Tumors

6

Xueying Ling and Hao Xu

1 Clinical Overview

1.1 Epidemiology

Metastatic tumors are the most common and accounts for about 10% of intracranial neoplasms. The tumors usually occur at ages of 50–70 years. Of patients with malignant tumors, 20–40% develop brain metastases, of which 70–75% are multiple brain metastases and located in the supratentorial region more often than in the subtentorial region. Lung cancer, breast cancer, and gastrointestinal cancer are common primary tumors, while urological cancer and skin cancer are infrequently seen. Sarcoma and germ cell tumor usually occur in children. The primary focus of the metastatic tumors cannot be identified in some patients. The malignant tumors that originated from the pelvis are prone to be a single metastatic tumor in the subtentorial region.

1.2 Pathology

Metastatic tumors usually occur at the gray-white matter junctions, more often at the areas supplied by the middle cerebral artery, and occasionally at the pituitary gland and cerebral ventricle.

There are three sources of metastases: through lung-blood circulation-brain; through direct invasion; and through the lymph space around spinal nerves and cranial nerves to cerebrospinal fluid circulation or through the vertebral vein to intracranial tissues.

Characteristics of gross morphology of metastases are as follows: multiple; vary in size; no capsule; prone to cystic necrosis or hemorrhage; and severe peritumoral edema.

When involved by metastasis, the meninges show general thickness and grayish white color.

1.3 Prognosis

Prognostic factors are the functional status of systemic organs and the nervous system, age, primary tumor status (location and extent of lesions, pathological type, and treatment response), the number and location of metastatic tumors, surgical excision, with/without extracranial metastasis, with/without recurrence, and the time interval between the appearance of the primary tumor and metastasis.

There are a relative long interval between the diagnosis of primary tumor and the occurrence of brain metastases and a relative long median survival in patients of age less than 60 years and females.

The mean survival time for untreated brain metastases is 1–2 months.

1.4 Clinical Management

Clinical manifestations of metastatic tumors are associated with the location and size of tumors as well as peritumoral edema and mainly include headache, nausea, and vomiting.

Clinical diagnosis is based on symptoms, history of primary tumors, and typical MRI findings.

Treatment plan may include medication, surgery, radiotherapy, and chemotherapy.

NCCN guidelines recommend a multidisciplinary team (MDT) approach for a reasonable management plan before treatment commences.

X. Ling · H. Xu (✉)
The First Affiliated Hospital of Jinan University, Guangzhou, Guangdong, China
e-mail: txh@jnu.edu.cn

Z. Yao, S. Li (eds.), *Atlas of PET/CT in Oncology - Volume 1*, https://doi.org/10.1007/978-981-99-1172-1_6

2 PET/CT Diagnostic Points

1. ^{18}F-FDG PET/CT The degree of FDG uptake varies, including ① the FDG uptake in lesions being higher than in normal gray matter; ② the FDG uptake in lesions being higher than in white matter while lower than in normal gray matter; ③ the FDG uptake in lesions being lower than in white matter; and ④ unremarkable distribution of brain FDG.

   Lesions with a high uptake of FDG are mostly nodular or annular and are often surrounded by regions of reduced metabolism or sparse areas due to cerebral edema.
2. CT Plain CT scan shows single or multiple nodular or annular intracerebral lesions with isodensity, mostly located in the cortex and subcortex. Contrast-enhanced CT scan shows nodular or mild to moderate annular enhancement. Peritumoral edema varies in degree. The metastases in the cortex, particularly in the centrum semiovale, can cause remarkable metastasis-related edema, showing "small tumor, large edema."
3. MRI Appearance T_1WI shows isointensity or slight hypointensity, and T_2WI shows hyperintensity and even higher signal intensity in lesions with cystic necrosis or heterogeneous intensity in lesions with hemorrhage. Contrast-enhanced T_1WI shows mild to moderate annular or nodular enhancement and can show tiny metastases without peritumoral edema. Nodular enhancement of the meninges suggests meningeal metastases.

3 Typical Cases

Case 1: A 35-year-old female complained of dizziness and headache, with nausea and vomiting after comprehensive treatment for the right lung adenocarcinoma. Metastatic tumors in the right occipital lobe were found on PET/CT (Fig. 6.1).

Case 2: A 47-year-old female underwent PET/CT examination after surgical resection of brain metastases in the right frontal lobe (Fig. 6.2).

Case 3: A 36-year-old female presented for follow-up after a comprehensive treatment for multiple systemic metastases after left breast cancer surgery (Fig. 6.3).

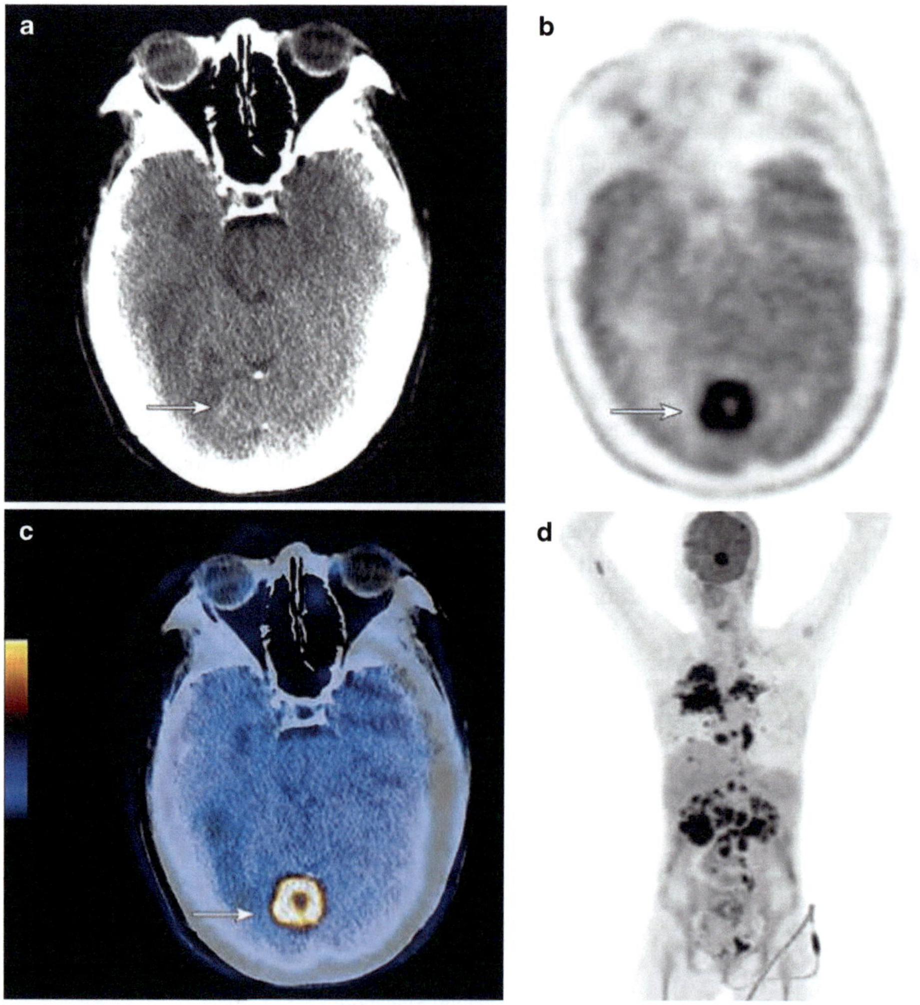

Fig. 6.1 ^{18}F-FDG PET/CT images of metastatic tumors. (**a**) Axial CT. (**b**) Axial PET. (**c**) Axial PET/CT. (**d**) PET MIP image. FDG PET/CT shows an isodensity lesion, with a hypodensity necrotic region in the central region and a ring-like increased FDG uptake (significantly higher than the cortical uptake), accompanied by severe edema. PET MIP image shows high FDG uptakes in the primary tumor of the right lung and multiple metastases

Fig. 6.2 ^{18}F-FDG PET/CT images of metastatic tumors. (**a**) Axial CT. (**b**) Axial PET. (**c**) Axial PET/CT. Metastatic tumors were noted in the right temporal and parietal lobes, showing nodular or annular lesions at the cortical medullary junction (white arrow) with isodensity and increased FDG uptake (close to the cortical uptake), with severe edema. (**d**) PET MIP image reveals primary tumor of the right lung and multiple systematic metastases with high FDG uptake. (**e**) Contrast-enhanced axial T_1WI. (**f**) Contrast-enhanced sagittal T_1WI. Contrast-enhanced T_1WI shows metastatic tumors with nodular or annular enhancement and can show more tiny metastases (white arrow)

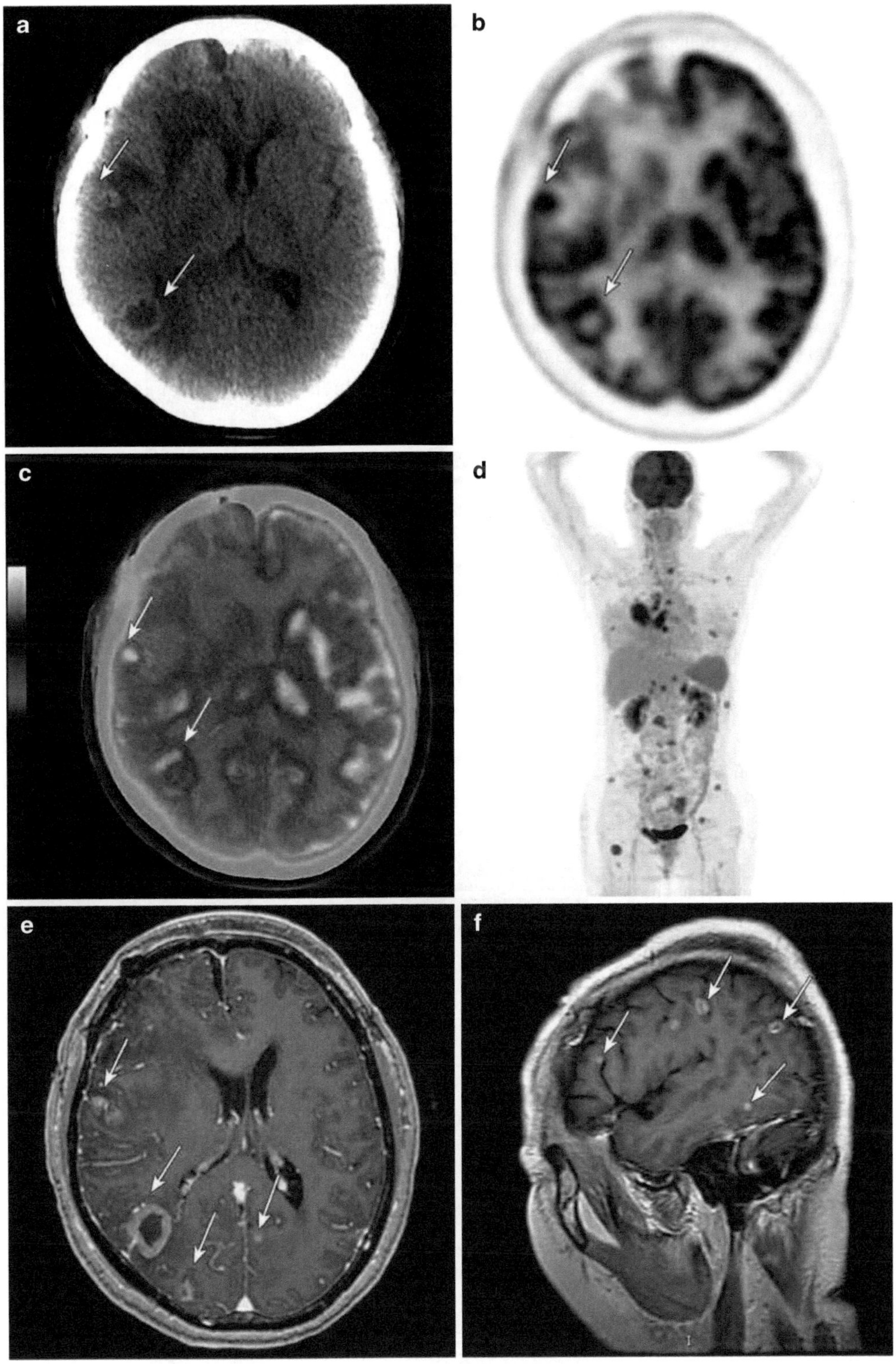

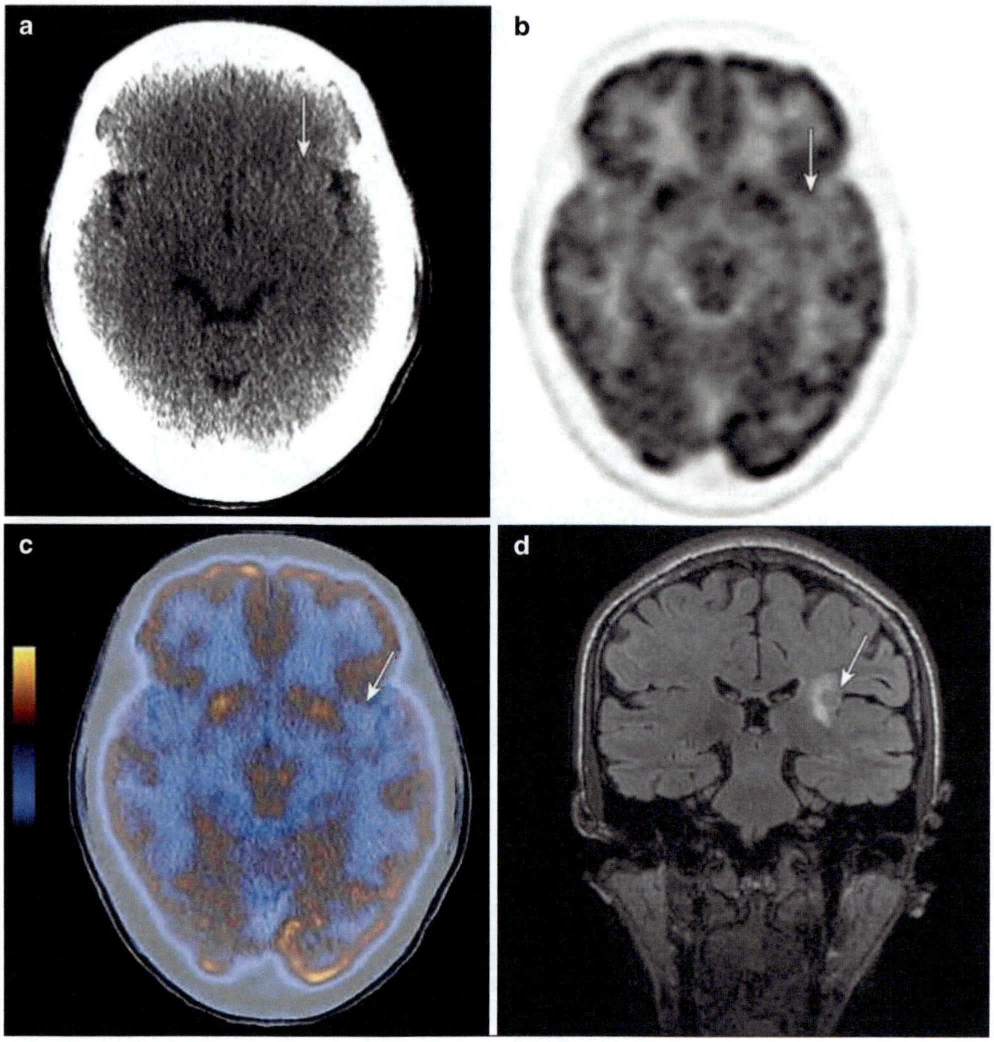

Fig. 6.3 ^{18}F-FDG PET/CT images of metastatic tumors. (**a**) Axial CT. (**b**) Axial PET. (**c**) Axial PET/CT. No abnormal density lesion was noted in the left insular lobe, and the FDG uptake in the local cerebral cortex is lower than that in the contralateral side. (**d**) Coronal T_2FLAIR. Metastatic tumor of isointensity was noted in the left insular lobe (white arrow), surrounded by hyperintensity edema

4 Rare Cases

A 34-year-old male presented with suspected meningeal metastases after right lung cancer surgery (Fig. 6.4).

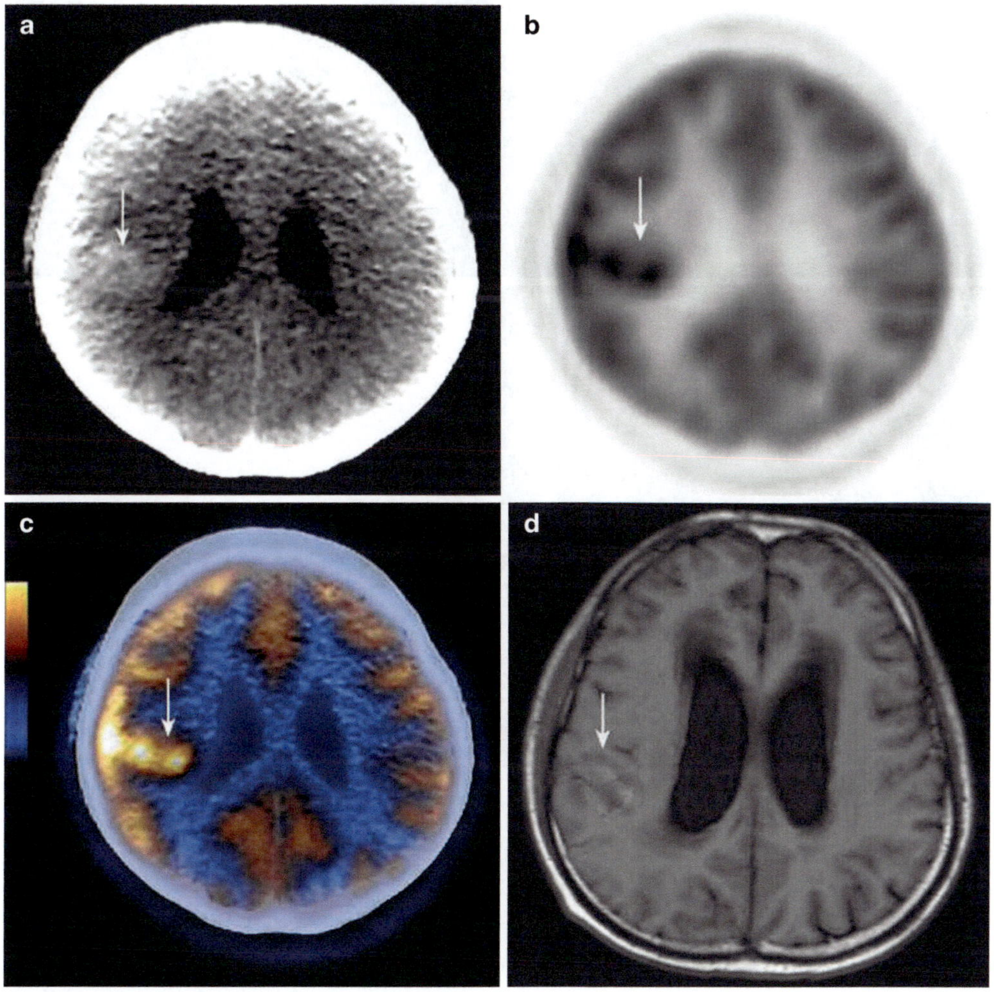

Fig. 6.4 ^{18}F-FDG PET/CT images of meningeal metastases. (**a**) Axial CT. (**b**) Axial PET. (**c**) Axial PET/CT. (**d**) Axial T_1WI. (**e**) Axial T_2WI. (**f**, **g**). Contrast-enhanced axial and sagittal T_1WI. PET/CT shows increased FDG uptake in the lesions with hyperdensity along the gyri (white arrow). T_1WI hyperintensity and T_2WI hypointensity in local meninges indicate hemorrhage in the lesions. Contrast-enhanced T_1WI shows more extensive meningeal metastases along the gyri

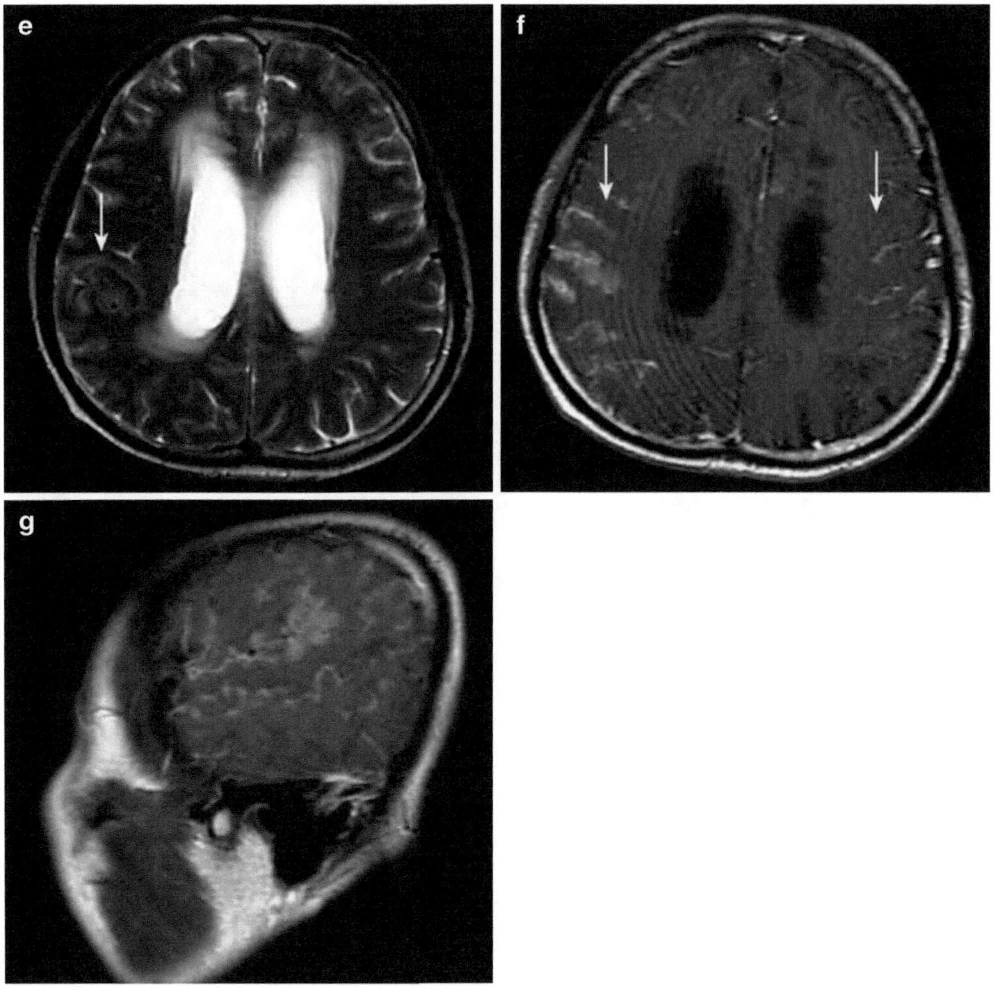

Fig. 6.4 (continued)

5 Differential Diagnosis

1. Glioblastomas: The appearance of solitary brain metastases is similar to that of glioblastomas, but most metastases occur at the cortical medullary junction. Also, in general, the history of malignant tumors or primary foci elsewhere in the body can be found in patients with metastases.
2. Brain abscess: After forming the wall of the abscess, the appearance of brain abscess is similar to that of cystic metastases, but on DWI, the pus of abscess shows a hyperintensity area, whereas cystic necrosis of the metastases shows a hypointensity area.
3. Meningiomas: Meningeal metastases should be differentiated from meningiomas. Most meningeal metastases are multiple, usually invade the skull, and have extracranial primary tumors (Fig. 6.5).

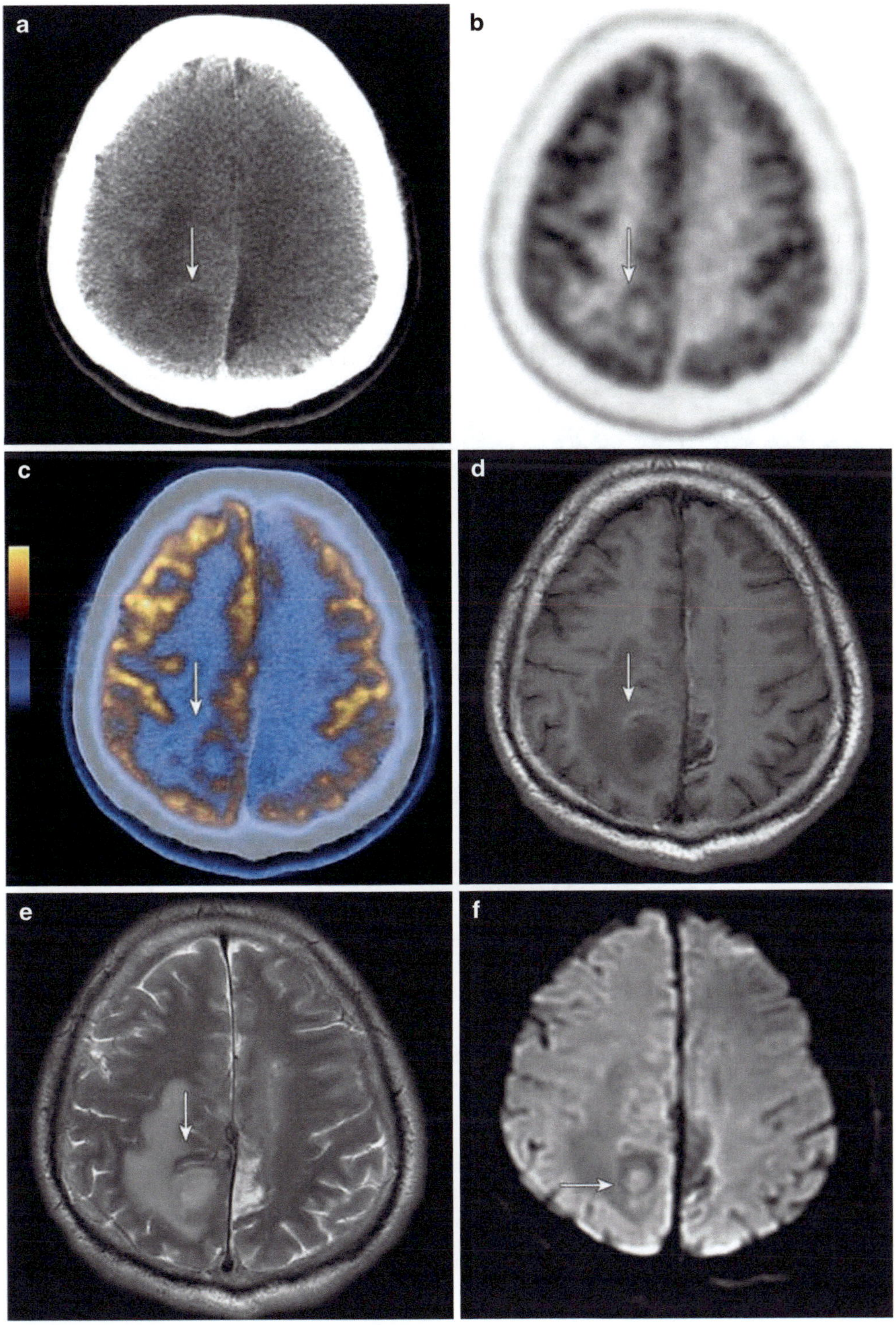

Fig. 6.5 ^{18}F-FDG PET/CT images of brain abscess. A 34-year-old male patient complained of dizziness, with right limb weakness and dysphonia. (**a**) Axial CT. (**b**) Axial PET. (**c**) Axial PET/CT. (**d**) Axial T_1WI. (**e**) Axial T_2WI. (**f**) Axial DWI. (**g**) Contrast-enhanced axial T_1WI. MRI shows an abscess in the right parietal lobe. PET/CT shows an oval lesion of mixed iso-hypodense and annular uptake of FDG (lower than the cortical uptake) in the right parietal lobe (white arrow). The wall of the abscess shows abnormal signal intensities at multiple levels on T_1WI and T_2WI. Pus shows higher signal intensity on DWI. Part of the cerebral falx is also enhanced after contrast agent administration (white arrow)

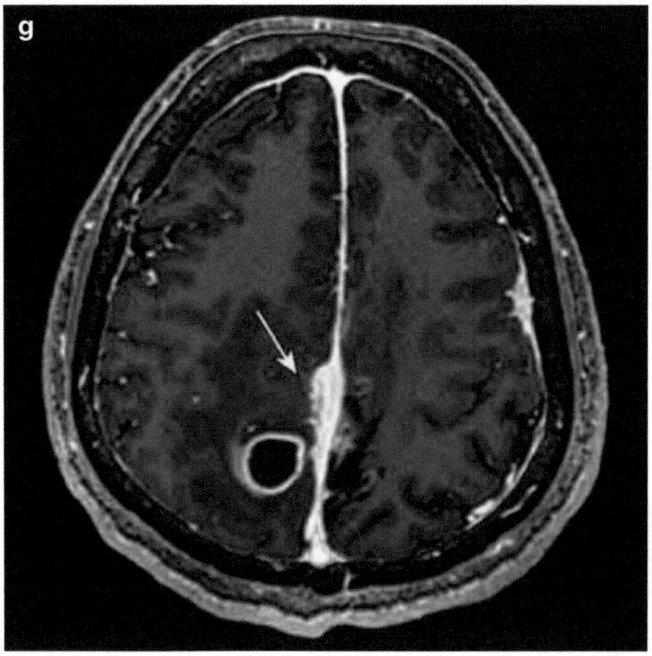

Fig. 6.5 (continued)

6 Summary

The main method for diagnosing brain metastases is contrast-enhanced MRI. ^{18}F-FDG PET/CT can detect cerebral metastases with increased FDG uptake, while whole body FDG PET/CT is helpful to detect primary tumors.

Part II

PET/CT of Nasopharyngeal and Oral Tumors

7 General Introduction of PET/CT of Nasopharyngeal Carcinoma

Xiaoping Lin, Shan Zheng, Wei Fan, and Weibing Miao

Head and neck tumors are clinically common, with various types and small proportions. Due to their location and complex surrounding structures, the tumors have a great impact on the human body's five sense organs and surrounding structures. At present, morphological and structural imaging, such as CT and MR, and endoscopy can only represent the changes in anatomical morphology or the surface of hollow organs. On the basis of observing the morphology and structure of the lesion, PET/CT can further represent the biological changes of tumor from the perspective of biochemical metabolism and perform qualitative and quantitative analysis on the primary lesion and metastasis, which is conducive to the location of primary lesion, clinical staging, efficacy evaluation, differential diagnosis of tumor recurrence/residual and changes after treatment, etc.

Head and neck tumors are mostly derived from epithelial tissues, and tumor proliferation is active. ^{18}F-FDG uptake is high in the primary lesion, metastatic lymph nodes, and advanced-stage distant metastatic lesions. Because of the heterogeneity of tumors, the distribution of ^{18}F-FDG in the same lesion may be inconsistent. If the radioactive background of the surrounding tissues is too high, the contrast between the tumor tissue and the surrounding normal tissues is not obvious, which makes it difficult to distinguish the tumor with the naked eye. Therefore, comprehensive analysis must be carried out in combination with the structural imaging characteristics of PET/CT. Radiopharmaceutical extravasation at the injection site can visualize the normal lymph nodes on the injection side. When ^{18}F-FDG PET/CT is performed within a short time after surgery or radiotherapy, the tissues in surgical site or radiotherapy area can accumulate ^{18}F-FDG and cause false positive findings. Besides, high ^{18}F-FDG uptake may also occur in some benign lesions and physiological processes. Granulation tissue repair and massive infiltration of lymphocytes may increase local regional metabolism. Obesity, diabetes, high blood sugar during imaging, insulin injection, or muscle tension may cause muscle to take in ^{18}F-FDG. Sympathetic nerve excitement before examination may cause brown fat to take in ^{18}F-FDG. Therefore, it is not accurate to judge the benign and malignant lesions only by the uptake of ^{18}F-FDG. When interpreting ^{18}F-FDG PET/CT, it is necessary to combine the medical history and correctly analyze the biological characteristics of the tumor, to make a scientific diagnosis.

X. Lin · W. Fan (✉)
Sun Yat-sen University Cancer Center, Guangzhou, Guangdong, China
e-mail: fanwei@sysucc.org.cn

S. Zheng · W. Miao
The First Affiliated Hospital of Fujian Medical University, Fuzhou, Fujian, China

1 Nasopharyngeal Carcinoma

Nasopharyngeal carcinoma is a malignant tumor derived from the covering epithelium of the nasopharynx. It occurs frequently in southern China and Southeast Asia. Guangdong Province is the area with the highest incidence of nasopharyngeal carcinoma, so it is also called "Canton tumor." Radiotherapy is the main treatment method, and concurrent chemoradiotherapy can improve the curative effect of nasopharyngeal carcinoma.

1.1 Anatomy

The nasopharynx is located between the base of skull and the soft palate, which connects the nasal cavity and the oropharynx. It can be divided into anterior, parietal, and posterior base walls and two symmetrical lateral walls. The anterior wall includes bilateral posterior nostrils and the posterior edge of the nasal septum of the midline. The parietal wall and posterior wall are connected with each other and inclined to form a circular arch; there is no clear anatomical boundary between the two walls, so it is often called the posterior parietal wall clinically, that is, from the upper edge of the posterior nostril back to the level of the soft palate; there are

Z. Yao, S. Li (eds.), *Atlas of PET/CT in Oncology - Volume 1*, https://doi.org/10.1007/978-981-99-1172-1_7

abundant lymphoid tissues under the mucosa to form the pharyngeal tonsils, which have obvious proliferation and form the proliferators in childhood.

The lymphatic tissue in the nasopharynx is very rich, which mainly drains into the retropharyngeal lymph nodes near the cervical atlas and then into the deep cervical lymph nodes, which mainly includes jugular vein lymph node chain, accessory nerve lymph node chain (located in the posterior cervical triangle), and transverse cervical arteriovenous lymph node chain (located in the supraclavicular fossa).

The parapharyngeal space is a deep fat space in the upper neck of the face and jaw, adjacent to the nasopharynx and oropharynx. The parapharyngeal space is formed by the styloid process and its attached muscles (styloid hyoid muscle, styloid tongue muscle, and styloid pharyngeal muscle) and multiple fasciae, which is symmetrical on both sides.

1.2 Epidemiology and Etiology

Nasopharyngeal carcinoma can occur in all age groups, but it is more common in 30–60 years old, accounting for 75–90%, with the male-to-female ratio of (2–3.8):1. The epidemiology of nasopharyngeal carcinoma is characterized by obvious regional clustering, racial and partial population susceptibility, family clustering, and relatively stable incidence.

The occurrence of nasopharyngeal carcinoma may be multi-factorial, and its carcinogenesis may involve multiple steps. Factors that may be related to the onset of nasopharyngeal carcinoma include genetic susceptibility, EB virus infection, environmental factors, and so on.

1.3 Pathology

The nasopharyngeal cavity is covered with a thin layer of mucosal epithelium, which is mainly composed of squamous epithelium, pseudostratified ciliated columnar epithelium, and transitional epithelium. There is often lymphocyte infiltration in the lamina propria, and there are serous and mucous glands in the submucosa.

More than 95% of nasopharyngeal carcinoma cells are poorly differentiated with high degree of malignancy. In 1991, the WHO classified nasopharyngeal carcinoma histologically into two major categories, squamous cell carcinoma or keratinizing squamous cell carcinoma (WHO I) and non-keratinizing carcinoma, the latter of which can be divided into differentiated non-keratinizing carcinoma (WHO II) and undifferentiated carcinoma or undifferentiated carcinoma of nasopharyngeal type (WHO III) according to the degree of differentiation of tumor cells.

1.4 Spread and Metastasis

Nasopharyngeal carcinoma often occurs in the lateral wall (especially pharyngeal recess) and posterior parietal wall of the nasopharynx.

Nasopharyngeal carcinoma not only invades upward by directly damaging the cranial base bone, but it can also infiltrate the intracranial space through natural openings or clefts such as the foramen lacerum, foramen ovale, foramen spinosum, internal carotid artery canal, or sphenoid and posterior ethmoid sinuses, affecting the cranial nerves. It invades forward into the nasal cavity, maxillary sinus, anterior ethmoid sinuses, and even into the orbit, either through intracranial, superior orbital fissure or optic canal, and pterygopalatine fossa. It can also infiltrate laterally into the parapharyngeal space, infratemporal fossa, and the muscles of mastication. Nasopharyngeal carcinoma infiltrates posteriorly into the soft tissues anterior to the cervical vertebrae, as well as the cervical vertebrae themselves. It can extend downward, involving the oropharynx and even the hypopharynx.

There is a rich network of lymphatic vessels under the nasopharyngeal mucosa, and lymphatic drainage can cross the midline to the contralateral neck. The cervical lymph node metastasis of nasopharyngeal carcinoma occurs early, and the metastasis rate is high. The location of lymph node metastasis is most common in the deep superior cervical lymph nodes under the digastric muscle, followed by the deep and middle cervical lymph nodes and the accessory nerve chain lymph nodes in the posterior triangle of the neck. The most common site of distant metastasis is the bone, followed by the lung and liver, and it often occurs in multiple organs at the same time.

1.5 Clinical Manifestations

The common symptoms and signs of nasopharyngeal carcinoma include nasal bleeding, nasal obstruction, headache, brain nerve damage, cervical lymph node enlargement, and distant metastasis.

1.6 Stage

1. Chinese Nasopharyngeal Carcinoma Staging, 2017 edition [American Joint Committee on Cancer (AJCC)/ Union for International Cancer Control, (UICC) 8th edition]

   T_x: The primary tumor cannot be estimated.

   T_0: No tumor is found, but there is EBV-positive cervical lymph node metastasis.

T_1: Confined to the nasopharyngeal cavity and oropharyngeal/nasal cavity, without invasion of parapharyngeal space.
T_2: Parapharyngeal space and/or adjacent soft tissues (medial pterygoid muscle, lateral pterygoid muscle, and anterior vertebral muscle) are invaded.
T_3: Bone structure of cervical vertebra, pterygoid structure, and/or paranasal sinus are involved.
T_4: Intracranial extension, the involvement of cranial nerves, hypopharynx, orbit, parotid gland, and/or extensive soft tissue infiltration beyond the lateral edge of the pterygoid muscle.
N_x: Regional lymph nodes cannot be estimated.
N_0: No regional lymph node metastasis.
N_1: Retropharyngeal lymph node metastasis (regardless of the number of sides) and/or lymph node metastasis in the unilateral neck and the area above the caudal border of the cricoid cartilage with the largest diameter ≤ 6 cm.
N_2: Bilateral cervical lymph node metastasis and lymph node metastasis extending above the caudal border of the cricoid cartilage with the maximum diameter ≤ 6 cm.
N_3: Maximum diameter of metastatic lymph node > 6 cm and lymph node metastasis extending below the caudal border of the cricoid cartilage.
M_0: No distant metastasis.
M_1: Distant metastasis.

2. Clinical stage
   Stage 0: $TisN_0M_0$.
   Stage I: $T_1N_0M_0$.
   Stage II: $T_{0-1}N_1M_0$, $T_2N_{0-1}M_0$.
   Stage III: $T_{0-2}N_2M_0$, $T_3N_{0-2}M_0$.
   Stage IV_a: $T_{0-3}N_3M_0$ or $T_4N_{0-3}M_0$.
   Stage IV_b: Any T, any N, M_1.

1.7 Treatment

Nasopharyngeal carcinoma is treated by radiotherapy-based comprehensive treatment. Surgical treatment is usually a rescue method for local lesions after chemoradiotherapy.

2 Laryngopharyngeal Carcinoma

Laryngopharyngeal carcinoma, also known as hypopharyngeal carcinoma, is a malignant tumor of the mucosal epithelium of the laryngopharynx. More than 95% of it is squamous cell carcinoma. Due to its special anatomical location, it is not easy to find early. It often has an infiltrative growth pattern and usually treated with radiotherapy and surgery-based comprehensive treatment.

2.1 Anatomy

The laryngopharynx is at the back of the larynx, between the level of the hyoid bone and the caudal border of the cricoid cartilage, which is equivalent to the third to sixth cervical vertebrae. The laryngopharynx is clinically divided into three anatomical regions: pyriform sinus, postcricoid region, and retropharyngeal wall. The postcricoid region is from the arytenoid cartilage and interarytenoid level to the caudal border of the cricoid cartilage, forming the anterior hypopharyngeal wall. The pyriform sinus is from the pharyngeal fold to the entrance of the esophagus, the outside is the lamina of the thyroid cartilage, and the inside is the hypopharyngeal side of the arytenoid fold, arytenoid cartilage, and cricoid cartilage. The posterior pharyngeal wall is from the level of the upper edge of the hyoid bone (or the bottom of the epiglottis) to the level of the caudal border of the cricoid cartilage.

2.2 Epidemiology and Etiology

The cause of laryngopharyngeal carcinoma is unknown. Studies have shown that the occurrence of laryngopharyngeal carcinoma is obviously related to excessive drinking and smoking and other factors such as reduced intake of vegetables and fruits, dental dysfunction, and exposure to occupational carcinogens.

2.3 Pathology

The histopathological morphology of laryngopharyngeal carcinoma is ulcerative, infiltrative, and exophytic type. The former two are more common. About 95% are squamous epithelial carcinoma, and others are rare. The incidence ratio of male to female is (12–25):11. The pyriform sinus carcinoma is the most common type of laryngopharyngeal carcinoma.

2.4 Spread and Metastasis

Different sites of the laryngopharyngeal carcinoma spread through different pathways. The posterior pharyngeal wall and pyriform sinus carcinoma can upward invade the oropharynx and downward invade the cervical esophagus. The tumor of postcricoid area can often invade the arytenoid cartilage and the cricoarytenoid joint, can downward invade the cervical esophagus, and can rarely invade the prevertebral fascia. The tumor of the lateral wall of the pyriform sinus mainly extends to the lateral wall of the pharynx, which can destroy the thyroid cartilage and cricoid cartilage. And the tumor of the medial wall easily extends to the laryngeal cavity and along the postcricoid area to the contralateral pyriform sinus. The paraglottic space and thyroid cartilage are the most vulnerable laryngeal structures, and the cricoid cartilage is less likely to be invaded. The tumor extends along the aryepiglottic fold and directly extends forward within the inner side of the thyroid cartilage lamina, invading the paraglottic space. It also extends inward and upward along the aryepiglottic fold, and invades the pre-epiglottic space in the upper part within the inner side of the thyroid cartilage lamina.

The tumor in this region often presents mucosal spread, especially at the junction of the pharynx and cervical esophagus. The submucosal lymphoid tissue is rich and accompanied by jumpy spread.

The cervical lymph node metastasis rate of laryngopharyngeal carcinoma is high, mainly unilateral, and common in II and III area, and then it can metastasize to IV, V, and VI area, and bilateral cervical lymph node metastasis can also occur.

In the late stage, hematogenous metastasis is the most common, in which the most frequent sites of metastasis include the lung, liver, and bone.

2.5 Clinical Manifestations

Clinically, it often manifests as a foreign body sensation in the retropharynx. The patient often feels that there is food residual in the pharynx after eating, which may be accompanied by pain and discomfort. Coughing, hoarseness, and cervical mass may appear in the late stage. The former is due to incomplete glottis closure caused by blockage of the lumps or invasion of the recurrent laryngeal nerve.

2.6 Stage

1. TNM stage

   T: Primary tumor.

   Tx: Primary tumor cannot be evaluated.

   Tis: Carcinoma in situ.

   T_1: The tumor is confined to an anatomical subregion of the hypopharynx, with a maximum diameter of <2 cm.

   T_2: The tumor invades more than one anatomical subregion or an adjacent structure of the hypopharynx, or the maximum diameter is 2–4 cm, without hemilaryngeal fixation.

   T_3: The maximum diameter of the tumor exceeds 4 cm or hemilaryngeal fixation.

   T_4: The tumor invades adjacent structures, such as the thyroid cartilage, cricoid cartilage, carotid artery, cervical soft tissue, prevertebral fascia and muscle, thyroid, or esophagus.

   N_0: No enlarged lymph nodes are palpated.

   N_1: A single lymph node on the same side with a diameter of <3 cm.

   N_2: A single lymph node on the same side with a diameter of 3–6 cm or multiple lymph nodes on the same side with a maximum diameter of < 6 cm.

   N_3: Lymph node diameter > 6 cm.

   M_0: No distant metastasis.

   M_1: Distant metastasis.

2. Clinical stage

   Stage I: $T_1N_0M_0$.

   Stage II: $T_2N_0M_0$.

   Stage III: $T_3N_0M_0$, $T_{1-3}N_1M_0$.

   Stage IV_a: $T_4N_{0-1}M_0$, $T_{1-4}N_2M_0$.

   Stage IV_b: $T_{1-4}N_3M_0$.

   Stage IV_c: Any T, any N, M_1.

2.7 Treatment

It is usually treated with radiotherapy and surgery-based comprehensive treatment. Radiotherapy or surgery alone can be used for stages T_1 and T_2, and surgery is suitable for stages T_3 and T_4, supplemented by radiotherapy or chemotherapy.

3 Laryngeal Carcinoma

Laryngeal carcinoma is a common malignant tumor of the head and neck. Surgery and radiotherapy are the main treatments for laryngeal carcinoma. While laryngeal carcinoma is radically cured, efforts should be made to preserve or rebuild the patient's vocal function and improve the quality of life of the patient.

3.1 Anatomy

The larynx is the respiratory channel and the vocal organ. It is at the level of the fourth to fifth cervical vertebra in the middle of the front of the neck. The upper part is connected to the aperture of the larynx and the laryngopharynx, and the lower part is connected to the trachea. The front is covered by skin, superficial cervical fascia, deep cervical fascia, and infrahyoid muscles. Both sides are in contact with cervical vessels, nerves, and lateral lobe of the thyroid.

1. Laryngeal boundary
   (a) Upper boundary: lingual surface of the epiglottis, free edge of the epiglottis, the aryepiglottic fold of two sides, and the arytenoid cartilage area of two sides.

(b) Lower boundary: caudal border of the cricoid cartilage.
(c) Anterior boundary: the thyrohyoid membrane, the anterior part of the thyroid cartilage, the cricothyroid membrane, and the arch of the cricoid cartilage.
(d) Posterior boundary: arytenoid area and cricoid cartilage plate.
(e) Lateral boundary: the outer edge of the epiglottis cartilage of two sides, aryepiglottic fold, the front part of the thyroid cartilage plate, and inner wall mucosa of the pyriform sinus.

2. Anatomical division of the larynx: The larynx is anatomically divided into the supraglottic portion, the glottic portion, and the subglottic portion.
   (a) Supraglottic portion: from the upper boundary of the larynx to the upper edge of the vocal cords is the supraglottic portion, including the lingual surface of the epiglottis, free edge of the epiglottis, laryngeal surface of the epiglottis, aryepiglottic fold of two sides, arytenoid cartilage area of two sides, ventricular cords of two sides, and laryngeal ventricle of two sides.
   (b) Glottic portion: the glottic portion includes vocal cords of two sides, the anterior commissure, and the posterior commissure.
   (c) Subglottic portion: the subglottic portion includes the area between the lower edge of the vocal cords and the caudal border of the cricoid cartilage.
3. Structure of the larynx: The structure of the larynx is complex, which consists of cartilage, joint, ligament, muscle, and mucosa.
   (a) Laryngeal cartilage: Laryngeal cartilage includes the unpaired thyroid cartilage, cricoid cartilage, and epiglottis cartilage as the structure and paired arytenoid cartilage, corniculate cartilage, and cuneiform cartilage attached to the structure.
   (b) Larynx joint and ligament: The laryngeal joint and ligament include the connection between the laryngeal cartilage, the cartilage, the hyoid bone, and the trachea. The joint includes the cricoarytenoid joint and cricothyroid joint. The laryngeal ligament includes the elastic cone (cricothyroid membrane), quadrangular membrane, thyrohyoid membrane, and tracheal ligament of the cricoid cartilage.
   (c) Laryngeal muscle: The laryngeal muscle mainly includes intrinsic laryngeal muscle and extrinsic laryngeal muscle. The intrinsic laryngeal muscles include three pairs of thyroarytenoid muscle, lateral cricoarytenoid muscle, and posterior cricoarytenoid muscle. The extrinsic laryngeal muscles are divided into suprahyoid muscles and infrahyoid muscles.
   (d) Laryngeal cavity: The laryngeal cavity is a cavity surrounded by the larynx wall, covered with mucosa, connected with the laryngopharyngeal mucosa on the upper side, and connected with the tracheal mucosa on the lower side. There are two pairs of mucosal folds running along the two side walls of the larynx, called the ventricular cord (false vocal cord) and the vocal cord (true vocal cord). The ventricle and vocal cords divide the laryngeal cavity into the laryngeal vestibule, the laryngeal ventricle, and the subglottic cavity. The epiglottis and true vocal cord are stratified squamous epithelium, and the rest are pseudostratified ciliated columnar epithelium.
   (e) Laryngeal space: There are three spaces in the larynx, namely, the pre-epiglottic space, the paraglottic space, and the Reinke space.
   (f) Lymphatic drainage of the larynx
      (i) Supraglottic portion: the lymphatic tissue is abundant, and the lymphatic capillary with superior laryngeal nerve passes through the thyrohyoid membrane and finally into the deep superior cervical lymph nodes (lymph nodes in area II) or passes through the ipsilateral cricothyroid membrane and thyroid lobe into the deep middle cervical lymph nodes (lymph nodes in area III).
      (ii) Glottic portion: almost no lymphatic system.
      (iii) Subglottic portion: the lymph tissue is less than that of the supraglottic portion, and lymph drains to the deep and middle cervical lymph nodes (lymph nodes in area III), deep inferior cervical lymph nodes (lymph nodes in area IV), or paratracheal lymph nodes (lymph nodes in area IV).

3.2 Epidemiology and Etiology

In recent years, the incidence of laryngeal carcinoma in China is increasing. Laryngeal carcinoma is common in people aged 50 to 69, and the incidence rate in men is significantly higher than in women.

The cause of laryngeal carcinoma is unknown. It is generally believed that the occurrence of laryngeal carcinoma is related to the following factors: smoking, viral infection (HPV), mutation and amplification of oncogenes such as *Ras* and *Myc*, inactivation of tumor suppressor gene *P53*, sex hormones, etc.

3.3 Pathology

The general pathological types of laryngeal carcinoma can be divided into ulcer type, cauliflower type, nodular type, and mass type. More than 90% of laryngeal carcinoma are squamous cell carcinoma, followed by carcinoma in situ, adenocarcinoma, and sarcoma. In the anatomical division of the larynx, laryngeal carcinoma in the glottic portion accounts for 55–65%, and the laryngeal carcinoma in the supraglottic portion accounts for 35–40%, and laryngeal carcinoma in the subglottic portion is less than 10%.

3.4 Metastasis

1. Cervical lymph node metastasis: The cervical lymph node metastasis of laryngeal carcinoma is related to the primary site of laryngeal carcinoma. Patients with the supraglottic carcinoma are prone to cervical lymph node metastasis due to the richness of blood vessels and lymphatic tissues, which are more common in the area II cervical lymph nodes of the ipsilateral jugular vein lymph node chain; glottic carcinomas rarely metastasize when they have not invaded outside the glottic portion; the lymph node metastasis rate of subglottic carcinoma is 13–20%.
2. Distant metastasis: The systemic metastasis rate is 5–10%. The lung is the most metastatic site, followed by the liver, bone, and skin. The distant metastasis rate of autopsy report can reach 30%.

3.5 Clinical Manifestations

The main clinical manifestations of patients with laryngeal carcinoma include hoarseness, foreign body sensation in the throat, cough and bloody sputum, dyspnea, and cervical mass. These manifestations vary with the location and stage of the tumor.

1. Supraglottic carcinoma: In the early stage, there may be no symptoms or only pharyngeal discomfort and foreign body sensation. As the disease progresses, sore throat may occur, which is aggravated when swallowing, hinders eating, and radiates to the ipsilateral ear. The tumor enlarges and festers, causing cough and bloody sputum. Hoarseness occurs when the tumor invades the glottic portion downward. Late-stage patients have dysphagia, dyspnea, and other symptoms.
2. Glottic carcinoma: Hoarseness appears in the early stage, which is progressively aggravating. Since the glottic portion is the narrowest part of the laryngeal cavity, when the glottic carcinoma grows to a certain size, it will cause laryngeal stridor and inspiratory dyspnea. The advanced patients may have sore throat, blood sputum, and other symptoms.
3. Subglottic carcinoma: In the early stage, the symptoms are not obvious. When the tumor enlarges and festers, there will be cough, bloody sputum, and so on. When the tumor invades the vocal cords, hoarseness occurs. When the tumor blocks the airway, dyspnea occurs.

3.6 Clinical Classification and Stage

UICC and AJCC revised the TNM clinical classification and stage of laryngeal carcinoma in 2010. The classification and stage are only applicable to cancer and should be confirmed histologically.

1. Anatomical division
   (a) Supraglottis: ① suprahyoid epiglottis (including epiglottis tip, lingual surface, and laryngeal surface); ② aryepiglottic fold; ③ arytenoid cartilage; ④ subhyoid epiglottis; ⑤ laryngeal ventricle; and ⑥ ventricular cord.
   (b) Glottis: ① vocal cords; ② anterior commissure; and ③ posterior commissure.
   (c) Subglottis: regional lymph node metastasis refers to the cervical lymph nodes.
2. TNM clinical classification
   (a) Primary tumor (T):
      T_x: The primary tumor cannot be estimated.
      T_0: No evidence of primary tumor.
      Tis: Carcinoma in situ.
   (b) Supraglottic type:
      T_1: The tumor is confined to a subregion of the supraglottis with normal vocal cord movement.
      T_2: The tumor invades more than one subregion of the supraglottis, invades the glottis, or invades beyond the supraglottic portion (root of tongue, epiglottic vallecula, inner wall mucosa of the pyriform sinus), without laryngeal fixation.
      T_3: The tumor is confined to the larynx, with vocal cord fixation, and/or the following sites are invaded, including the postcricoid area, the pre-epiglottic space, the paraglottic space, and/or the thyroid cartilage inner plate.
      T_{4a}: The tumor invades the thyroid cartilage and/or invades extralaryngeal tissues (such as the trachea, cervical soft tissue including deep extrinsic lingual muscles, ribbon muscles, thyroid, or esophagus).
      T_{4b}: Invade the prevertebral fascia, wrap the carotid artery, or invade the mediastinal structure.
   (c) Glottic type:
      T_1: The tumor invades the vocal cords (can invade the anterior or posterior commissure), and the vocal cord movement is normal.
      T_{1a}: The tumor is confined to one vocal cord.
      T_{1b}: The tumor invades both vocal cords.

T_2: The tumor invades the supraglottis or subglottis, and/or vocal cord movement is restricted.
T_3: Confined to the larynx with vocal cord fixation and/or invade the paraglottic space and/or thyroid cartilage inner plate.
T_{4a}: The tumor invades the thyroid cartilage and/or invades extralaryngeal tissues (such as the trachea, cervical soft tissue including deep extrinsic lingual muscles, ribbon muscles, thyroid, or esophagus).
T_{4b}: Invade the prevertebral fascia, wrap the carotid artery, or invade the mediastinal structure.

(d) Subglottic type:
T_1: The tumor is confined to the subglottis.
T_2: The tumor invades the vocal cords, and the vocal cord movement is normal or restricted.
T_3: The tumor is confined to the larynx with the vocal cord fixation.
T_{4a}: The tumor invades the cricoid cartilage or thyroid cartilage and/or invades extralaryngeal tissues (such as the trachea, cervical soft tissue including deep extrinsic lingual muscles, ribbon muscles, thyroid, or esophagus).
T_{4b}: Invade the prevertebral fascia, wrap the carotid artery, or invade the mediastinal structure.

(e) Regional lymph nodes (N):
N_x: It cannot be evaluated whether there is regional lymph node metastasis.
N_0: No regional lymph node metastasis.
N_1: A single ipsilateral lymph node metastasis, with a diameter $\leq$ 3 cm.
N_2: A single ipsilateral lymph node metastasis, with a diameter > 3 cm but $\leq$6 cm, multiple ipsilateral lymph node metastasis with a maximum diameter < 6 cm, or bilateral or contralateral lymph node metastasis, with a maximum diameter $\leq$ 6 cm.
N_{2a}: A single ipsilateral lymph node metastasis, with a diameter > 3 cm but $\leq$ 6 cm.
N_{2b}: Multiple ipsilateral lymph node metastasis with a maximum diameter $\leq$ 6 cm.
N_{2c}: Bilateral or contralateral lymph node metastasis, with a maximum diameter $\leq$ 6 cm.
N_3: Maximum diameter of metastatic lymph node > 6 cm.

(f) Systemic metastasis (M):
M_x: Cannot evaluate whether there is distant metastasis.
M_0: No distant metastasis.
M_1: Distant metastasis (the location of metastasis should also be indicated).

3. Clinical stage
Stage 0: $T_{is}N_0M_0$.
Stage I: $T_1N_0M_0$.
Stage II: $T_2N_0M_0$.
Stage III: $T_3N_0M_0$, $T_{1-3}N_1M_0$.
Stage IV_a: $T_{4a}N_0M_0$, $T_{4a}N_1M_0$, any T, N_2M_0.
Stage IV_b: Any T, N_3M_0, T_{4b}, any N, M_0.
Stage IV_c: Any T, any N, M_1.

3.7 Treatment

Surgery and radiotherapy are the main treatment for laryngeal carcinoma. Surgery (including laser therapy) and radiotherapy are the main treatment for local early laryngeal carcinoma (T_1 and T_2 lesions); surgery in combination with radiotherapy and chemotherapy is used for locally advanced laryngeal carcinoma (T_3 and T_4 lesions).

Chemotherapy is the main comprehensive treatment or palliative treatment for advanced laryngeal carcinoma. In addition, molecular targeted drugs for the treatment of laryngeal carcinoma include cetuximab (C225), gefitinib (Iressa), erlotinib (Tarceva), etc. Molecular targeted drugs in combination with radiotherapy or chemotherapy have achieved good results.

4 Salivary Gland Tumor

The salivary gland is divided into large type and small type. There are three pairs of large salivary glands, namely, parotid, submandibular, and sublingual glands; hundreds of small salivary glands are mainly distributed under the mucosa of the oral cavity, nasal sinus, and trachea.

4.1 Local Anatomy

1. Anatomy of the parotid gland: It is located on the side of the face and is a single gland, but it is often divided into deep and shallow lobes by the facial nerve; the shallow lobe is larger and irregular in shape, located on the superficial surface of the posterior part of the masseter muscle, up to the zygomatic arch, and down to the lower edge of the mandible; the deep lobe is smaller, is upward adjacent to the cartilage of the external auditory canal, and extends inward around the posterior edge of the ascending ramus of the mandible, adjacent to the parapharyngeal space.
2. Anatomy of the submandibular gland: It is divided into two parts: deep and shallow: the shallow part is larger; the deep part starts from the inner side of the shallow part, passes through the gap between the mandibular hyoid muscle and the hyoglossus muscle to the sublingual area, and connects with the posterior end of the sublingual gland.

3. Anatomy of the sublingual gland: The sublingual gland is prolate in shape. It is composed of many small glands. It is in sublingual area, and its back end connects with the extension of the submandibular gland. There are two types of output tubes: large and small.

4.2 Epidemiology and Etiology

The incidence of parotid gland tumors is the highest among salivary gland tumors, accounting for about 80%. Submandibular gland tumors account for 10%, and sublingual gland tumors account for 1%. Among parotid gland tumors, benign tumors are in the majority, while malignant tumors are in the minority; among submandibular gland tumors, the incidence of benign and malignant tumors is similar; among sublingual gland tumors, the incidence of malignant tumors is high, and that of the benign tumors is low. Warthin tumor (lymphomatous papillary cystadenoma or adenolymphoma) and eosinophilic adenoma almost only occur in the parotid gland; among benign tumors, pleomorphic adenoma (mixed tumor) has the highest incidence, followed by Warthin tumor; among malignant tumors, mucoepidermoid carcinoma has the highest incidence, followed by adenoid cystic carcinoma.

The cause of salivary gland tumor is not clear.

4.3 Pathology and Clinical Features

Salivary gland tumors mainly come from ductal glandular epithelial cells or myoepithelial cells or both. Serous or mucinous acini rarely develop tumors. The common pathological types of benign tumors and malignant tumors are described.

1. Pleomorphic adenoma: Also known as mixed tumor, is the most common type of salivary gland tumors. Among the three pairs of large salivary glands, the parotid gland is the most common, the submandibular gland is the second, and the sublingual gland is very rare. It can also occur in the small salivary gland.
2. Warthin tumor: Almost all occur in the parotid gland, and most of them are located in the lower pole of the parotid gland; very few cases occur in the submandibular glands, and it rarely occurs in the small salivary glands of the oral cavity. It is more common in males, accounting for 85–90%. Most of them are aged 50–60. It may have the characteristics of bilateral parotid gland involvement and multiple primary lesions. If the operation is not handled properly, it can reappear locally.
3. Mucoepidermoid carcinoma: Among the large salivary gland tumors, it accounts for 5–10%, of which 90% occur in the parotid gland and the rest in the submandibular gland. Among small gland tumors, it accounts for 4–20%, and it is most common in palatine gland. This disease usually occurs at the age of 40–50, and it is more common in women than in men. Mucoepidermoid carcinoma is of varying degrees of malignancy. In low-grade malignancy, the course of disease is longer and the growth is more limited, which presents as a progressive, painless, and enlarged mass. In moderate- and high-grade malignancy, the course of disease is short and the growth is rapid, and the tumor is fixed by adhesion to surrounding tissues, maybe accompanied by pain and ulcers.
4. Adenoid cystic carcinoma: May occur in the submandibular gland and parotid gland, but more common in the small salivary gland. Most patients are aged 30–50, and there is no significant difference between the incidence of men and women. The tumor grows slowly and is locally aggressive, with a high recurrence rate after surgery.
5. Malignant mixed tumor: Refers to a type of mixed tumor with both benign and malignant components. The malignant component can be primary or from malignant transformation of mixed tumor, the latter is more common, and sometimes both can exist. The age of onset of tumors was around 50 years old, tumors are more common in male, and more than half of them occur in the parotid gland. Malignant mixed tumor, which is malignant at the beginning, generally grows fast, with local pain or numbness. The tumor is hard and often infiltrates into deep tissues or adheres to the skin. Another type of malignant transformation from benign mixed tumor generally has a longer course of disease, and the recent tumor growth accelerates and enlarges with larger mass as the clinical manifestation.
6. Acinic cell carcinoma: It is a low-grade malignant tumor, accounting for about 3% of salivary gland tumors. It mainly occurs in the parotid gland, with a few in the submandibular and small salivary glands. Most of the patients are aged 30–50, with male patients slightly more than the female patients. Tumors often grow slowly. The main clinical manifestations are symptoms of mass and nervous system involvement. The disease develops slowly and lymph node metastasis is rare. The tumor is less destructive locally, but can recur locally or repeatedly. It occasionally metastasizes, and hematogenous metastasis is more common. Patients with lung metastasis can live with tumor for a long time, and patients with extrapulmonary metastasis have a very poor prognosis. Because adenoid cystic carcinoma has the characteristics of strong local invasiveness and spreading along the neurovascular bundle, the positive rate of surgical margin is high. The curative effect of comprehensive treatment is better than that of surgery alone. Radiation therapy in

comprehensive treatment may improve the survival time of patients.

7. Adenocarcinoma: At present, there are still great differences in the classification criteria of adenocarcinoma pathology. Except for the abovementioned cancers, all glandular origin is classified as adenocarcinoma. There are different histologic types such as tubular, papillary, and poorly differentiated. The differentiation is quite different and the prognosis is also different.
8. Squamous cell carcinoma: Primary squamous cell carcinoma of the salivary gland is rare. It mostly occurs in the parotid gland and submandibular gland and rarely in the sublingual gland and other small salivary glands. Most of the patients are middle-aged and elderly men with high degree of malignancy. The lymphatic and hematogenous metastases are more likely to occur, and the prognosis is poor.

4.4 Stage

TNM stage of malignant tumors of the large salivary gland

1. Primary tumor (T)

   T_x: The primary tumor cannot be evaluated.

   T_0: No evidence of the existence of the primary tumor.

   T_1: The maximum diameter of the tumor is ≤2 cm, without extraparenchymal (glandular) expansion.

   T_2: The maximum diameter of the tumor is >2 cm and ≤4 cm, without extraparenchymal (glandular) expansion.

   T_3: The maximum diameter of the tumor is >4 cm, with extraparenchymal (glandular) expansion.

   T_{4a}: The tumor invades the skin, mandible, external auditory canal, and/or facial nerve.

   T_{4b}: The tumor invades the cranial base and alar plate and/or wraps the internal carotid artery.
2. Regional lymph nodes (N)

   N_x: It cannot be evaluated whether there is regional lymph node metastasis.

   N_0: No regional lymph node metastasis.

   N_1: A single ipsilateral lymph node metastasis, with a diameter ≤ 3 cm.

   N_2: A single ipsilateral lymph node metastasis, with a diameter > 3 cm but ≤ 6 cm, multiple ipsilateral lymph node metastasis with a maximum diameter ≤ 6 cm, or bilateral or contralateral lymph node metastasis, with a maximum diameter ≤ 6 cm.

   N_{2a}: A single ipsilateral lymph node metastasis, with a diameter > 3 cm but ≤ 6 cm.

   N_{2b}: Multiple ipsilateral lymph node metastasis with a maximum diameter ≤ 6 cm.

   N_{2c}: Bilateral or contralateral lymph node metastasis, with a maximum diameter ≤ 6 cm.

   N_3: Maximum diameter of metastatic lymph node > 6 cm.
3. Distant metastasis (M)

   M_x: Cannot evaluate whether there is distant metastasis.

   M_0: No distant metastasis.

   M_1: Distant metastasis.
4. Clinical stage

   Stage I: $T_1N_0M_0$, $T_2N_0M_0$.

   Stage II: $T_3N_0M_0$.

   Stage III: T_1N_1M, $T_2N_1M_0$.

   Stage IV_a: $T_{4a}N_0M_0$, $T_{4a}N_1M_0$, $T_1N_2M_0$, $T_2N_2M_0$, T_3N_2M, $T_aN_2M_0$, any T, N_2M_0.

   Stage IV_b: T_{4b}, any N, M_0, any T, N_3M_0.

   Stage IV_c: Any T, any N, M_1.

4.5 Treatment

Surgery is the main treatment for salivary gland tumors. Surgery plus radiotherapy may be considered for patients with advanced stage. Complete resection of the tumor by first operation is the key to cure.

5 Oral Malignant Tumor

5.1 Clinical Overview

Oral malignant tumor is one of the top 10 malignant tumors in incidence in the world. Oral cancer generally refers to squamous cell carcinoma, accounting for more than 95% of oral malignant tumors. Other malignant tumors that occur in oral mesenchymal tissues or hematopoietic tissues and malignant tumors from small salivary glands are included in their corresponding chapters, which are not discussed in this chapter.

According to the data from China, oral cancer accounts for 1.9% to 3.5% of all malignant tumors in the body and 4.7% to 20.3% of malignant tumors in the head and neck region, ranking second among malignant tumors in the head and neck, second only to nasopharyngeal cancer. It is more common in individuals aged 40 to 60, with a higher incidence in males than females (male-to-female ratio of 2~3:1). The main risk factors for oral cancer are smoking and drinking, and others are betel nut chewing, ultraviolet rays, X-rays, chronic irritation and injury, human papillomavirus (especially HPV16), etc. According to the latest classification of the International Agency for Research on Cancer, oral squamous cell carcinoma includes tongue cancer, gingival carcinoma, mouth floor carcinoma, buccal carcinoma, carcinoma of the palate, and lip carcinoma. Among them, tongue cancer is the most common, followed by gingival carcinoma, mouth floor carcinoma, and buccal carcinoma.

In recent years, some progress has been made in the basic research and treatment of oral cancer, but the survival rate has not been significantly improved. The current treatment methods for oral malignant tumors include surgery, radiotherapy, and chemotherapy, of which surgery is the most important.

5.2 Gist of PET/CT Image Acquisition

The preparations for PET/CT examination of patients with oral malignant tumor are basically the same as those for conventional tumor PET/CT imaging. It should be emphasized that such patients should avoid speaking and chewing as much as possible before the examination. Some scholars suggest that patients should take sitting position after injection of imaging agent to improve the imaging effect of oral lesions.

The following points should be noted when PET/CT acquisition is performed:

1. Ask the patient to remove metal foreign bodies such as dentures, ear studs, necklaces, etc. before the examination.
2. After the whole-body examination, instruct the patients to place their hands on both sides of their thighs, and collect oral local image to improve the matching of PET image and CT image, and reduce the PET image attenuation and CT artifact caused by arm lifting.
3. Instruct patients to avoid swallowing and coughing as much as possible during the image acquisition process. Some scholars have reported that instructing patients to open their mouth when performing oral local acquisition can effectively improve image quality.

5.3 Overview of PET/CT Diagnosis of Oral Malignant Tumors

Since it is easy to obtain pathological biopsy specimens, the clinical diagnosis of oral malignant tumor is not difficult. The main application value of PET/CT in oral malignant tumors lies in clinical stage, prognosis, development of therapeutic plan, and efficacy evaluation.

The 2017 version of the AJCC Oral Cancer TNM staging criteria emphasizes the importance of depth of invasion (DOI) for tumor T staging. Among the existing imaging methods, MRI has become the first choice for evaluating tumor T staging due to its superior tissue resolution. Although the tissue resolution of PET/CT images is not as good as that of MRI, some studies have shown that its sensitivity in the diagnosis of primary head and neck malignant tumors (including oral malignant tumors) is higher than that of MRI. In addition, PET/CT can also be used as the first choice for some patients contraindicated for MRI (such as those with difficult-to-remove dentures or metal foreign bodies). PET/CT has higher diagnostic efficiency in N staging of tumor, especially for suspicious lymph nodes with short diameter > 1 cm. Many studies have shown that the sensitivity, specificity, and accuracy of PET/CT in the diagnosis of metastatic lymph nodes are 62%–88%, 97%–99%, and 82%–96%, respectively, higher than other imaging methods. Since whole-body images can be obtained in one examination, PET/CT has obvious advantages in evaluating the M staging of oral malignant tumors. Moreover, PET/CT examinations in patients with oral malignant tumors can sometimes accidentally find second primary malignant tumors. Based on the above reasons, PET/CT also has important clinical application value in the selection of treatment regimen of oral malignant tumor and efficacy evaluation. Some studies recommend that PET/CT follow-up should be carried out at 12 weeks after treatment and the accuracy is the highest at this time. Recent studies have shown that certain parameters of ^{18}F-FDG PET/CT imaging, such as maximum standard uptake value (SUVmax), metabolic tumor volume (MTV), total lesion glycolysis (TLG), etc., may have a certain value in predicting the prognosis of oral malignant tumors, but the cutoff values of various parameters reported in these studies are quite different, such as SUVmax from 4.0 to 19.3, MTV from 6.0 to 7.7, and TLG from 18.3 to 71.4, so there is no unified reference values.

PET/CT also has certain limitations in the diagnosis of oral malignant tumors: the normal physiological uptake and non-specific uptake of oral cavity often lead to false positive; it is not as good as MRI in identifying cystic degeneration and necrotic lymph nodes and assessing peripheral nerve invasion; false-negative results can be caused when the lesion is small or FDG uptake is low; inflammatory hyperplastic lymph nodes and metastatic lymph nodes are sometimes difficult to distinguish; local infection or local inflammation caused by radiotherapy and non-specific inflammation caused by surgery may lead to false positives in diagnosis.

8 PET/CT of Nasopharyngeal Carcinoma

Xiaoping Lin and Wei Fan

1 Clinical Overview

Nasopharyngeal carcinoma originates from the covering epithelium of the nasopharynx, and more than 95% are poorly differentiated with high degree of malignancy. In 1991, the WHO classified nasopharyngeal carcinoma histologically into two major categories, squamous cell carcinoma or keratinizing squamous cell carcinoma (WHO I) and non-keratinizing carcinoma, the latter of which can be divided into differentiated non-keratinizing carcinoma (WHO II) and undifferentiated carcinoma or undifferentiated carcinoma of nasopharyngeal type (WHO III) according to the degree of differentiation of tumor cells.

Nasopharyngeal carcinoma often occurs in the lateral wall (especially pharyngeal recess) and posterior parietal wall of the nasopharynx. The adjacent structures of the nasopharynx are complex. It is necessary to fully understand the local invasion pathway of the nasopharynx in order to accurately describe the PET/CT signs of local invasion of nasopharyngeal carcinoma. Nasopharyngeal carcinoma not only invades upward by directly damaging the cranial base bone, but it can also infiltrate the intracranial space through natural openings or clefts such as the foramen lacerum, foramen ovale, foramen spinosum, internal carotid artery canal, or sphenoid and posterior ethmoid sinuses, affecting the cranial nerves. It invades forward into the nasal cavity, maxillary sinus, anterior ethmoid sinuses, and even into the orbit, either through intracranial, superior orbital fissure or optic canal, and pterygopalatine fossa. It can also infiltrate laterally into the parapharyngeal space, infratemporal fossa, and the muscles of mastication. Nasopharyngeal carcinoma infiltrates posteriorly into the soft tissues anterior to the cervical vertebrae, as well as the cervical vertebrae themselves. It can extend downward, involving the oropharynx and even the hypopharynx.

The cervical lymph node metastasis of nasopharyngeal carcinoma occurs early, and the metastasis rate is high. There is a rich network of lymphatic vessels under the nasopharyngeal mucosa, and lymphatic drainage can cross the midline to the contralateral neck. Cervical lymph node metastasis is closely related to the occurrence of distant metastasis – with the increase of cervical lymph node metastasis, the probability of distant metastasis increases significantly. The most common site of distant metastasis is the bone, followed by the lung and liver, and it often occurs in multiple organs at the same time.

Radiotherapy is the main treatment for nasopharyngeal carcinoma. For patients with advanced disease, comprehensive chemotherapy can improve the curative effect, and surgery can also be used for tumor recurrence or residual lesions.

The ^{18}F-FDG metabolism of nasopharyngeal carcinoma lesions shows high proliferation. Lymph node metastasis and distant metastasis both show increased ^{18}F-FDG uptake, and tumor necrosis may show sparse or defective radioactive distribution.

2 PET/CT Diagnostic Points

2.1 General Diagnostic Points

1. Have a clinical history, such as nosebleed, cervical lymph node enlargement, elevated EBV, etc.
2. Nasopharyngeal space-occupying lesion.
3. When nasopharyngeal lesions invade the brain nerves, corresponding symptoms may occur.

X. Lin · W. Fan (✉)
Sun Yat-sen University Cancer Center, Guangzhou, Guangdong, China
e-mail: fanwei@sysucc.org.cn

Z. Yao, S. Li (eds.), *Atlas of PET/CT in Oncology - Volume 1*, https://doi.org/10.1007/978-981-99-1172-1_8

2.2 CT Diagnostic Points

1. The nasopharyngeal mucosa is locally thickened. The lesion can be seen on the upper wall, posterior parietal wall, and bilateral walls. The normal symmetrical structure is lost. The shape of lesion is mostly flat or nodular, with clear boundary and uniform or slightly high density.
2. When the lesion is large, it can occupy and deform the nasopharyngeal cavity.
3. The pharyngeal recess on the affected side becomes shallow or disappears. The lesion can directly destroy the cranial base bone when extending upwards, or it can invade the intracranial space through natural openings or clefts such as the foramen lacerum, foramen ovale, foramen spinosum, internal carotid artery canal, or sphenoid and posterior ethmoid sinuses. It may invade the cavernous sinus and the inferior pole of the temporal lobe. When extending forward, it invades the nasal cavity, maxillary sinus, and anterior ethmoid sinuses, and further infiltrates into the orbit. It can also invade the orbit through intracranial routes, superior orbital fissure, optic canal, or pterygopalatine fossa. The lesion can infiltrate laterally into the parapharyngeal space, infratemporal fossa, and the muscles of mastication. It infiltrates posteriorly into the soft tissues anterior to the cervical vertebrae and the cervical vertebrae themselves. It can extend downward, involving the oropharynx and even the hypopharynx.
4. Enlarged lymph nodes may appear on the ipsilateral or the contralateral posterior pharynx, or they can skip the retropharyngeal lymph nodes and metastasize directly to bilateral cervical and distant lymph nodes. When the postpharyngeal lymph nodes are >0.8 cm, the submandibular lymph nodes are >1.5 cm, and the other cervical lymph nodes in other areas of the neck are >1 cm, it is usually indicated as metastatic lymph nodes. Metastatic lymph nodes may be accompanied by necrosis or extracapsular invasion, manifested as irregular or fuzzy edges of lymph nodes, striated infiltration into adjacent fat, and unclear borders with adjacent carotid arteries or cranial nerves.

2.2.1 ^{18}F-FDG PET Diagnostic Points

1. The primary lesion of the nasopharynx, metastatic lymph nodes, and distant metastasis show metabolically active changes.
2. The lesions of the nasopharynx are small, or due to partial volume effect, the local metabolism is slightly active. In some patients, the local metabolism is not significantly different from the surrounding normal tissues after the biopsy tumor tissue is clamped.
3. Retropharyngeal lymph nodes are easy to fuse with nasopharyngeal lesions. It is helpful to identify them by enhanced CT on the same PET/CT scan.
4. When nasopharyngeal lesions invade the skull base and intracranial structures, we should pay attention to the morphological and structural changes due to the similar radioactive distribution with the surrounding normal brain tissue. If necessary, we should carry out the same-machine enhanced CT scan to distinguish them.

3 Typical Cases

1. Early-stage nasopharyngeal carcinoma: Male patient, 40 years old. Pathology: Undifferentiated non-keratinizing nasopharyngeal carcinoma ($T_1N_0M_0$, stage I) (Fig. 8.1)
2. Locally advanced nasopharyngeal carcinoma: Female patient, 30 years old. Pathology: Undifferentiated non-keratinizing nasopharyngeal carcinoma and extensive invasion of the skull base with bilateral cervical lymph node metastasis ($T_4N_3M_1$, stage IV) (Figs. 8.2, 8.3, 8.4, and 8.5)
3. Systemic advanced nasopharyngeal carcinoma: Male patient, 58 years old. Pathology: Undifferentiated non-keratinizing nasopharyngeal carcinoma, with multiple metastases to the bilateral cervical lymph nodes, liver, and lung ($T_4N_2M_1$, stage IV_b) (Figs. 8.6, 8.7, 8.8, 8.9, and 8.10)

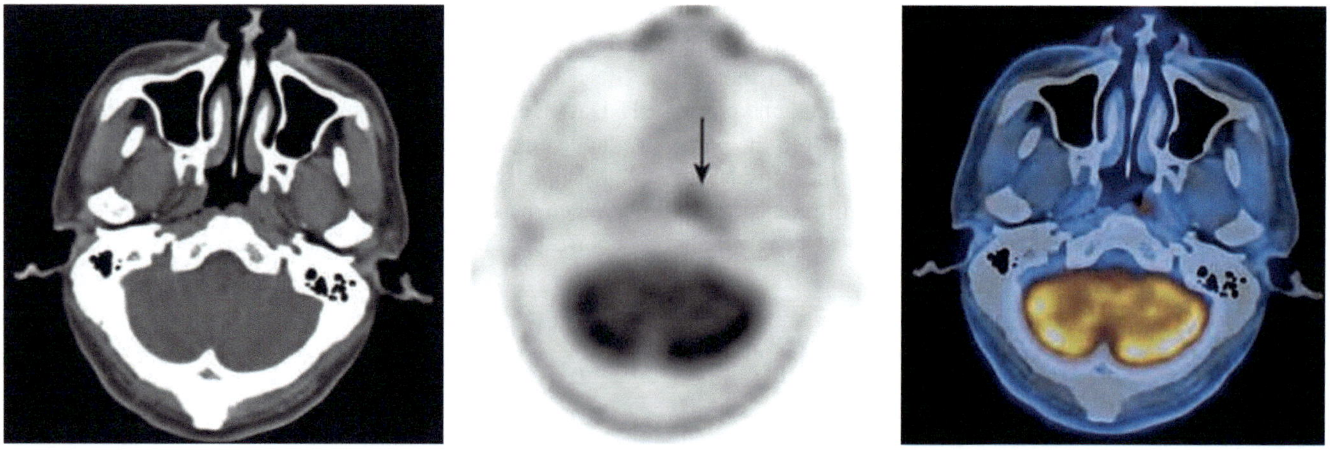

Fig. 8.1 FDG PET/CT image of early nasopharyngeal carcinoma. The mucosa of the pharyngeal recess on the left side of the nasopharynx was thickened and there was increased focal FDG uptake with SUVmax 6.2 (arrow), and the left pharyngeal recess became shallow

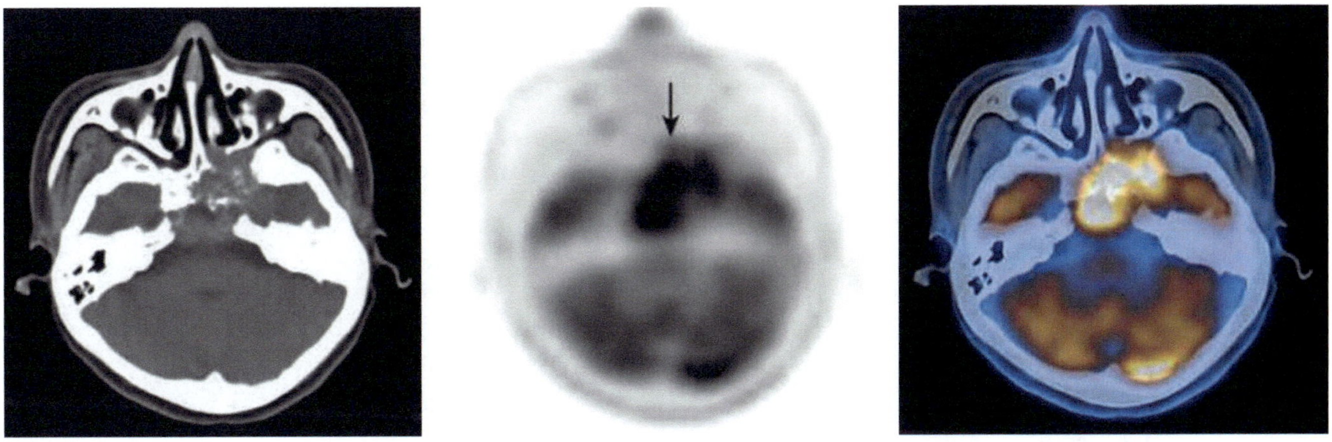

Fig. 8.2 FDG PET/CT image of locally advanced nasopharyngeal carcinoma. The mucosa of the upper wall, posterior parietal wall, and bilateral walls of the nasopharynx was thickened, and there was intense FDG uptake with SUVmax 10.6 (arrow). The lesions of the left foramen lacerum, foramen ovale, left sphenoid sinus, left ethmoid sinus, and sella turcica invaded the skull base, including the left petrous apex, clivus, medial and lateral plate and basilar part of the left pterygoid process, basilar part of the right pterygoid process, basilar part of the sphenoid bone, body of the sphenoid bone, and great wing of the left sphenoid bone, invading the left pterygopalatine fossa, the prepontine cistern, the left cavernous sinus, and the left inferior pole of the temporal lobe

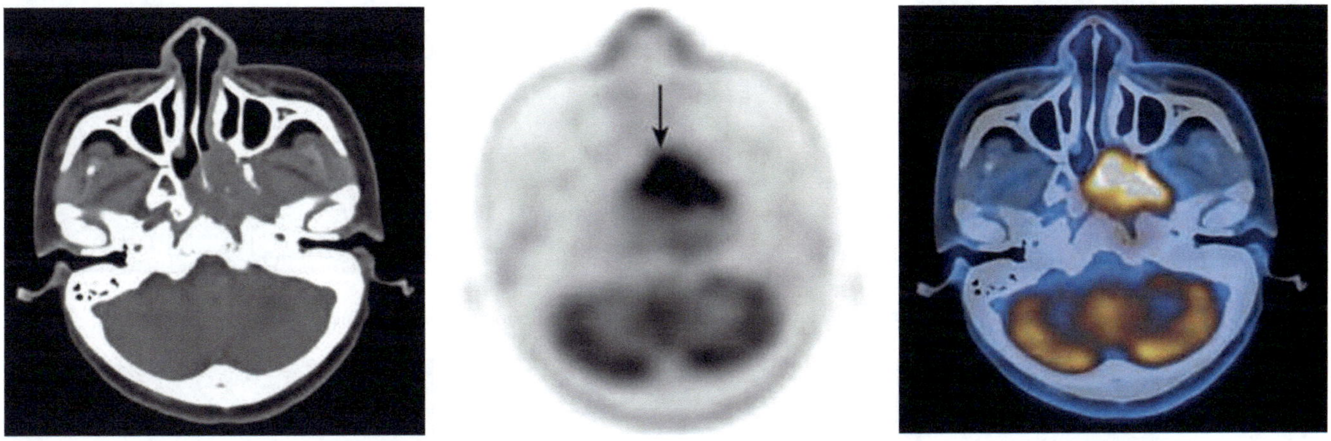

Fig. 8.3 FDG PET/CT image of locally advanced nasopharyngeal carcinoma. Nasopharyngeal lesions invaded bilateral posterior nostrils

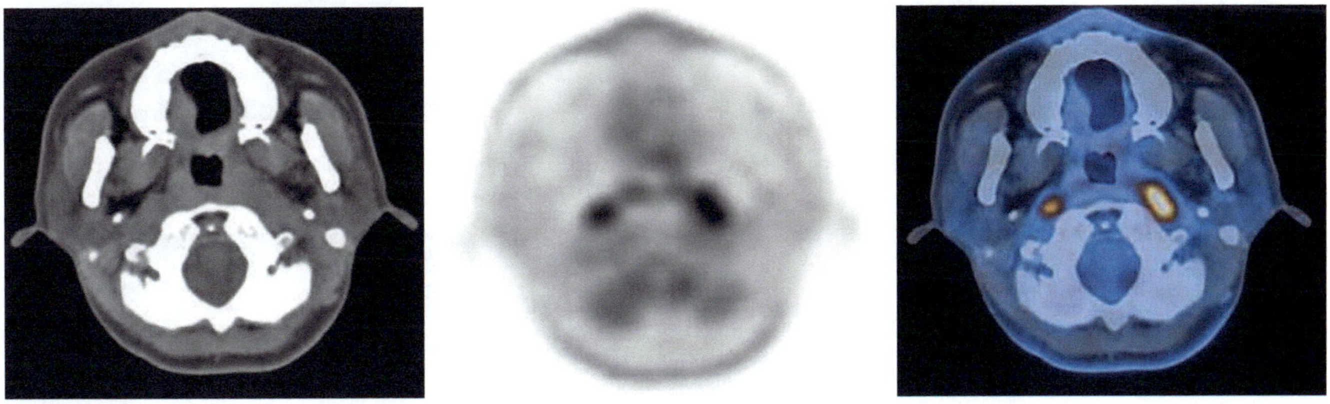

Fig. 8.4 Lymph node metastasis of nasopharyngeal carcinoma. Multiple bilateral retropharyngeal lymph nodes showed high uptake of FDG with SUVmax 11.2 (size 1.0 cm × 1.2 cm)

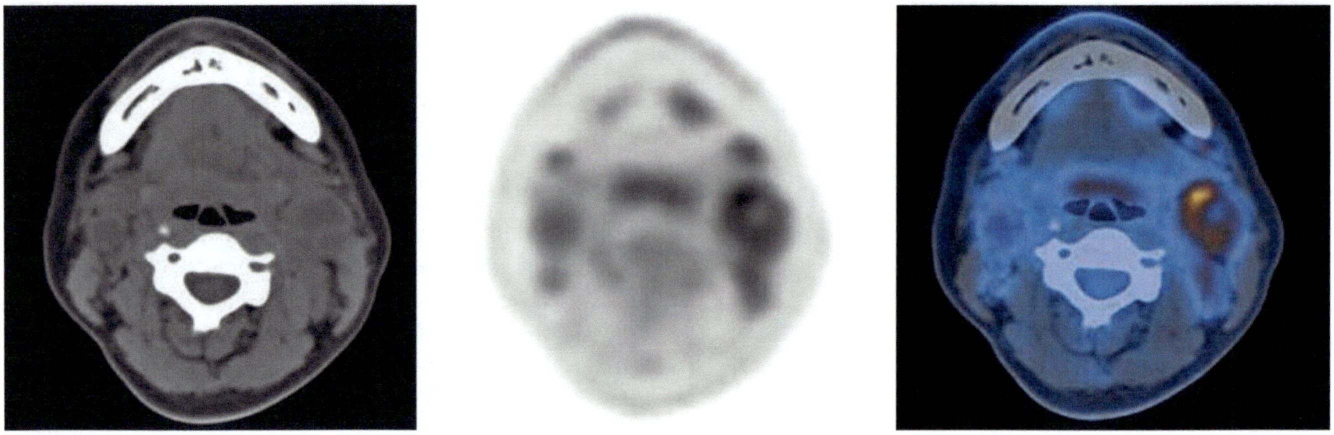

Fig. 8.5 FDG PET/CT image of lymph node metastasis of nasopharyngeal carcinoma. Multiple lymph nodes in bilateral level II and left level III showed increased FDG uptake (SUVmax 13.4). Some nodes exhibit partial fusion with the largest one measuring 2.2 cm × 3.1 cm, and internal necrotic changes were visible

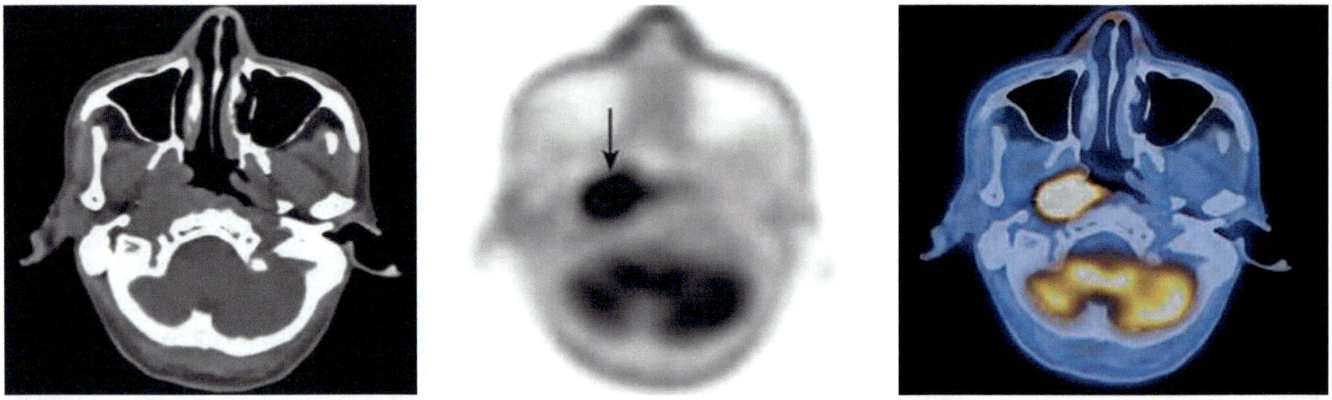

Fig. 8.6 FDG PET/CT image of right nasopharyngeal carcinoma. Nasopharyngeal carcinoma lesions are metabolically active (arrow)

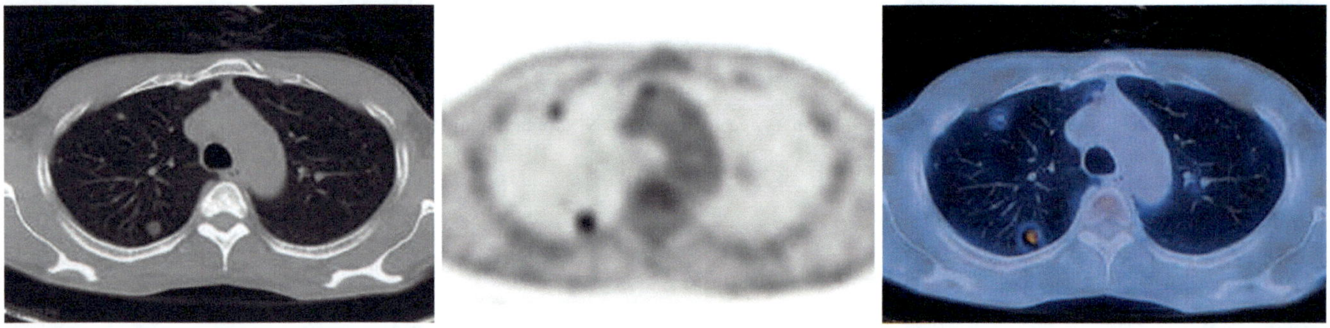

Fig. 8.7 FDG PET/CT image of lung metastasis of nasopharyngeal carcinoma. Metabolism of multiple metastases in lungs was active: pulmonary metastases can show vacuolar changes

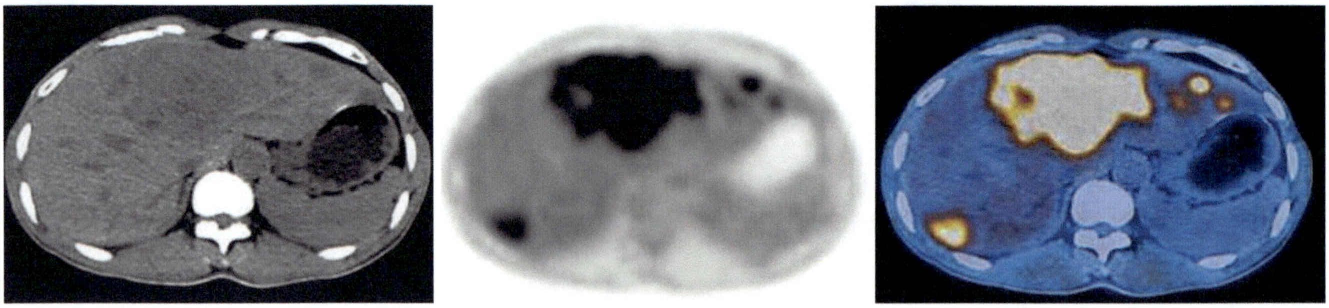

Fig. 8.8 FDG PET/CT image of liver metastases of nasopharyngeal carcinoma. Intense FDG uptake in the liver had multiple metastases

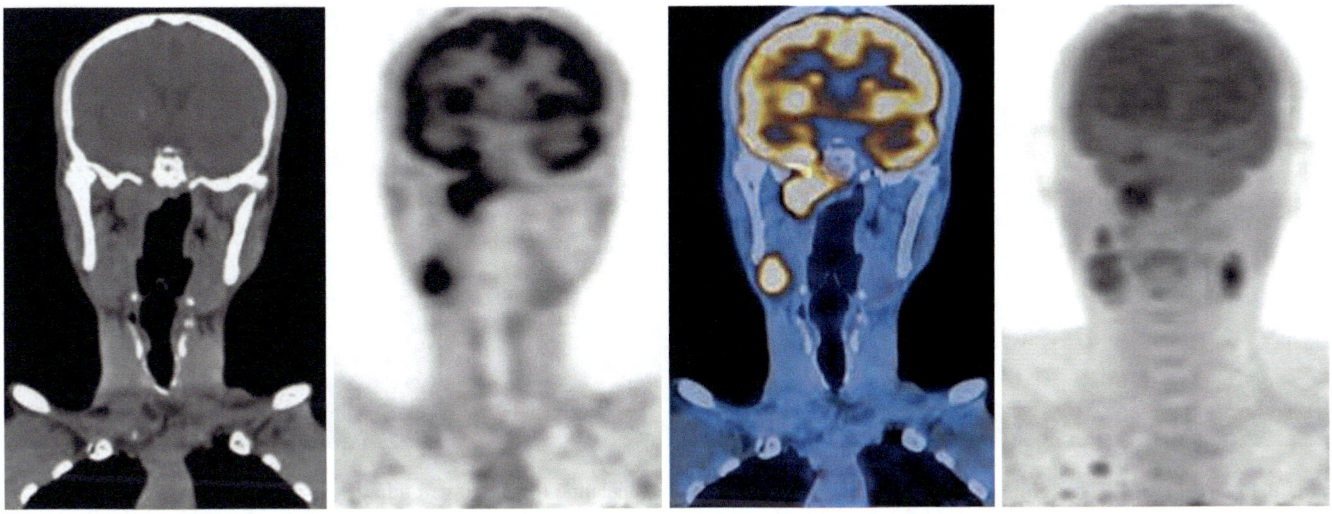

Fig. 8.9 FDG PET/CT image of lymph node metastasis of nasopharyngeal carcinoma. Increased FDG uptake in multiple metastatic lymph nodes on both sides of the neck

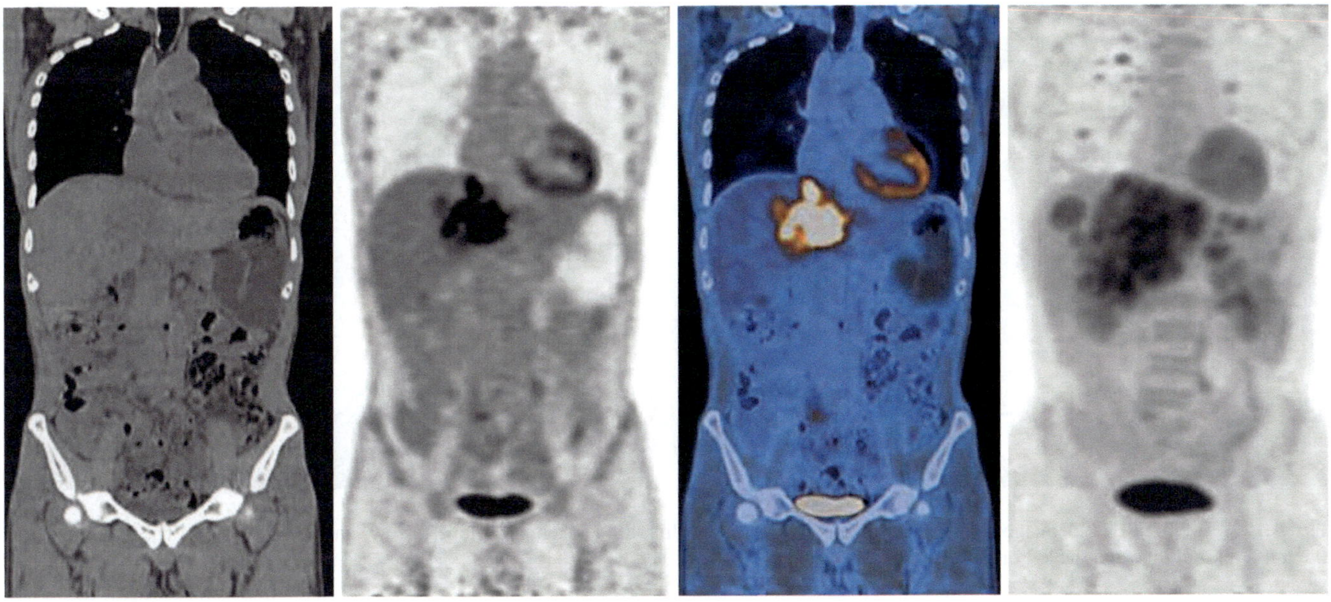

Fig. 8.10 FDG PET/CT images of liver metastasis of nasopharyngeal carcinoma. The coronal image of the body showed multiple liver and lung metastases with high metabolism

4 Rare Cases

1. Nasopharyngeal carcinoma extensively invades the skull base structure with left temporal lobe edema. Male patient, 30 years old. Pathology: Undifferentiated non-keratinizing nasopharyngeal carcinoma, extensively invading the skull base structure with lymph node metastasis ($T_4N_2M_0$, stage IV_a) (Figs. 8.11, 8.12, 8.13, 8.14, and 8.15).
2. Left adrenal metastasis of nasopharyngeal carcinoma and comparison before and after treatment: Male patient, 62 years old. Pathology: Undifferentiated non-keratinizing nasopharyngeal carcinoma, left adrenal metastasis of nasopharyngeal carcinoma, and comparison before and after treatment (Figs. 8.16 and 8.17).
3. Single lung metastasis after treatment of nasopharyngeal carcinoma: Female patient, 64 years old, with single lung metastasis after treatment of nasopharyngeal carcinoma. Pathology: The frozen paraffin section (left upper pulmonary nodule) showed poorly differentiated carcinoma. Combined with the results of immunohistochemistry and in situ hybridization, it was consistent with lymphoepithelioma-like carcinoma. Since the patient had a history of nasopharyngeal carcinoma, it was considered as metastasis of nasopharyngeal carcinoma (Fig. 8.18).

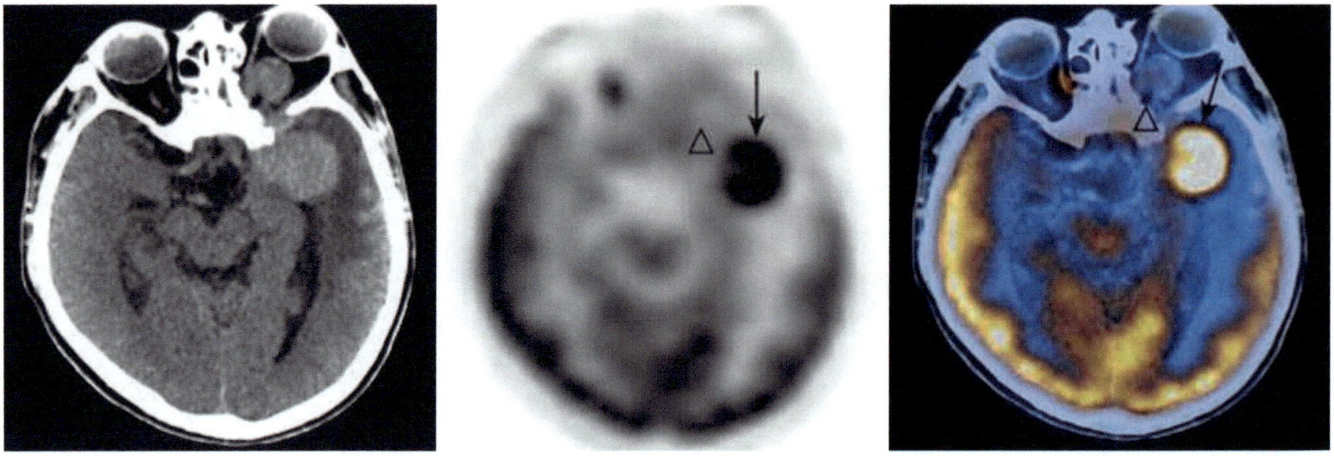

Fig. 8.11 ^{18}F-FDG PET/CT image of nasopharyngeal carcinoma invading the left temporal lobe (arrow) and left orbit (△). The mucosa of the upper wall, posterior parietal wall, and bilateral walls of the nasopharynx was thickened, and FDG uptake intense increased with SUVmax 15.3 (arrow). The lesion invaded the left temporal lobe, left cavernous sinus, left orbital apex, left posterior eyeball, and left pterygopalatine fossa, left carotid artery, sphenoid sinus, small wing of the left sphenoid bone, great wing of the left sphenoid bone, basilar part of the sphenoid bone, bilateral pterygoid process, vomer, occipital clivus, bilateral longus capitis muscle, bilateral tensor veli palatini muscle and levator veli palatini muscles, left lateral pterygoid muscle, and left retropharyngeal space

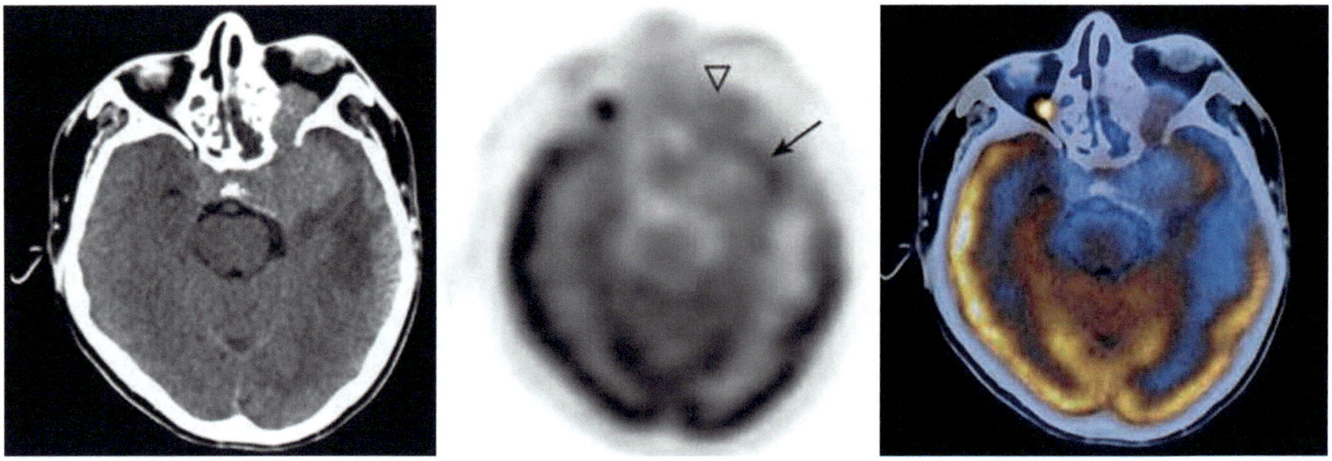

Fig. 8.12 ^{18}F-FDG PET/CT image of nasopharyngeal carcinoma invading the left temporal lobe (arrow) and left orbit (△). The lesion invaded the left temporal lobe and the left orbit

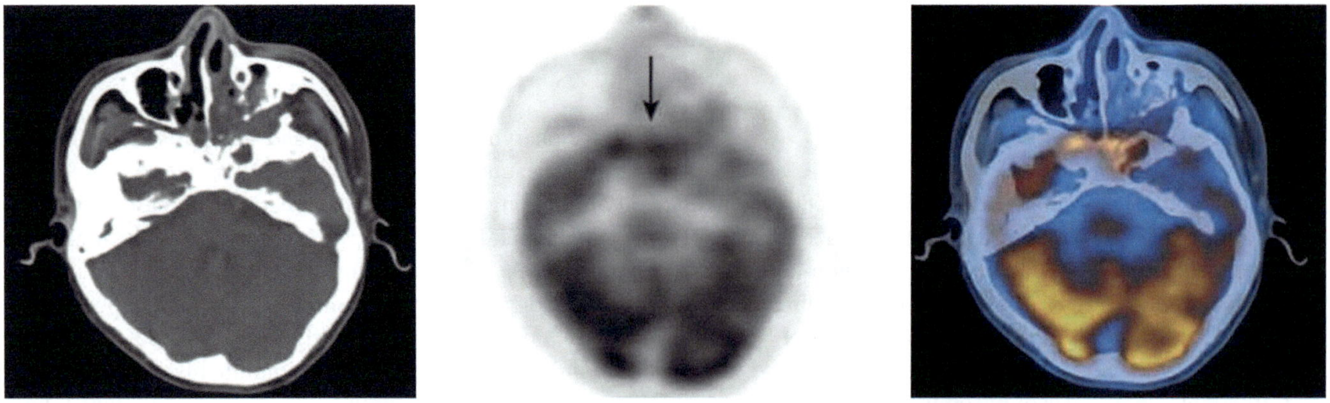

Fig. 8.13 Nasopharyngeal carcinoma involving the skull base (arrow). The lesion invaded the bone of the skull base

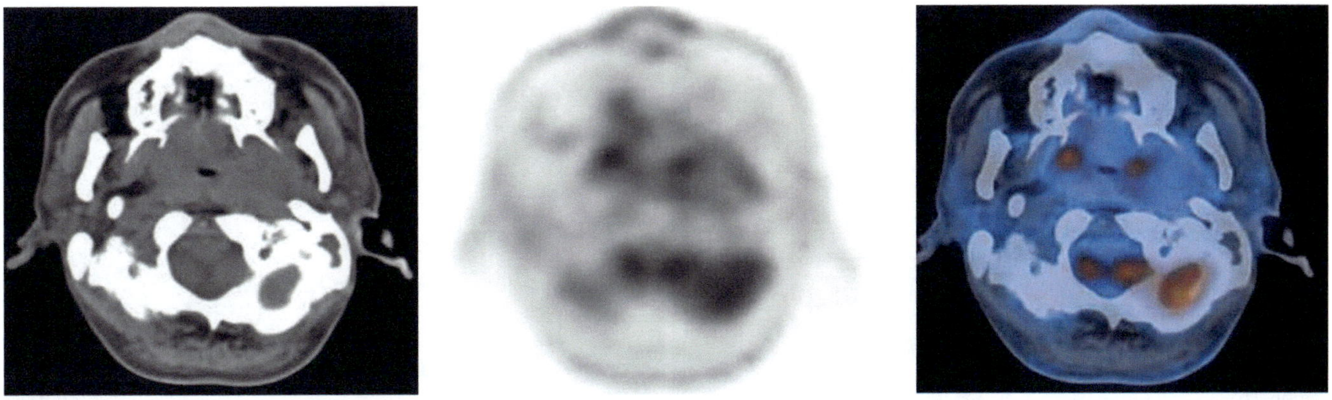

Fig. 8.14 FDG PET/CT image of nasopharyngeal carcinoma invading the oropharynx. The lesion invaded the nasopharynx and oropharynx

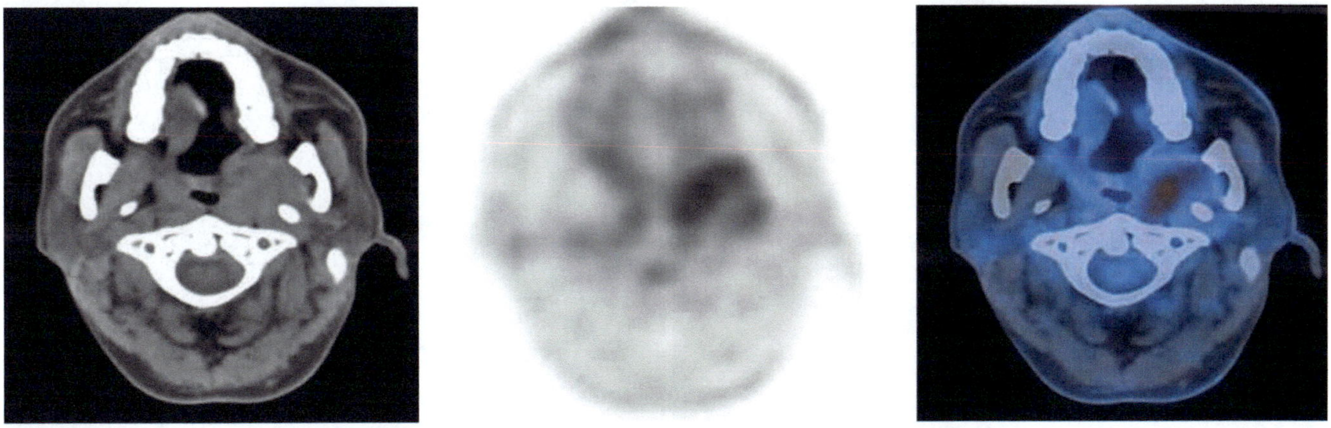

Fig. 8.15 FDG PET/CT image of lymph node metastasis of nasopharyngeal carcinoma. Increased FDG uptake (SUVmax 5.9) in the enlarged lymph nodes in the left cervical II and Va area; the largest one was 1.9 cm × 3.4 cm in size

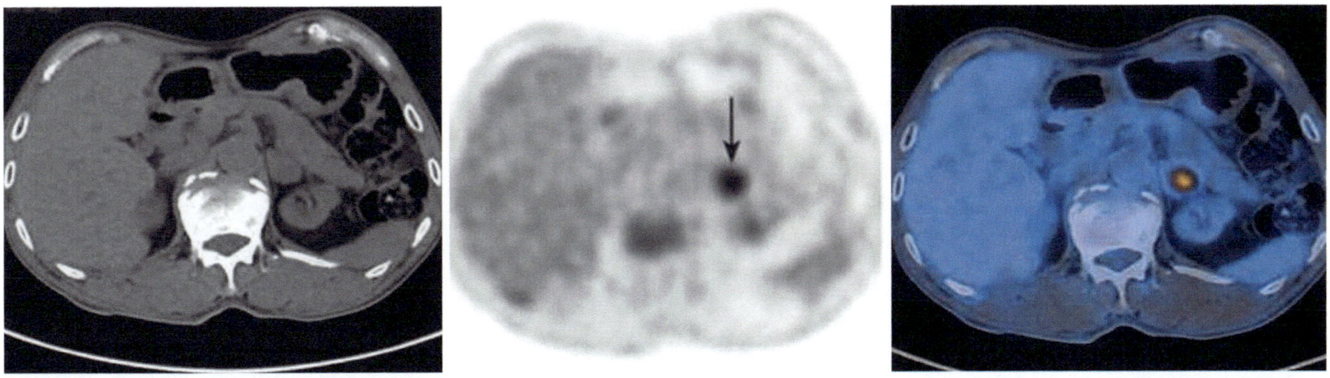

Fig. 8.16 PET/CT images of left adrenal metastasis of nasopharyngeal carcinoma (arrow) before treatment. PET/CT before treatment showed increase FDG uptake in the round soft tissue nodules in the left adrenal gland. The lesion's SUVmax is 7.4 and size 2.0 cm × 2.1 cm

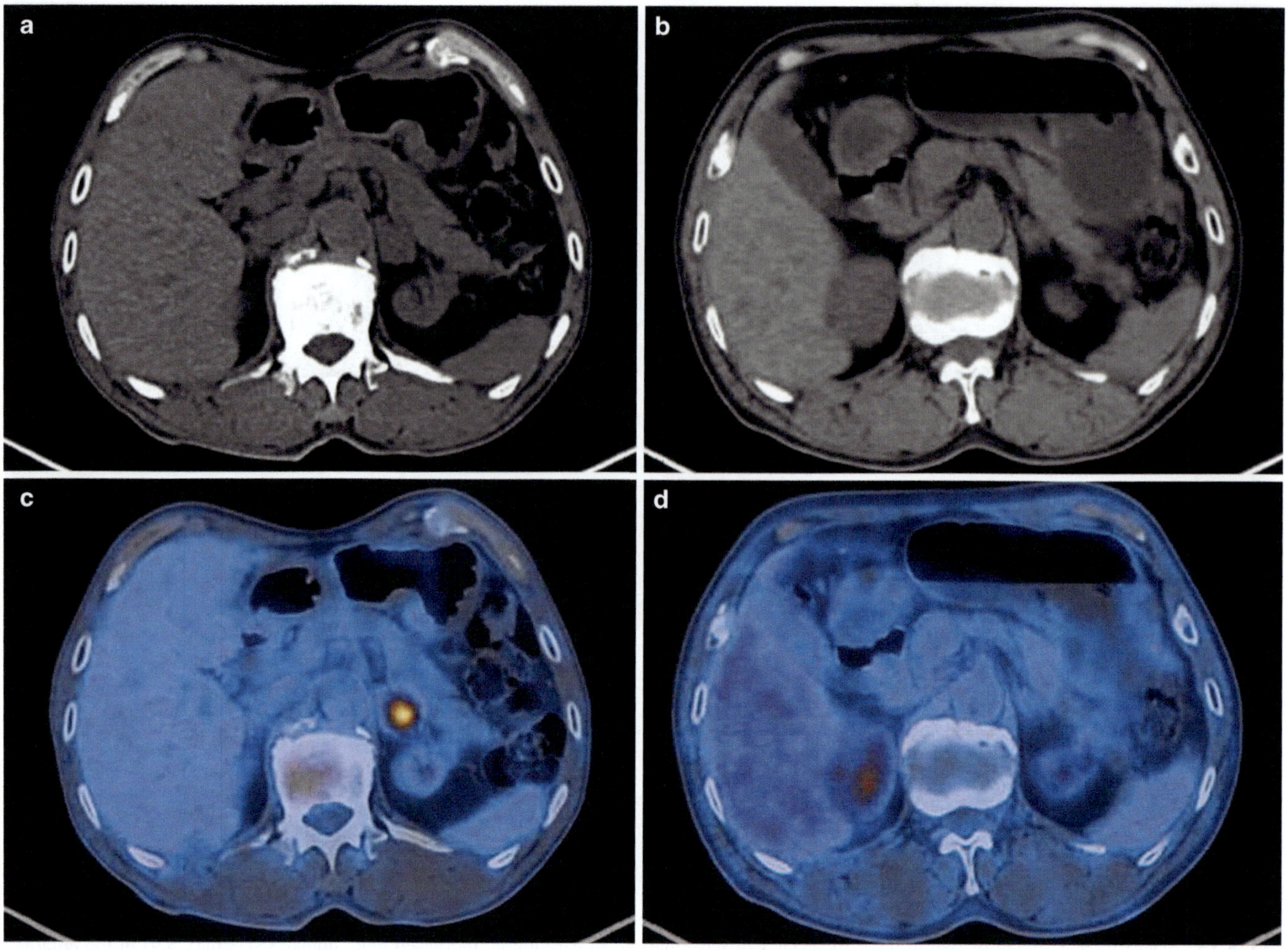

Fig. 8.17 PET/CT images before and after left adrenal metastasis of nasopharyngeal carcinoma. PET/CT showed that after treatment, the left adrenal gland became slightly thickened with normal radioactive distribution, compared with high uptake of FDG in it before treatment (**a** and **c** were before treatment, and **b** and **d** were after treatment, compared with the images on the same level)

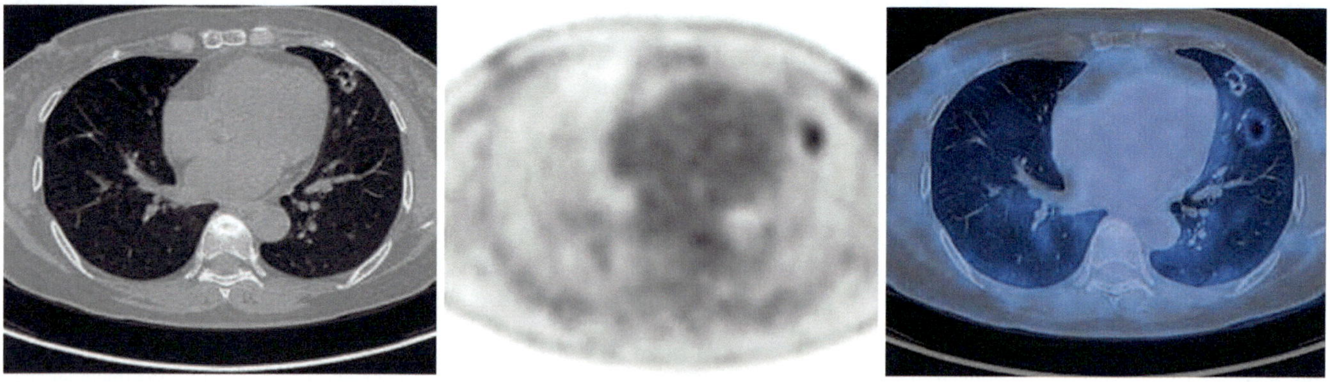

Fig. 8.18 FDG PET/CT cross-sectional images of single pulmonary metastasis after treatment of nasopharyngeal carcinoma. After radiotherapy for nasopharyngeal carcinoma and radiochemotherapy for mediastinal lymph node metastasis: there is no obvious thickening or abnormal FDG uptake in the mucosa of the nasopharyngeal walls, and bilateral pharyngeal recess was present. Increased FDG uptake in the cavity with irregular thickened wall in the lower tongue segment of the left upper lung was found, with SUVmax 4.2 and the size 1.0 cm × 1.8 cm

5 Differential Diagnosis

5.1 Nasopharyngeal Lymphoma

It occurs in the mucosal lymphatic tissue near the pharyngeal tonsils on the posterior parietal wall of the nasopharynx and the tonsils of the Eustachian tube. It grows diffusely along the surface of the nasopharynx wall, tends to "grow flatly," and even spreads to the oropharynx, nasal cavity, and sinuses, but generally does not invade the deep submucosa; the structural image shows a thickened nasopharyngeal wall or a soft tissue mass with a clear outline. When the lesion area is large, it can grow diffusely around, and the density is more uniform. Nasopharyngeal carcinoma usually invades the surrounding deep structures and skull base at an early stage, the fat space in the parapharyngeal space is blurred or completely occupied by tumors, and the edges of the mass are not clear. Nasopharyngeal carcinoma often invades the surrounding tissues, with which the boundary is not clear. It can invade and destroy the sphenoid bone, petrous bone, clivus, and other skull base bone structures. It can invade the skull along the cavernous sinus and foramen lacerum. Their biological behaviors have their own characteristics, and there is a certain regularity in the invasion of surrounding structures. This difference is helpful to the differential diagnosis.

1. Diffuse large B-cell lymphoma: Female patient, 55 years old. Pathology: Diffuse large B-cell lymphoma (Figs. 8.19 and 8.20)
2. Mantle cell lymphoma: Male patient, 67 years old. Pathology: Mantle cell lymphoma and nasopharyngeal and systemic multiple lymph node infiltration (Figs. 8.21 and 8.22)
3. Extranodal NK/T-cell lymphoma: Male patient, 57 years old. Pathology: Nasopharyngeal NK/T-cell lymphoma (Fig. 8.23)

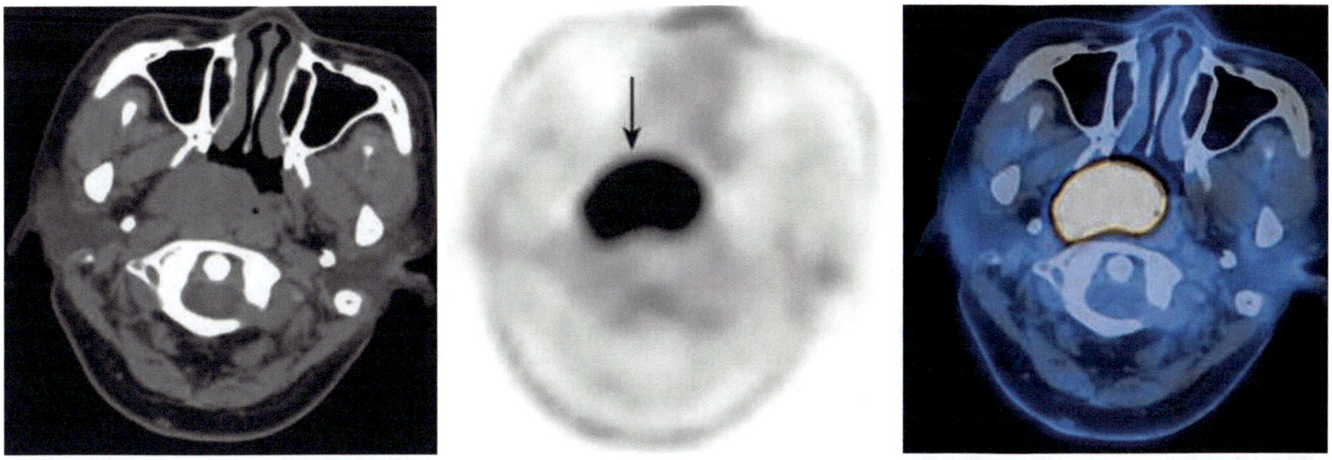

Fig. 8.19 Lymphoma of the posterior parietal wall of the nasopharynx (arrow). The soft tissue mass on the right part of the posterior parietal wall and the right-side wall of the nasopharynx showed high FDG uptake (arrow) with SUVmax 43.8 and the size 2.5 cm × 4.0 cm

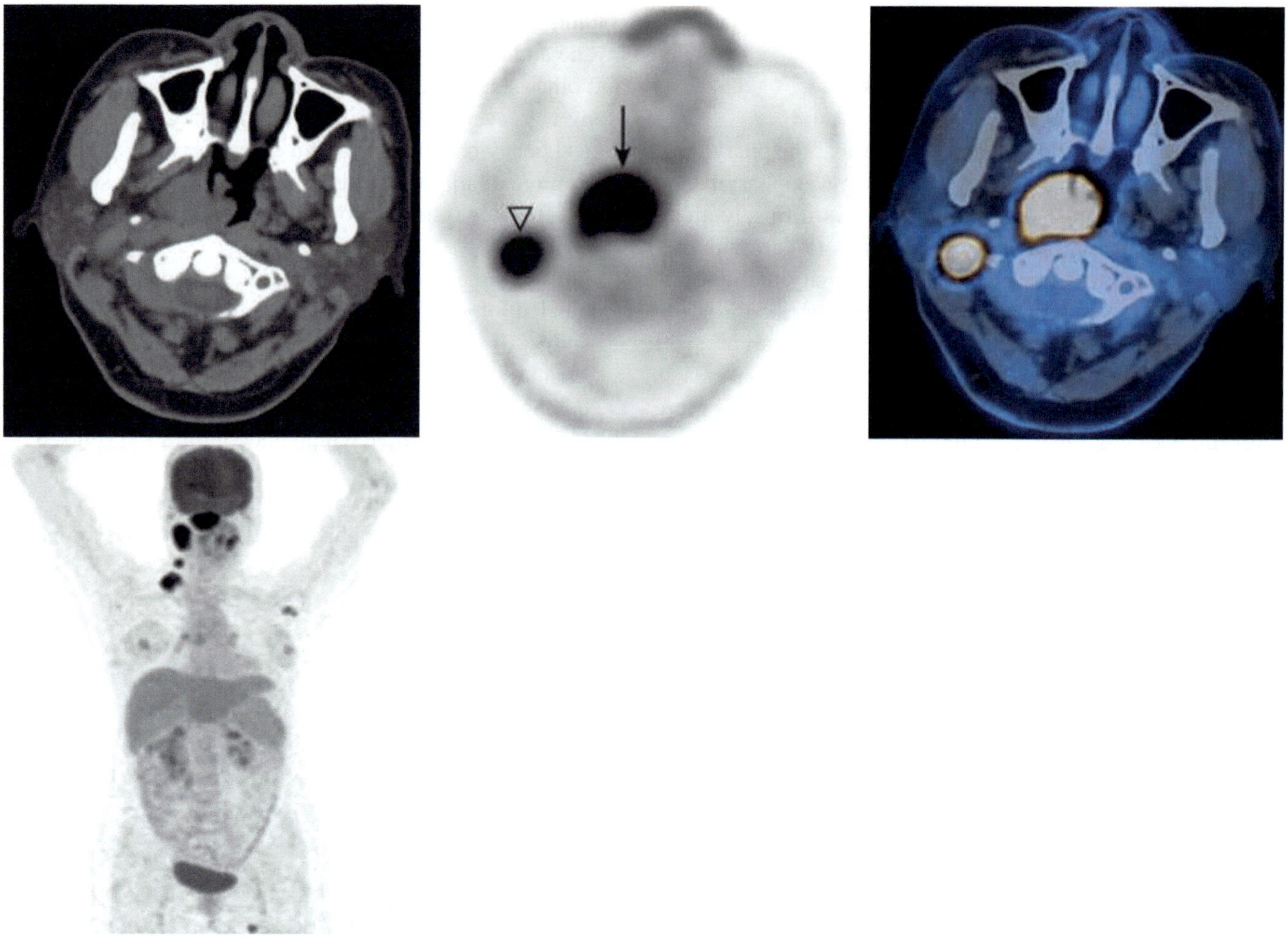

Fig. 8.20 PET/CT image of nasopharyngeal lymphoma. Multiple lymph nodes in the bilateral cervical II region and the right cervical III–V area showed high FDG uptake (Δ). The SUVmax was about 50.4, with partial lymph node fusion. The largest one was about 1.9 cm × 2.2 cm (MIP image also showed active metabolism of left axillary lymph nodes)

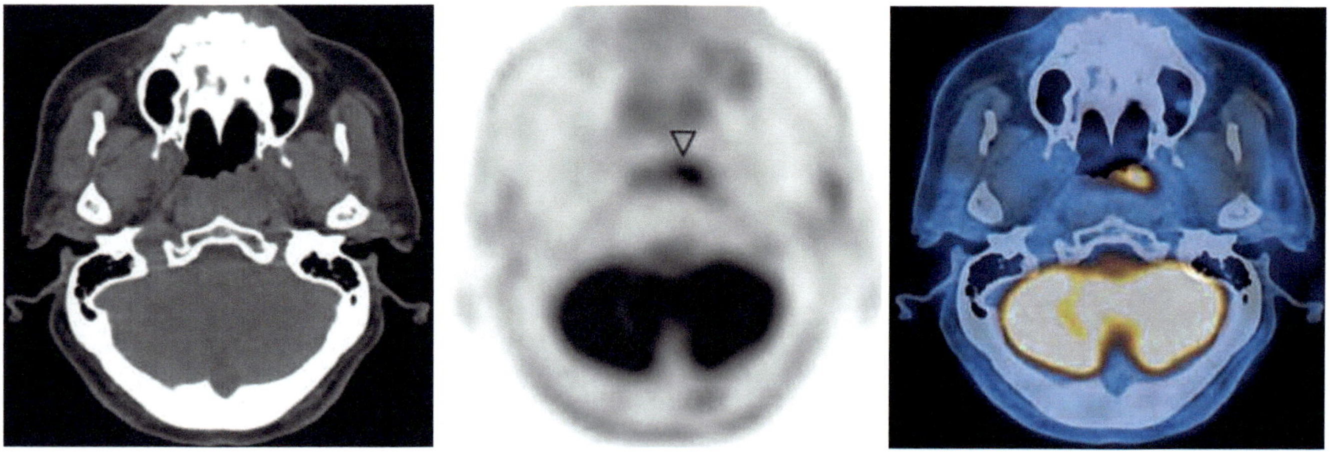

Fig. 8.21 PET/CT image of nasopharyngeal lymphoma. The mucosa of the upper wall, posterior parietal wall, and left-side wall of the nasopharynx was slightly thickened, and FDG uptake increased with SUVmax 11.0 (△)

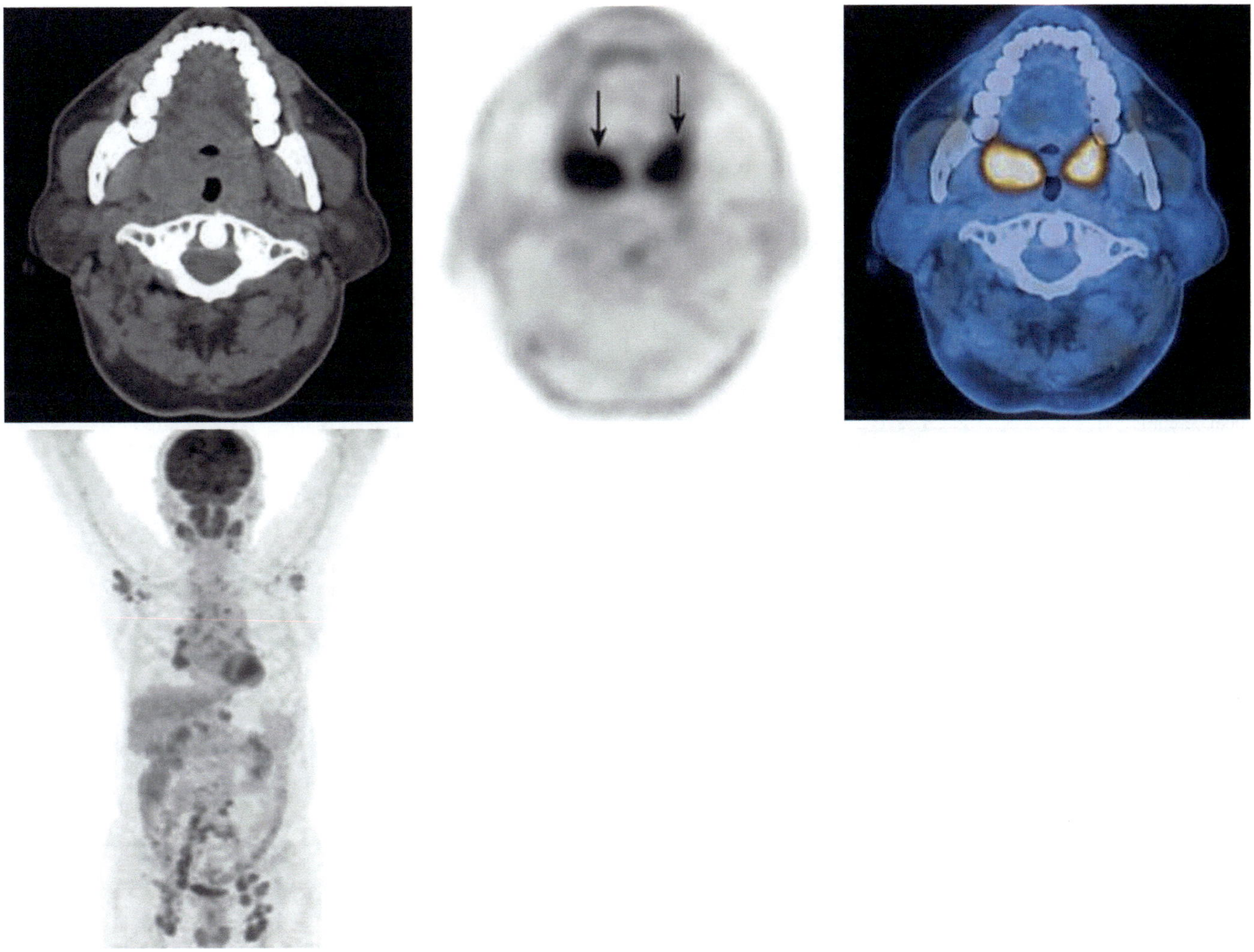

Fig. 8.22 PET/CT image of nasopharyngeal lymphoma. Increased FDG uptake (SUVmax 14.2) were noted in bilateral tonsils that were enlarged (arrows). PET MIP image also showed multiple hypermetabolic lymph nodes throughout the body

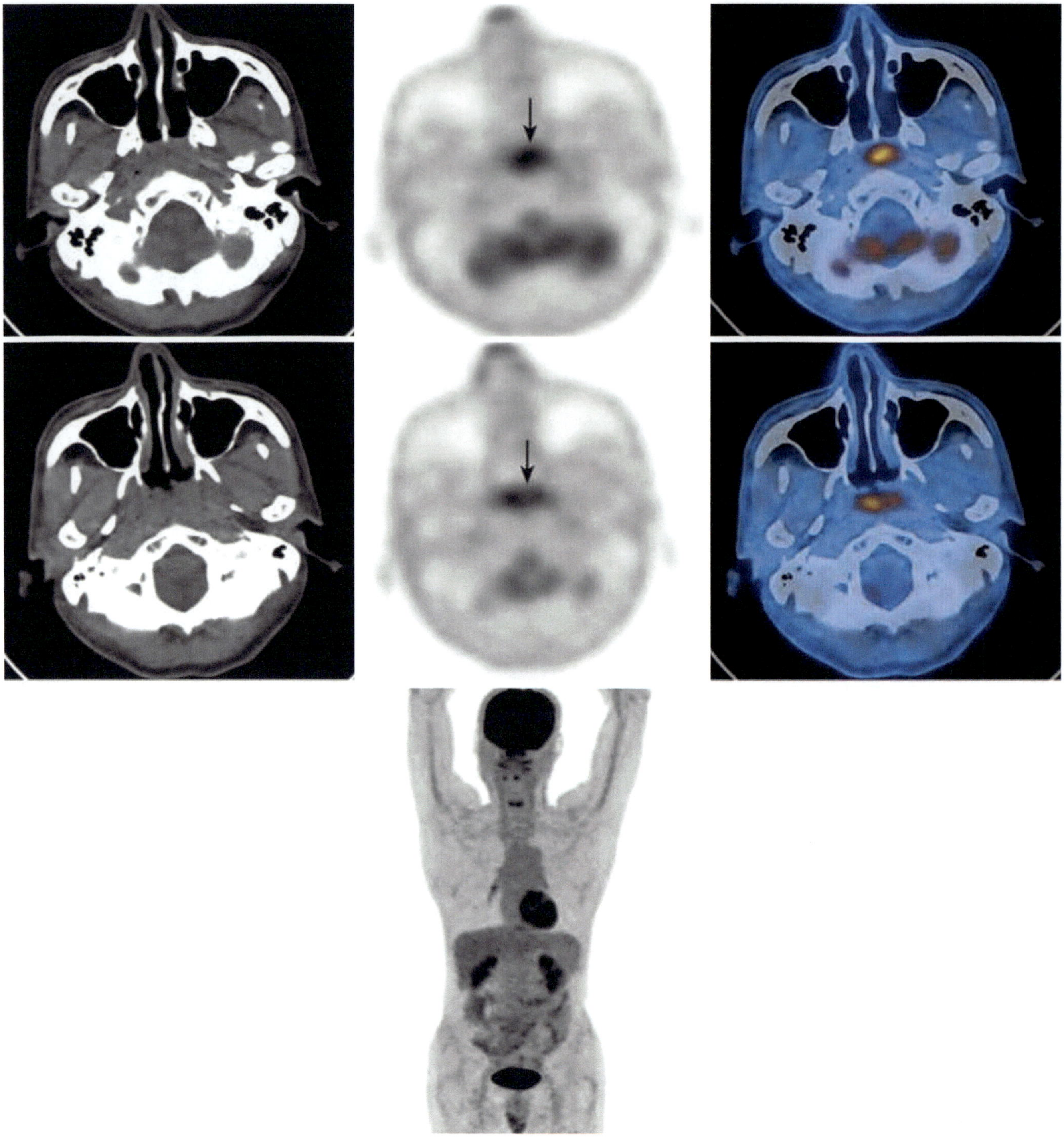

Fig. 8.23 PET/CT image of nasopharyngeal lymphoma. The soft tissue on the upper wall and the posterior parietal wall of the nasopharynx showed high FDG uptake with SUVmax 9.1 (arrow)

5.2 Adenoidal Hypertrophy

The lymphatic tissue contained in the posterior wall of the nasopharynx, called adenoids, gradually grows up after birth, reaches a peak at 6–7 years old under normal physiological conditions, and then shrinks with age and degenerates to an adult state at 14–15 years old. But sometimes it can last to adulthood. The residual nasopharyngeal lymphoid tissue is sometimes similar to the tumor. The main differentiation points include age, tissue morphology, and invasion of surrounding structures. Generally, the lymphatic tissue is in the superficial area, does not involve the underlying muscles, and is not accompanied by necrosis. ^{18}F-FDG PET generally shows an increased metabolism homogeneously.

1. Adenoidal hypertrophy: Male patient, 3 years old (Fig. 8.24)
2. Adenoidal hypertrophy: Male patient, 5 years old (Fig. 8.25)

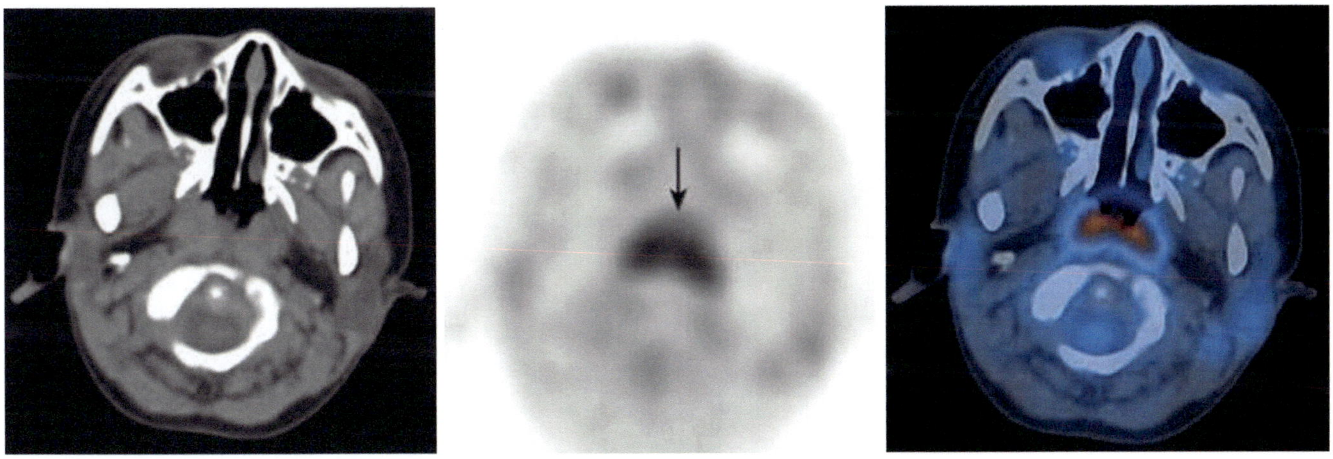

Fig. 8.24 PET/CT image of adenoidal hypertrophy in the nasopharynx. The soft tissue of the nasopharynx was thickened, located under the mucosa, and the local uptake of FDG was significantly increased (arrow)

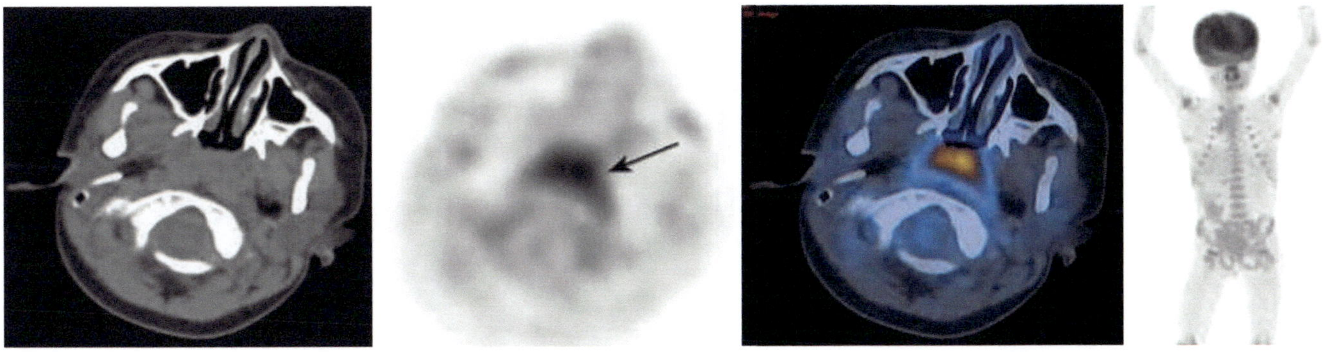

Fig. 8.25 PET/CT image of adenoidal hypertrophy. Typical adenoidal hypertrophy; local FDG uptake increased significantly (arrow)

6 Summary

Nodular high uptake of FDG in the nasopharynx, accompanied by asymmetric thickening of the nasopharynx wall or soft tissue masses are typical manifestations of nasopharyngeal carcinoma. At the same time, attention should be paid to whether there are invasion of surrounding tissue structure and lymph node metastasis. If the FDG uptake in the nasopharyngeal cavity is symmetrical, and there is no mucosal thickening or the mucosal thickening is uniform on the structural image, nasopharyngeal lymphoma, or adenoid, inflammation should be considered. Nasopharyngeal endoscopy is helpful to identify.

PET/CT can simultaneously obtain whole-body PET functional metabolism images, CT anatomical images, and PET/CT fusion images, which helps to determine the range of the nasopharyngeal primary lesion and regional lymph nodes, the location and range of distant metastases, and the clinical staging; determine the biological target area of nasopharyngeal carcinoma; improve the accuracy of radiotherapy, thereby reducing the radiation damage of normal tissue; identify the recurrence, residual, or changes of tumor after treatment; evaluate and monitor the therapeutic effect of tumor; and assist the development and adjustment of treatment plan.

9 PET/CT of Malignant Tumors of Nasal Cavity and Paranasal Sinus

Xiaoping Lin and Wei Fan

Among all malignant tumors of the nasal cavity and paranasal sinus, 50–65% occurs in the maxillary sinus, 15–30% occurs in the nasal cavity, 10–25% occurs in the ethmoid sinus, and 0.1–4.0% occurs in the frontal sinus and sphenoid sinus. Malignant tumors of the nasal cavity and paranasal sinus are mostly malignant epithelial tumors, which refer to cancers that occur in the respiratory area of the nasal cavity and paranasal sinus. Squamous cell carcinoma is the most common, and adenocarcinoma is rare (often occurring in the ethmoid sinus). Non-epithelial-derived tumors are mainly olfactory neuroblastoma and malignant melanoma.

The nasal cavity and paranasal sinus lesions of epithelial and non-epithelial-derived tumors show high metabolism on ^{18}F-FDG PET. Lymph node metastasis and distant metastasis are both manifested as high ^{18}F-FDG uptake, while the tumor with necrosis may be manifested as reduced or lack of metabolism.

1 Epithelial-Derived Malignant Tumors

1.1 Clinical Overview

The common early symptoms are nasal congestion, increased secretion, and/or epistaxis, which are similar to those of rhinitis, sinusitis, and benign epithelial tumors. When the medical treatment is ineffective, the symptoms appear repeatedly, or symptoms occur unilaterally, the tumor should be highly suspected.

X. Lin · W. Fan (✉)
Sun Yat-sen University Cancer Center, Guangzhou, Guangdong, China
e-mail: fanwei@sysucc.org.cn

1.2 PET/CT Diagnostic Points

1.2.1 General Diagnostic Points

1. There is a clinical history, for example, nasal carcinoma can cause pain, and maxillary sinus carcinoma is often accompanied by infection and may have submandibular swelling and active inflammatory lymph nodes palpated.
2. Intranasal mass can be seen in nasal carcinoma.
3. When the lesions of the nasal cavity and paranasal sinus invade the brain nerve, the corresponding symptoms may occur.
4. It is usually unilateral.

1.2.2 CT Diagnostic Points

Nasal carcinoma is manifested as an iso-dense mass in the nasal cavity and enlarged nasal cavity. When the tumor is large, it can invade the outer wall of the nasal cavity and invade the maxillary sinus or ethmoid sinus. It can further damage the orbital wall and enter the orbit. The advanced tumor can enter the oral cavity through the hard palate downward, and invade the nasal septum inward and involve the contralateral nasal cavity, and upward destroy the ethmoid plate and enter the intracranial space and involve the structure of the anterior cranial fossa. Necrosis can be seen inside the tumor.

In the early stage, maxillary sinus carcinoma grows in the sinus mucosa and often occurs in the lower half of the maxillary sinus. The enlargement of the tumor can invade the sinus wall and the structure outside the sinus. The tumor often destroys the anterior wall and invades the maxillofacial soft tissue or the gingival buccal sulcus, invades the nasal cavity through the sinus wall, involves the pterygopalatine fossa through the posterior wall, and invades the orbit through the upper wall. Maxillary sinus carcinoma often involves the ethmoid sinus. It can upward invade the orbit and can involve skull base. When it invades outward, it can involve the zygoma and infratemporal fossa. The bone destruction of the

Z. Yao, S. Li (eds.), *Atlas of PET/CT in Oncology - Volume 1*, https://doi.org/10.1007/978-981-99-1172-1_9

sinus wall is the main point of identification. In the late stage, lymph node metastasis may occur, mostly to superficial cervical lymph nodes (such as submaxillary lymph nodes and preauricular lymph nodes), cervical lymph nodes in II area, and retropharyngeal lymph nodes. Distant metastasis mostly occurs in the late stage.

Ethmoid sinus carcinoma typically manifests as an irregular soft tissue tumor in the ethmoid sinus, with irregular edges and iso-density. When the tumor is small, only the bone in the ethmoid sinus septum is destroyed. When the mass is large, it inward involves the nasal cavity and forms a soft tissue mass in the nasal cavity, which can destroy the middle turbinate, the upper turbinate, and even the nasal septum. The mass can outward invade the maxillary sinus and downward destroy the inner wall of the orbit to the orbit, which is manifested as orbital soft tissue mass and displacement of extraocular muscle and optic nerve due to compression. It can upward invade the anterior cranial fossa.

1.2.3 ^{18}F-FDG PET Diagnostic Points

1. The primary lesions of the nasal cavity and paranasal sinus, metastatic lymph nodes, and distant metastases show hypermetabolic changes.
2. Tumors of the nasal cavity and paranasal sinus are often accompanied by nasal secretions and sinusitis, and the inflammation is generally less hypermetabolic than tumors.
3. When the lesions of the nasal cavity and paranasal sinus invade the skull base and intracranial space structure, the hypermetabolic active lesion involves the intracranial.
4. Ocular muscles generally show increased physiological uptake, and when the tumor invades the orbit, the boundary between the tumor and the adjacent ocular muscles is not clear. If necessary, same-machine enhanced CT can help determine the range of invasion.

1.2.4 Typical Cases

1. Squamous cell carcinoma of the left nasal cavity: Male patient, 51 years old. Pathology: Poorly differentiated squamous cell carcinoma of the left nasal cavity (Fig. 9.1)
2. Squamous cell carcinoma of the right nasal cavity: Male patient, 54 years old. Pathology: Moderately to poorly differentiated squamous cell carcinoma of the right nasal cavity (Figs. 9.2, 9.3, 9.4, and 9.5)
3. Squamous cell carcinoma of the left maxillary sinus: Female patient, 56 years old. Pathology: Differentiated squamous cell carcinoma of the left maxillary sinus (Fig. 9.6)
4. Undifferentiated carcinoma of the right sphenoethmoidal recess: Male patient, 34 years old. Pathology: Undifferentiated carcinoma of the right undifferentiated carcinoma of the right sphenoethmoidal recess (Fig. 9.7)

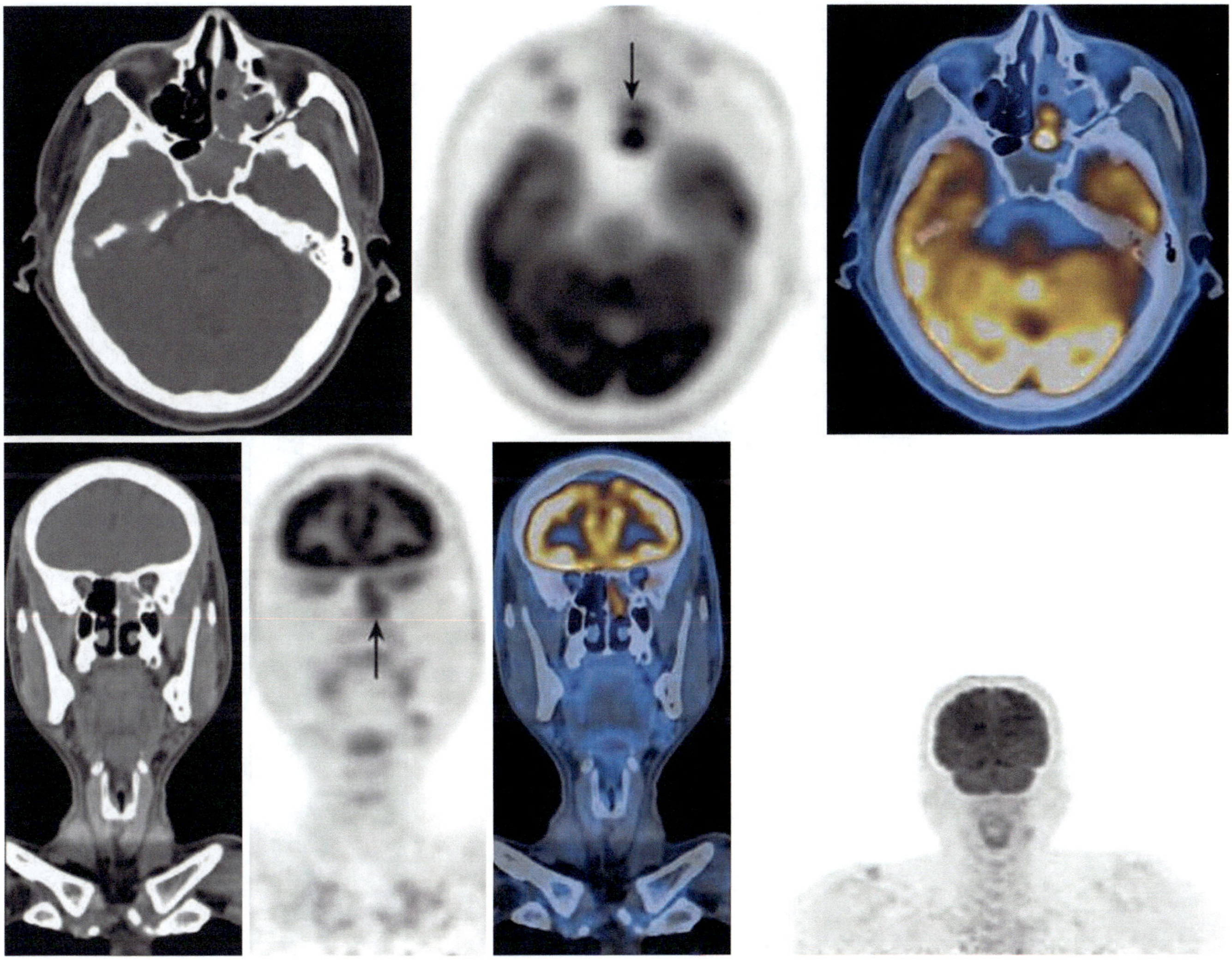

Fig. 9.1 PET/CT image of poorly differentiated squamous cell carcinoma of the left nasal cavity. PET/CT showed increased FDG uptake (SUVmax 15.2) in the soft tissue nodules of the left nasal cavity (arrow); its size was 1.2 cm × 2.0 cm. It invaded the posterior part of the left upper and middle turbinate, nasal septum, left pterygopalatine fossa, left medial bone wall of the maxillary sinus, left ethmoid sinus, and sphenoid sinus (including the ethmoid sinus plate and sphenoid bone)

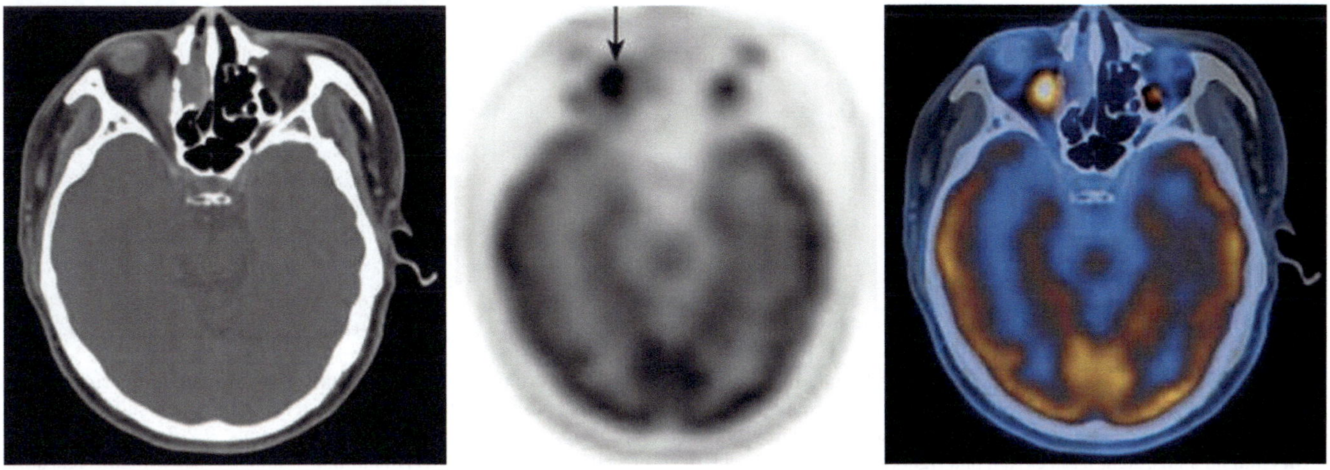

Fig. 9.2 PET/CT cross-sectional image of moderately to poorly differentiated squamous cell carcinoma of the right nasal cavity

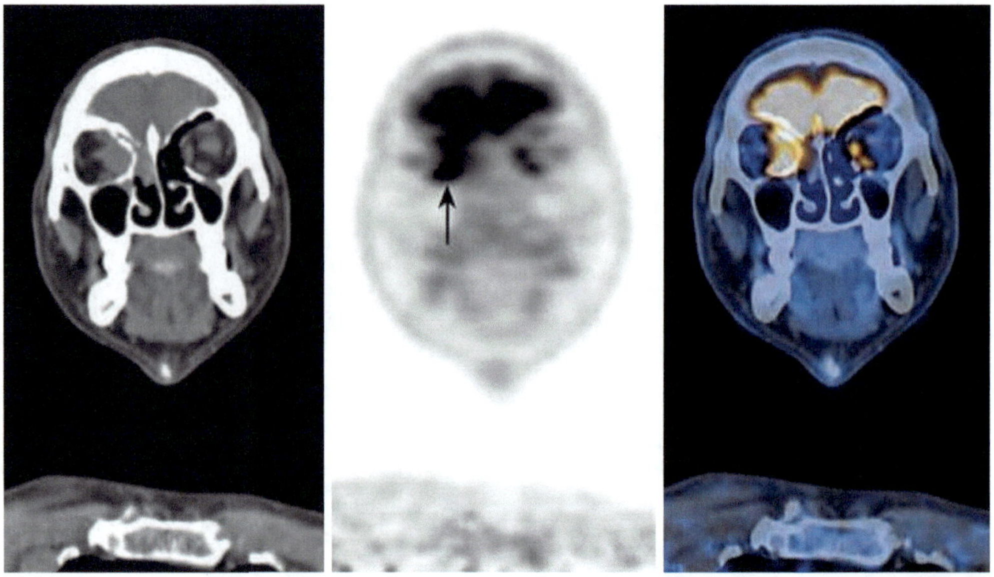

Fig. 9.3 PET/CT coronal image of moderately to poorly differentiated squamous cell carcinoma of the right nasal cavity

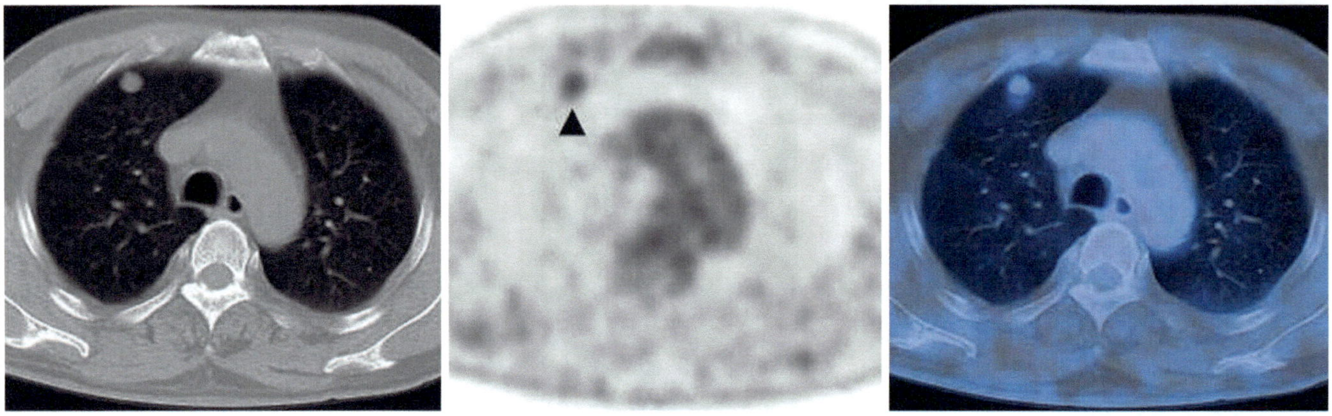

Fig. 9.4 PET/CT cross-sectional image of the right lung metastasis (▲) of moderately to poorly differentiated squamous cell carcinoma of the right nasal cavity

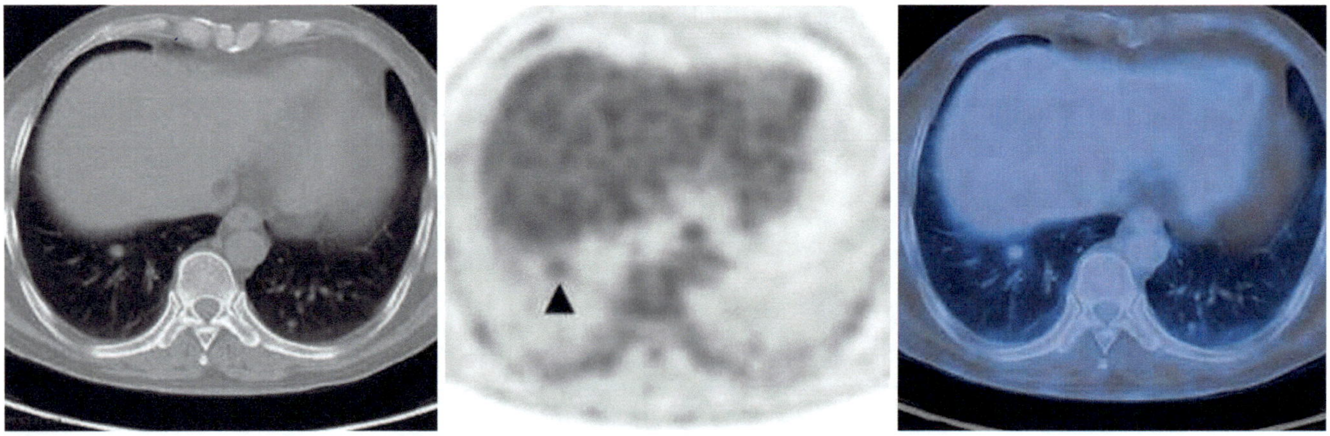

Fig. 9.5 PET/CT cross-sectional image of the right lung metastasis of moderately to poorly differentiated squamous cell carcinoma of the right nasal cavity. Increased FDG uptake in the soft tissue mass (arrow) in the right ethmoid sinus, right nasal cavity, and right orbit (inside the back of the eyeball); its size was 2.4 cm × 3.2 cm. It invaded the right medial rectus muscle, the inner wall of the right orbital bone, the inner upper wall of the right orbital bone, and the bone of the top wall of the right maxillary sinus, pushed on the right optic nerve, causing it to shift to the right and having an unclear boundary with it (Figs. 9.2 and 9.3). Increased FDG uptake (SUVmax 4.1) in multiple round nodules with different sizes in both lungs (▲); the biggest one's size was 1.2 cm × 1.3 cm. Part of the nodules was not clearly separated from the pleura (Figs. 9.4 and 9.5)

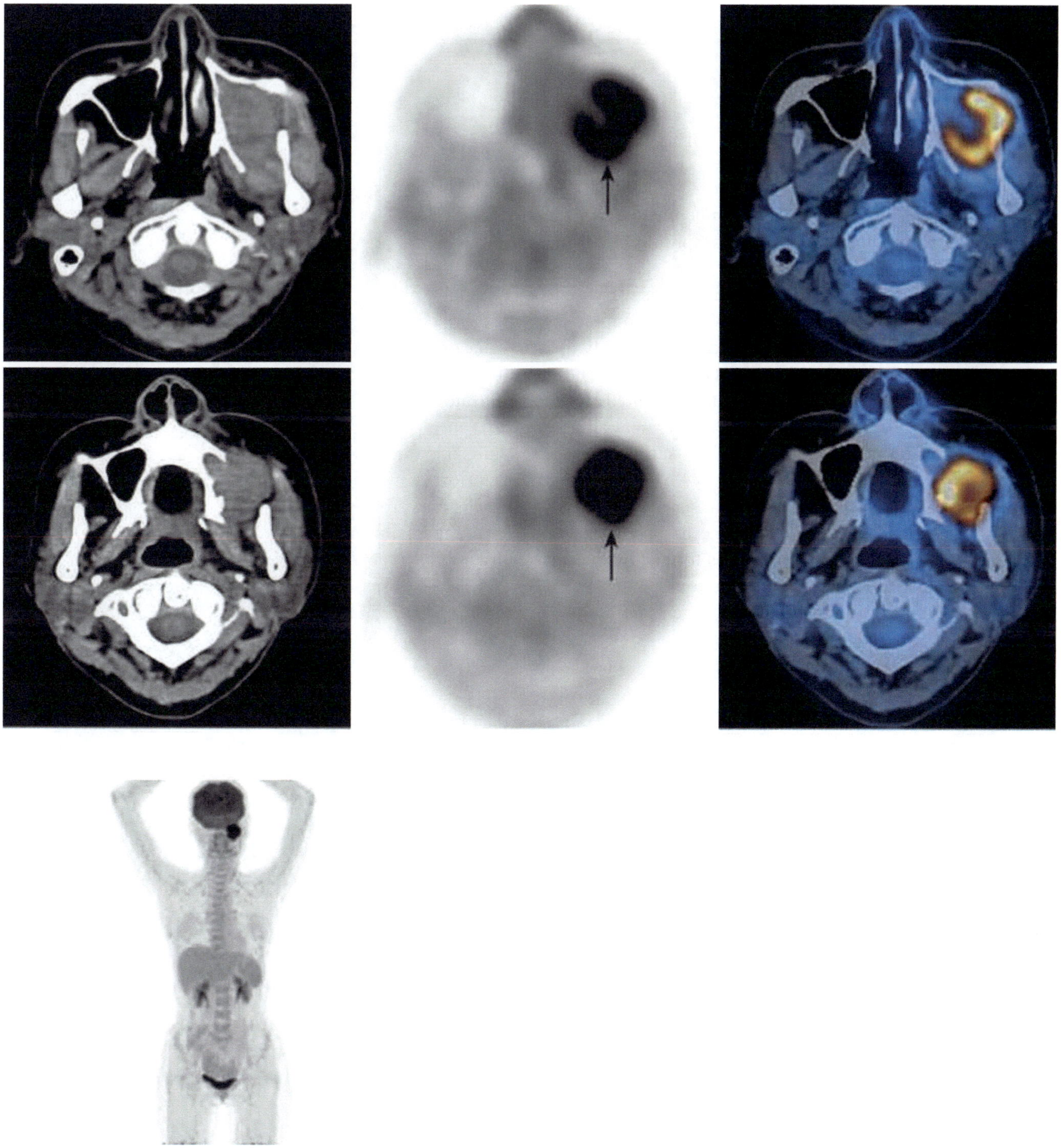

Fig. 9.6 PET/CT cross-sectional images of squamous cell carcinoma of the left maxillary sinus. Intense FDG uptake in the soft tissue mass in the left maxillary sinus cavity; its SUVmax was 19.0 and size 3.0 cm × 3.8 cm. The lesion invaded the inner wall and anterior wall of the left maxillary sinus, the left maxillary alveolar bone, and the pterygopalatine fossa, left pterygoid process, left infratemporal fossa, left lateral pterygoid muscle, left masseter muscle, and left temporal muscle

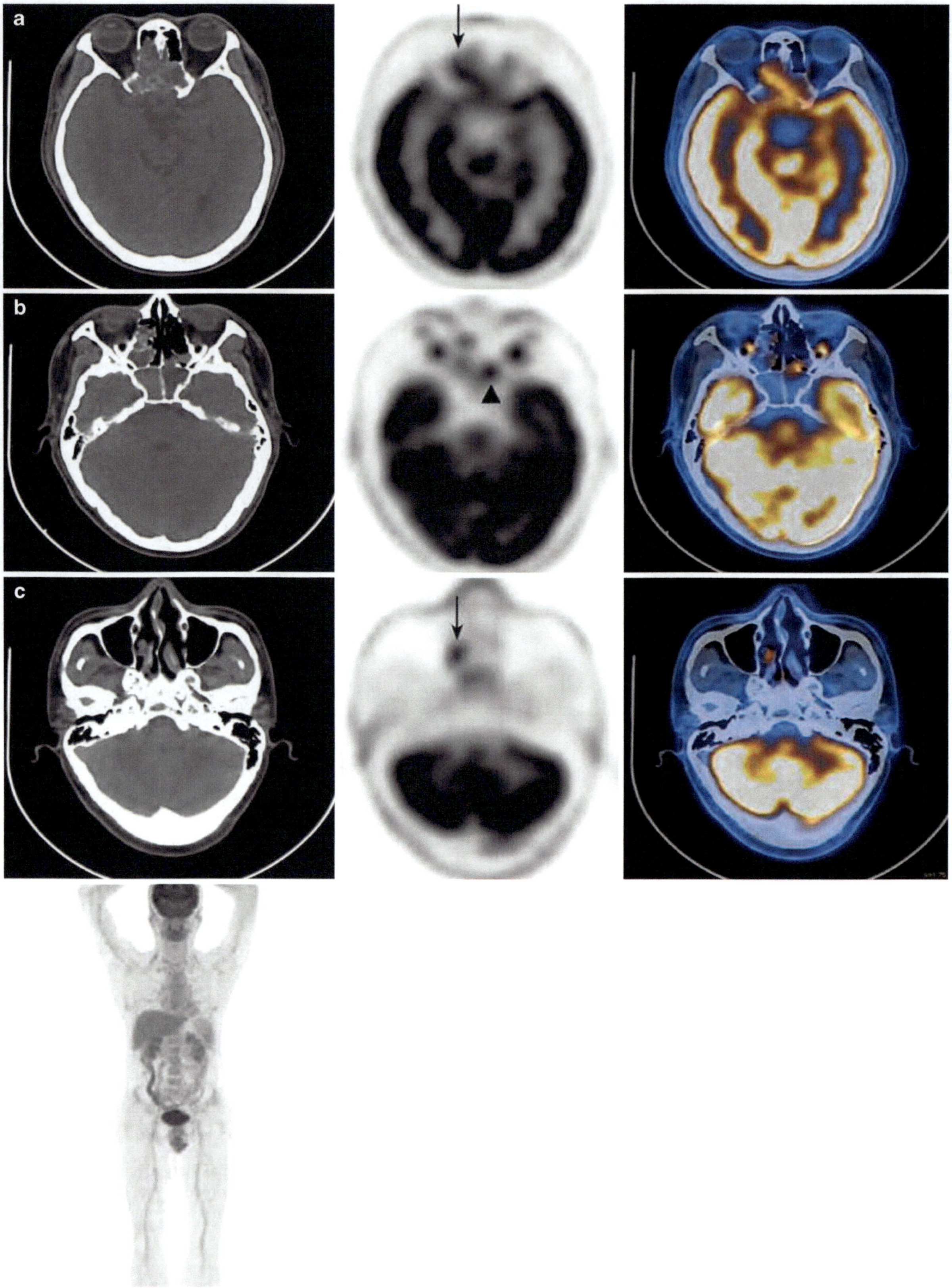

Fig. 9.7 PET/CT image of undifferentiated carcinoma of the left sphenoethmoidal recess. The soft tissue in the ethmoid sinus was hypermetabolic with SUVmax 10.8. The main body of the lesion was located in the right ethmoid sinuses (**a**, **c**), it invaded the left side of the sphenoid sinus (▲) (**b**), and the boundary between the lesion and the bilateral middle turbinate was unclear. There was no obvious damage to the bone of the sinus wall

2 Olfactory Neuroblastoma

2.1 Clinical Overview

Olfactory neuroblastoma usually occurs in the location of the olfactory epithelium, that is, the top of the nasal cavity, cribriform plate, superior turbinate, and upper part of the nasal septum. It can also occur in the lower nasal cavity, ethmoid sinus, and maxillary sinus. There were two peaks in the age of onset, 10–20 years old and 50–60 years old, and slightly more female patients. Olfactory neuroblastoma tends to spread in the submucosa and intracranial space. It can spread to intracranial space in early stage, but does not invade the dura mater of the anterior cranial fossa. When the tumor is small, it can fill one side of the nasal cavity and ethmoid sinus; when it is larger, it can fill the bilateral nasal cavity. When the tumor is large, it can involve the nasopharynx, paranasal sinus, dura mater, and even frontal lobe. It is more common to metastasize to cervical lymph nodes, while other sites include the parotid gland, skin, lung, bone, liver, eyeball, spinal cord, spinal canal, etc.

2.2 PET/CT Diagnostic Points

2.2.1 General Diagnostic Points

1. Have a clinical history, such as nasal congestion and epistaxis, followed by anosmia and headache. When it invades the orbit, it causes exophthalmos and visual impairment.
2. Space-occupying lesions of the nasal cavity.
3. When the lesions of the nasal cavity invade the brain nerve, the corresponding symptoms may occur.
4. It can be involved unilaterally or bilaterally.

2.2.2 CT Diagnostic Points

In the early stage, the tumor is confined to the nasal cavity and ethmoid sinus. The typical site is the anterior superior nasal cavity. The base is located in the cribriform plate area. Most of them are uniform and iso-dense, and a few may have cystic change and/or calcification. When the mass is large, it fills the entire nasal cavity, and the bone of the ethmoid sinus wall and the bone of the middle and lower turbinate are destroyed. The orbital invasion is characterized by destruction of the orbital wall bone and orbital mass. The lesion can upward invade the anterior cranial fossa, which is manifested as an irregular mass in the anterior cranial fossa, with thickening and obvious enhancement of the frontal dura mater.

2.2.3 ^{18}F-FDG PET Diagnostic Points

1. The lesions of the nose and paranasal sinus, metastatic lymph nodes, and distant metastases show metabolically active changes.
2. The lesions are small, or due to partial volume effect, the local metabolism is slightly highly active.
3. When it is accompanied by nasal secretions and sinusitis, the inflammatory part is generally not metabolically active.
4. When the lesions invade the skull base and intracranial structures, attention to the morphological and structural changes should be paid, due to the similar radioactive distribution of FDG between the lesion and the normal brain tissue surrounding the lesion. If necessary, the enhanced CT scan by PET/CT will be helpful to distinguish them.

2.3 Typical Cases

1. Olfactory neuroblastoma of the nasal cavity and paranasal sinus before and after treatment: Male patient, 48 years old. Pathology: Olfactory neuroblastoma of the nasal cavity (Figs. 9.8 and 9.9)
2. Olfactory neuroblastoma of the right nasal cavity with lymph node metastasis: Female patient, 56 years old. Pathology: Poorly differentiated olfactory neuroblastoma in the right pharyngeal recess (Figs. 9.10, 9.11, 9.12, and 9.13)

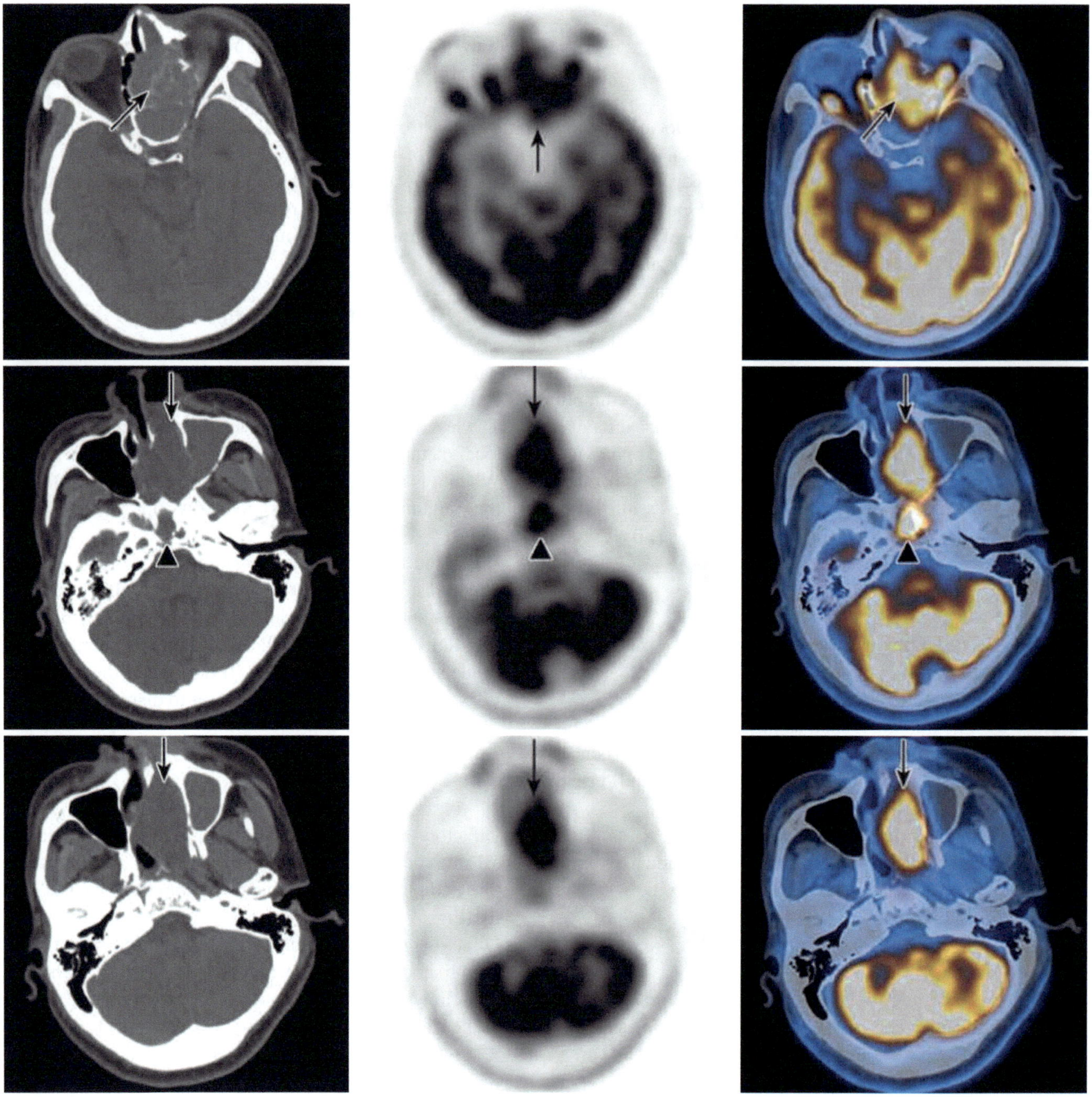

Fig. 9.8 PET/CT cross-sectional images of olfactory neuroblastoma of the nasal cavity and paranasal sinus before treatment. Increased FDG uptake in irregular soft tissue masses in the nasal cavity, ethmoid sinus, and sphenoid sinus were noted, with SUVmax 14.1. The lesion invaded the left maxillary sinus and the left retrobulbar muscles. The left inferior rectus muscle and left medial straight muscle were swelled with SUVmax 8.2. The nasal septum, left orbital bone, sphenoid bone, and clivus (▲) bone were destroyed, with SUVmax 13.2

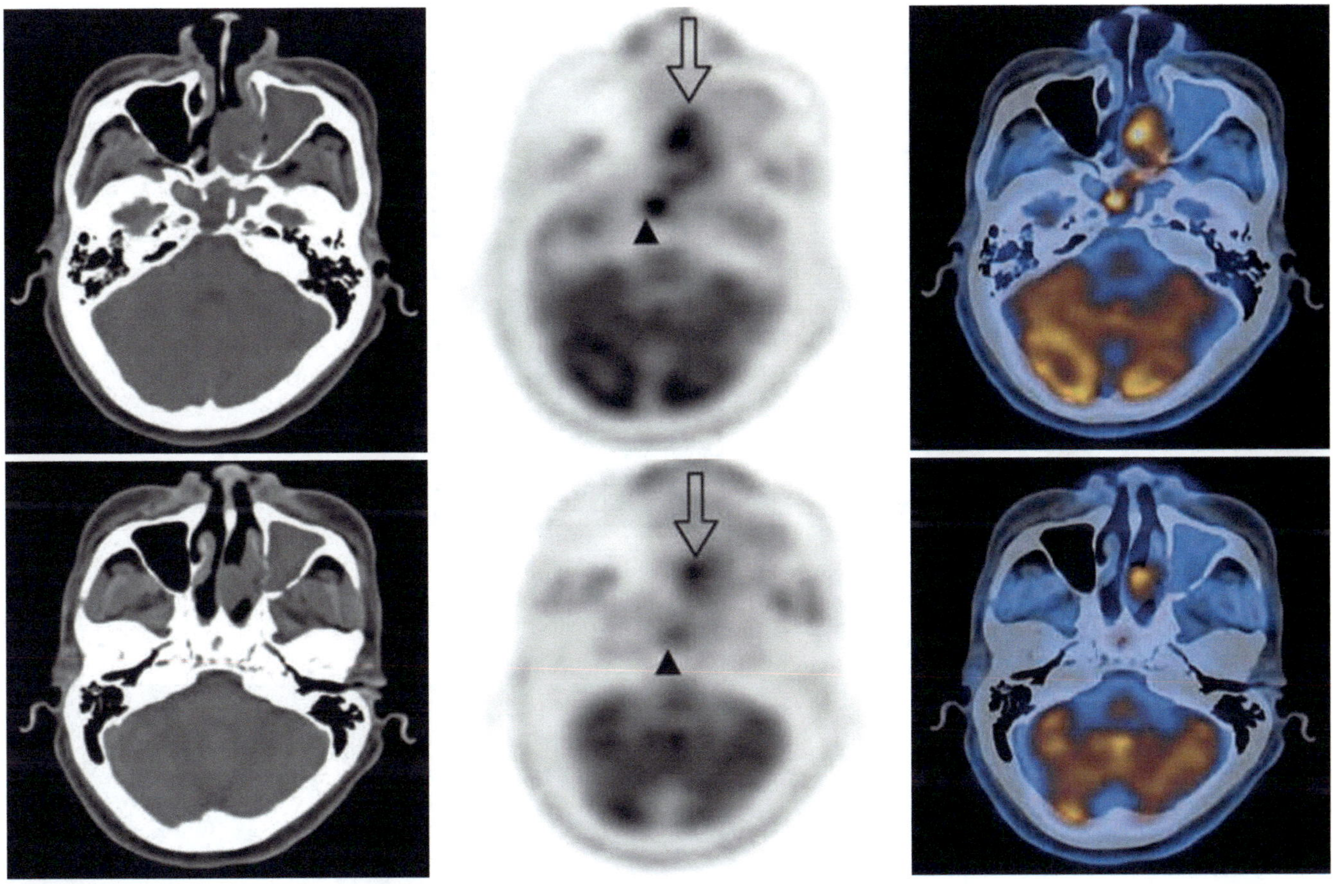

Fig. 9.9 PET/CT cross-sectional images of olfactory neuroblastoma of the nasal cavity and paranasal sinus after chemotherapy. After two courses of chemotherapy, PET/CT showed that the metabolic activities of soft tissue masses (arrow) in the ethmoid sinus, sphenoid sinus, and left nasal cavity were slightly reduced, with SUVmax from 14.1 reduced to 11.5, and the size measured on the largest layer was 3.2 cm × 4.1 cm. After treatment, the lesions invading in the frontal lobe, left pterygopalatine fossa, medial wall of the left maxillary sinus, sphenoid base, occipital clivus (▲), and nasal septum were significantly reduced, and the metabolic activity was decreased

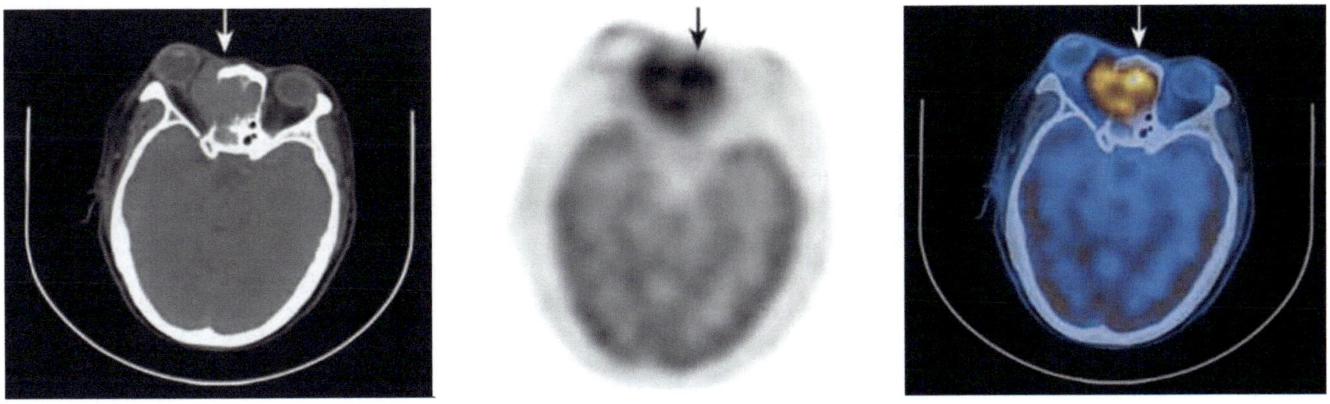

Fig. 9.10 PET/CT cross-sectional image of olfactory neuroblastoma in the right nasal cavity

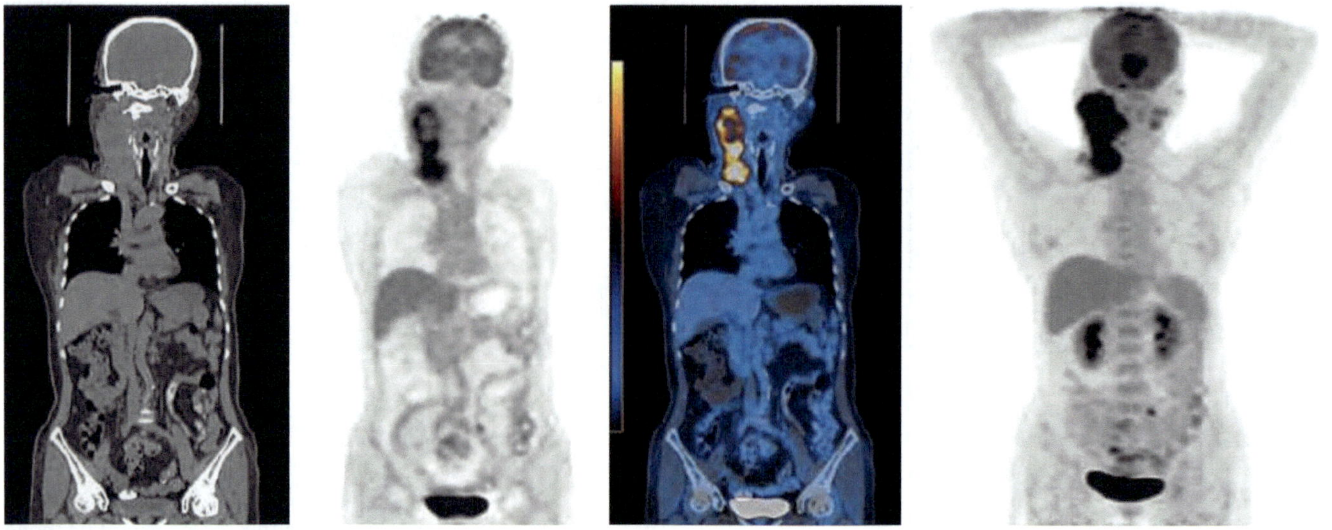

Fig. 9.11 PET/CT coronal image of olfactory neuroblastoma in the right nasal cavity. The soft tissue mass in the right nasal cavity was hypermetabolic with SUVmax 11.6 and size 4.2 cm × 4.3 cm. The lesion invaded the ethmoid sinus, bilateral frontal sinus, sphenoid sinus, right frontal lobe, and right medial rectus muscle through the inner wall of the right orbit (Figs. 9.10 and 9.11)

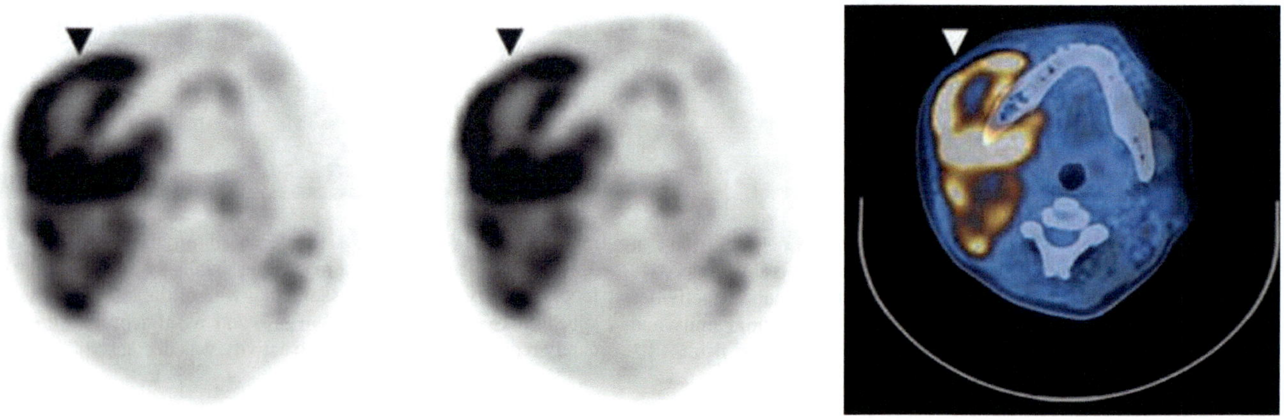

Fig. 9.12 PET/CT cross-sectional images of right nasal olfactory neuroblastoma invading the subcutaneous soft tissue of the cheek. The subcutaneous soft tissue of the right cheek had intense FDG uptake with SUVmax 14.1 and size 3.1 cm × 6.7 cm

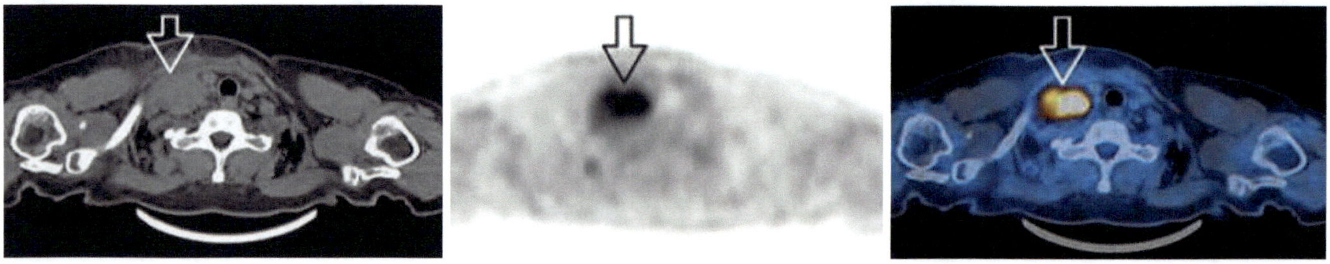

Fig. 9.13 PET/CT cross-sectional image of cervical lymph node metastasis of olfactory neuroblastoma in the right nasal cavity. Increased FDG uptake in multiple enlarged lymph nodes in the bilateral cervical I–V area (open arrow)

2.4 Rare Cases

Olfactory neuroblastoma with intracranial invasion: Male patient, 42 years old. Pathology: Olfactory neuroblastoma of the right ethmoid sinus, grade IV (Figs. 9.14, 9.15, and 9.16)

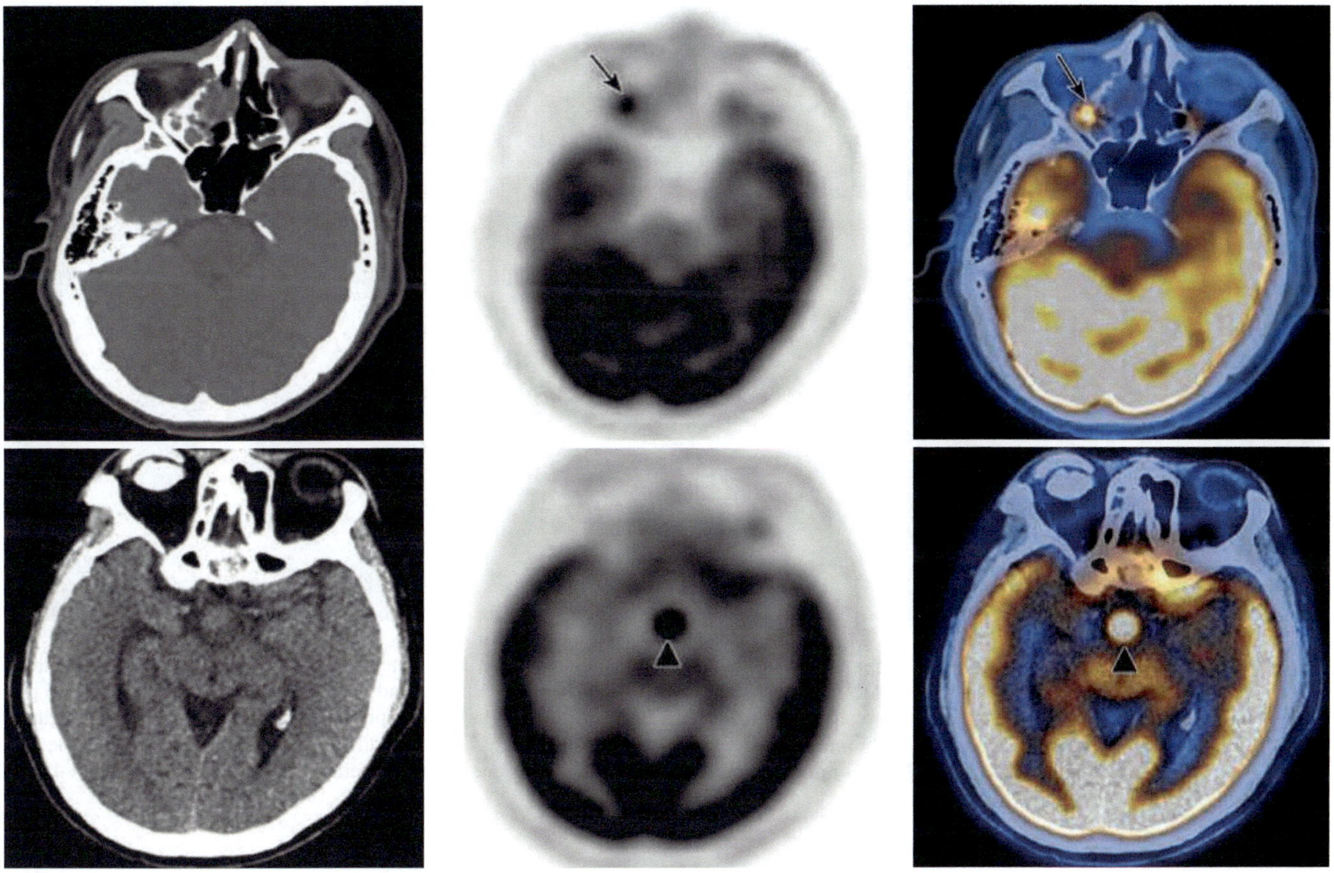

Fig. 9.14 PET/CT cross-sectional images of ethmoid sinus olfactory neuroblastoma (arrow) invading the medulla oblongata (▲)

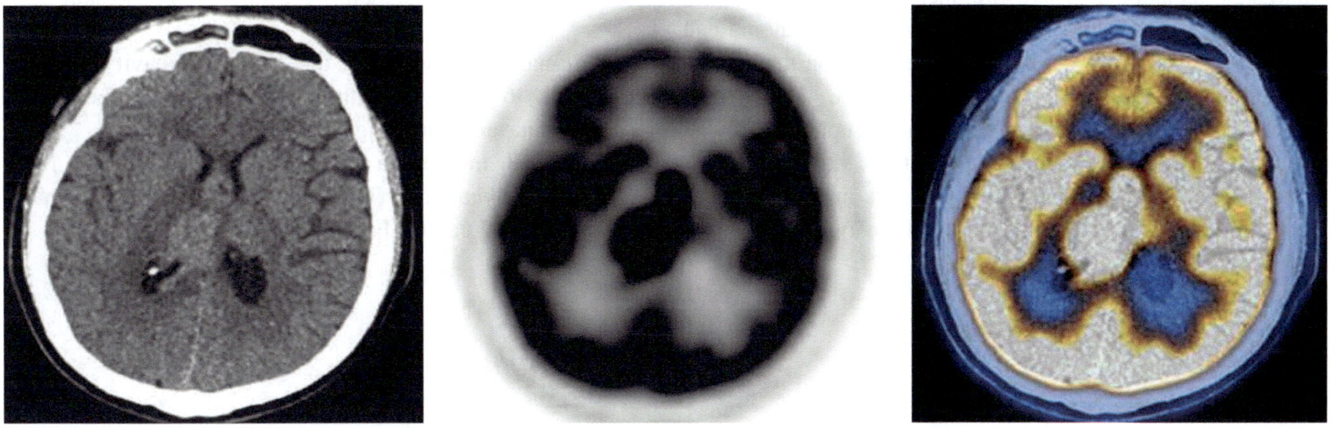

Fig. 9.15 PET/CT cross-sectional image of ethmoid sinus olfactory neuroblastoma invading the ventricle, suprasellar cistern, and pituitary stalk

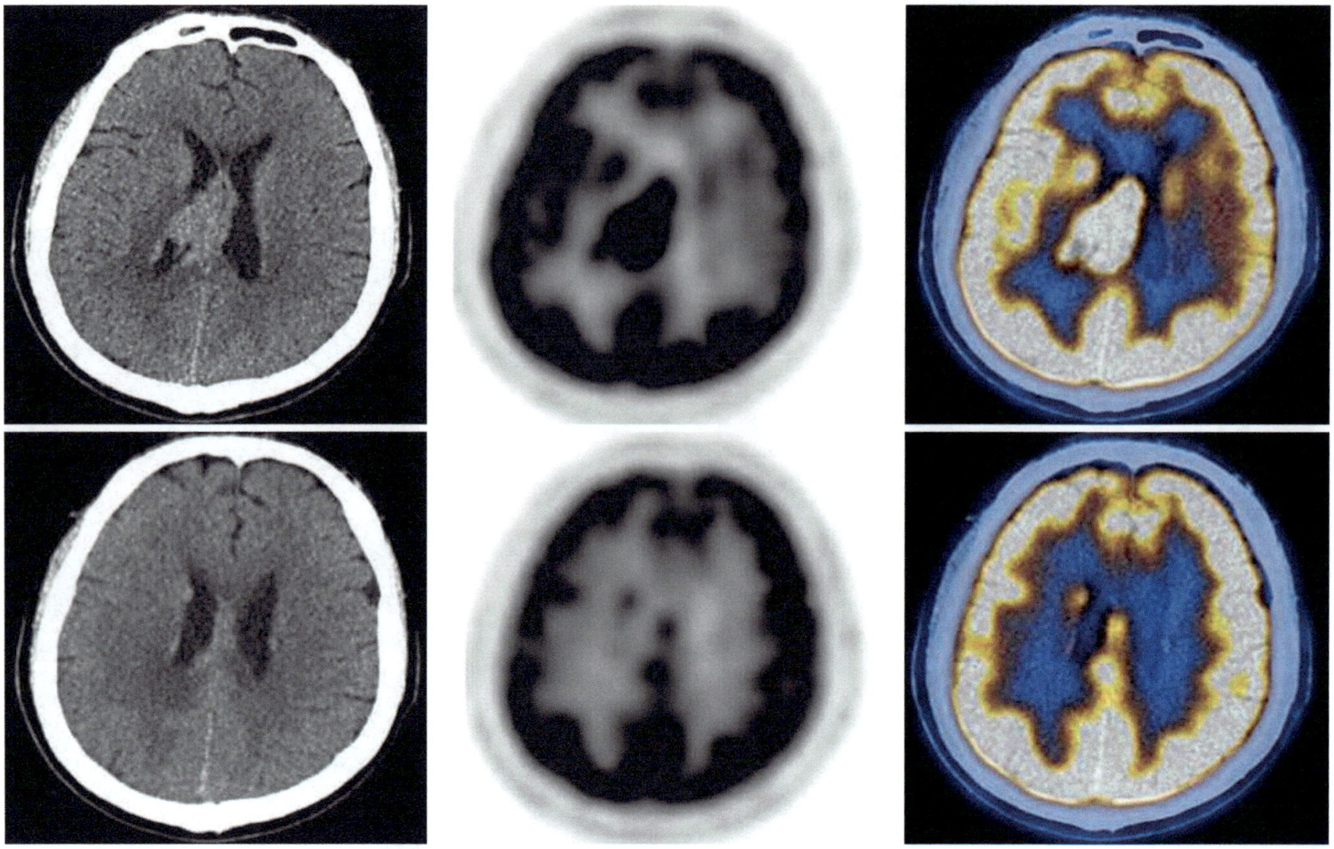

Fig. 9.16 PET/CT cross-sectional images of ethmoid sinus olfactory neuroblastoma invading the ventricle. Increased FDG uptake (SUVmax 13.0) in the soft tissue shadow of the right anterior and middle ethmoid sinus; its boundary was unclear, accompanied by ethmoid sinusitis (Fig. 9.14a). Intense FDG uptake (SUVmax 22.8) in multiple nodules and masses within the bilateral ventricles (Fig. 9.16), third ventricle (Figs. 9.14b and 9.15), ependyma of the fourth ventricle, septum pellucidum, suprasellar cistern, pituitary stalk, and surface of the medulla oblongata (Figs. 9.14, 9.15, and 9.16). The largest one was in the septum pellucidum and the right lateral ventricle with size 2.6 cm × 4.4 cm

2.5 Differential Diagnosis

Malignant melanoma: There are melanocytes in the nasal mucosa of normal adults. Primary malignant melanoma can occur in the nasal cavity, which is more common than in the paranasal sinus. Malignant melanoma of the nasal cavity mostly occurs in the anterior part of the nasal septum, followed by the middle turbinate and inferior turbinate. Malignant melanoma of the paranasal sinus mostly occurs in the maxillary sinus. Malignant melanoma of the nasal cavity and paranasal sinus is easy to invade the anterior cranial fossa through the skull base and often metastasize to the cervical lymph nodes. The distant metastasis is mainly the lung, brain, and skin.

1. Malignant melanoma of the left nasal cavity: Female patient, 46 years old. Pathology: Malignant melanoma of the left nasal cavity (Figs. 9.17 and 9.18)
2. Malignant melanoma of the left nasal cavity: Male patient, 52 years old. Pathology: Malignant melanoma of the left nasal cavity (Figs. 9.19 and 9.20)

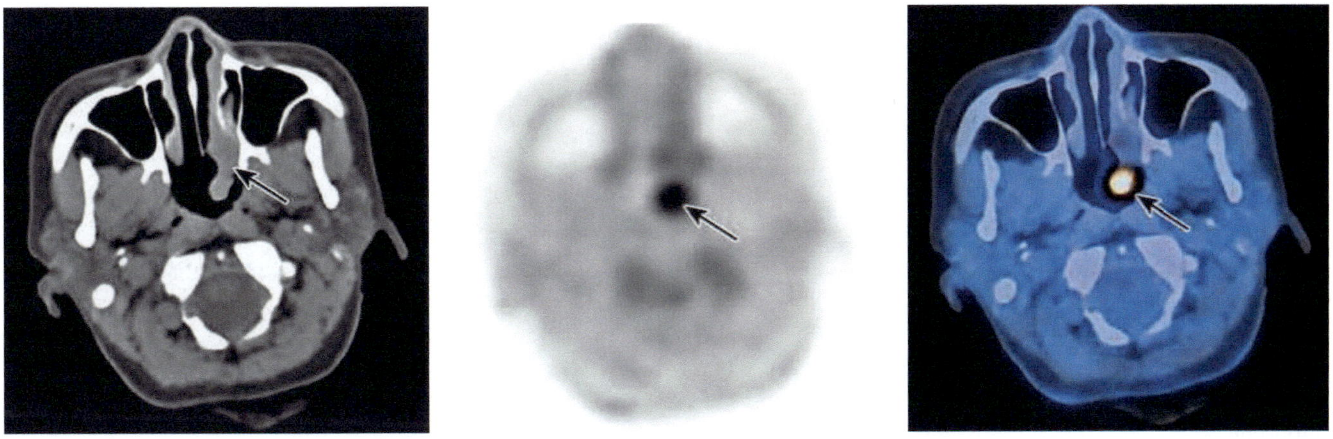

Fig. 9.17 PET/CT cross-sectional image of malignant melanoma in the left nasal cavity

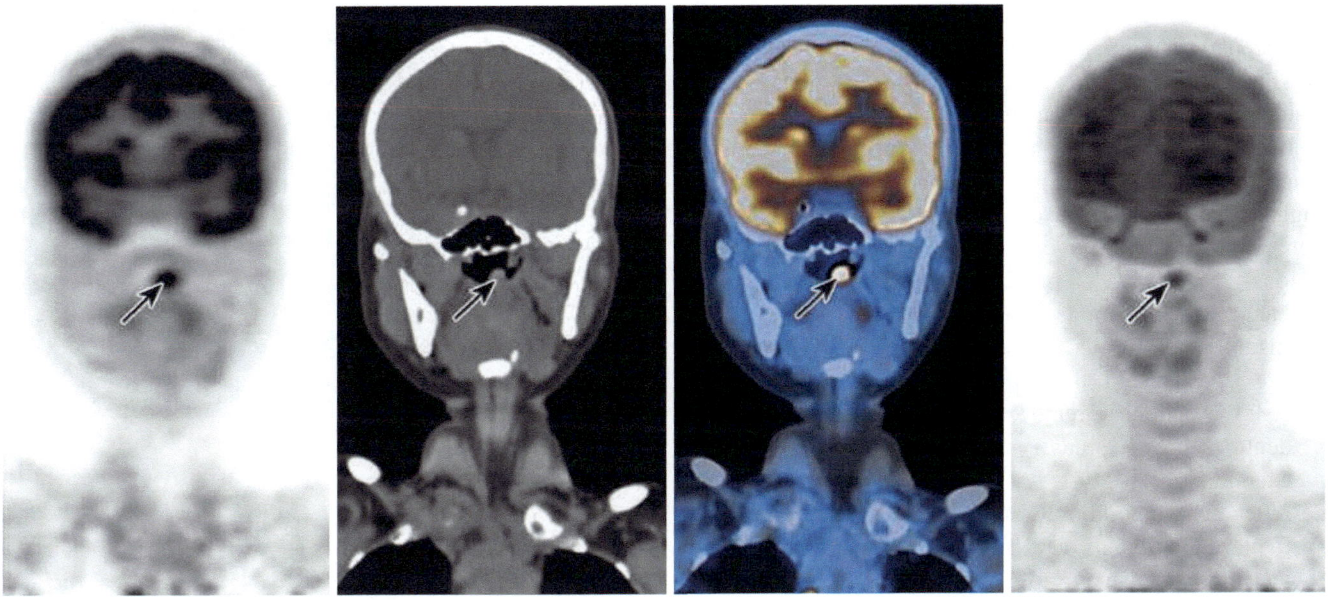

Fig. 9.18 PET/CT coronal and PET MIP image of malignant melanoma of the left nasal cavity. Increased FDG uptake in soft tissue nodules in the left nasopharynx, with SUt 15.4 and size 1.0 cm × 1.4 cm. The front edge of the lesion was connected to the back of the left inferior turbinate (Figs. 9.17 and 9.18)

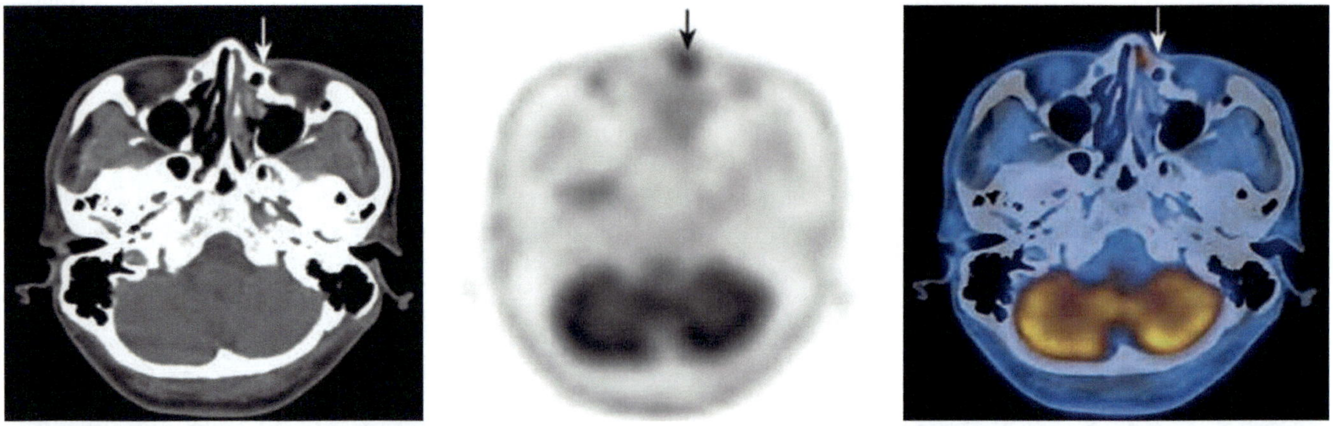

Fig. 9.19 PET/CT cross-sectional image of malignant melanoma of the left nasal cavity

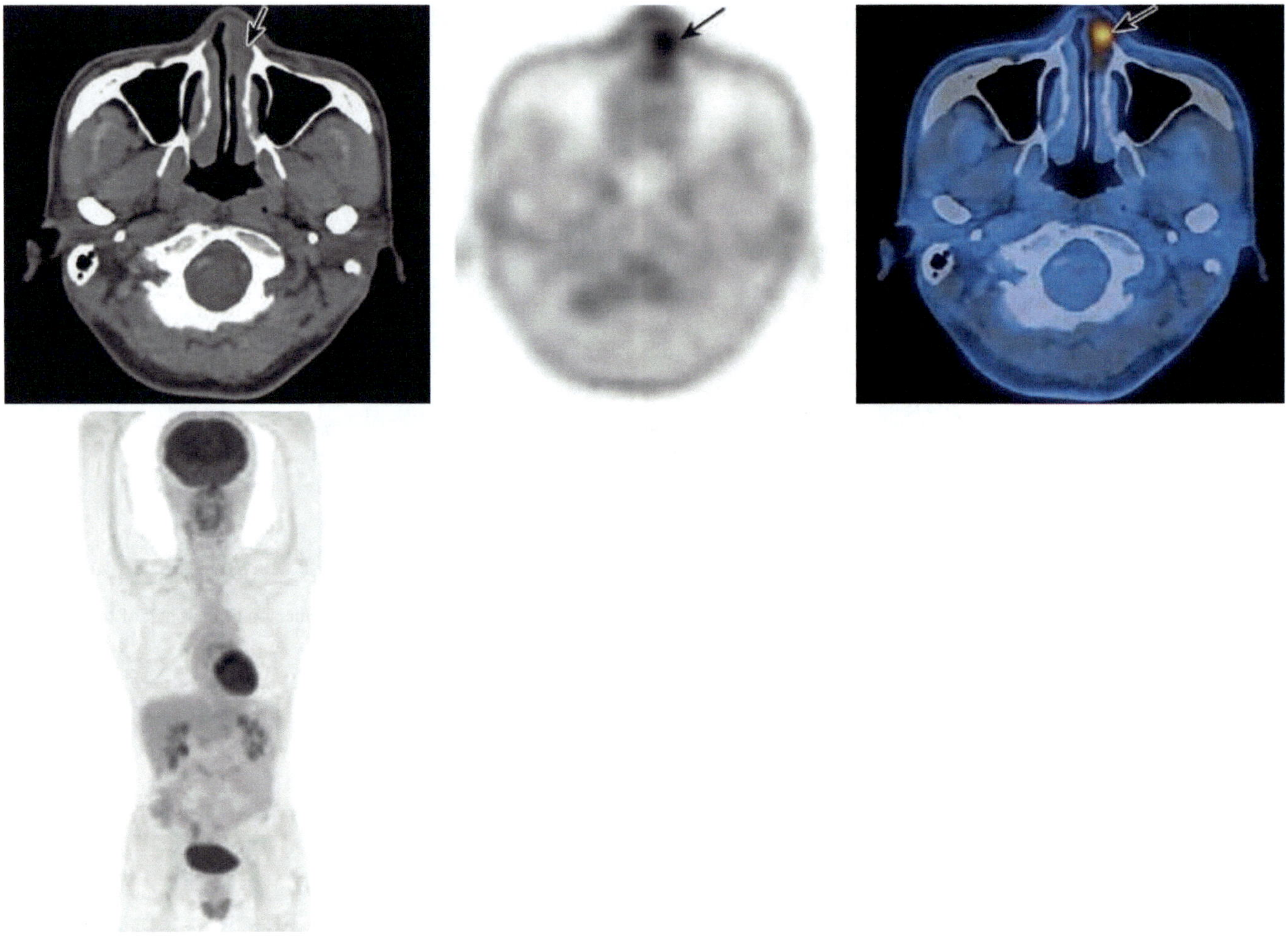

Fig. 9.20 PET/CT cross-sectional and PET MIP image of malignant melanoma of the left nasal cavity. The mucosa of the left anterior part of the nasal cavity was thickened, and the radioactive uptake was significantly increased (arrow), with SUVmax 7.2. The lesion invaded the anterior part of the nasal septum, the anterior part of the left inferior turbinate, the left nasal dorsum, and the left nasal bone (Figs. 9.19 and 9.20)

2.6 Summary of This Chapter

Most of the malignant tumors of the nasal cavity and paranasal sinus are malignant epithelial tumors, among which squamous cell carcinoma is the most common and adenocarcinoma is rare. The tumors of non-epithelial origin are mainly olfactory neuroblastoma. These tumors are typically characterized by abnormal increased FDG uptake in soft tissue masses or nodule in the nasal cavity and/or paranasal sinus. At the same time, attention should be paid to whether there are invasion of surrounding tissue structure and lymph node metastasis. Nasal and sinus epithelial-derived tumors and olfactory neuroblastoma need to be differentiated from tumors with significantly increased metabolic activity in the nasal cavity, such as malignant melanoma, lymphoma, etc.

^{18}F-FDG PET/CT can observe not only the FDG uptake but also the morphology of tumor. It is a one-time examination and whole-body imaging. It is superior to other imaging examinations in finding the primary lesions. It can detect the primary lesions and metastases at an early stage and provide help for differential diagnosis and prognosis.

PET/CT of Laryngopharyngeal Malignant Tumors

10

Xiaoping Lin and Wei Fan

1 Laryngopharyngeal Carcinoma

1.1 Clinical Overview

Hypopharyngeal carcinoma, also known as hypopharyngeal carcinoma, is a malignant tumor of the laryngopharyngeal mucosa epithelium. More than 95% of them are squamous cell carcinoma. Undifferentiated carcinoma and adenocarcinoma are rare. Soft tissue sarcoma and melanoma are occasionally seen. The incidence of laryngopharyngeal cancer is relatively low, with more male patients than female patients. Laryngopharyngeal carcinoma includes piriform sinus carcinoma, postcricoid carcinoma, and retropharyngeal wall carcinoma. Piriform sinus carcinoma is the most common, and postcricoid carcinoma is rare. Piriform sinus carcinoma and retropharyngeal wall carcinoma are more common in men, and postcricoid carcinoma is more common in women. Laryngopharyngeal carcinoma is mainly exogenous and infiltrating, often accompanied by ulcers on the surface. The clinical manifestations include retropharyngeal foreign body sensation, swallowing obstruction, pain and discomfort, coughing, hoarseness, and cervical mass.

Piriform sinus carcinoma that occurs in the lateral wall can invade the posterior wing of the thyroid cartilage, rarely invade the larynx, or spread to the opposite side. When it occurs on the medial wall, it may be accompanied by involvement of the postcricoid region, which mainly damages the internal laryngeal structure in the early stage, or spreads directly under the mucosa, invading the laryngeal ventricle and vocal cords through the ipsilateral paraglottic space or spreading to the opposite side through the postcricoid region. The tumor occupies the whole pyriform sinus, and the inner and outer walls may be invaded at the same time, and it may be accompanied by postcricoid involvement. Postcricoid carcinoma usually infiltrates around submucosa and causes hypopharyngeal stenosis. Retropharyngeal carcinoma may invade the oropharynx upward and esophageal entrance downward. Hypopharyngeal squamous cell carcinoma is less differentiated than laryngeal squamous cell carcinoma and has a poor prognosis. It is often accompanied by cervical lymph node metastasis, which is mainly unilateral, is common in II and III regions, and can later metastasize to IV, V, and VI regions, or bilateral lymph node metastasis can also occur. In the late stage, hematogenous metastasis is the most common, and lung, liver, and bone metastases are more common.

The ^{18}F-FDG metabolism of laryngopharyngeal carcinoma lesions showed high proliferation. Lymph node metastasis and distant metastasis both show increased ^{18}F-FDG uptake, and tumor necrosis may show sparse or defective radioactive distribution.

X. Lin · W. Fan (✉)
Sun Yat-sen University Cancer Center, Guangzhou, Guangdong, China
e-mail: fanwei@sysucc.org.cn

Z. Yao, S. Li (eds.), *Atlas of PET/CT in Oncology - Volume 1*, https://doi.org/10.1007/978-981-99-1172-1_10

1.2 PET/CT Diagnostic Points

1.2.1 General Diagnostic Points

1. Have a clinical history, such as pharyngeal discomfort, hoarseness, dyspnea, etc.; bloody sputum may appear in the late stage.
2. Laryngopharyngeal space-occupying lesion.
3. It may be unilateral, bilateral, or annular involvement.

1.2.2 CT Diagnostic Points

1. The laryngopharyngeal mucosa is thickened, or the mass appears, which may deform the larynx and even block the airway.
2. Pyriform sinus carcinoma is mostly located at the bottom of the pyriform sinus. In the early stage, the mucosa of the pyriform sinus is swollen and thickened, or the pyriform sinus is full. When the lesions are significantly enlarged, the pyriform sinus is deformed and narrowed or even disappears, with mass protruding from the surface and expanding in a circular shape, which make the arytenoid epiglottis fold thicken and the paralaryngeal space stenosis disappear.
3. The tumor can directly invade the vocal cords, causing vocal cord pyknosis.
4. Postcricoid carcinoma and retropharyngeal wall carcinoma are common in protruding type, located in the upper part of the pyriform sinus, manifested by thickening exceeding 1 cm or soft tissue mass at the prevertebral soft tissue.
5. The postcricoid carcinoma is likely to invade the surrounding cartilage and the lower cervical esophagus.
6. The enlarged tumor may invade the adjacent structures: The retropharyngeal wall carcinoma may upward invade the parapharyngeal space, leading to the destruction of the laryngeal cartilage; backward invade into the retropharyngeal soft tissue; and downward invade the esophagus, causing the thickening of the entrance tube wall.

1.2.3 ^{18}F-FDG PET Diagnostic Points

1. The laryngopharyngeal primary lesion, metastatic lymph nodes, and distant metastases show changes of increased FDG uptake.
2. Due to partial volume effect, the small lesions may only show slightly high FDG uptake. In some cases, there are no significant differences between the metabolism of the local and that of the normal tissues surrounding it after the biopsy of tumor tissue.
3. Physiological high FDG uptake on one side of the vocal cord may occur in patients with hoarseness (also manifested as vocal cord tension on CT), and symmetrically physiological increased FDG uptake at the retropharyngeal wall may be observed in a crying child. Before giving diagnosis, it is better to know well the patient's status during PET/CT examination, carefully adjust image brightness, and determine if it matches well between CT and PET.

1.3 Typical Cases

1. Right piriform sinus carcinoma: Male patient, 61 years old. The cervical lymph nodes were enlarged, and then the primary tumor was being looked for. PET/CT found the right pyriform sinus carcinoma; pathological biopsy: the right pyriform sinus tumor biopsy was moderately to poorly differentiated squamous cell carcinoma (Figs. 10.1 and 10.2).
2. Postcricoid carcinoma: Male patient, 64 years old. Pathology: Moderately differentiated squamous cell carcinoma in the postcricoid region (Fig. 10.3).
3. Laryngopharyngeal carcinoma invaded the thyroid: Male patient, 60 years old. Pathology: Differentiated squamous cell carcinoma in the left pyriform sinus (Figs. 10.4, 10.5, 10.6, and 10.7).

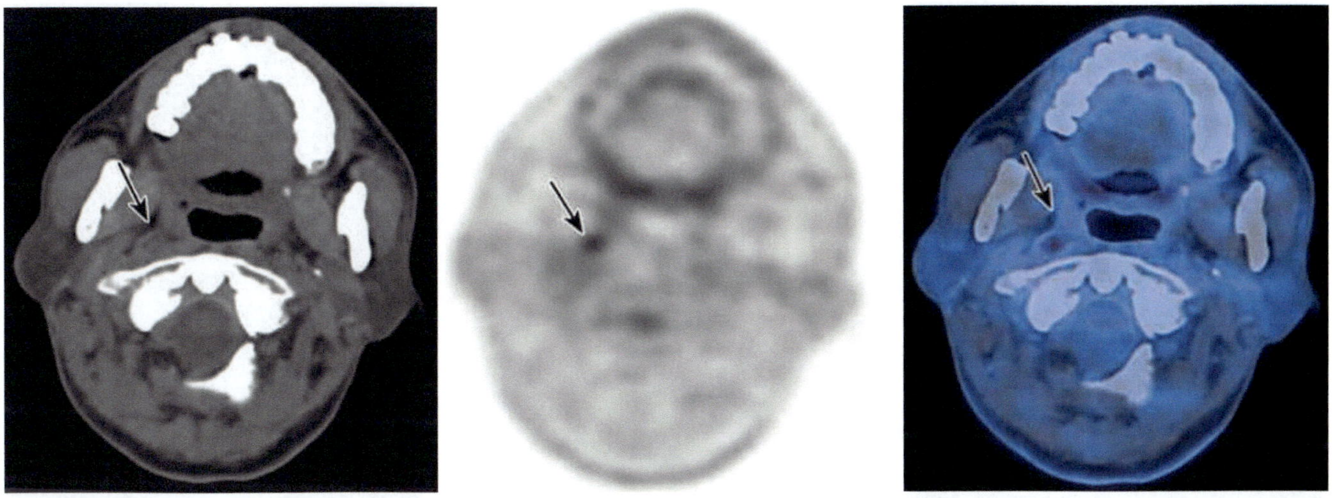

Fig. 10.1 PET/CT cross-sectional image of the right pyriform sinus carcinoma. Increased FDG uptake (SUVmax 8.5) in the mucosa of the right pyriform sinus

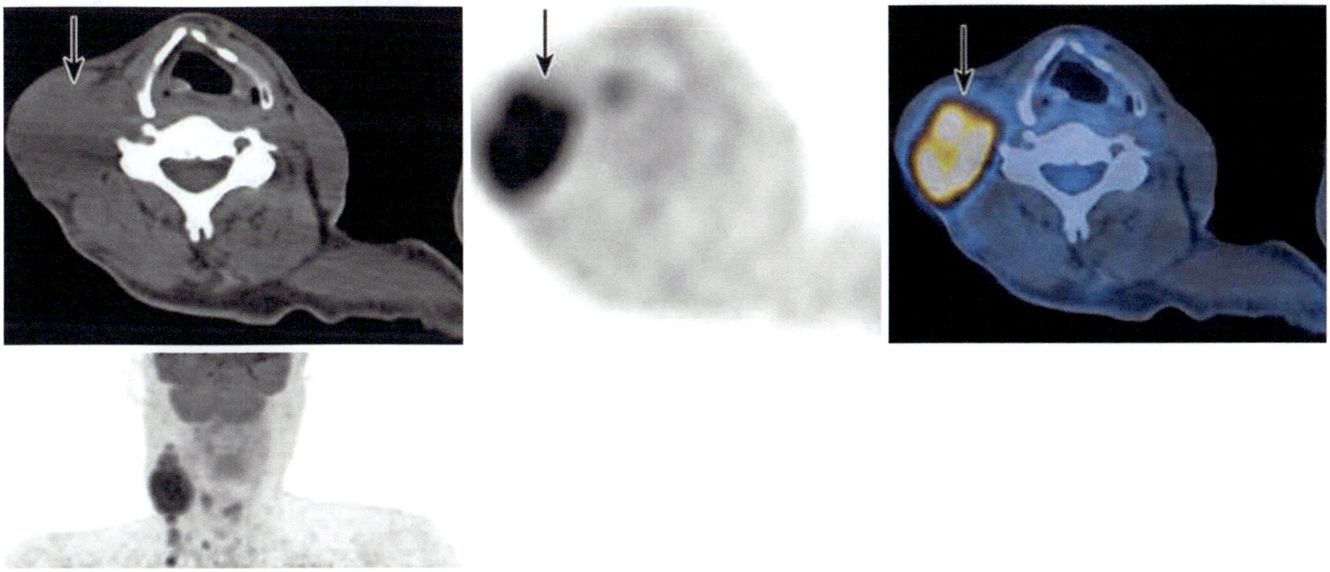

Fig. 10.2 PET/CT cross-sectional image of lymph node metastasis of the right pyriform sinus carcinoma. Intense FDG uptake (SUVmax 19.1) in multiple enlarged lymph nodes in the right cervical II–IV regions; the biggest one was 3.3 cm × 5.1 cm in size and partly fused into a mass, wrapping the right carotid sheath (arrow)

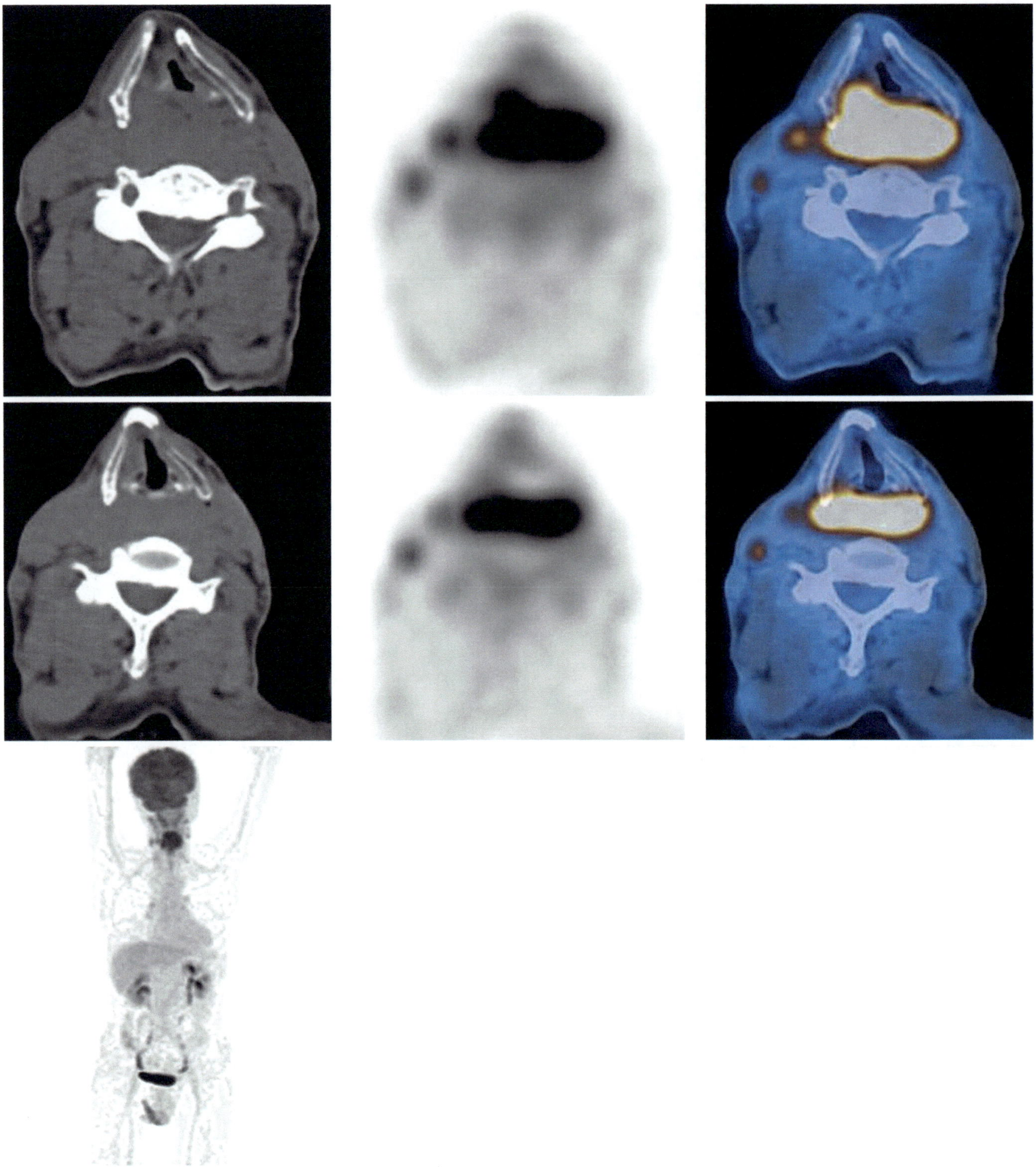

Fig. 10.3 PET/CT cross-sectional image of squamous cell carcinoma of the postcricoid region. The thickened posterior wall of the laryngopharynx formed a soft tissue mass with increased FDG uptake (SUVmax 11.4) soft tissue mass. The lesions invaded the right part of the epiglottis, right piriform recess, right arytenoid epiglottis fold, right paralaryngeal space, arytenoid area, postcricoid region, cervical esophagus, right thyroid cartilage, and cricoid cartilage

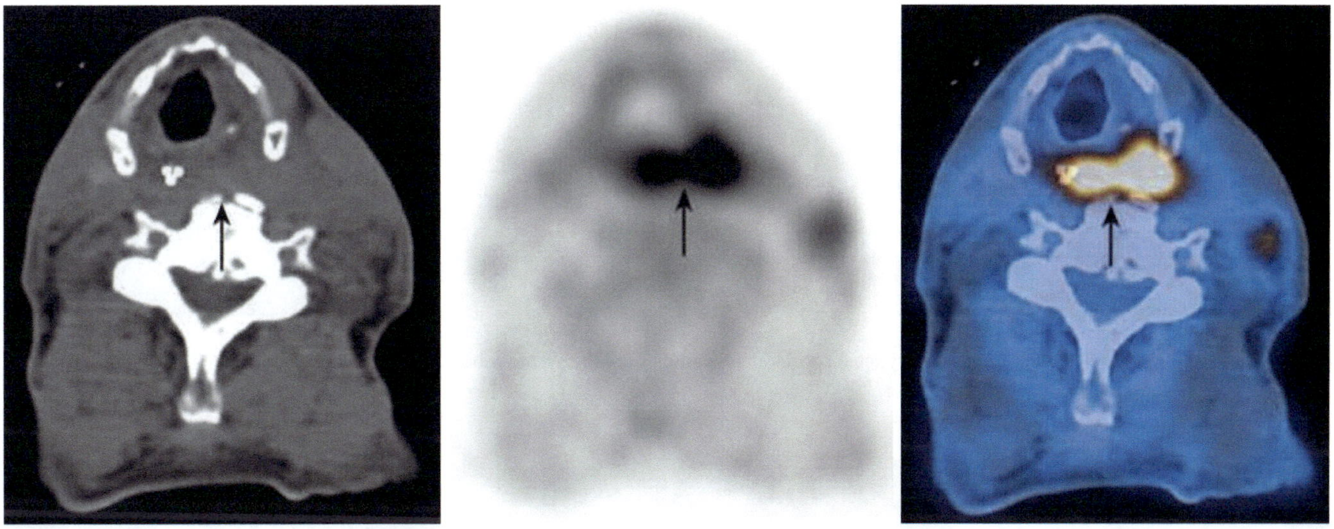

Fig. 10.4 PET/CT cross-sectional image of laryngopharyngeal carcinoma

Fig. 10.5 PET/CT coronal image of laryngopharyngeal carcinoma

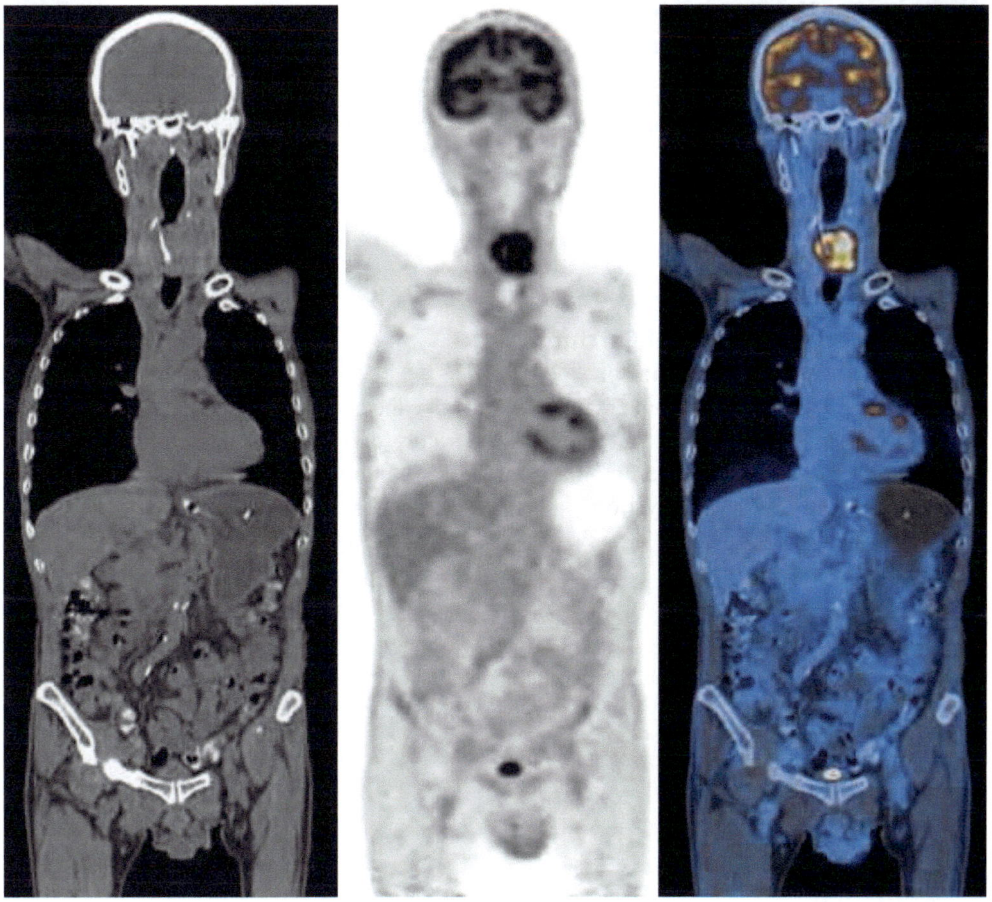

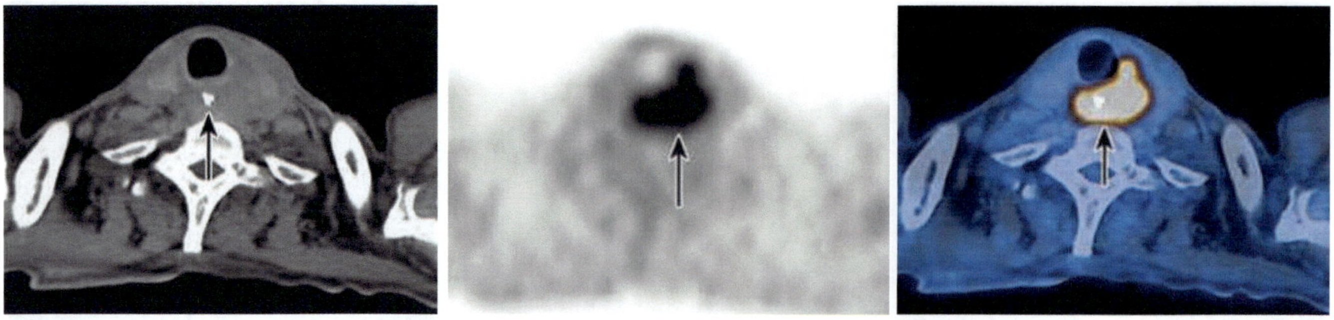

Fig. 10.6 PET/CT cross-sectional image of laryngeal carcinoma invading the left thyroid lobe

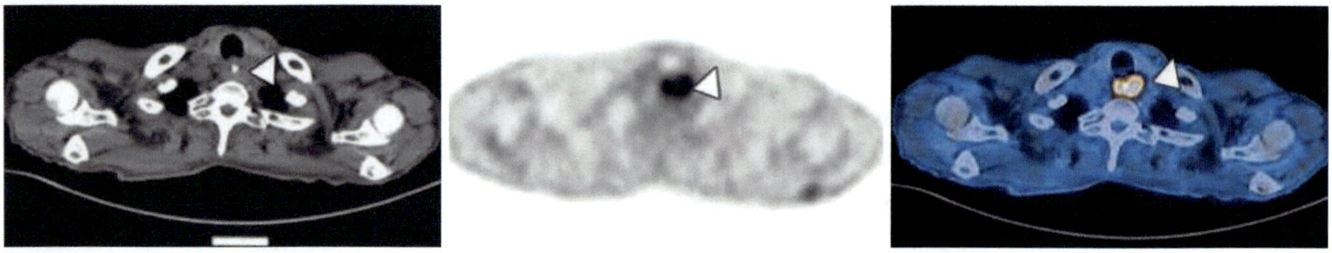

Fig. 10.7 PET/CT cross-sectional image of laryngopharyngeal carcinoma invading the esophagus. Increased FDG uptake in irregular soft tissue masses (arrows) in the posterior wall of the hypopharynx and the postcricoid region; its SUVmax was 12.9 and size 3.0 cm × 3.7 cm × 6.2 cm (Figs. 10.4 and 10.5). It invaded the cervical esophagus downward (Fig. 10.7) and invaded the left lobe of the thyroid gland (Δ) (Fig. 10.6)

1.4 Rare Cases

1.4.1 Laryngopharyngeal Carcinoma with Esophageal Cancer

1. Laryngopharyngeal carcinoma with esophageal cancer: Male patient, 52 years old. Pathology: Moderately differentiated squamous cell carcinoma in the left aryteno-epiglottic fold and the left pyriform sinus and esophageal cancer 30–34 cm away from the incisors (Figs. 10.8 and 10.9)
2. Pyriform sinus carcinoma with esophageal cancer: Male patient, 41 years old. Pathology: Moderately differentiated squamous cell carcinoma of the laryngopharynx and moderately differentiated squamous cell carcinoma of the esophagus (Figs. 10.10, 10.11, and 10.12)

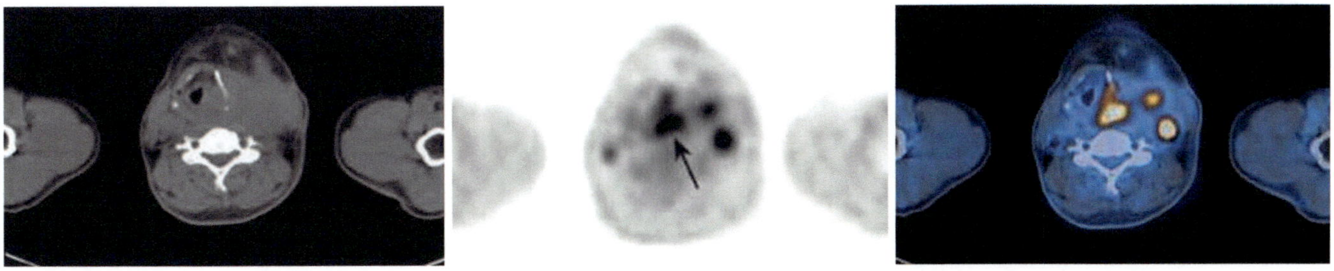

Fig. 10.8 PET/CT cross-sectional image of laryngopharyngeal carcinoma. Increased FDG uptake (SUVmax 13.3) in the soft tissue mass in the left wall of the laryngopharynx (arrow); its size was 3.1 cm × 3.5 cm. The mass pushed the laryngopharynx to the right and invaded the left pyriform sinus, left arytenoepiglottic fold, left hyoid bone, left thyroid cartilage, left arytenoid cartilage, left epiglottic space, and left parapharyngeal space. The boundary between the mass and the left enlarged lymph node was unclear

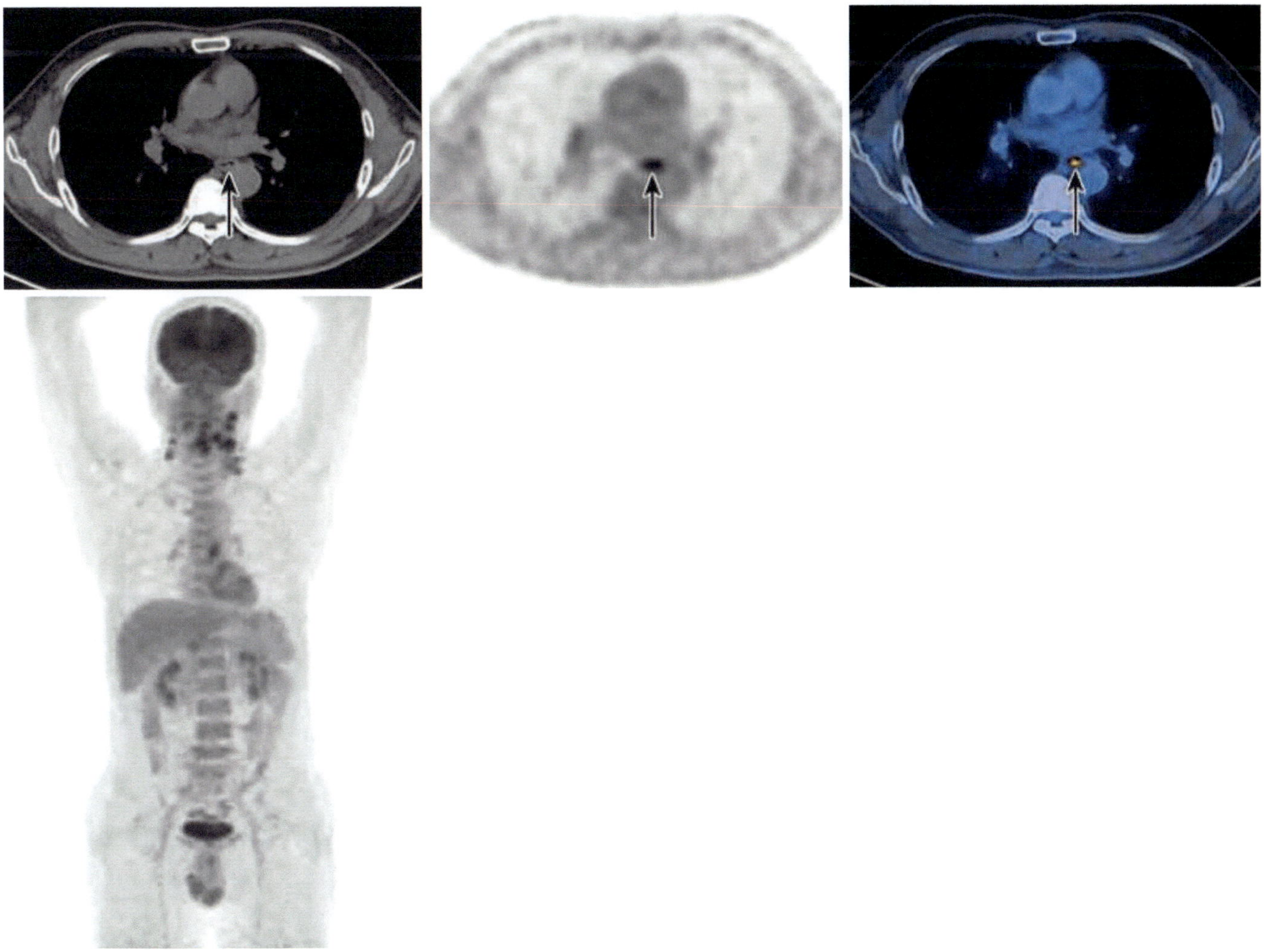

Fig. 10.9 PET/CT cross-sectional image and PET MIP image of esophageal cancer. It is the same PET/CT image of the same patient as Fig. 10.8. The wall of the middle esophagus was inhomogeneously thickened and FDG uptake increased (arrow). Its SUVmax was about 9.8 and the thickest part was about 0.6 cm. The PET MIP image comprehensively shows the lesions with increased metabolic activity in laryngopharyngeal carcinoma, cervical lymph node metastasis, and middle esophageal cancer

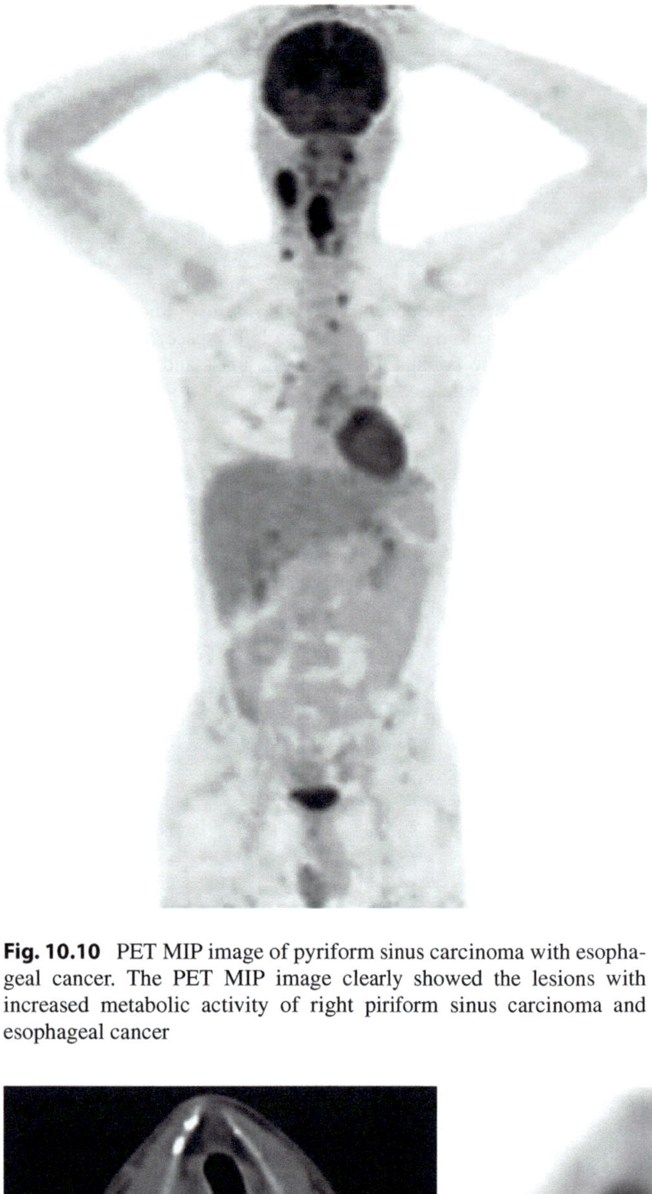

Fig. 10.10 PET MIP image of pyriform sinus carcinoma with esophageal cancer. The PET MIP image clearly showed the lesions with increased metabolic activity of right piriform sinus carcinoma and esophageal cancer

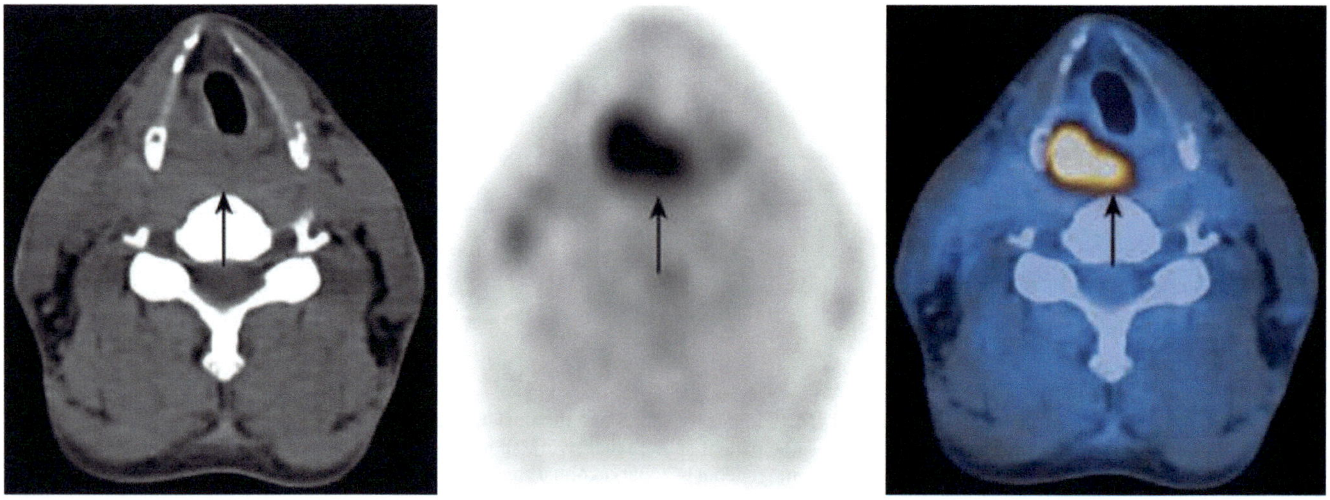

Fig. 10.11 PET/CT cross-sectional image of the right pyriform sinus carcinoma. Intense FDG uptake (SUVmax 17.4) in the soft tissue nodules of the right pyriform sinus (arrow), with size 1.6 cm × 1.9 cm. It invaded the right part of the epiglottis, the right arytenoepiglottic fold, the posterior wall of the laryngopharynx, the postcricoid region, the right parapharyngeal space, and the right arytenoid cartilage and involved the esophageal entrance

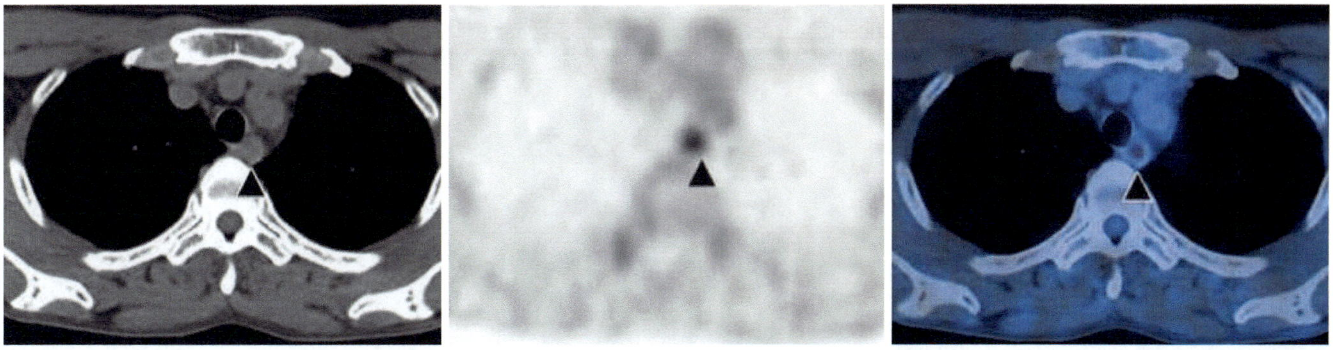

Fig. 10.12 PET/CT cross-sectional image of esophageal cancer. It is the same PET/CT image of the same patient as Fig. 10.11. Increased FDG uptake (SUVmax 4.8) in the local thickened wall of the upper and middle esophagus. Its thickness was 0.8 cm and peripheral fat space was still clear (▲)

1.4.2 Laryngopharyngeal Carcinoma with Binary Tumor

Pyriform sinus carcinoma with lung adenocarcinoma: Male patient, 60 years old. Pathology: Moderately differentiated squamous cell carcinoma of the right pyriform sinus and highly to moderately differentiated adenocarcinoma of the left upper lung (Figs. 10.13, 10.14, and 10.15)

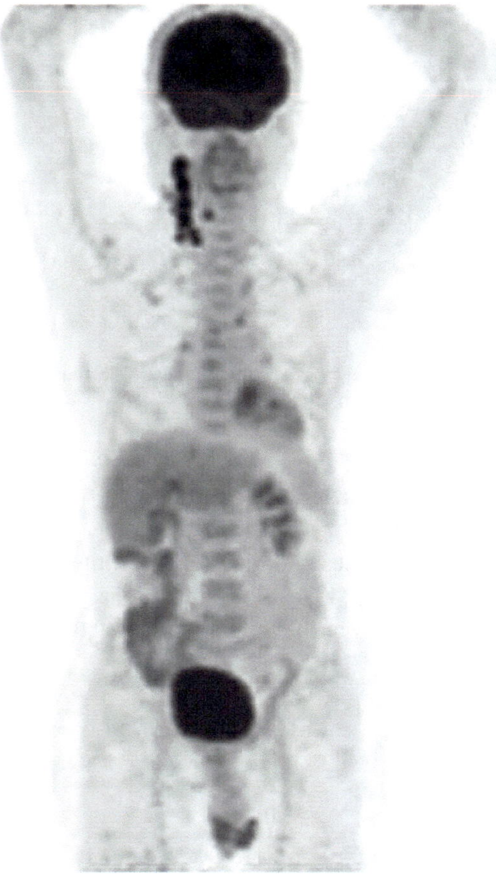

Fig. 10.13 PET MIP image of pyriform sinus carcinoma with lung adenocarcinoma. PET MIP image showed increased FDG uptake in piriform sinus carcinoma and intense FDG uptake in the right cervical metastatic lymph nodes, and the accompanied lung adenocarcinoma had no increased metabolic activity on the MIP image

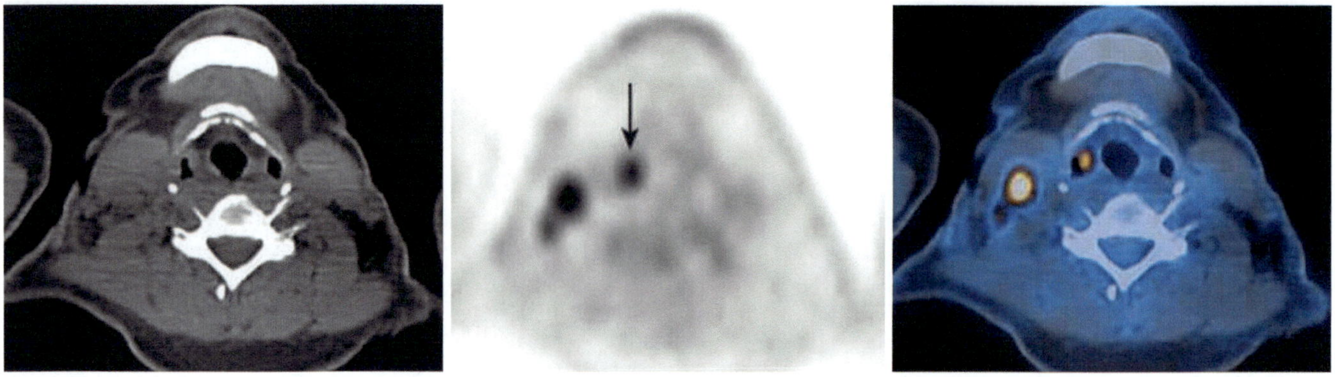

Fig. 10.14 PET/CT cross-sectional image of pyriform sinus squamous cell carcinoma. Increased FDG uptake in the soft tissue nodules of the right pyriform sinus (arrow); its SUVmax was 7.0, and its size was 0.6 cm × 0.8 cm, involving the right aryepiglottic fold

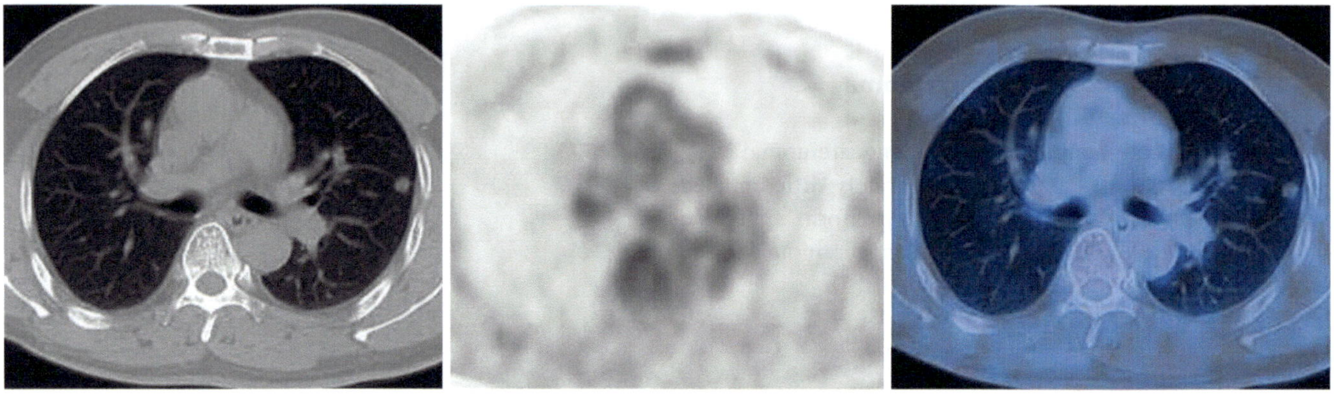

Fig. 10.15 PET/CT cross-sectional image of left lung adenocarcinoma. Normal FDG uptake in the soft tissue nodules in the upper left lung; its size was about 0.7 cm × 0.8 cm

1.4.3 Metastatic Carcinoma of the Laryngopharynx

Multiple metastases and recurrences in the laryngopharynx and whole body 4 years after nasopharyngeal carcinoma treatment: A 57-year-old female patient with multiple metastases and recurrences in the laryngopharynx and whole body 4 years after nasopharyngeal carcinoma treatment. Pathology: Metastatic nasopharyngeal carcinoma of the laryngopharynx and metastatic nasopharyngeal carcinoma of the liver (Figs. 10.16, 10.17, 10.18, and 10.19)

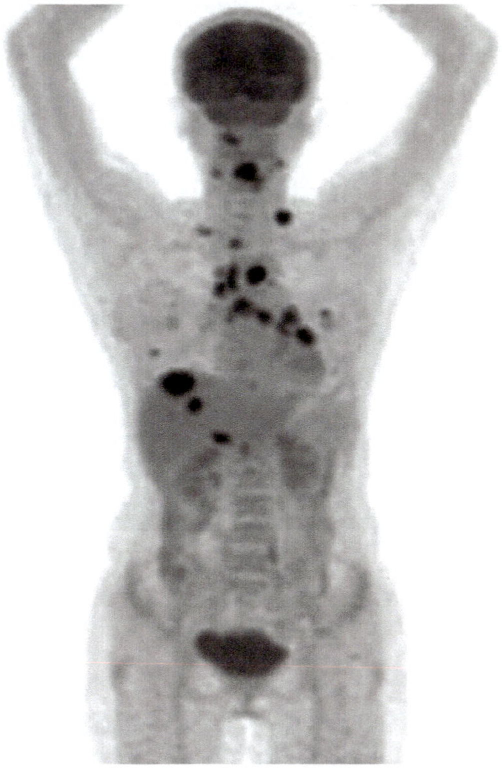

Fig. 10.16 PET MIP of multiple metastatic tumors such as laryngopharyngeal metastasis after treatment of nasopharyngeal carcinoma. The PET MIP image showed that the local lesions of nasopharyngeal carcinoma had been completely relieved and the metabolic activity had returned to normal. However, there were many metastases with significantly increased metabolic activity in the body, laryngopharyngeal metastasis, liver metastasis, and lymph node metastasis

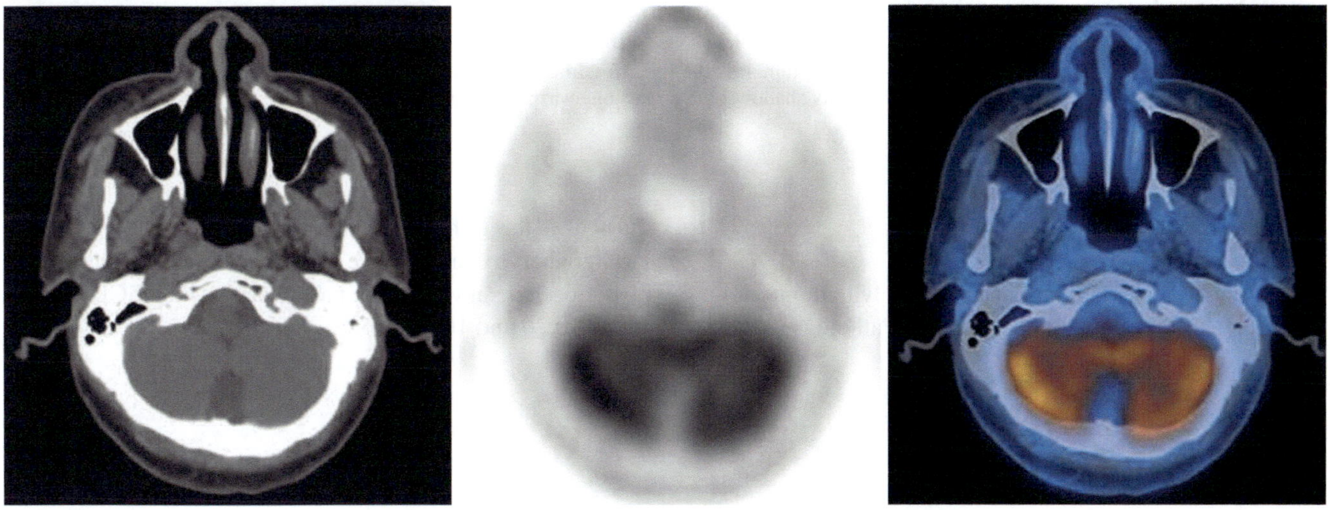

Fig. 10.17 PET/CT cross-sectional image of complete remission of the primary tumor after treatment of nasopharyngeal carcinoma. After nasopharyngeal treatment, the primary tumor of nasopharyngeal carcinoma had no obvious abnormalities

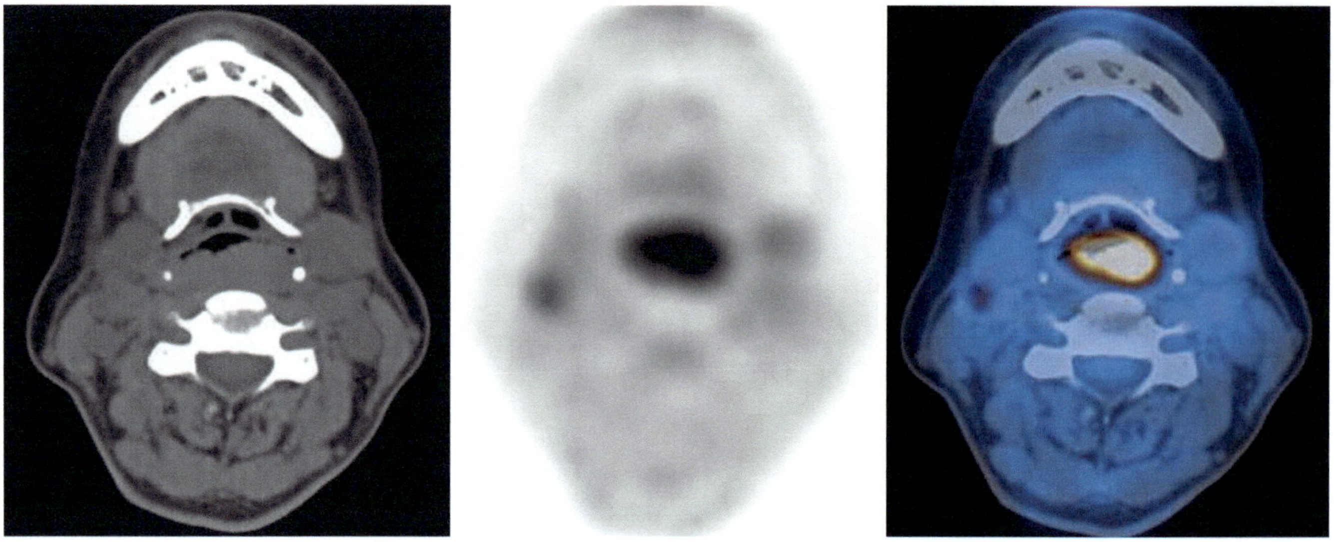

Fig. 10.18 PET/CT cross-sectional image of metastatic carcinoma of the laryngopharynx. It is the same patient's PET/CT image as Fig. 10.17. Increased FDG uptake (SUVmax 18) in the thickened posterior wall of the laryngopharynx. It invaded the bilateral pyriform sinus, bilateral arytenoepiglottic fold, left upper corner of the thyroid cartilage, and prevertebral space

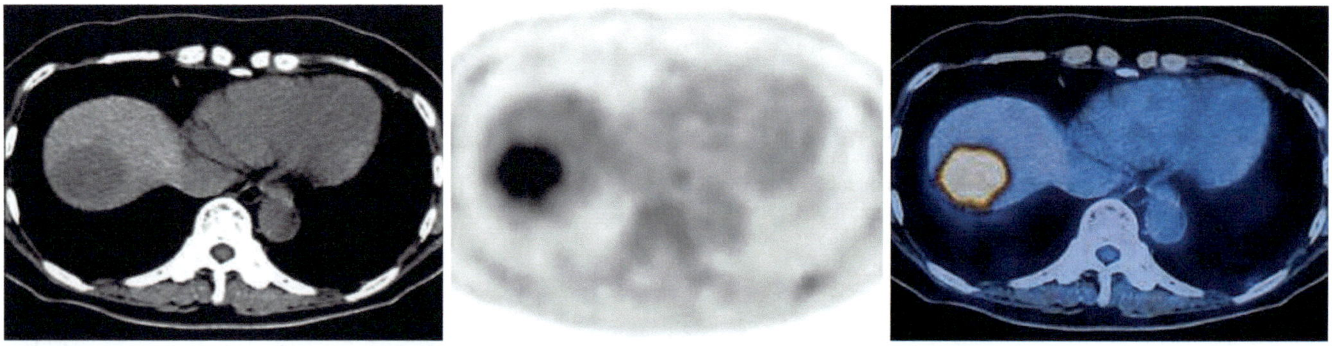

Fig. 10.19 PET/CT cross-sectional image of metastatic tumor of the liver. It is the same patient's PET/CT image as Fig. 10.17. Intense FDG uptake (SUVmax 20.5) in several round-like low-density shadows; the largest one was about 3.6 cm × 3.9 cm in size

1.5 Differential Diagnosis

Laryngopharyngeal diffuse large B-cell lymphoma among lymphomas: Male patient, 64 years old. Pathology: Mucosal mass near the right pyriform sinus on the right wall of the laryngopharynx and diffuse large B-cell lymphoma on the posterior parietal wall of the nasopharynx, non-GCB subtype (Figs. 10.20 and 10.21)

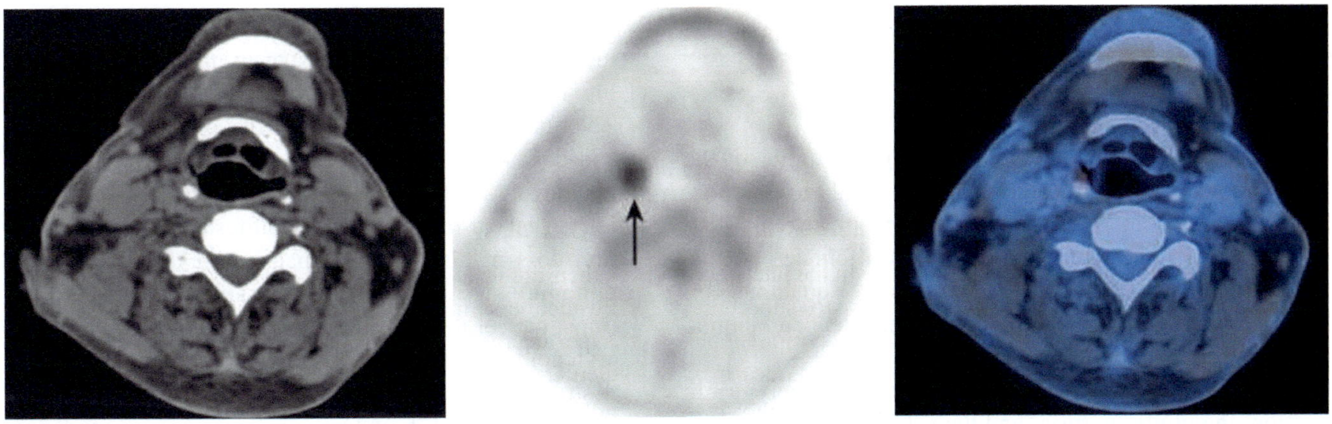

Fig. 10.20 PET/CT cross-sectional image of lymphoma of the right wall of the laryngopharynx. Increased FDG uptake in the slightly thickened mucosa of the right pyriform sinus; the SUVmax was 5.7

Fig. 10.21 PET/CT coronal image of head and neck lymphoma. The PET/CT image is of the same patient as Fig. 10.20. The mucosa of the upper wall, posterior parietal wall, and bilateral wall of the nasopharynx was thickened with FDG uptake increased (SUVmax 19). The lesion invaded the bilateral tensor veli palatini muscle, bilateral parapharyngeal space, right retropharyngeal space, right posterior portion of the middle turbinate, bilateral foramen lacerum, and skull base bone (basilar part of the sphenoid bone, basilar part of the bilateral pterygoid process, basilar part of the occipital bone, and bilateral petrous apex)

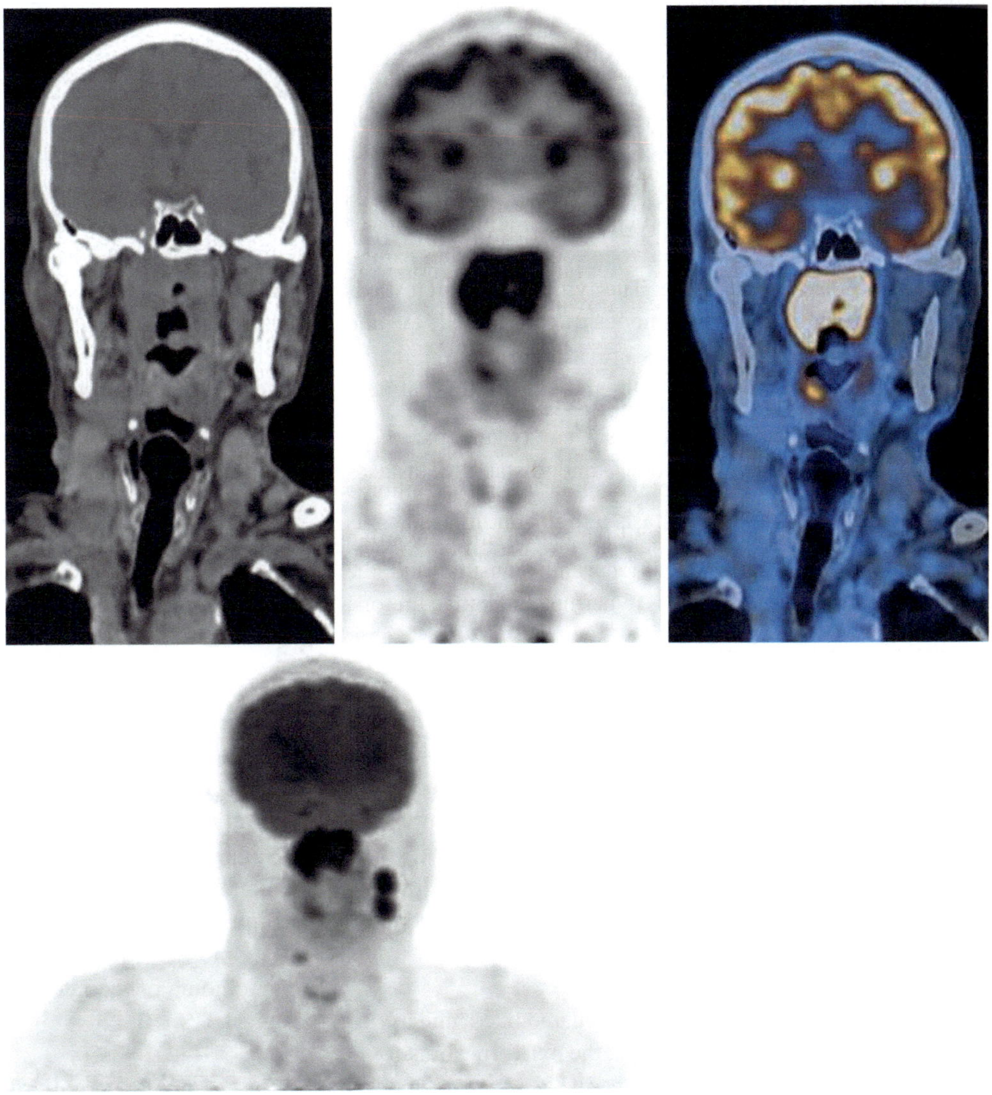

2 Laryngeal Carcinoma

2.1 Clinical Overview

Laryngeal carcinoma is a common malignant tumor of the head and neck, and its incidence is second only to nasopharyngeal carcinoma. It is common in people aged 50 to 69 years old, with more male patients than female patients. More than 90% of laryngeal carcinomas are squamous cell carcinoma, followed by carcinoma in situ, adenocarcinoma, and sarcoma.

The larynx is anatomically divided into the supraglottic portion, the glottic portion, and the subglottic portion. The supraglottic portion includes the lingual surface of the epiglottis, free edge of the epiglottis, laryngeal surface of the epiglottis, arytenoepiglottic fold of two sides, arytenoid cartilage area of two sides, ventricular cords of two sides, and laryngeal ventricle of two sides. The lymph node metastasis is more common in the lymph nodes of the cervical II area. The glottic portion includes vocal cords of two sides, the anterior commissure, and the posterior commissure. The tumor rarely metastasizes when it does not invade outside the glottis. The subglottic portion includes the area between the lower edge of the vocal cords and the caudal border of the cricoid cartilage. The lymph node metastasis is more common in the lymph nodes of cervical III, IV, and VI regions. Distant metastases are more common in the lungs, followed by the liver, bone, and skin. The treatment of laryngeal carcinoma is mainly surgery and radiotherapy.

The increased ^{18}F-FDG uptake in laryngeal carcinoma lesions and lymph node metastasis and distant metastasis is common. Decreased or defective FDG uptake in the necrotic part of tumor can be seen.

2.2 PET/CT Diagnostic Points

2.2.1 General Diagnostic Points

1. Have a clinical history, such as pharyngeal discomfort, hoarseness, dyspnea, etc.; bloody sputum may appear in the late stage.
2. Laryngopharyngeal space-occupying lesion.
3. It may be unilateral, bilateral, or annular involvement.

2.2.2 CT Diagnostic Points

1. Vocal cords are thickened, deformed and fixed, and asymmetrical. When the mass is large, the pyriform sinus fossa can be narrowed and blocked, and the airway can be deviated; when the arytenoepiglottic fold is invaded, it appears as local thickening, with asymmetrical sides.
2. The lesion can be localized or diffuse, and when it involves surrounding soft tissues, it may lead to thickening, interstitial turbidity, and density of soft tissues.
3. The tumor may forward involve the anterior commissure and downward invade the subglottis. In severe cases, it may involve the contralateral vocal cords.
4. Laryngeal cartilage invasion, manifested as bone destruction, loss of dissolution, expansion or displacement by tumor pressure, and calcified or ossified hyaline cartilage (most part of the thyroid cartilage, cricoid cartilage, and arytenoid cartilage) edge, is not smooth, indicating bone destruction; epiglottic cartilage is elastic cartilage, which is not visible on CT, and its invasion is not easy to judge.
5. The paralaryngeal structure is involved, and when the anterior horn of the cricothyroid membrane or thyroid cartilage is completely dissolved, the prelaryngeal soft tissue will be involved.

2.2.3 ^{18}F-FDG PET Diagnostic Points

1. The laryngeal lesions, metastatic lymph nodes, and distant metastases are hypermetabolic.
2. Due to partial volume effect, there is only slightly increased FDG uptake in small lesion.
3. In addition to the lesions on the surface of the laryngeal cavity, it can also show the submucosal and deep occult lesions.
4. Physiological increased FDG uptake on one side of the vocal cord may occur in patients with hoarseness (also manifested as vocal cord tension on CT), while symmetrically physiological increased FDG uptake at the retropharyngeal wall may also occur in crying children. It is better to know well the patient's status during examination before diagnosis.

2.3 Typical Cases

1. Glottic carcinoma: Male patient, 59 years old. Pathology: Moderately differentiated squamous cell carcinoma of the right vocal cord (Fig. 10.22)
2. Glottic carcinoma: Male patient, 64 years old. Pathology: Squamous cell carcinoma of the anterior edge of the bilateral vocal cords and anterior commissure (Fig. 10.23)
3. Supraglottic carcinoma: Male patient, 54 years old. Pathology: Moderately differentiated squamous cell carcinoma of the lateral wall of the left fold (Figs. 10.24 and 10.25)

The metabolic activity of the left supraglottic carcinoma and the left cervical metastatic lymph nodes was significantly increased.

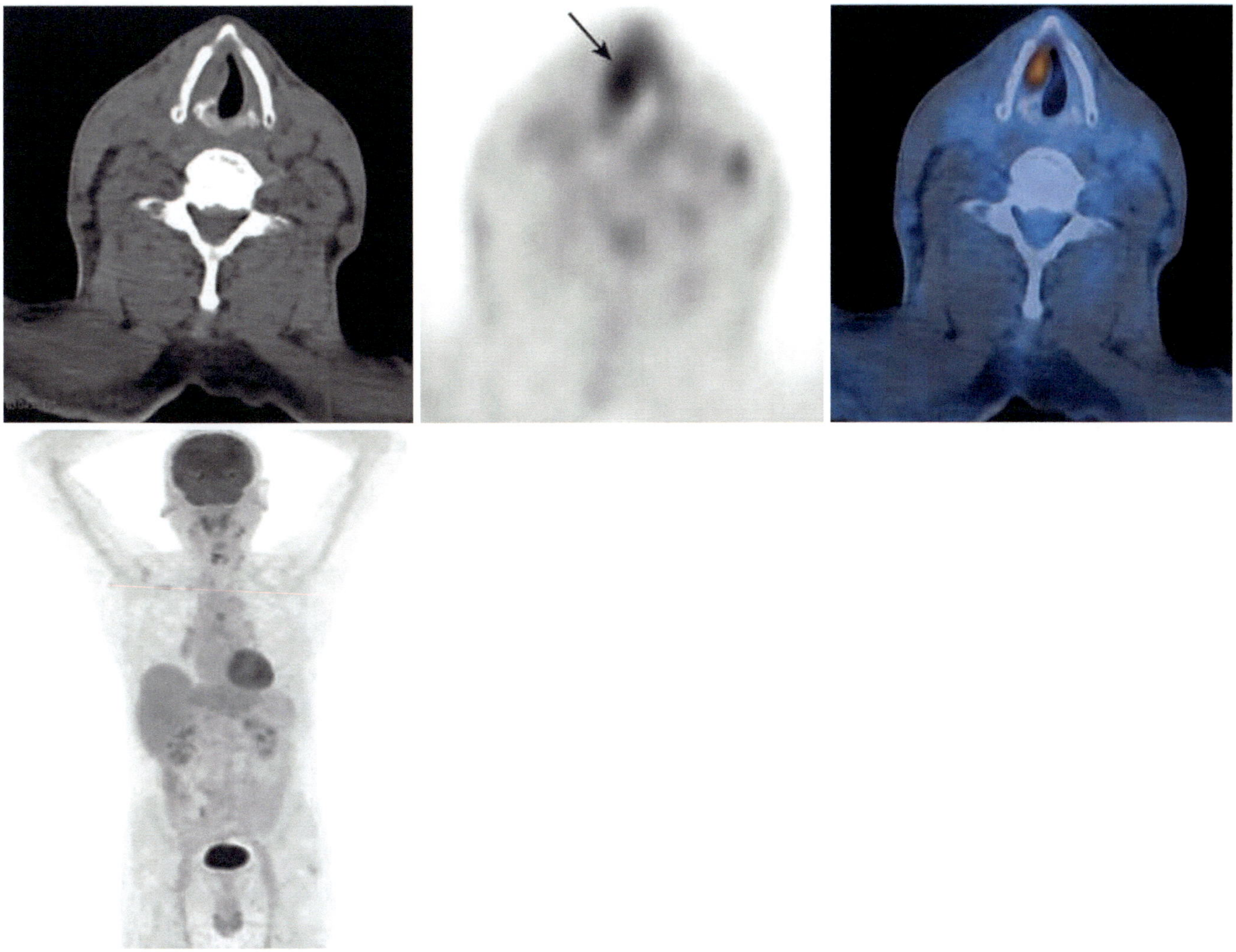

Fig. 10.22 PET/CT cross-sectional image and PET MIP image of glottic carcinoma. Increased FDG uptake in the nodule of the right vocal cord (arrow). The nodule's SUVmax was 8.0 cm, and size 0.6 cm × 1.1 cm. The lesion involved the anterior commissure and right part of the thyroid cartilage

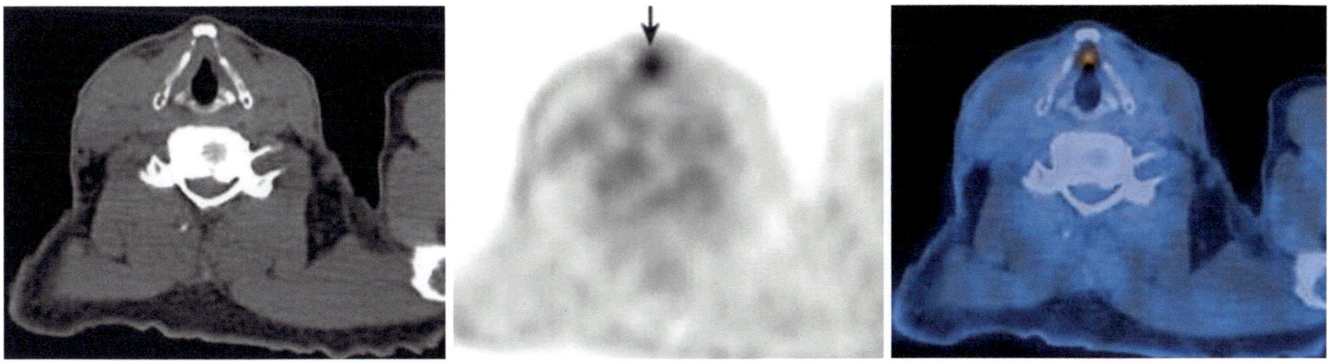

Fig. 10.23 PET/CT cross-sectional image of glottic carcinoma. Increased FDG uptake in the small nodules of soft tissue in the anterior edge of the bilateral vocal cords and the anterior commissure; its SUVmax was 6.0 and size 0.6 cm × 0.8 cm (arrow)

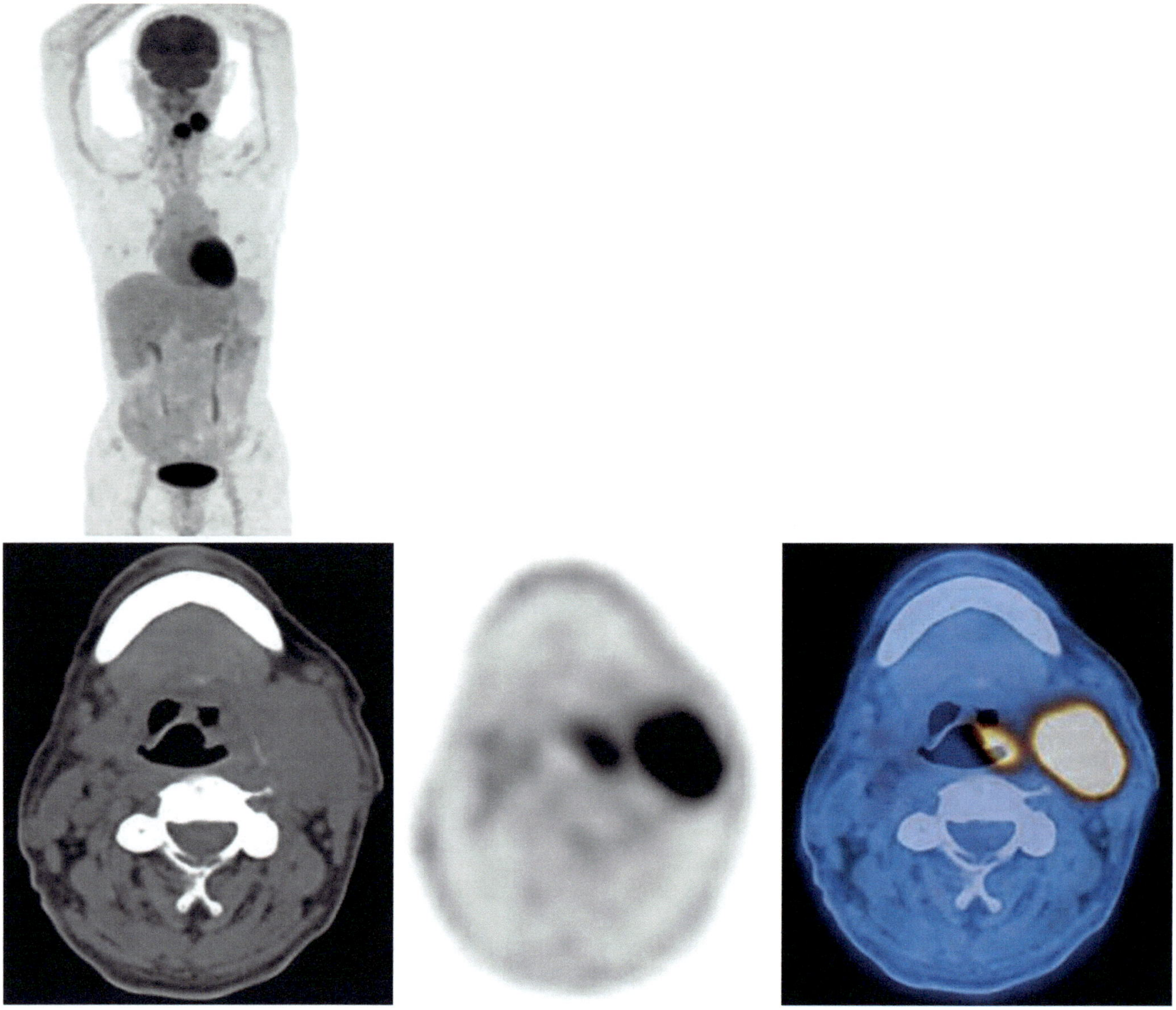

Fig. 10.24 PET MIP image of supraglottic carcinoma with cervical lymph node metastasis

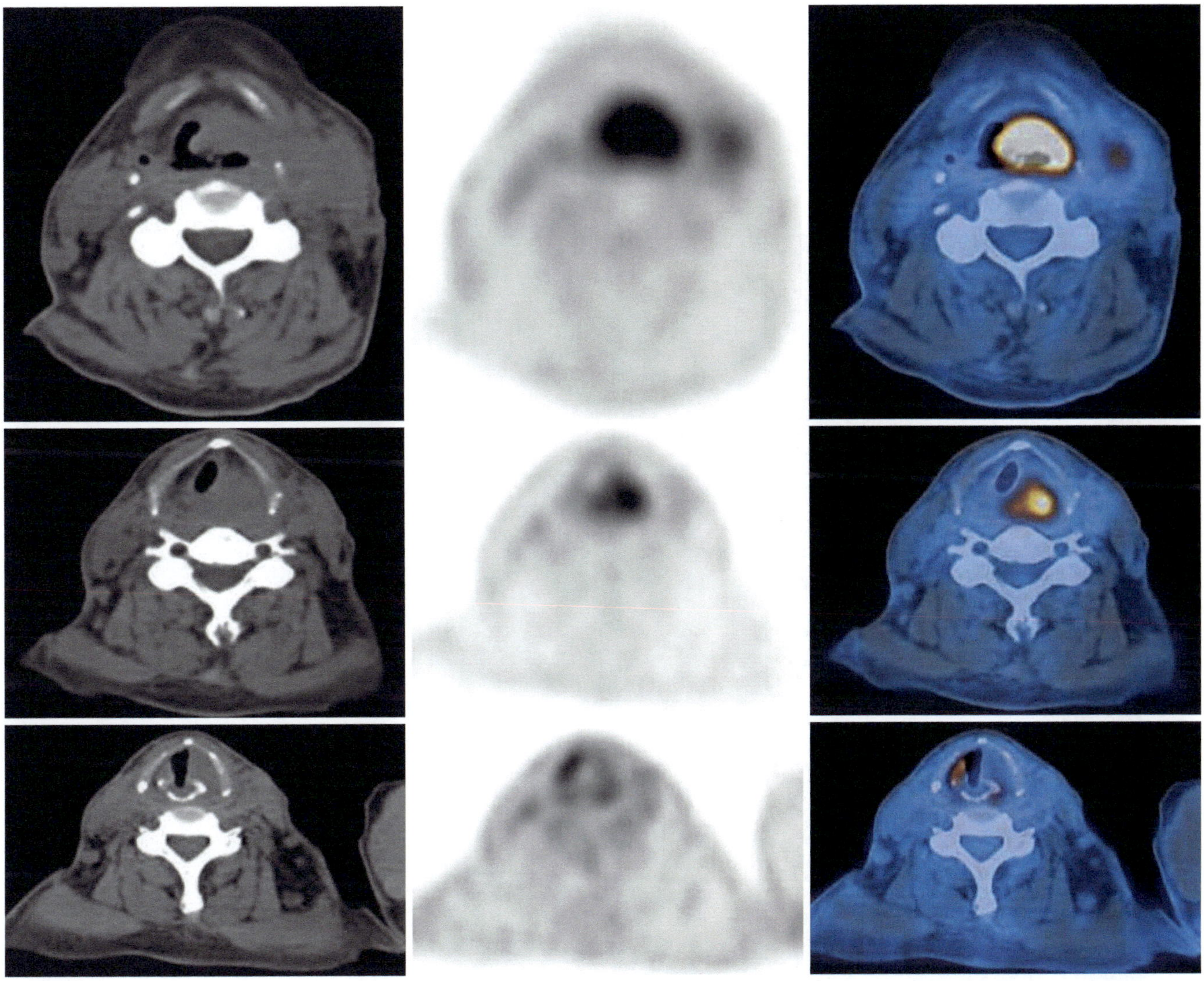

Fig. 10.25 PET/CT cross-sectional images of supraglottic carcinoma. Intense FDG uptake in the irregular soft tissue mass in the left supraglottic portion protruded into the laryngopharynx and the laryngeal vestibule; its SUVmax was 25.7 and size 2.5 cm × 2.7 cm. The lesion invaded the left portion of the epiglottis, the left laryngeal valley, the pre-epiglottic space, the left arytenoepiglottic fold, the left pyriform recess, and the left parapharyngeal space. The left vocal cord was loose and there was increased FDG uptake (SUVmax 7.1) in the right vocal cord. Intense FDG uptake in the enlarged lymph nodes in the left cervical II and III regions, with SUV22.9 and size 2.7 cm × 3.5 cm (Fig. 10.23)

2.4 Summary of This Chapter

Laryngopharyngeal carcinoma includes piriform sinus carcinoma, postcricoid carcinoma, and retropharyngeal wall carcinoma. Piriform sinus carcinoma is the most common, and postcricoid carcinoma is rare. Hypopharyngeal squamous cell carcinoma is less differentiated than laryngeal squamous cell carcinoma and has a poor prognosis. It is often accompanied by cervical lymph node metastasis, or bilateral lymph node metastasis can also occur. In the late stage, hematogenous metastasis is the most common, and lung, liver, and bone metastases are more common. Laryngopharyngeal cancer can be accompanied by multicenter tumors such as esophageal cancer. Laryngeal carcinoma is a common malignant tumor of the head and neck, its incidence is second only to nasopharyngeal carcinoma, and it is often accompanied by cervical lymph node metastasis; distant metastases are more common in the lungs, followed by the liver, bone, and skin. The typical manifestations of laryngopharyngeal carcinoma and laryngeal carcinoma are both significantly increased uptake of ^{18}F-FDG. Laryngopharyngeal carcinoma and laryngeal carcinoma need to be differentiated from diseases with significantly increased metabolic activity of the larynx, such as lymphoma.

^{18}F-FDG PET/CT can show the metabolic characteristics of laryngeal carcinoma cells and the distribution of systemic lesions based on the morphological changes of the lesions. It can identify the primary, recurrent, and residual lesions. It can provide comprehensive information for the staging of laryngeal carcinoma, help to detect the curative effect, and predict the prognosis.

PET/CT of Oral Malignant Tumors

11

Shan Zheng, Shaoming Chen, and Weibing Miao

1 Tongue Cancer

1.1 Clinical Overview

Tongue cancers are mostly squamous cell carcinomas, and lateral 1/3 of the tongue is the most common site of tongue cancers. Adenocarcinoma is rare, mostly in the root of the tongue. Sometimes, lymphoepithelial carcinoma and undifferentiated carcinoma can also occur in the root of the tongue. The cause of tongue cancer is still unclear. Most believe that the occurrence of tongue cancer is related to local trauma (residual root, crown, and sharp ridge), smoking, and drinking. Some environmental factors such as heat, chronic damage, ultraviolet rays, X-ray, and other radioactive substances may also be carcinogenic factors. Besides, neuropsychiatric factors, endocrine factors, immune status, and genetic factors are also related to the occurrence of tongue cancer. Tongue cancer is more common in men than women. The diagnosis of tongue cancer is not difficult. It mainly depends on pathological biopsy, which should be distinguished from traumatic ulcer and tuberculous ulcer. The treatment method is surgery-based comprehensive treatment. Generally, the primary lesion resection and cervical lymph node dissection are performed, with radiotherapy or chemotherapy before or after surgery. The 5-year survival rate of tongue cancer after comprehensive treatment is about 60%. Whether there is cervical lymph node metastasis is the most important factor affecting the prognosis.

S. Zheng · S. Chen · W. Miao (✉)
The First Affiliated Hospital of Fujian Medical University, Fuzhou, Fujian, China

1.2 PET/CT Diagnostic Points

Most of the tongue cancer lesions show uniform or inhomogeneous abnormal increased FDG uptake. The density and shape of the tongue can be abnormal: the lesion shows relatively uniform soft tissue density, which is similar to the tongue muscle and often difficult to distinguish from the normal tongue tissue. When the lesion is large, soft tissue mass shadow can be formed, and enhanced scanning can show different degrees of enhancement; morphological changes are manifested as asymmetric lingual margin, swelling of the affected side, and displacement of the lingual septum. Cervical metastatic lymph nodes are generally located on the affected side, but bilateral metastasis is also possible. The imaging findings are enlarged lymph nodes with inhomogeneous density reduction. Sometimes, they can fuse with each other, and their FDG uptake is significantly increased.

1.3 Typical Cases

1. Tongue cancer with lymph node metastasis in the cervical IIA area: A 71-year-old male patient with ulcer of the left ventral surface of the tongue with mass for more than 5 months. Pathology: Highly differentiated squamous cell carcinoma of the left tongue with lymph node metastasis in the left cervical IIA area (Fig. 11.1)
2. Tongue cancer with lymph node metastasis in the left cervical IB area: A 54-year-old male patient with left tongue ulcer for more than 4 months. Pathology: Moderately differentiated squamous cell carcinoma of the left tongue with lymph node metastasis in the left cervical region IB (Fig. 11.2)

Z. Yao, S. Li (eds.), *Atlas of PET/CT in Oncology - Volume 1*, https://doi.org/10.1007/978-981-99-1172-1_11

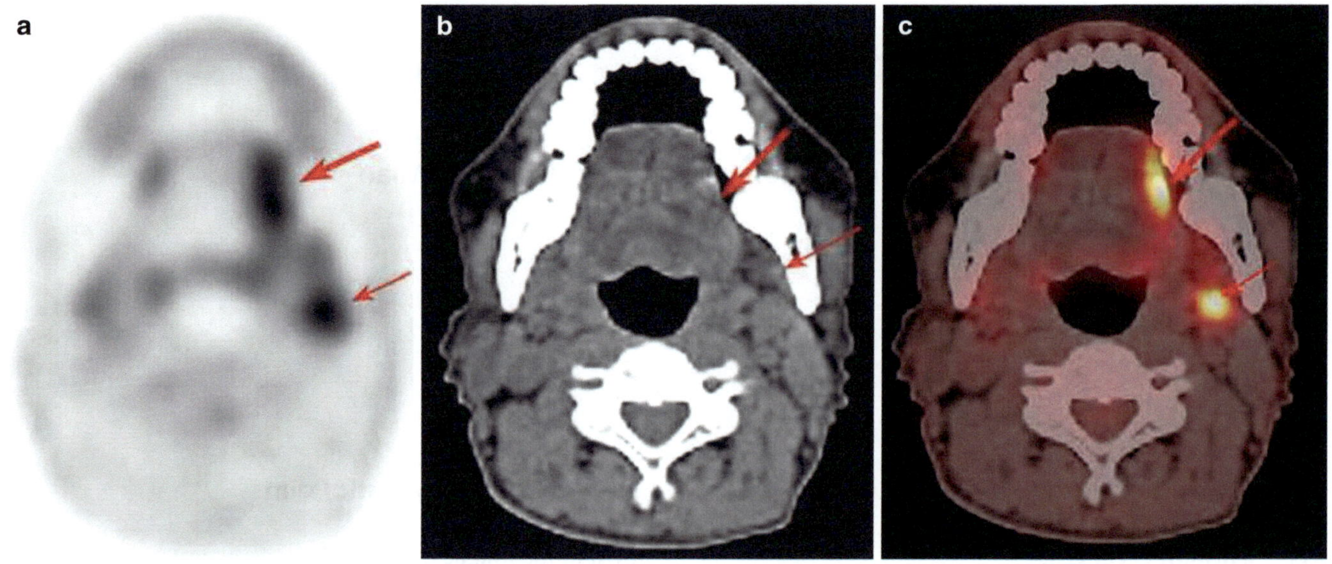

Fig. 11.1 FDG PET/CT images of tongue cancer with lymph node metastasis in the left cervical IIA area. PET/CT imaging showed a strip of abnormally hypermetabolic lesion on the left edge of the tongue; the size was about 2.6 cm × 1.4 cm × 1.5 cm. SUVmax was about 18.5; CT images showed slightly higher-density soft tissue shadows at the corresponding sites, with unclear boundary (thick arrows). Enlarged lymph nodes with abnormal hypermetabolism were found in the left cervical IIA area. The short diameter was about 1.1 cm and the SUVmax was 18.6 (thin arrow)

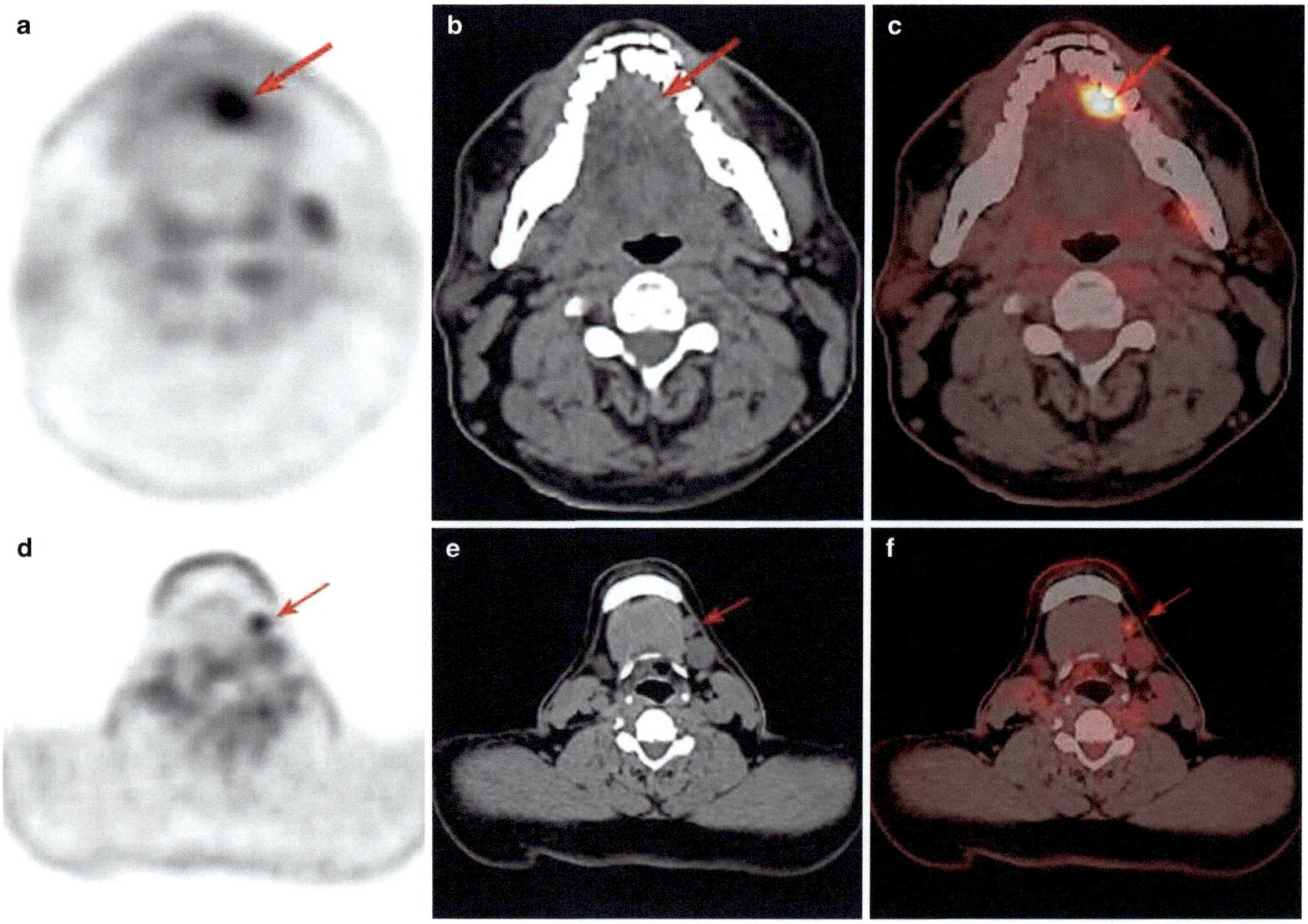

Fig. 11.2 FDG PET/CT images of tongue cancer with lymph node metastasis in the left cervical IB area. (**a–c**). PET/CT imaging showed an abnormal increased FDG uptake in lesion on the left front edge of the tongue, with a size 1.8 cm × 1.3 cm × 1.1 cm and SUVmax 5.1. The CT image showed iso-density and unclear boundary at the corresponding site. (**d–f**). Small lymph nodes with increased FDG uptake were observed in the left cervical IB area, with a short diameter of about 0.8 cm and SUVmax of 3.9

1.4 Differential Diagnosis

1. Papilloma Benign tumor, which usually occurs on the edge of tongue tip and rarely on the dorsum of the tongue and back of the tongue. They present as small papillae on the surface of the tongue, usually protruding, white in color with clear boundary. The imaging manifestations are soft tissue masses with clear edges and no base infiltration, and PET imaging shows low metabolism.
2. Mixed tumors Mostly benign tumors, but they can be transformed to be malignant or primary malignant. The tongue is shortened and deformed, movement is restricted, and the surface of the tongue mucosa is normal. The imaging manifestations are that the lesion is relatively localized, with light degree of enhancement on contrast CT and normal or slightly increased FDG uptake on PET, and most patients' cervical lymph nodes are not enlarged.
3. Inflammatory lesions No masses are formed, and the lesions are scattered with exudation.

1.5 Summary

Most of tongue cancer is squamous cell carcinoma, and the diagnosis mainly depends on biopsy pathology. PET/CT imaging shows that increased FDG uptake in most of the tongue cancer lesions is uniform or inhomogeneous; cervical metastatic lymph nodes are generally located on the affected side, but bilateral metastasis is possible, with abnormally increased FDG uptake.

2 Gingival Carcinoma

2.1 Clinical Overview

Gingival carcinoma is second only to tongue cancer in oral cancer. However, in recent years, it has shown a downward trend year by year. There are more male patients than female patients. Older age, smoking, drinking, hyperglycemia, low-income families, family history of tumor, eating habits, oral disease history, HPV infection, and so on are the risk factors of gingival carcinoma. Gingival carcinoma is mostly highly differentiated squamous cell carcinoma, which is clinically ulcerative or exophytic. Among them, ulcerative type is more common. The diagnosis of gingival carcinoma is not difficult, and it mainly depends on pathological biopsy. Early gingival carcinoma needs to be differentiated from gingivitis, periodontitis, and gingival tuberculosis, while in the late stage, it should be differentiated from primary maxillary sinus carcinoma and mandibular primary malignant tumor. Since gingival carcinoma often invades the bone in the early stage, the treatment is mainly surgical operation, and radiotherapy and chemotherapy are the auxiliary or palliative means of comprehensive treatment. The 5-year survival rate of gingival carcinoma after comprehensive treatment is high, more than 60%. The prognosis of lower gingival carcinoma is better than that of upper gingival carcinoma.

2.2 PET/CT Diagnostic Points

Gingival carcinoma usually occurs in the lower gingiva. The lesion with abnormally increased FDG uptake can be observed in the gingival area. Soft tissue-occupying lesion can be observed in the corresponding site. It often invades the alveolar bone and adjacent jaw bone, with osteolytic bone destruction and rough edges. Mandibular gingival carcinoma often metastasizes to the submandibular and submental lymph nodes of the affected side and then to the deep cervical lymph nodes, while the maxillary gingival carcinoma often metastasized to the submaxillary and deep cervical lymph nodes of the affected side, showing enlarged lymph nodes with high metabolism and uniform or inhomogeneous density, and some of them could fuse with each other.

2.3 Typical Cases

Right mandibular gingival carcinoma with lymph node metastasis in the cervical I area: A 73-year-old female patient with a mass and numbness in the right mandibular gingiva for 2 months. Pathology: Highly to moderately differentiated squamous cell carcinoma of the right lower gingiva with multiple lymph node metastasis in the left cervical IB area (Fig. 11.3)

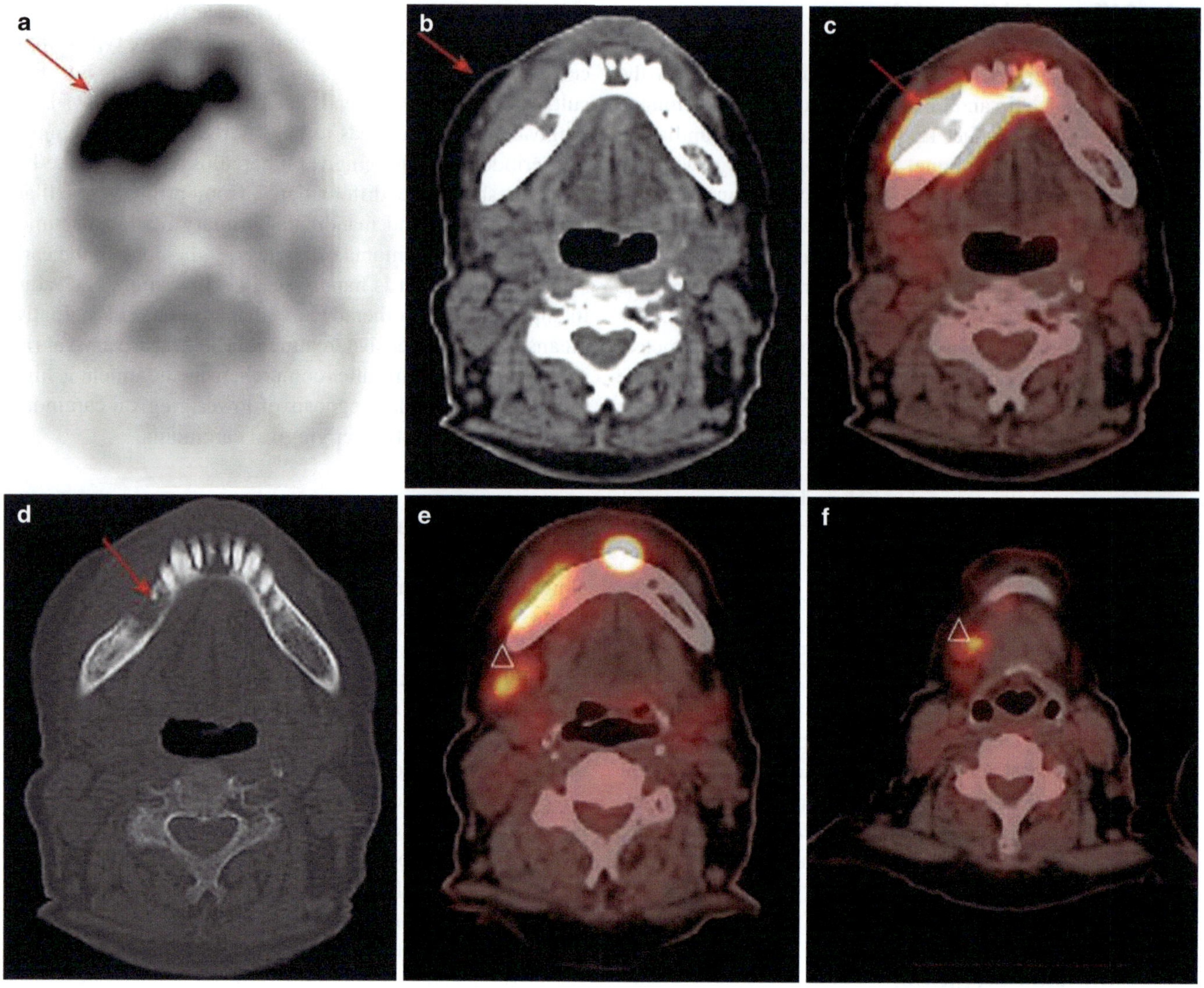

Fig. 11.3 FDG PET/CT images of right mandibular gingival carcinoma with lymph node metastasis in the cervical I area. (**a–d**) PET/CT imaging showed intense FDG uptake in the right lower-mid gingiva, with size 6.5 cm × 3.1 cm × 2.5 cm and SUVmax 21.1. A soft tissue mass was observed in the corresponding site, with unclear boundary and bone absorption and destruction adjacent to the mandible (arrow). (**e**, **f**) There were multiple abnormal lymph nodes with increased FDG uptake in the right cervical I area. The larger one had a short diameter of 1.2 cm and SUVmax 8.6 (Δ)

2.4 Differential Diagnosis

Gingival carcinoma needs to be differentiated from benign gingival lesions.

Benign lesions mainly manifested as a slight thickening of the ipsilateral gingiva, no invasion of adjacent soft tissue and bone, and no lymph node metastasis. PET/CT imaging generally shows low metabolism in lesion. Although some benign lesions show high metabolism in early stage, they can be distinguished from gingival carcinoma by delayed PET imaging. The degree of hypermetabolism in benign lesions will be unchanged or decreased on delay PET imaging than that on early PET imaging, while the hypermetabolic degree in gingival carcinoma lesions usually will be further increased on delay PET imaging.

2.5 Summary

Gingival carcinoma mostly occurs in the lower gingiva, mainly squamous cell carcinoma, and more men than women. PET/CT imaging shows the lesion has abnormal hypermetabolism, and soft tissue occupies in the corresponding site of the gingiva. It often invades the alveolar bone and adjacent jaw bone, with osteolytic bone destruction and rough edges.

3 Carcinoma of Mouth Floor

3.1 Clinical Overview

Mouth floor carcinoma refers to squamous cell carcinoma that occurs in the mucosa of the mouth floor. In Western countries, mouth floor carcinoma is very common, second only to tongue cancer. In China, it ranks at the bottom of oral cancer. Mouth floor carcinoma usually occurs at the age of 40–60, mostly in men. The cause may be related to smoking and drinking. Mouth floor carcinoma is common in the anterior floor of the mouth on both sides of the tongue frenulum, and ulcers or masses may appear locally. Due to the small area of the mouth floor, it is easy to invade the tongue frenulum to the opposite side and forward invade the gingiva and mandible. The cervical lymph node metastasis is very likely to occur in the mouth floor carcinoma, which is reported in the literature to account for 40%–70%. Early-stage mouth floor carcinoma needs to be differentiated from ulcerative diseases, and invasive mouth floor carcinoma needs to be differentiated from sublingual adenocarcinoma, and pathological biopsy should be used for diagnosis. Surgery is the main treatment, and the patient with advanced cancer is treated with preoperative chemotherapy, surgery, and postoperative radiotherapy. The 5-year survival rate of mouth floor carcinoma is lower than that of tongue cancer, about 50% on average, and the prognosis of the advanced stage is worse.

3.2 PET/CT Diagnostic Points

It commonly occurs in the anterior mouth floor on both sides of the tongue frenulum. The soft tissue mass of the mouth floor can be observed, with high metabolism, uniform density, and irregular edge. It can invade the mandible. Late-stage lesion can deep invade the muscles of the mouth floor and invade the mandible. It is often accompanied by cervical lymph node metastasis, especially the anterior mouth floor carcinoma close to the midline that is prone to have bilateral cervical lymph node metastasis, it is most likely to invade the submental and submandibular lymph nodes, and in the late stage, it mostly metastasizes to the deep upper cervical lymph nodes.

3.3 Typical Cases

Mouth floor squamous cell carcinoma: Male patient, 54 years old. A mass on the left mouth floor was found for more than 1 month. Pathology: Highly to moderately differentiated squamous cell carcinoma of the left mouth floor (Fig. 11.4)

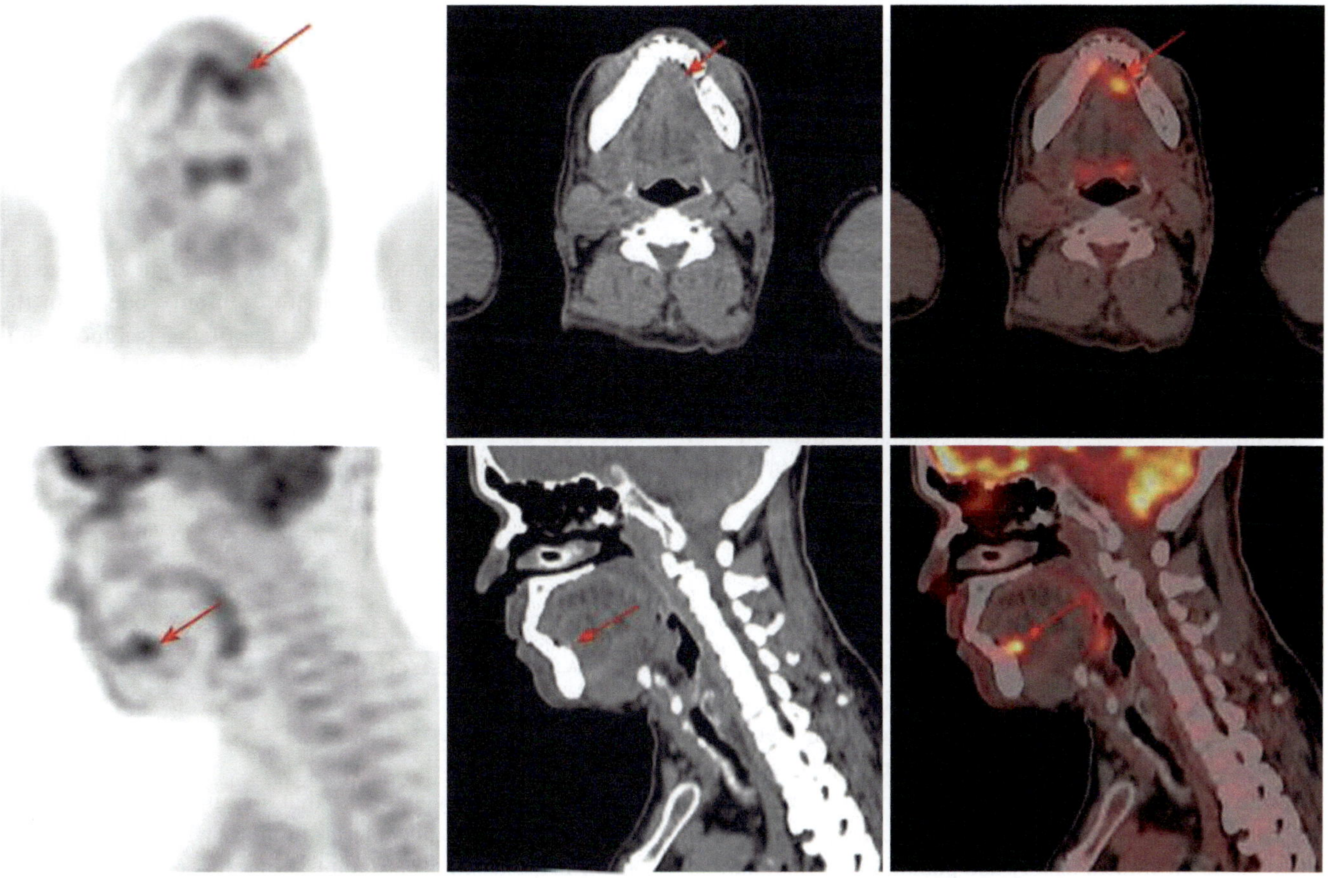

Fig. 11.4 FDG PET/CT images of mouth floor squamous cell carcinoma. PET/CT showed abnormally increased FDG uptake in the left mouth floor, with the size of 2.1 cm × 0.9 cm × 0.6 cm and SUVmax of 6.9. A shadow of iso-density was seen in the corresponding site with unclear boundary. No metastasis was observed in other parts

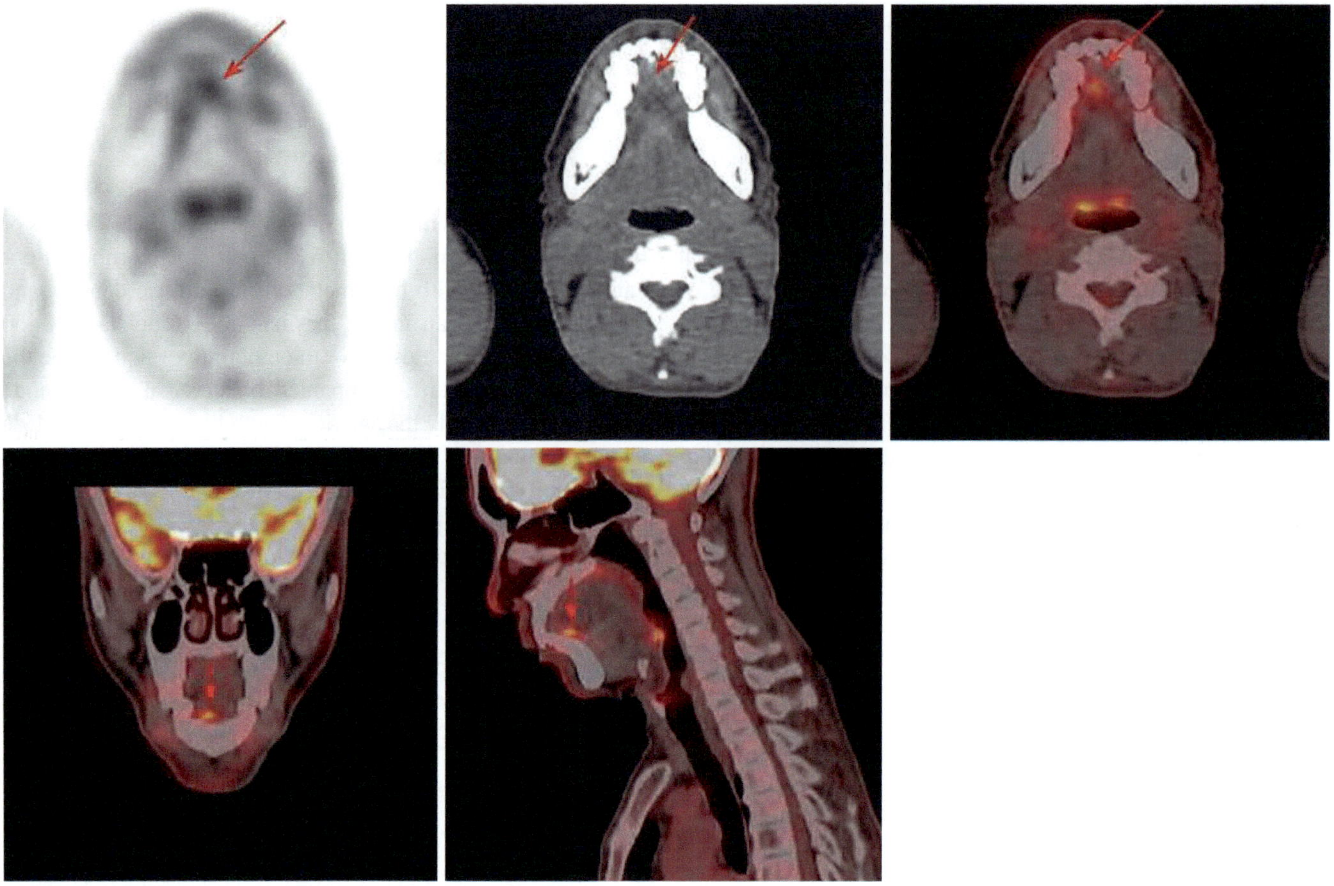

Fig. 11.5 FDG PET/CT images of mouth floor carcinoma. PET/CT imaging showed increased FDG uptake in a small nodular in the middle of the mouth floor, with a diameter of about 1.0 cm and SUVmax of 4.6; the CT image was not able to show the soft tissue lesion at the corresponding site

3.4 Atypical Cases

Some mouth floor carcinomas are easy to be missed due to their small size and proximity to the sublingual gland, so it is necessary to be carefully identified.

Mouth floor carcinoma: A 58-year-old male patient with ulceration of the mouth floor remaining for more than 4 months. Pathology: Highly differentiated squamous cell carcinoma of the mouth floor, with no metastasis to the cervical lymph nodes (Fig. 11.5)

3.5 Differential Diagnosis

Mouth floor carcinoma needs to be differentiated from traumatic ulcers and diffuse floor inflammation. Invasive mouth floor carcinoma needs to be differentiated from sublingual adenocarcinoma. Most of the mucosa of the latter is intact in the early stage, and the vascular dilatation of the mucosa can be seen in the late stage, but ulcer rarely occurs. It can be identified based on clinical history and pathological examination.

3.6 Summary

Mouth floor carcinoma usually occurs at the age of 40–60 years, mostly in men. It commonly occurs in the anterior mouth floor on both sides of the tongue frenulum. Increased FDG uptake, uniform density, and irregular edge in the soft tissue mass of the mouth floor can be observed on PET/CT. It can invade the mandible. Some mouth floor carcinomas are easy to be missed on PET imaging due to their small size and proximity to the sublingual gland, so it is necessary to be carefully identified.

4 Buccal Carcinoma

4.1 Clinical Overview

Traditionally, only cancers that originate in the buccal mucosa are called buccal carcinomas, while those of skin origin are classified as facial skin cancers. Buccal carcinoma is also one of the common oral cancers, ranking the second or third in China; in South Asia, especially in southern India, it accounts for more than 50% of oral cancer; in Europe and America, it only accounts for 2%–10%. The buccal carcinoma mostly occurs at the age of 50–59 years old, mostly in men. Most are squamous cell carcinoma, and a few are adenocarcinoma and malignant pleomorphic adenoma. The cause and pathogenesis of buccal carcinoma are not fully clear. People frequently chewing areca nut have a higher incidence than the general population. Buccal carcinoma often occurs near the molar area, which is ulcerative or exophytic. It grows fast and infiltrates deep, passing through the buccal muscles and skin. It can ulcerate and spread to the upper and lower gingiva and jaw. Clinically, patients with buccal carcinoma often have obvious precancerous lesions, among which the most common are oral leukoplakia and oral submucosal fibrosis. The diagnosis of buccal carcinoma is not difficult, mainly depending on biopsy. Surgery-based comprehensive treatment is usually adopted. The 5-year survival rate is more than 50%. Patients with distant metastasis have a poor prognosis.

4.2 PET/CT Diagnostic Points

PET imaging shows abnormally high metabolic lesion in the buccal mucosa, most common in the posterior part of the upper and lower teeth; CT images generally show local soft tissue thickening, which can protrude into the mouth to form soft tissue mass with the development of the disease, invading the buccal muscles and masticatory muscles. Advanced tumor can penetrate the buccal skin, form a sinus, and invade the upper and lower gingiva and jawbone. In terms of metastatic lymph nodes, the submandibular lymph nodes are most involved, with high metabolism and enlarged lymph nodes. PET/CT imaging helps to understand the extent of lesion involvement, find distant metastatic lesions, and assist in the development of treatment plan and prognosis assessment.

4.3 Typical Cases

Right buccal carcinoma: A 76-year-old female patient with a right buccal ulcer for more than 3 months. Pathology: Moderately differentiated squamous cell carcinoma of the right cheek (Fig. 11.6)

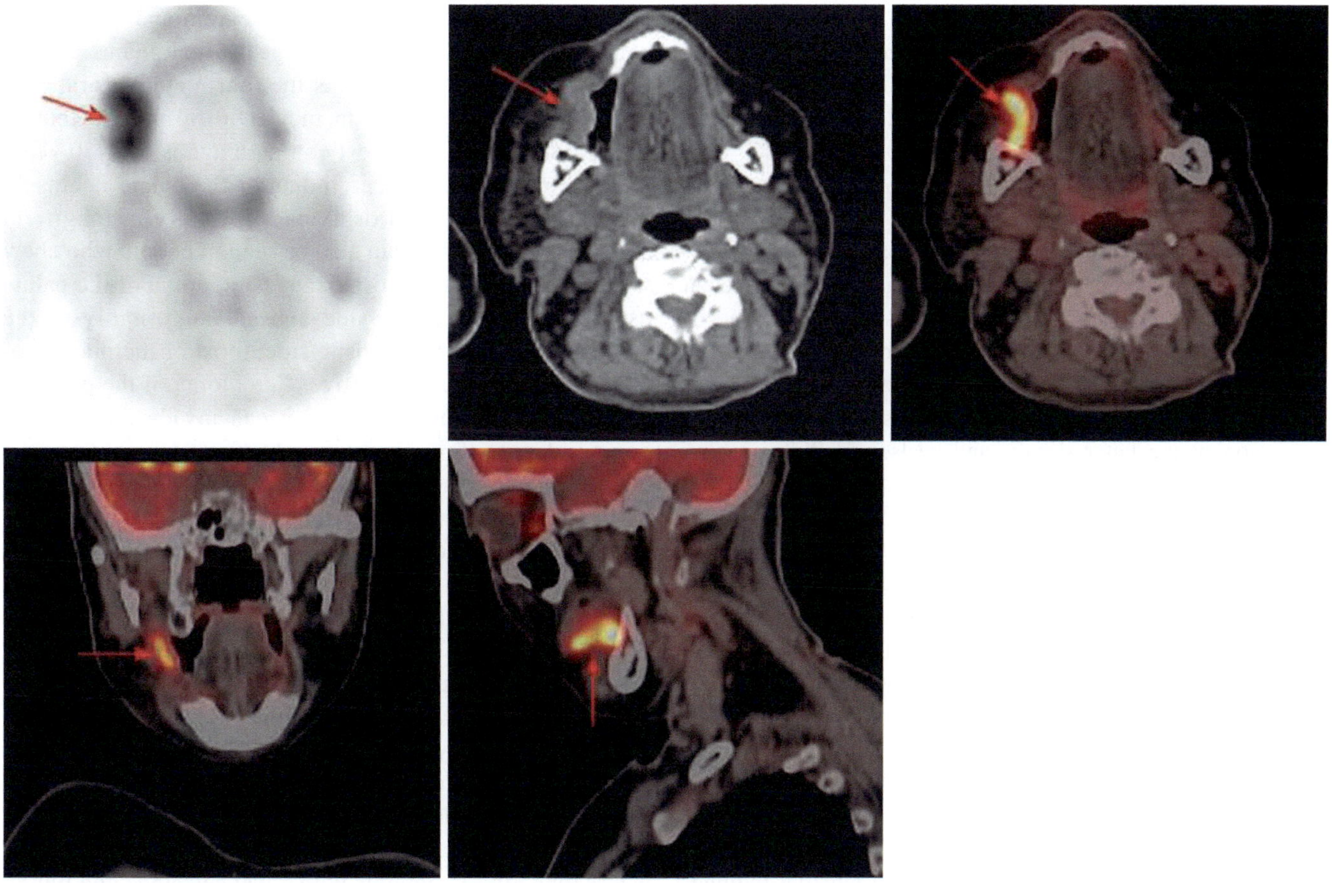

Fig. 11.6 FDG PET/CT images of right buccal carcinoma. PET/CT showed intense FDG uptake in an irregular lesion in the right buccal region, with size 3.0 cm × 1.6 cm × 3.2 cm and SUVmax 15.4, and the soft tissue was thickened at the corresponding site

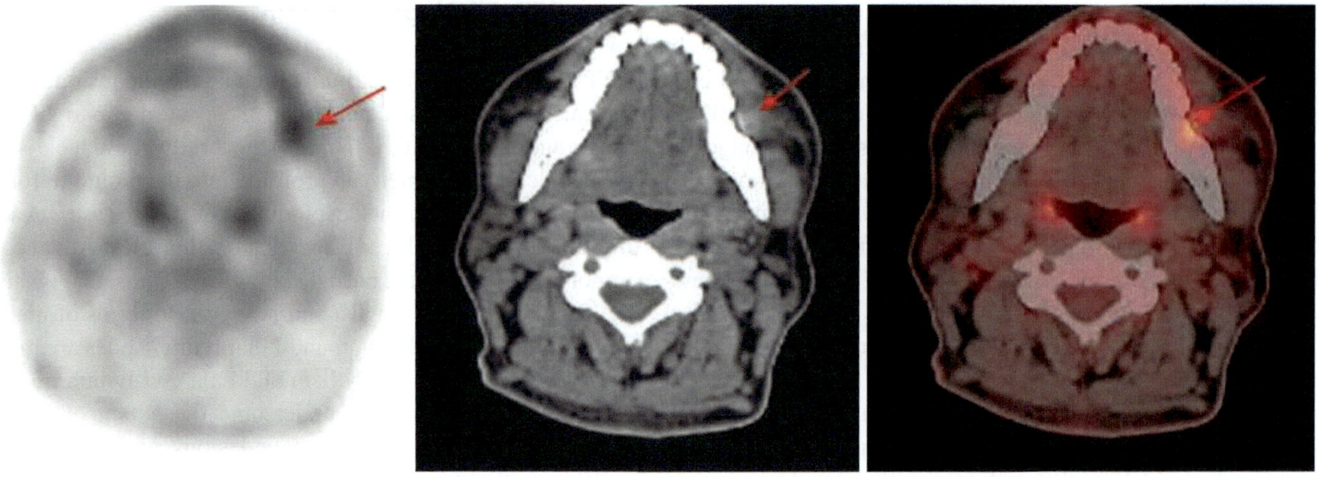

Fig. 11.7 FDG PET/CT images of left buccal carcinoma. PET/CT imaging showed increased FDG uptake in the left cheek, with unclear boundary, size 1.4 cm × 1.0 cm, and SUVmax 4.8. CT scan showed the soft tissue at the corresponding site was slightly swollen and the adjacent alveolar bone was not absorbed and destroyed

4.4 Atypical Cases

Some buccal carcinomas may be unclear when the lesions are small, so they need to be carefully identified.

Left buccal carcinoma: A 61-year-old male patient with left buccal ulcer and mass for more than 1 year. Pathology: Highly differentiated squamous cell carcinoma of the left cheek (Fig. 11.7)

4.5 Differential Diagnosis

The erosive ulcer of early buccal mucosa cancer should be differentiated from premalignant lesions such as oral leukoplakia and erosive lichen planus. Biopsy can assist in early diagnosis. It should also be differentiated from chronic mucosal ulcer, especially traumatic ulcer caused by chronic stimulation such as residual crown and residual root. After the stimulus is removed, the lesion of the latter shrinks and heals, and PET imaging shows that the degree of FDG metabolism also decreases.

4.6 Summary

Buccal carcinoma is mainly squamous cell carcinoma, which often occurs near the molar area and may have obvious precancerous lesions or precancerous conditions. PET imaging shows abnormally hypermetabolic lesion in the buccal mucosa, most common in the posterior part of the upper and lower teeth; soft tissue at the corresponding site is thickened, which can protrude into the mouth to form soft tissue mass; PET/CT imaging can also help to evaluate whether the buccal and masticatory muscles are invaded.

5 Carcinoma of the Palate

5.1 Clinical Overview

Carcinoma of the palate mainly refers to squamous cell carcinoma of the hard palate, and carcinoma of the soft palate belongs to oropharyngeal malignant tumor. Carcinoma of the palate ranks the fourth among oral cancers. It is more common in men, with a male-to-female ratio of about 3:2. The most common age is over 50 years old. The occurrence of carcinoma of the palate is closely related to smoking and drinking, especially in long-term and heavy smokers; it can also be seen in people who chew tobacco and add other stimulants. Carcinoma of the palate usually starts from one side and spreads rapidly to the alveolar side and the opposite side; most of them are exophytic and a few are ulcerative. Carcinoma of the palate is likely to invade the bone, and it can invade the palatine bone and pass through the nasal cavity or penetrate the maxilla to enter the maxillary sinus. In the late stage, the soft palate, palatal gingiva, and alveolar process could be affected. Lymph node metastasis mainly involves the submandibular lymph nodes and deep upper cervical lymph nodes, and contralateral lymph node metastasis can occur in the late stage. The diagnosis of palate carcinoma is not difficult, and the pathological diagnosis can be obtained directly by biopsy. Carcinoma of the palate needs to be differentiated from syphilis and nasal NK/T-cell lymphoma. Surgery is the main treatment for carcinoma of the palate. The effect of radiotherapy is often unsatisfactory. The 5-year survival rate is about 60%. The 5-year survival rate is less than 30% in patients with advanced stage and lymph node metastasis.

5.2 PET/CT Diagnostic Points

FDG uptake is mild in the normal palate, which is evenly distributed and symmetrical on the left and right sides. Squamous cell carcinoma of the palate shows increased focal FDG uptake, with localized protrusion of the soft tissue or enlargement of the soft palate and irregular surface, and in some patients, destruction of the hard palate or alveolar bone can occur. Carcinoma of the palate may have early lymph node metastasis, which is manifested as increased metabolism in enlarged lymph nodes. It mainly invades the submandibular lymph nodes and the deep upper cervical lymph nodes and sometimes may involve the retropharyngeal lymph nodes.

5.3 Typical Cases

Carcinoma of the hard palate: A 70-year-old male patient with a mass on his right upper palate found for 3 years. Pathology: Moderately differentiated squamous cell carcinoma of the right upper palate and benign lymph nodes in the right cervical II area (Fig. 11.8)

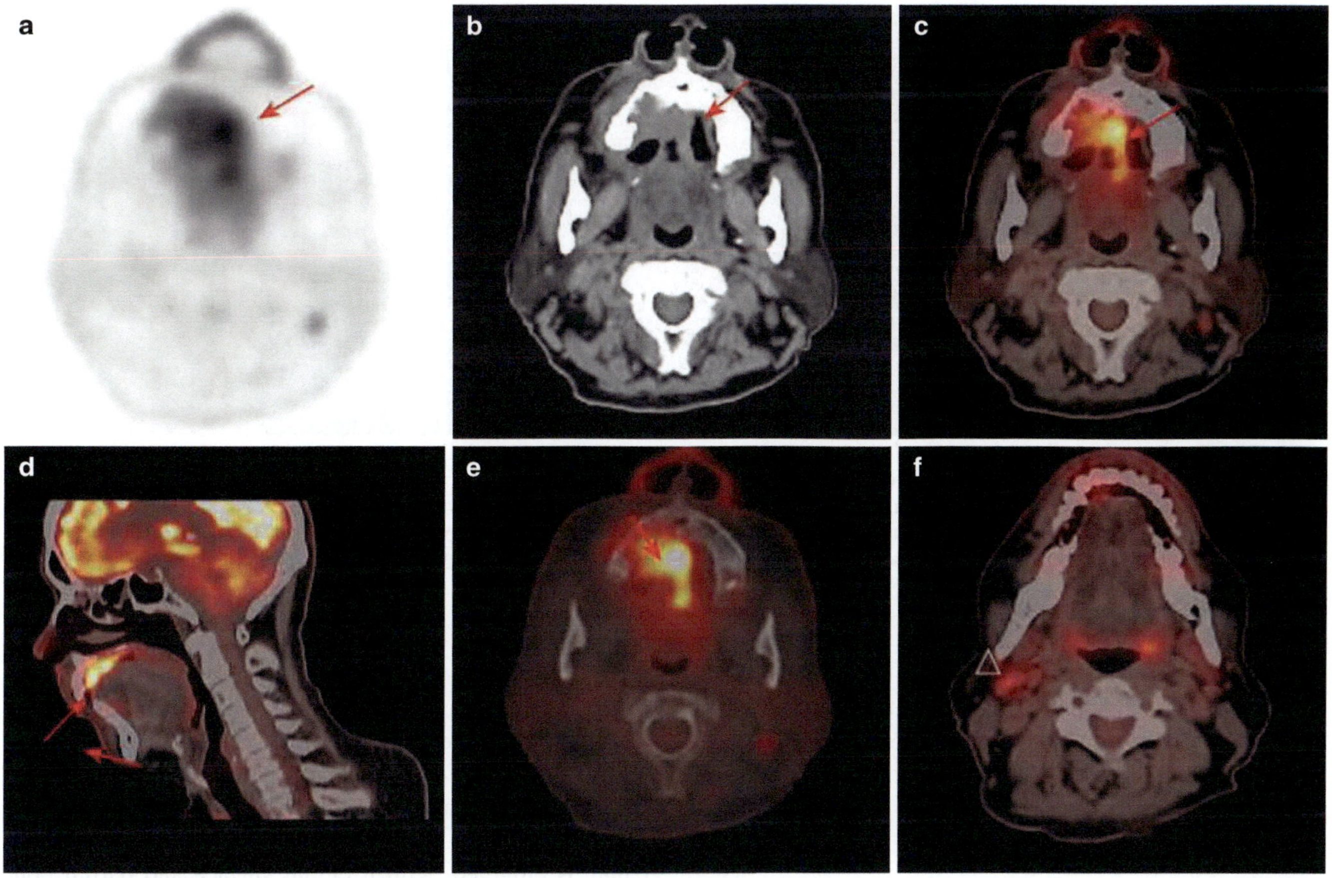

Fig. 11.8 FDG PET/CT images of carcinoma of the hard palate. (**a–d**) PET/CT imaging showed intense FDG uptake (SUVmax 15.4) in an irregular abnormal lesion (arrow) on the right upper hard palate, invading the maxilla and right cheek, with a range of about 5.5 cm × 4.3 cm × 2.3 cm. (**e**) Local bone destruction of the maxilla (arrow). (**f**) A prolate lymph node with increased metabolism in the right cervical II area with a short diameter of about 0.6 cm and SUVmax of 6.5 (Δ)

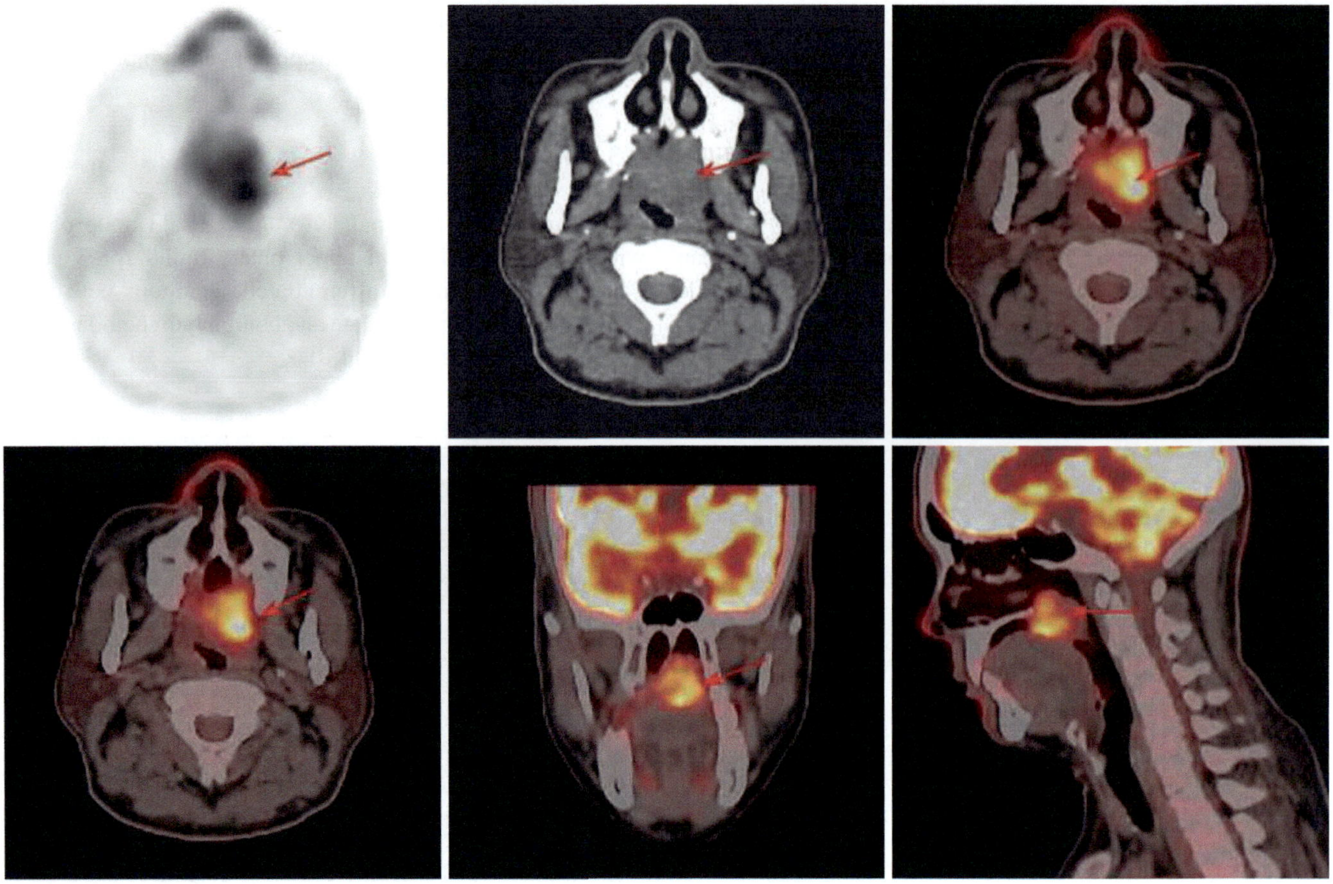

Fig. 11.9 FDG PET/CT images of moderately differentiated mucoepidermoid carcinoma of the palate. PET/CT imaging showed abnormal hypermetabolism in the mass on the left side of the palate, involving the left posterior nostril, the left side wall of the nasopharynx, and the right palate, with a range of about 3.2 cm × 2.9 cm × 3.5 cm and SUVmax of 9.0; CT images showed an irregular soft tissue mass at the corresponding site; the nasopharyngeal cavity was narrowed. The left pharyngeal recess and the opening of Eustachian tube disappeared

5.4 Rare Cases

Rare malignant epithelial tumors and mucoepidermoid carcinoma of the palate. Moderately differentiated mucoepidermoid carcinoma of the palate: A 48-year-old male patient with a palatal mass found for half a year (Fig. 11.9)

5.5 Differential Diagnosis

Carcinoma of the palate needs to be differentiated from mixed palate tumors. The latter mostly are benign, but can transform to be malignant; its lesion is relatively localized and regular, with uniform density, normal local mucosa, and normal FDG uptake. There are neat edges when the palatine bone is compressed by mixed palate tumors. There are no cervical enlarged lymph nodes with significantly increased FDG uptake in most patients with mixed palate tumors.

5.6 Summary

Carcinoma of the palate mainly refers to squamous cell carcinoma of the hard palate, which is more common in men and at the age of more than 50 years old. The PET/CT imaging shows that the lesion is obviously hypermetabolic and the soft tissue of the palate is locally raised or the soft palate is enlarged, with irregular surface and partial bone destruction of the hard palate or alveolar bone. PET/CT examination can sensitively detect metastatic lymph nodes and bone destruction and assess the extent of lesion involvement.

6 Carcinoma of the Lip

6.1 Clinical Overview

Carcinoma of the lip refers to the cancer that occurs in the red lip mucosa and the joint of the mouth corner (i.e., the mucosa within 1 cm from the cleft of the mouth), which is more common in Western countries. Carcinoma of the lip mostly occurs in outdoor workers such as farmers, fishermen, and workers who have been exposed to ultraviolet rays for a long time. Moreover, smoking and some other local stimulation factors are also related to the occurrence of lip cancer. It is more likely to occur in men, most of them are over 40 years old, and almost all are squamous cell carcinomas. Carcinoma of the lip mostly occurs in the lower lip, often located in the mucosa of the edge of the red edge between the middle and outer 1/3 of the lower lip. In the early stage, it is herpetic scab mass, or the local mucosa is thickened, then followed by crater-like ulcers or cauliflower-like mass. Carcinoma of the lip grows slowly and generally has no symptoms. Later, it could spread to the surrounding skin and mucous membrane and at the same time infiltrates into the deep muscle tissue. In the advanced stage, it may spread to the oral vestibule and jawbone. The diagnosis depends on pathological biopsy. The treatment of carcinoma of the lip mainly adopts surgery-based comprehensive treatment, which has a good prognosis. Reports have shown that its 3-year, 5-year, and 10-year survival rates are 90.0%, 85.7%, and 76.6%, respectively.

6.2 PET/CT Diagnostic Points

Carcinoma of the lip usually occurs in 1/3 of the middle and outer parts of the lower lip. In the early stage, it is manifested as thickened lip soft tissue with increased abnormal metabolism, and irregular soft tissue masses can be seen in the advanced stage of the disease, some of which are cauliflower-like, and it invades the cheeks, with obvious high metabolism. Carcinoma of the lip is well differentiated, and its metastasis rate is less than other oral cancers, and the metastasis occurs late. Carcinoma of the lower lip usually metastasizes to the submental and submandibular lymph nodes, while carcinoma of the upper lip metastasizes to the preauricular, parotid, submandibular, and deep cervical lymph nodes. A very small number of patients in advanced stage have distant metastases. If the lesion is small in the early stage, the PET/CT examination may show false negative.

6.3 Typical Cases

Carcinoma of the right lip with lymph node metastasis in the right cervical IB area: A 57-year-old male patient with ulceration of the right lower lip for more than 2 months (Fig. 11.10). Pathology: Squamous cell carcinoma

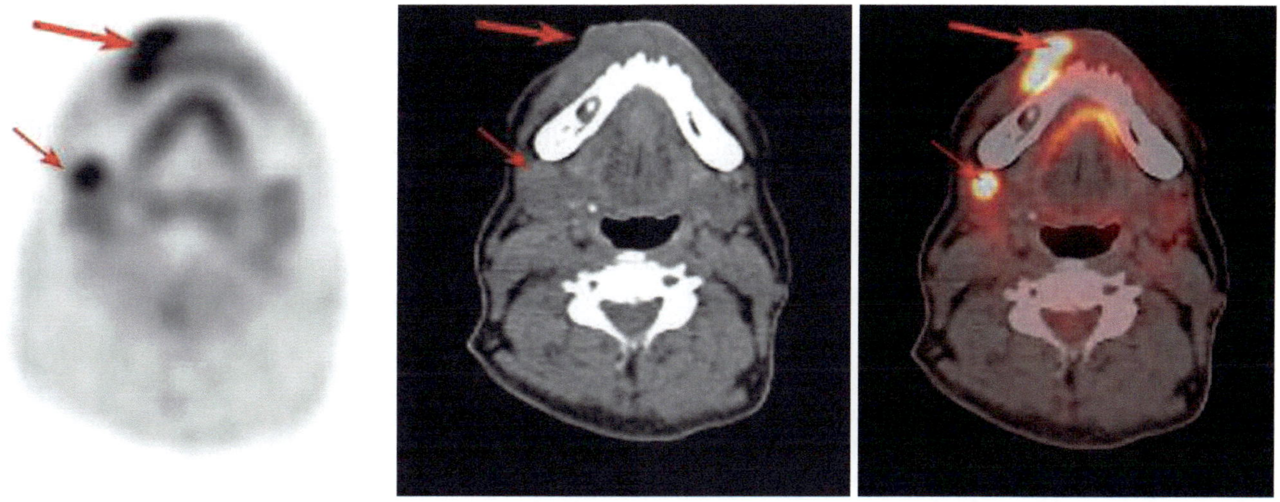

Fig. 11.10 PET/CT imaging showed increased FDG uptake in the lesion of the right lower lip, with a size of 3.8 cm × 1.9 cm × 2.5 cm and SUVmax 15.3. The lesion posteriorly involved the inferior gingiva and the CT image showed irregular soft tissue mass in the corresponding site (thick arrow). Increased FDG uptake in enlarged lymph nodes were found in the right level IB, with the size of 1.6 cm × 1.8 cm and SUVmax 11.4 (thin arrow)

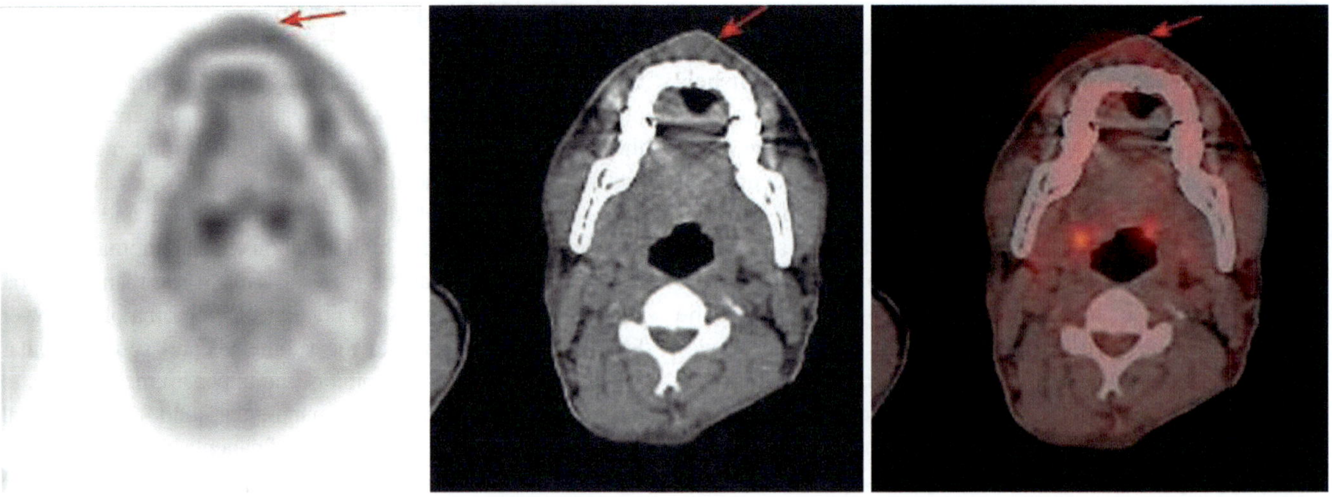

Fig. 11.11 FDG PET/CT images of adenoid cystic carcinoma of the upper lip. PET/CT imaging showed that the soft tissue of the upper lip was slightly thickened and no lesion with abnormal increased metabolism was found

6.4 Rare Cases

Adenoid cystic carcinoma can also occur in the lips, but it is rare.

Adenoid cystic carcinoma of the upper lip: A 52-year-old male patient with a mass on the upper lip for 1 year. Pathology: Adenoid cystic carcinoma (tubular type) (Fig. 11.11)

6.5 Differential Diagnosis

Early carcinoma of the lip should be differentiated from chronic cheilitis. The latter usually shows chapped, parakeratosis, erosion, exudation and bleeding of the lip mucosa. Furthermore, carcinoma of the lip should be differentiated from benign lesions such as keratoacanthoma, papilloma, and syphilitic chancre. The PET/CT imaging shows normal or low FDG uptake in the latter and no cervical lymph node with significantly increased metabolism.

6.6 Summary

Almost all carcinomas of the lip are squamous cell carcinomas, which mostly occur in the mucosa of the red edge between the middle and outer 1/3 of the lower lip. The PET/CT imaging shows that in the early stage, it is manifested as thickened lip soft tissue with abnormal increased metabolism and irregular soft tissue masses can be seen in the advanced stage of the disease, some of which are cauliflower-like, and it invades the cheeks.

12 PET/CT of Carcinoma of the Parotid Gland

Xiaoping Lin and Wei Fan

1 Clinical Overview

Benign salivary gland tumors usually have a long course of disease, while malignant tumors generally grow faster and have a shorter course. However, the course of low-grade malignant tumors can be as long as several years. The location and nature of the mass can be used as the basis for clinical diagnosis of the primary site of the tumor, as well as benign and malignant tumors. The tumor from the parotid gland should be considered for the mass before, under, and behind the earlobe. If the mass has no adhesion or activity with surrounding tissues, it is usually considered as benign tumor; if the mass is hard, adheres to surrounding tissues or even fixed, and has facial nerve and other nerve involvement symptoms, malignant tumor should be considered. Malignant tumors often cause pain.

It is common that there is increased ^{18}F-FDG uptake in parotid carcinoma lesions, lymph node metastasis, and distant metastasis, while decreased or defective FDG uptake can be found in the necrotic part of the tumor.

2 PET/CT Diagnostic Points

2.1 General Diagnostic Points

1. With clinical history, the growth rate of lesion is generally fast. If the facial nerve is invaded, facial paralysis will occur; local persistent pain may occur; the involvement of the masticatory muscles may cause mouth opening disturbance.
2. Enlargement of cervical lymph nodes: When the tumor has lymph node metastasis, the enlarged lymph nodes can be palpated in the deep upper, middle, and lower parts of the neck (II–IV areas).

2.2 CT Diagnostic Points

1. Parotid carcinoma is manifested as a soft tissue mass with unclear boundary and irregular outline. The adjacent fat or envelope disappears. There may be a necrotic area in the center. The tumor may develop outside the envelope and may invade the surrounding muscle tissue and even the subcutaneous and skin.
2. Cervical lymph node metastasis may occur. The metastatic lymph node may be accompanied by necrosis, or it may invade outside the envelope, which is manifested as irregular or fuzzy margins of lymph nodes, streaky infiltration to adjacent fat, and unclear boundaries with adjacent carotid arteries or cranial nerves.

2.3 ^{18}F-FDG PET Diagnostic Points

1. Increased FDG uptake in the primary lesions of the parotid gland, metastatic lymph nodes, and distant metastases.
2. Due to partial volume effect, the small lesion may manifest a slightly increased FDG uptake.
3. Parotid carcinoma lesions can be fused with cervical metastatic lymph nodes. It is helpful to differentiate them by enhanced CT.

3 Typical Cases

Carcinoma of the right parotid gland: Male patient, 68 years old. Pathology: Poorly differentiated carcinoma of the right parotid gland, which was consistent with salivary duct carcinoma (Figs. 12.1 and 12.2)

X. Lin · W. Fan (✉)
Sun Yat-sen University Cancer Center,
Guangzhou, Guangdong, China
e-mail: fanwei@sysucc.org.cn

Z. Yao, S. Li (eds.), *Atlas of PET/CT in Oncology - Volume 1*, https://doi.org/10.1007/978-981-99-1172-1_12

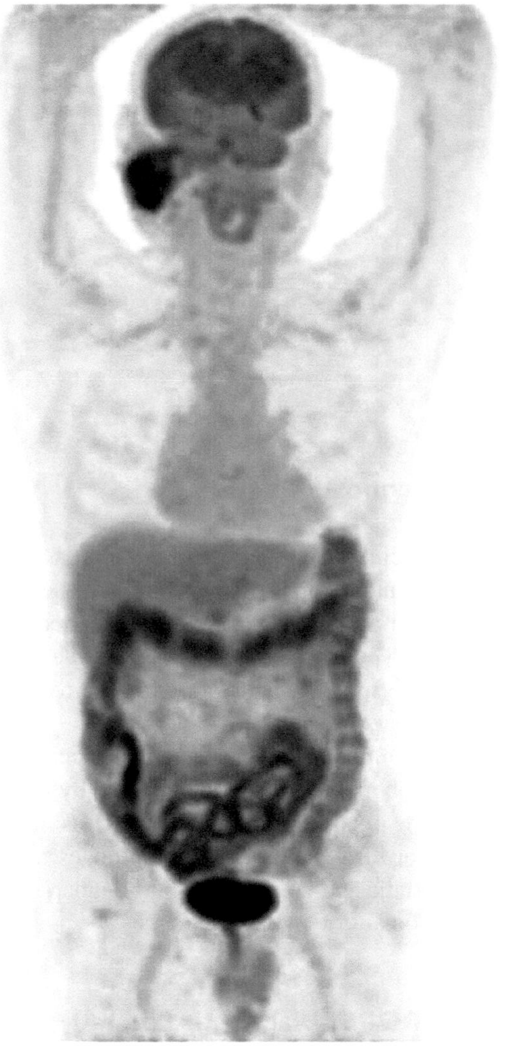

Fig. 12.1 PET MIP image of right parotid carcinoma. PET MIP image showed the lesion of salivary duct carcinoma of the right parotid gland was a mass, with inhomogeneous significantly increased FDG uptake

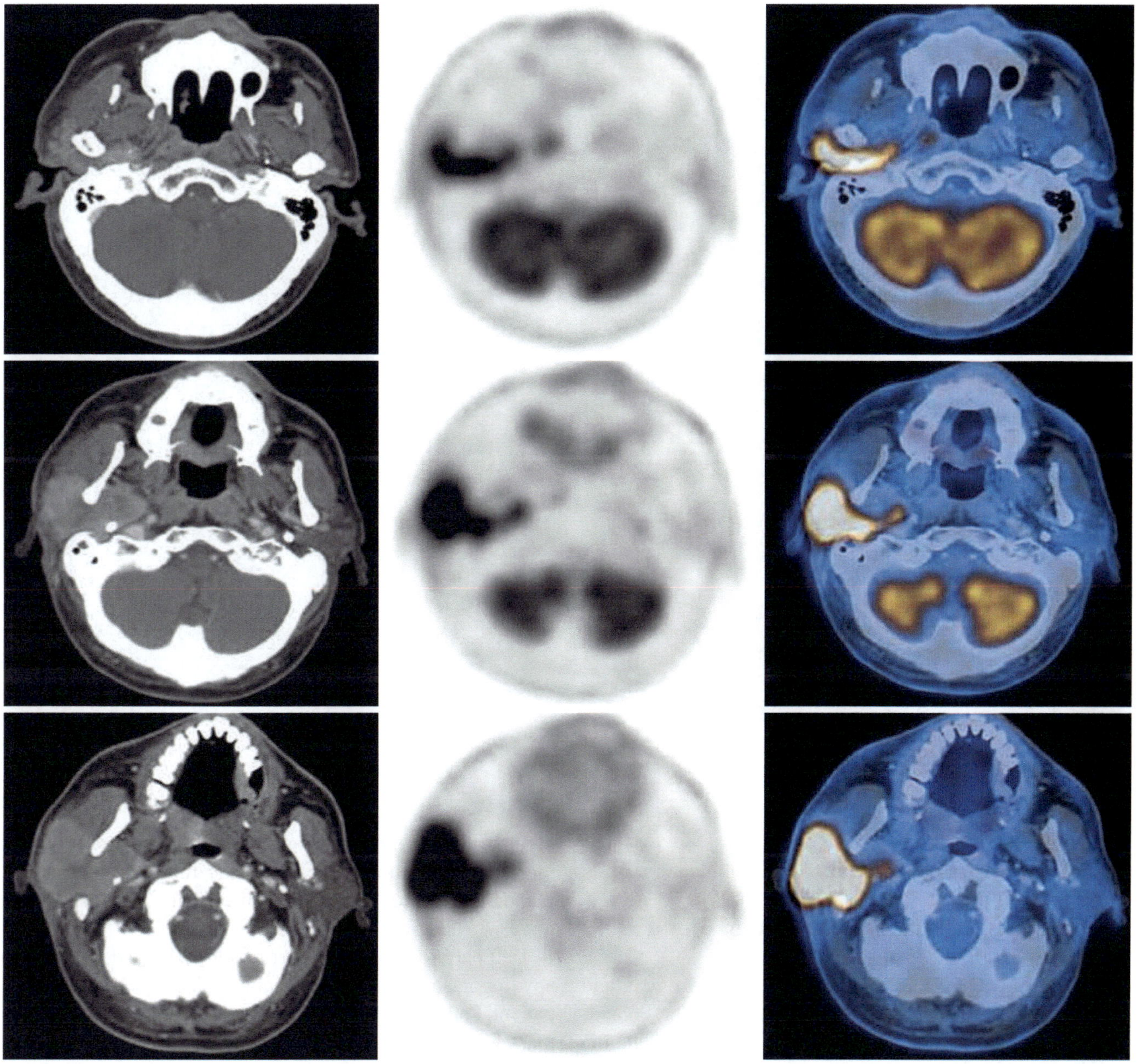

Fig. 12.2 PET/CT (same-machine enhanced CT) cross-sectional images of right parotid carcinoma. Increased FDG uptake in the lobulated soft tissue mass in the right parotid gland; its SUVmax was 17.7 and size 4.6 cm × 5.4 cm. There were low-density necrotic and small punctate calcification areas in the mass; FDG uptake was decreased in these areas. The enhanced CT scan showed obviously inhomogeneous enhancement in the mass. The lesion invaded the right parapharyngeal fat space, and the boundary with the right masseter, right pterygoid muscle, and right sternocleidomastoid muscle was not clear. It wrapped the right mandibular branch and styloid process and pushed the blood vessels in the right carotid sheath area

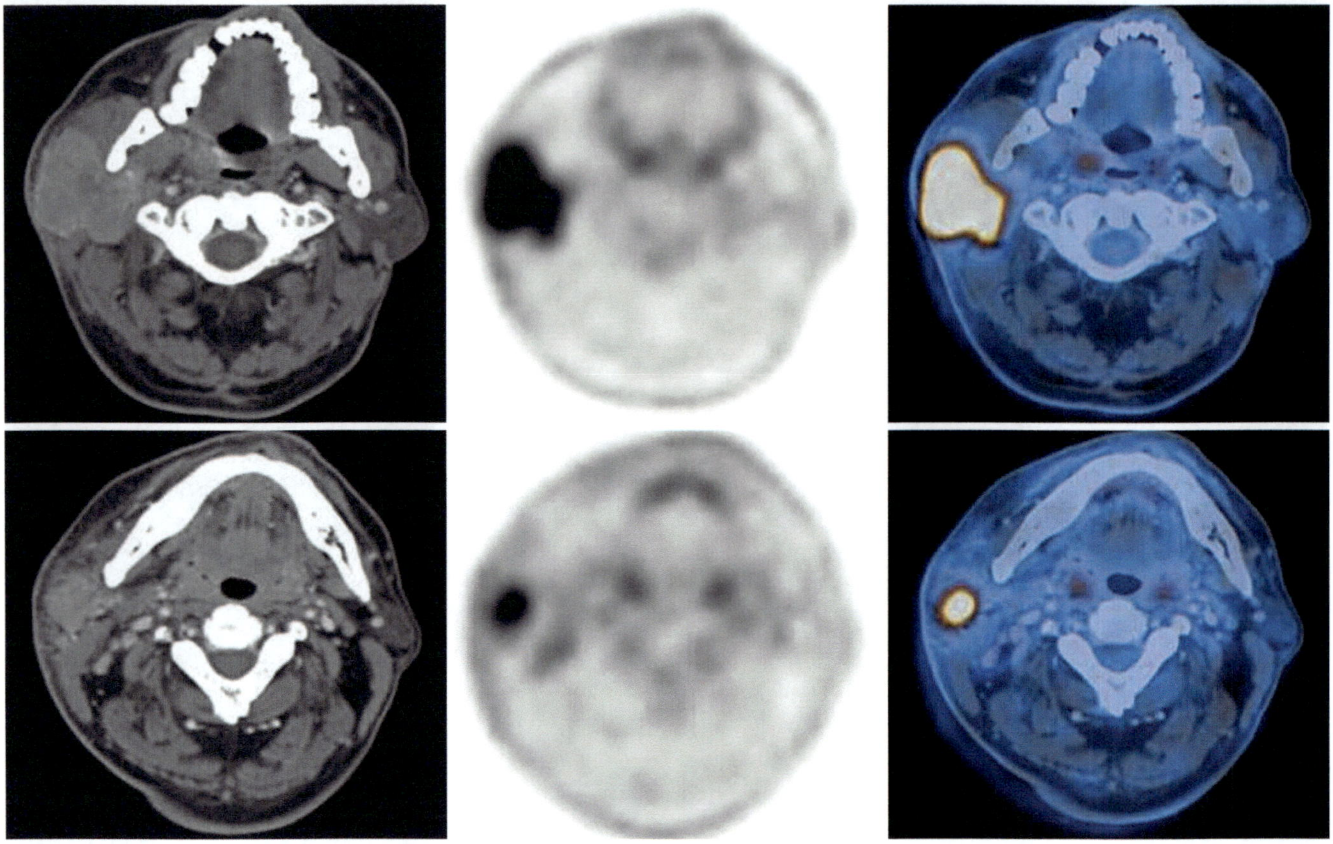

Fig. 12.2 (continued)

4 Differential Diagnosis

4.1 Metastatic Tumor of the Parotid Gland

It is rare, but when there is a mass in the parotid gland area, the possibility of metastasis should also be considered. Squamous cell carcinoma and malignant melanoma are the most likely metastatic tumor to the parotid gland, which should be judged in combination with the medical history and general examination. PET/CT generally shows increased FDG uptake in metastatic tumor in the parotid gland, and tumor sometimes fuses with cervical lymph nodes.

Left parotid metastasis after radiotherapy and chemotherapy for nasopharyngeal carcinoma: A 45-year-old female patient. Pathology: The pathologic result of left parotid gland mass was conformed to be the same as lymph node metastasis of undifferentiated non-keratinizing carcinoma (Figs. 12.3, 12.4, 12.5, and 12.6).

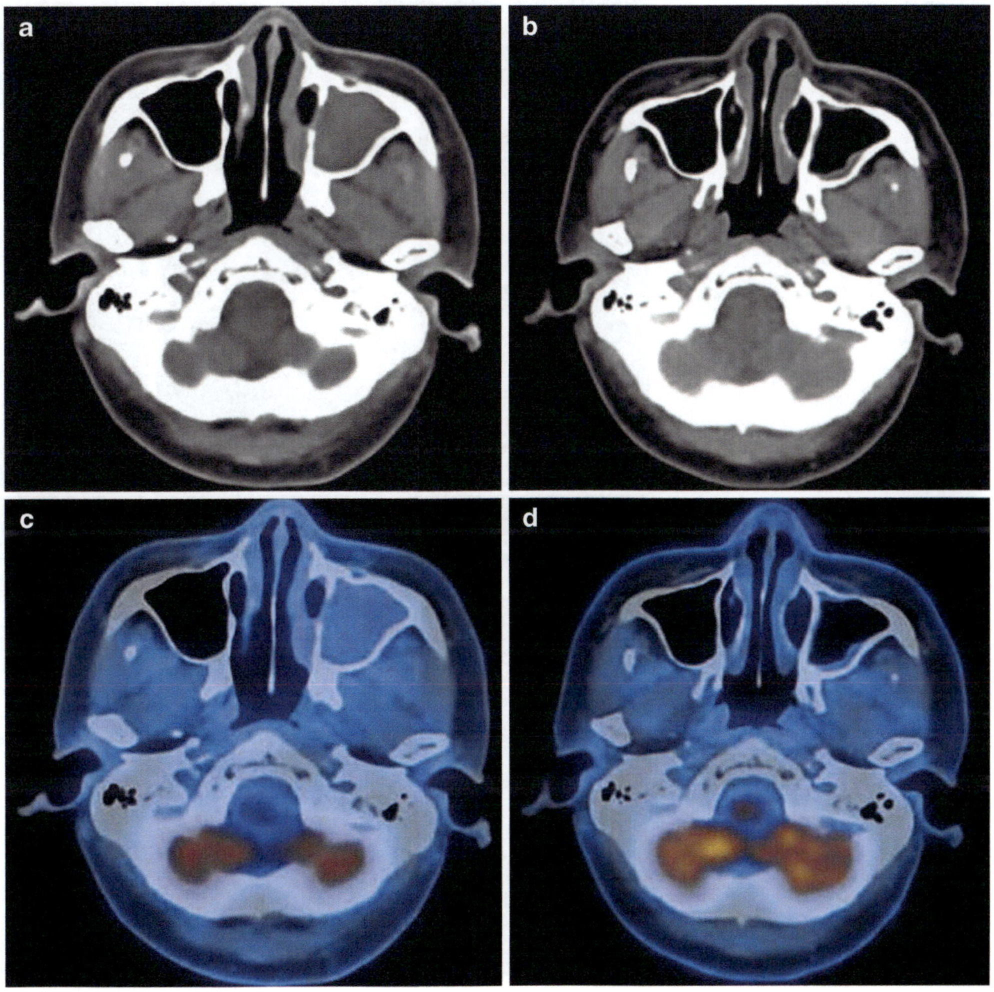

Fig. 12.3 PET/CT cross-sectional images of the follow-up of local complete remission after radiotherapy and chemotherapy for nasopharyngeal carcinoma. Nasopharyngeal carcinoma post-radiotherapy and chemotherapy: the mucosa of the nasopharyngeal upper wall, posterior parietal wall, and left wall of the nasopharynx was slightly thickened and without obvious abnormality FDG uptake. Figure **a** and Figure **c** are half a year earlier than Figure **b** and Figure **d**, respectively

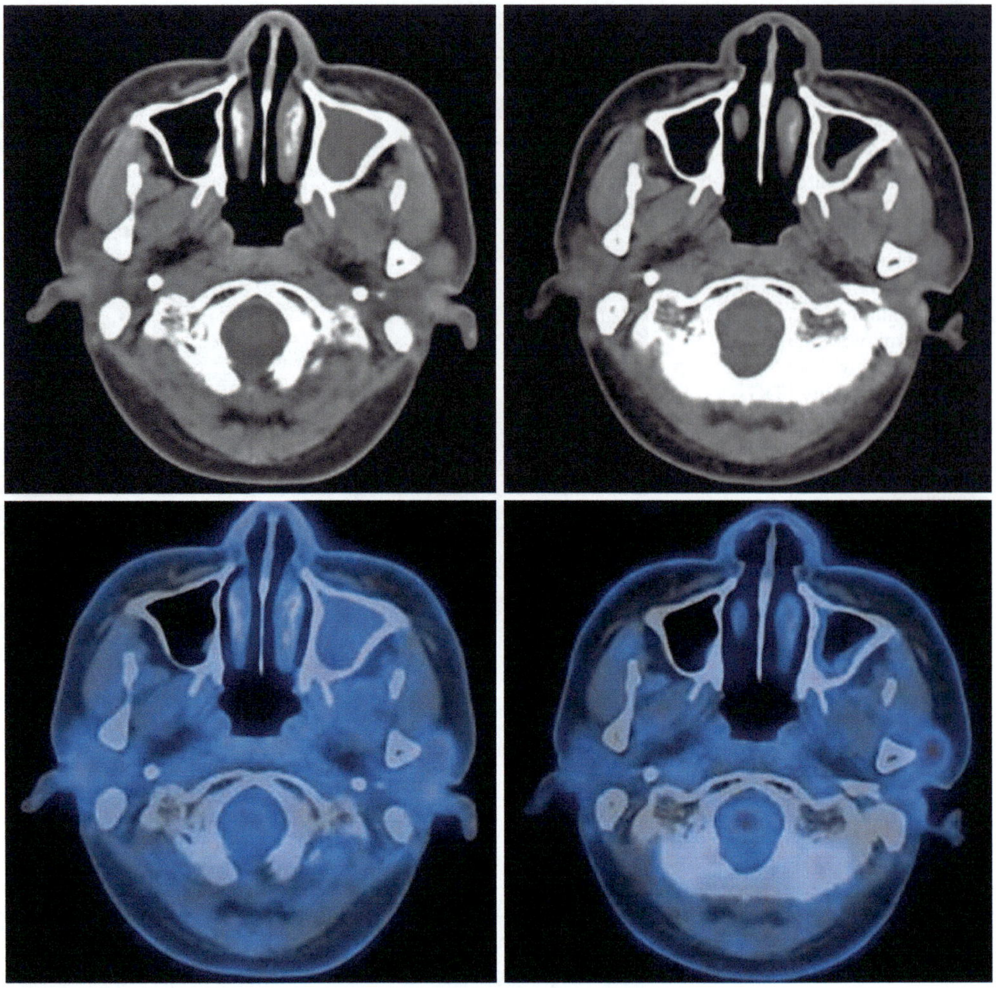

Fig. 12.4 PET/CT cross-sectional images of follow-up left parotid metastasis (1)

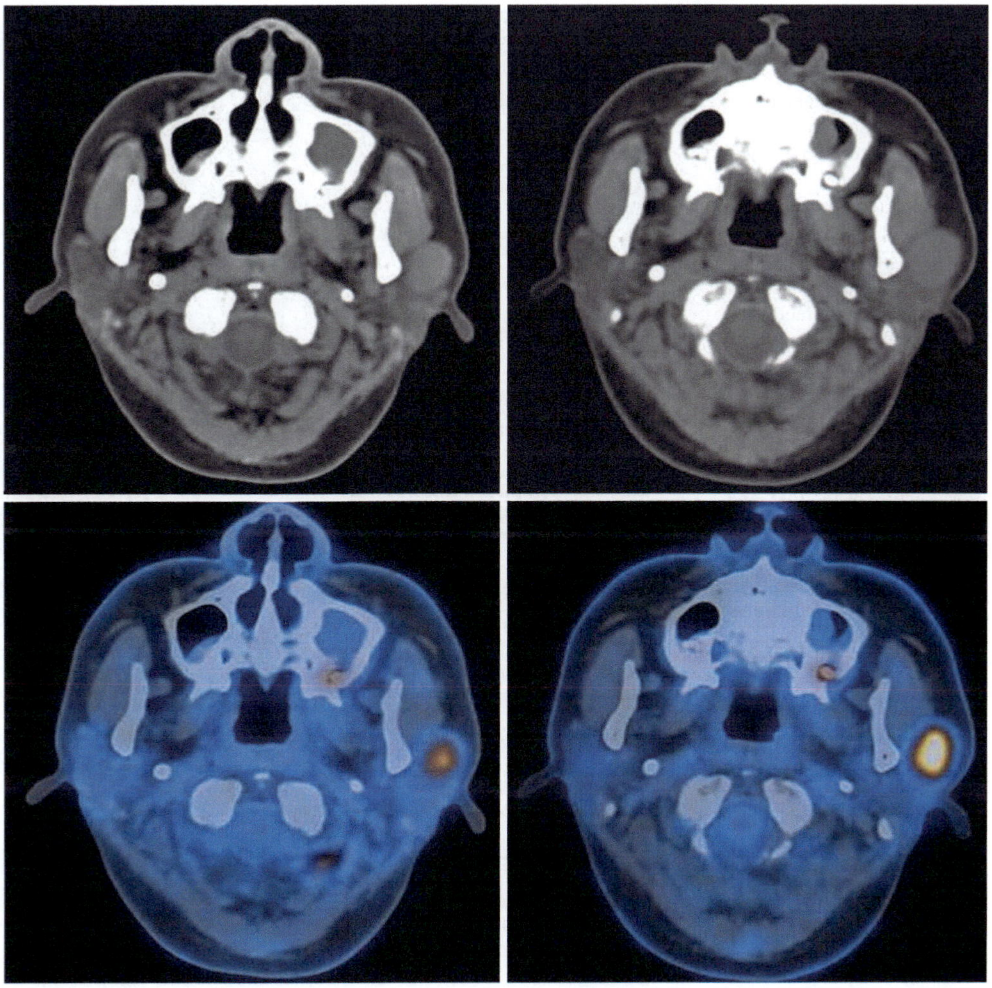

Fig. 12.5 PET/CT cross-sectional images of follow-up left parotid metastasis (2)

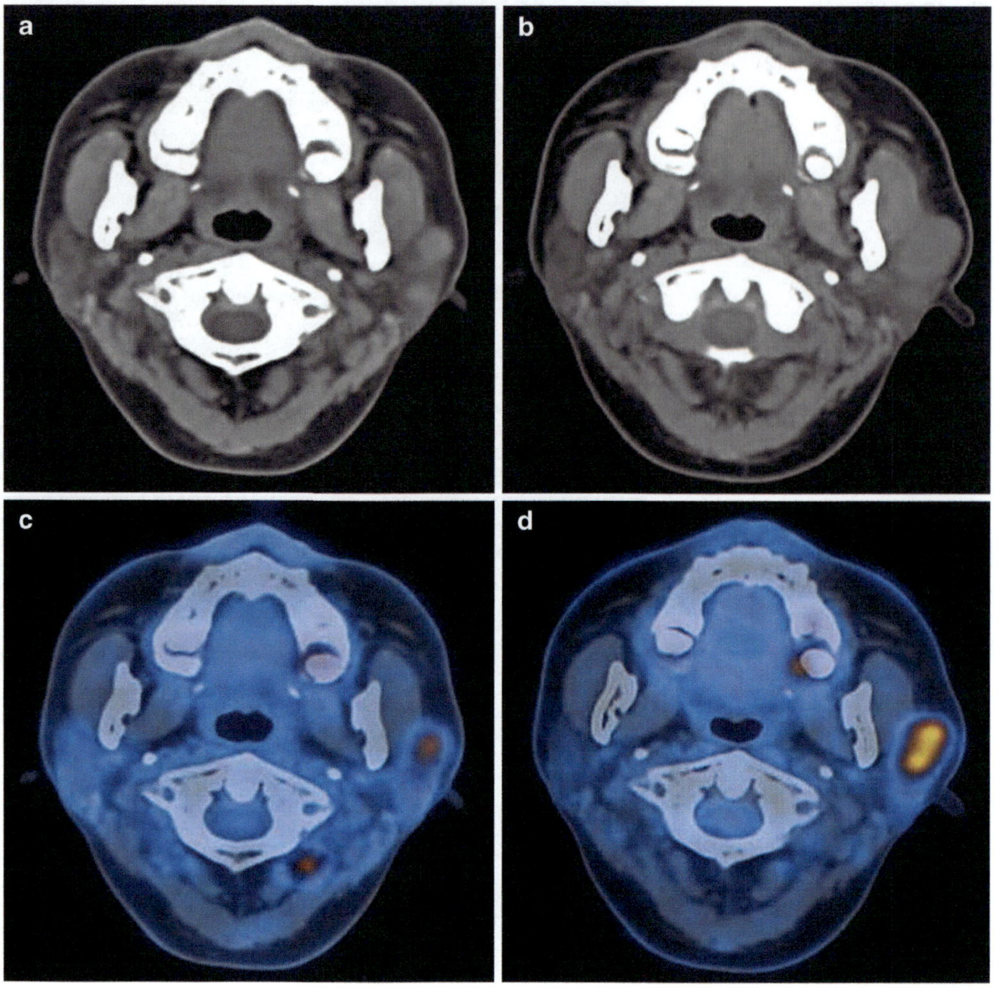

Fig. 12.6 PET/CT cross-sectional images of follow-up left parotid metastasis (3). Increased FDG uptake in several high-density nodules on the left parotid gland, with SUVmax 7.9 and 1.5 cm × 2.0 cm in size. Half a year later, inhomogeneous increased FDG uptake in the slightly high-density nodules in the left parotid gland was observed, their SUVmax was 11.4, and the size of the largest nodule was 1.8 cm × 2.5 cm (Figs. 12.4, 12.5, and 12.6 are all level images of the parotid gland in cross section of the PET and fusion images of this case). (All figures of this case are after treatment of nasopharyngeal carcinoma; Fig. **a** and Fig. **c** are half a year earlier than Fig. **b** and Fig. **d**, respectively)

4.2 Lymphoma

Rarely, it can be parotid infiltration of systemic lymphoma, or it can be primary lymphoma of the parotid gland. PET/CT generally shows increased FDG uptake in soft tissue mass of the parotid gland.

Left parotid lymphoma: An 18-year-old male patient. Pathology: Lymph nodes in the left parotid gland conform to non-Hodgkin's lymphoma, B cell (follicular lymphoma, grade II/FL II; children follicular lymphoma) (Fig. 12.7).

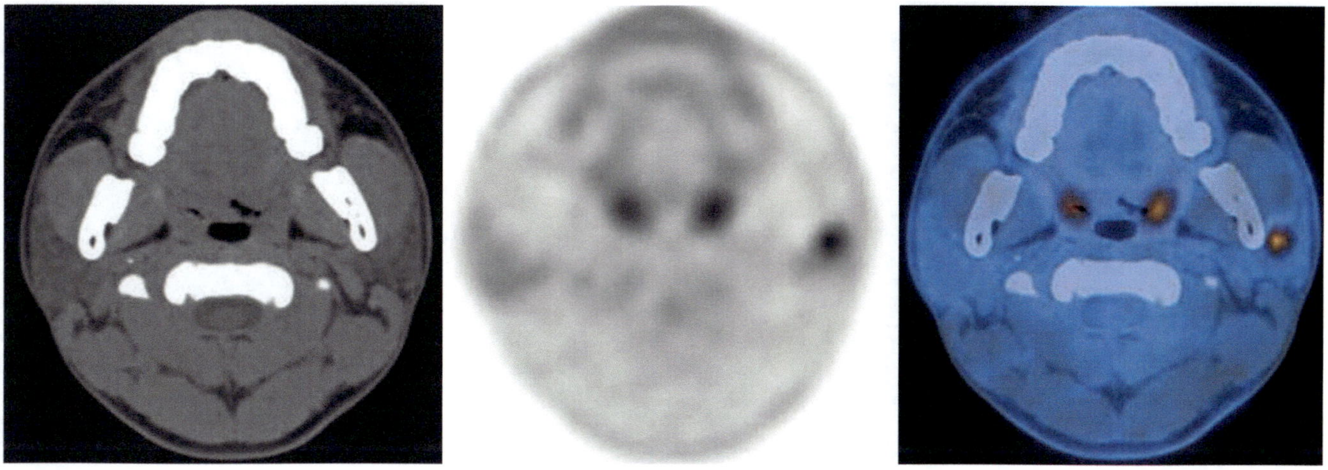

Fig. 12.7 PET/CT cross-sectional image of left parotid lymphoma. Increased FDG uptake in the nodule in the left parotid gland; its SUVmax was 10.1 and size was 0.8 cm × 0.9 cm

4.3 Benign Lesions of the Parotid Gland

Mixed tumor of the parotid gland manifests as a round or oval soft tissue density mass in the parotid gland, with smooth edges and a clear boundary with the surrounding normal parotid gland tissue. When there is cystic change, liquid density may appear. Warthin tumor can show lobulation and multiple vesicles. PET/CT usually shows nodule of soft tissue in the parotid gland with clear boundary and focal increased FDG uptake slightly higher than or close to the background.

1. Warthin tumor of the left parotid gland (active metabolism): A 56-year-old male patient. Pathology: Lymphomatous papillary cystadenoma of the left parotid gland (Warthin tumor) (Fig. 12.8)
2. Warthin tumor of the left parotid gland (slightly active metabolism): A 66-year-old male patient. Pathology: Lymphomatous papillary cystadenoma of the left parotid gland (Warthin tumor) (Fig. 12.9)

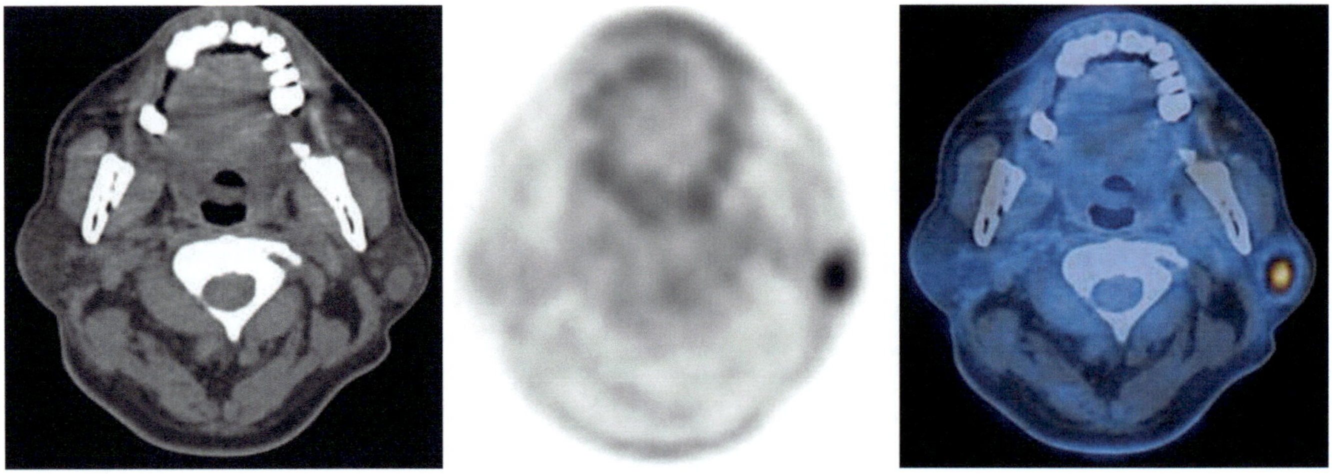

Fig. 12.8 PET/CT cross-sectional image of Warthin tumor in the left parotid gland. Increased FDG uptake in the soft tissue density nodule in the superficial lobe of the left parotid gland; its SUVmax was 10.8 and size 1.1 cm × 1.4 cm. It was round-shaped, with lower density in the central area. The edge of the nodules was clear

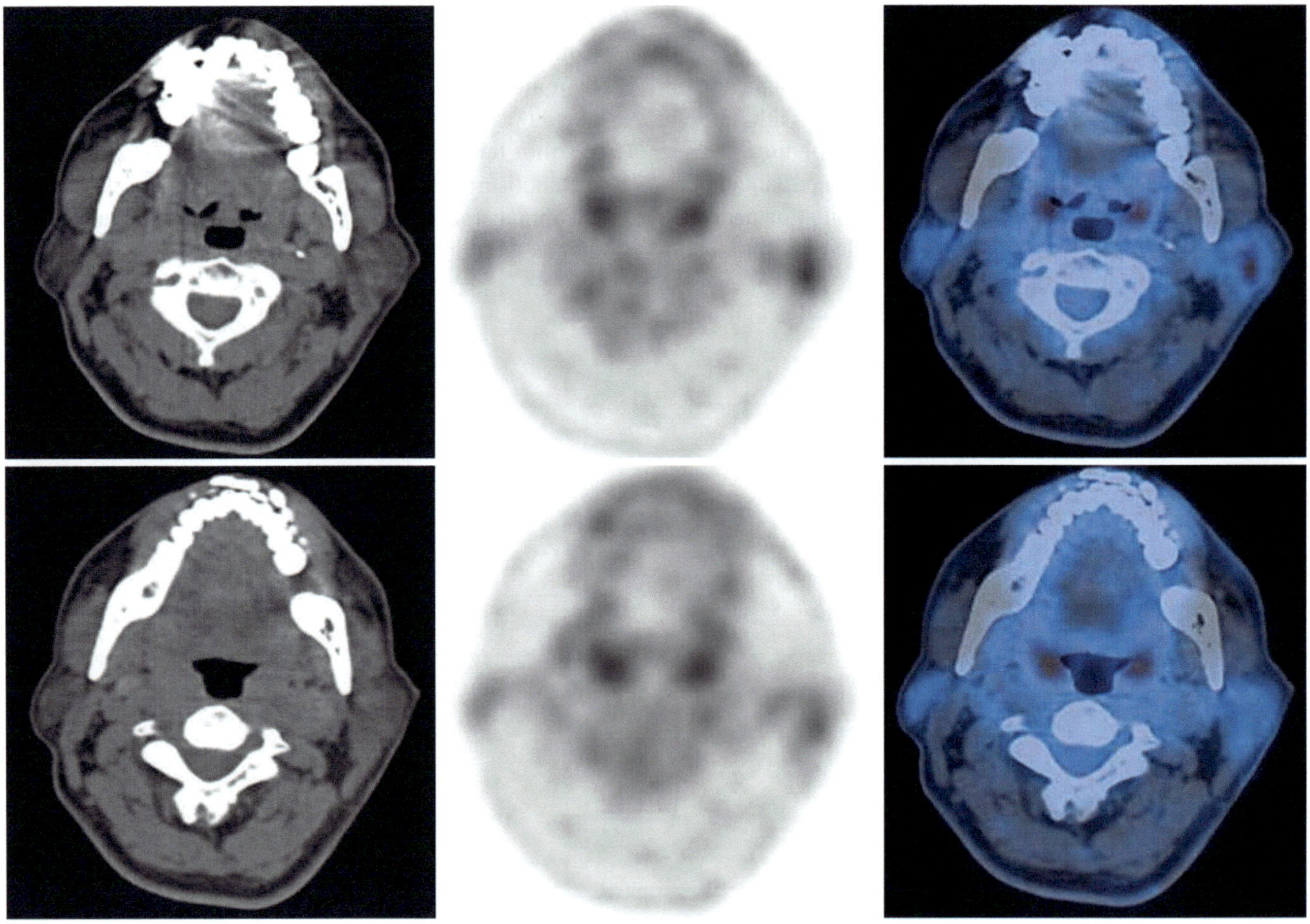

Fig. 12.9 PET/CT cross-sectional image of Warthin tumor in the left parotid gland. The FDG uptake of several nodules in the left parotid gland was moderately increased, its SUVmax was 5.4, and the size of the largest one was 1.1 cm × 1.2 cm

5 Summary

Parotid carcinoma is a common malignant tumor of the salivary gland, and surgery is the main treatment. Increased FDG uptake in the nodule or mass in the parotid area is a typical manifestation of parotid adenocarcinoma. It should be noticed whether the tumor invades the tissue surrounding itself and whether there is lymph node metastasis or not. If the FDG uptake in parotid nodules is close to the background, the density of the structure image is uniform, and the boundary is clear, benign parotid lesions can be considered. If FDG uptake in the parotid nodules is increased and the boundary is clear, Warthin tumor should be excluded.

PET/CT can simultaneously obtain whole-body PET functional metabolism images, CT anatomical images, and PET/CT fusion images, which is helpful for staging TNM, observing the curative effect, assisting the development and adjustment of the treatment plan, and follow-up.

Part III

PET/CT of Ocular Tumors

General Introduction of PET/CT of Ocular Tumors

13

Guoren Yang, Xiaoli Lan, and Tingting Lu

1 Overview

Ocular tumor can occur in each tissue component of the eye and not only can be directly spread from adjacent structures but also can be transferred through blood. Among ophthalmic tumors, primary tumors are the most common, followed by secondary tumors. Based on different tissues, tumors can be classified as eyeball tumor, lacrimal gland tumor, optic nerve tumor, orbital tumor, and metastatic tumor. The eyeball is composed of the sclera, pigment layer, and retina, which is filled with lens and vitreous body and where no tumor may occur because of their component of water and protein. Ocular tumors and neoplastic lesions mainly occur in the sclera, pigment layer, and retina, where the retinoblastoma and choroidal melanoma are the common tumors. The lacrimal gland is located in the outer upper lacrimal fossa of the orbit, which is divided into the superficial palpebral lobe and deep orbital lobe. The tumors account for 7%–13% of orbital tumors, mainly pleomorphic adenomas. The optic nerve is part of the cerebral nerve, similar to white matter histology is of axon fiber bundle of neurons and nerve glial tissues. Primary tumors originating from the optic nerve are mostly optic glioma and optic nerve sheath meningioma. The orbit is composed of the frontal bone, ethmoid bone, lacrimal bone, sphenoid bone, zygomatic bone, palatine bone, and maxilla, adjacent to the sinus, anterior cranial fossa, and middle cranial fossa. The orbit is in a rectangular pyramidal shape, with the anterior margin of the orbit facing outward and the orbital tip pointing backward. The walls of the orbit are of different thickness, and the superior wall is adjacent to the anterior cranial fossa. The medial wall is the thinnest and adjacent to the superior ethmoid labyrinth. The dacryocyst fossa in front of the wall is communicated with the nasal cavity through the nasolacrimal duct, and the upper margin of the medial wall has the anterior ethmoidal foramen and the posterior ethmoidal foramen. The lateral wall is the thickest, and between the posterior part and the inferior orbital wall is the inferior orbital fissure connecting with the inferior temporal fossa and the pterygopalatine fossa, and between the lateral wall and the superior orbital wall is the superior orbital fissure connecting with the middle cranial fossa. There are accessory structures such as the eyeball and extraocular muscle, lacrimal gland, blood vessel, and nerve in orbit, with fat filling between each tissue. Orbital tumors are classified into orbital wall tumors and intraorbital tumor. The tumors originating from the orbital wall include osteoma, osteosarcoma, chondrosarcoma, and abnormal proliferation of bone fibers. Most of the tumors originating in the orbit are vasogenic tumors, and cavernous hemangioma and lymphangioma are relatively common.

2 Examination Techniques

2.1 X-Ray

There are anterior and posterior orbital radiography, lateral orbital radiography, optic foramen radiography, and dacryocyst dacryocystography. However, due to the popularity of CT, X-ray examination has been rarely applied.

2.2 CT

Conventional cross-sectional and coronal scanning is used, with a thickness of 3–5 mm, including the entire orbit. Soft tissue window is often used. HRCT scanning technology for patient with trauma is used with 2 mm thickness and bone algorithm reconstruction.

G. Yang (✉) · T. Lu
Shandong Cancer Hospital, Jinan, Shandong, China

X. Lan
Union Hospital, Tongji Medical College, Huazhong University of Science and Technology, Wuhan, Hubei, China

Z. Yao, S. Li (eds.), *Atlas of PET/CT in Oncology - Volume 1*, https://doi.org/10.1007/978-981-99-1172-1_13

2.3 MRI

There are many imaging parameters and sequences, which can be diagnosed according to the difference in relaxation time between different tissues of the eye and between tissues and lesions. The commonly used imaging sequences are T_1WI, T_2WI, etc.

2.4 PET/CT Examination

The glucose analogue ^{18}F-FDG is mainly used as an imaging agent, and the tissue concentration degree of ^{18}F-FDG reflects its glucose utilization ratio. Most of the tumors show increased ^{18}F-FDG uptake due to its high expression of glucose transporter (GLUT) and increased intracellular hexokinase activity.

1. Preparation and precautions for patient examination
   (a) The patient fasted for at least 4 h before receiving the radioactive tracer, including parenteral nutrition and intravenous fluids containing glucose. Drinking plain water 2 h prior to the examination is encouraged for adequate hydration to reduce background in blood pools and soft tissues on PET image and to reduce radiation as well.
   (b) It is better that the patient's blood glucose is in normal range.
2. Radioactive tracer injection can be based on the 0.10–0.14 mCi/kg standard. The general principle is to reduce the amount of the radioactive tracer as much as possible, and the injection dose shall fit the need of acquisition time.
3. After intravenous injection of radionuclides, the patients are allowed to have a rest of 60 min in a quiet and light-free environment, and then their bladder is emptied for examination. The patient is in supine position for acquiring images, and the orbital line is vertical to the couch. Different from conventional PET/CT examination, folded hands of the patient are placed on the abdomen to avoid radio-sclerosis artifacts caused by lifting hands on the head and neck, which may affect the observation of lesions.

14 Ocular Tumors

Guoren Yang, Xiaoli Lan, Jie Zhang, Tingting Lu, Congxia Chen, and Zhiming Yao

1 Ocular Lymphoma

1.1 Clinical Overview

Ocular lymphoma is one of the most common malignant tumors of the orbit, accounting for about 10.3% of orbital malignant tumors. It often occurs in middle-aged and elderly people, with slightly more in women. In most cases, the disease progresses slowly, mainly with non-Hodgkin lymphoma (NHL), accounting for 1–2% of all NHL and 5–15% of peripheral NHL, whose prevalence has been rising in recent years. Ocular lymphoma mainly consists of extranodal marginal zone lymphoma and a small amount of follicular lymphoma, diffuse large B-cell lymphoma, mantle cell lymphoma, and lymphoplasmacytic lymphoma.

Ocular lymphoma can involve orbital, extraocular muscle, conjunctiva, eyelid, lacrimal gland and lacrimal sac, etc. The clinical manifestations are often related to the site and structure of the lymphoma involved. The treatment of ocular lymphoma is based on histopathological findings and lesion infiltration. Local radiotherapy or temporary observation can be selected for lesions confined to the orbit, and intervention can be performed until the disease progresses and requires chemotherapy.

G. Yang · T. Lu
Shandong Cancer Hospital, Jinan, Shandong, China

X. Lan (✉) · J. Zhang
Union Hospital, Tongji Medical College, Huazhong University of Science and Technology, Wuhan, Hubei, China

C. Chen
Beijing Hospital, National Center of Gerontology, Institute of Geriatric Medicine, Chinese Academy of Medical Sciences, Beijing, China
e-mail: Congxia.Chen@sysucc.org.cn

Z. Yao
Department of Nuclear Medicine, Beijing Hospital, National Center of Gerontology, Institute of Geriatric Medicine, Chinese Academy of Medical Sciences, Beijing, China

1.2 PET/CT Diagnostic Points

1.2.1 General Diagnosis

1. It tends to occur among the middle-aged and elderly people.
2. Orbital space-occupying lesions are more common.
3. Mostly single eye is involved.
4. The patient may have a prominent eyeball, palpable mass, ptosis, diplopia, and other clinical manifestations.

1.2.2 CT Diagnostic Points

1. There are ocular soft tissue density masses, often showing as soft tissue mass inside the orbit and also as eyelid swelling, thickening of extraocular muscles, and other signs.
2. Adjacent structures may be involved, and orbital apex involvement is more common.
3. No significant change in the bone is found around ocular lesions.

1.2.3 FDG PET Diagnostic Points

1. FDG uptake level in ocular lymphoma is associated with the pathological type of lesion. Low-grade lymphomas such as MALT usually have slightly increased or low FDG uptake, resulting in the possibility of false negative in PET/CT examination. MALT is usually limited to the eyes. Diffuse large B-cell lymphoma (DLBCL) involves the eye and many other parts of the body as well, with significantly increased FDG uptake in its lesions.
2. FDG PET can be used to determine the size of lesions and systemic involvement and is an excellent tool of staging lymphoma.

1.3 Typical Cases

Case 1: Male patient, 53 years old, presented with painless mass of the left eye for more than 5 months (Fig. 14.1).

Z. Yao, S. Li (eds.), *Atlas of PET/CT in Oncology - Volume 1*, https://doi.org/10.1007/978-981-99-1172-1_14

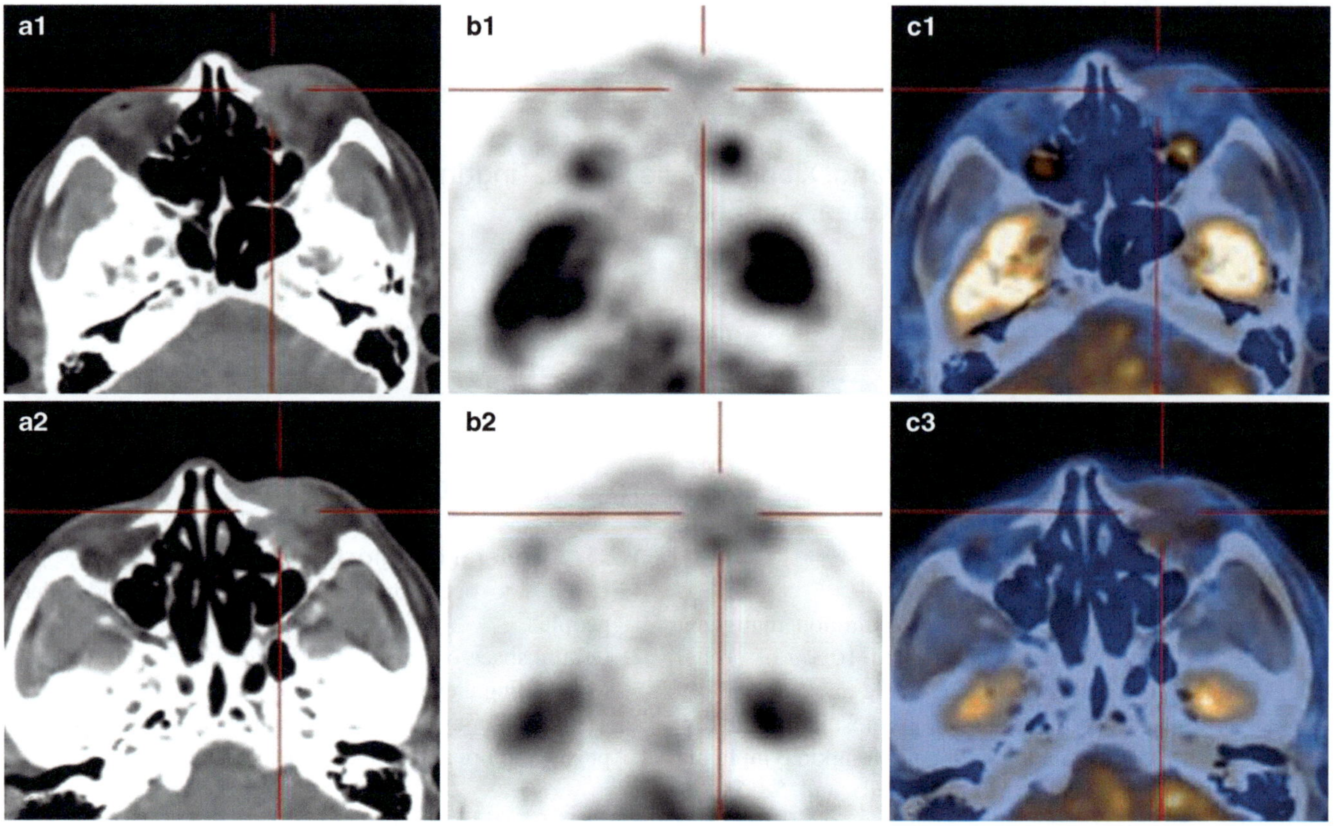

Fig. 14.1 FDG PET/CT images of MALT in the left orbit. (**a1** and **a2**) Cross-sectional CT images showed soft tissue density shadow in the left medial orbital wall, and there was no obvious destruction of the adjacent bone (criss-cross). (**b1** and **b2**) Cross-sectional FDG PET images showed diffuse increased FDG uptake in ocular lesions (SUVmax 5.0). (**c1** and **c2**) Cross-sectional PET/CT fusion images

Reminder: The orbit is a common site of ocular lymphoma, and low-grade lymphomas such as MALT usually have low FDG uptake, and some lesions may be false negative.

Case 2: Male patient, 47 years old, with "gradual decrease in vision in the right eye" (Fig. 14.2)

Reminder: FDG uptake in ocular DLBCL is intense, and other parts of the body are often involved by DLBCL.

Case 3: Female patient, 82 years old. The patient had oropharyngeal MALT lymphoma 6 years ago, received radiotherapy and chemotherapy, and recovered. In 2018, surgery was performed due to left orbital mass, and the specific pathology was unknown. After surgery, she had impaired vision and ptosis of the left eye. 3 weeks ago she complained a mass in the right eyelid, accompanied with impaired vision of the right eye (Fig. 14.3).

Case 4: Male patient, 73 years old. The patient complained of left ocular proptosis accompanied with spilling tears for about 2 months. On April 3, 2018, plain MRI scan of the orbit revealed that the left orbital muscle cone was occupied. On May 8, 2018, needle biopsy of the left orbital mass indicated NHL, consistent with diffuse large B-cell lymphoma, with nonspecific type, which was the source of activated B cells (Fig. 14.4).

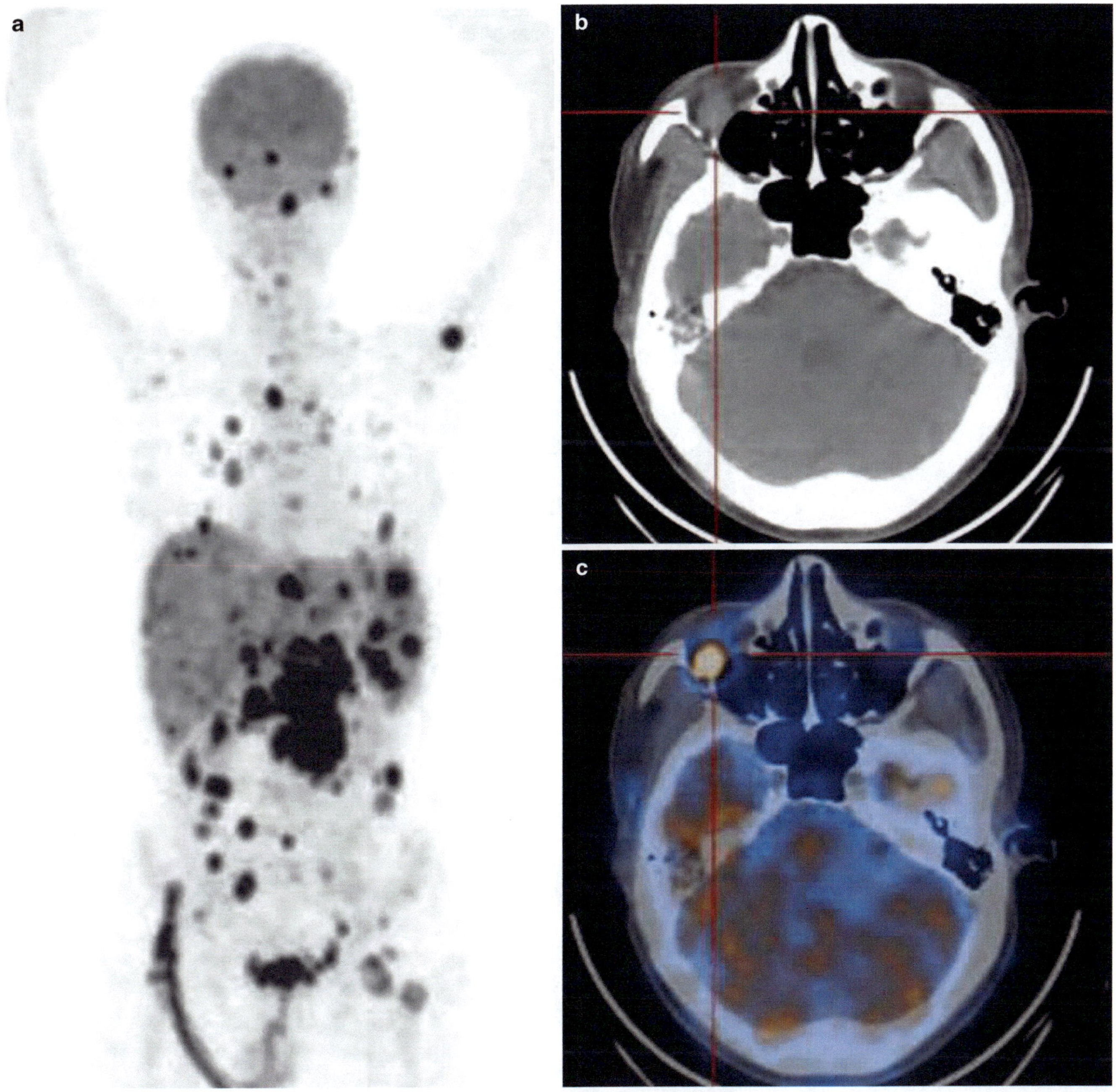

Fig. 14.2 PET/CT images of DLBCL of the right orbit. (**a**) FDG PET MIP images, in which multiple lesions with increased FDG uptake were observed in the whole body, some of which were fused into clumps. (**b**) Cross-sectional CT image showed soft tissue density nodules (cruciform) in the inferior wall of the right orbital posterior region, and no obvious destruction of the adjacent bone was seen. (**c**) Cross-sectional PET/CT fusion images showed intense FDG uptake (SUVmax 18.4) in lesions. FDG PET/CT showed multiple soft tissue density nodules of the right orbit, pituitary gland, systemic lymph nodes, bilateral lungs, liver and spleen, bilateral adrenal gland, and others were partially fused into masses with hypermetabolism. Some of the wall of the stomach and small intestine thickened, and FDG uptake increased. Focal FDG increase in lesions was found in the bone; the bone density in these lesions did not change significantly. The patient was definitely diagnosed as DLBCL by liver biopsy. PET/CT defined the clinical stage and could provide a good basis for the selection of clinical treatment

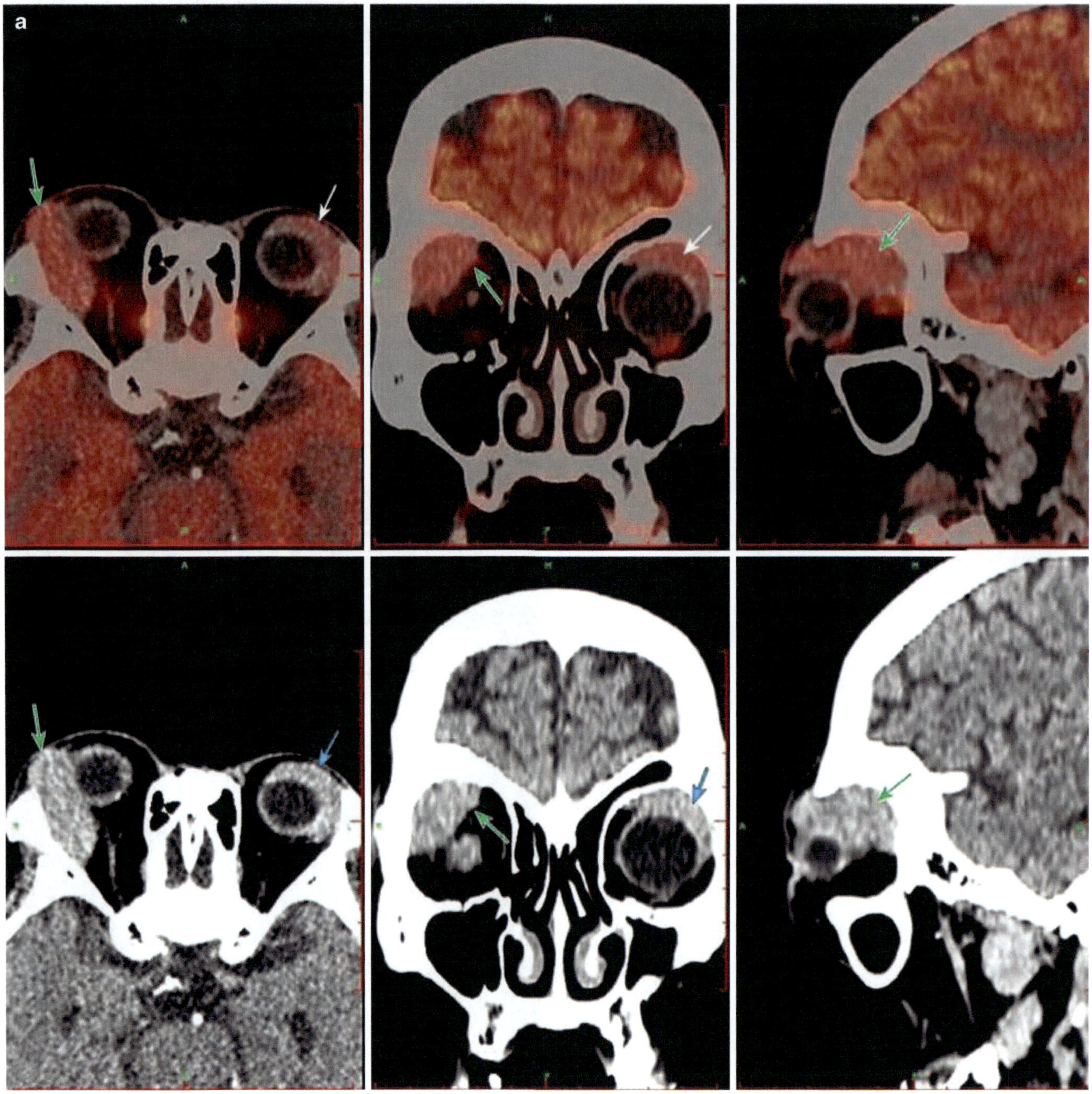

Fig. 14.3 FDG PET/CT images of MALT lymphoma of double orbital. (**a**) The upper and lower rows were the cross section, coronal plane, and sagittal plane of PET/CT fusion images and CT images, respectively. (**b**) Coronal plane of PET/CT fusion image. FDG PET/CT showed soft tissue masses in the orbit above both eyeballs (arrow); the mass curved around the eyeball, with unclear boundary with the tear gland, eyelid, and wall of the eyeball; the right side was more obvious; and the metabolic activity of the mass was significantly increased (SUVmax 9.6) and the maximum cross section about 1.9 cm × 3.7 cm (this case was provided by Dr. Xiuling Shen and Dr. Zhiming Yao, Beijing Hospital)

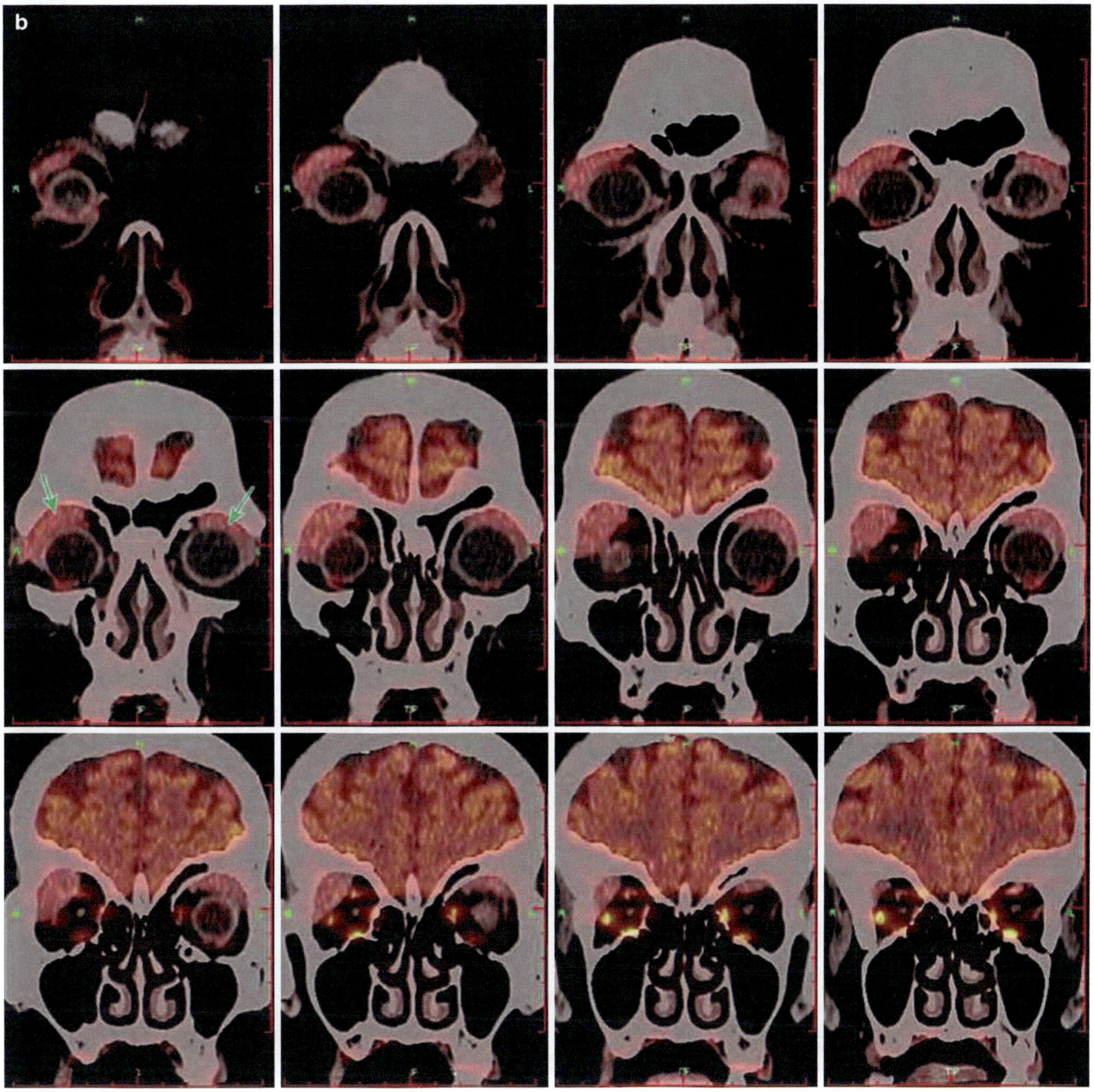

Fig. 14.3 (continued)

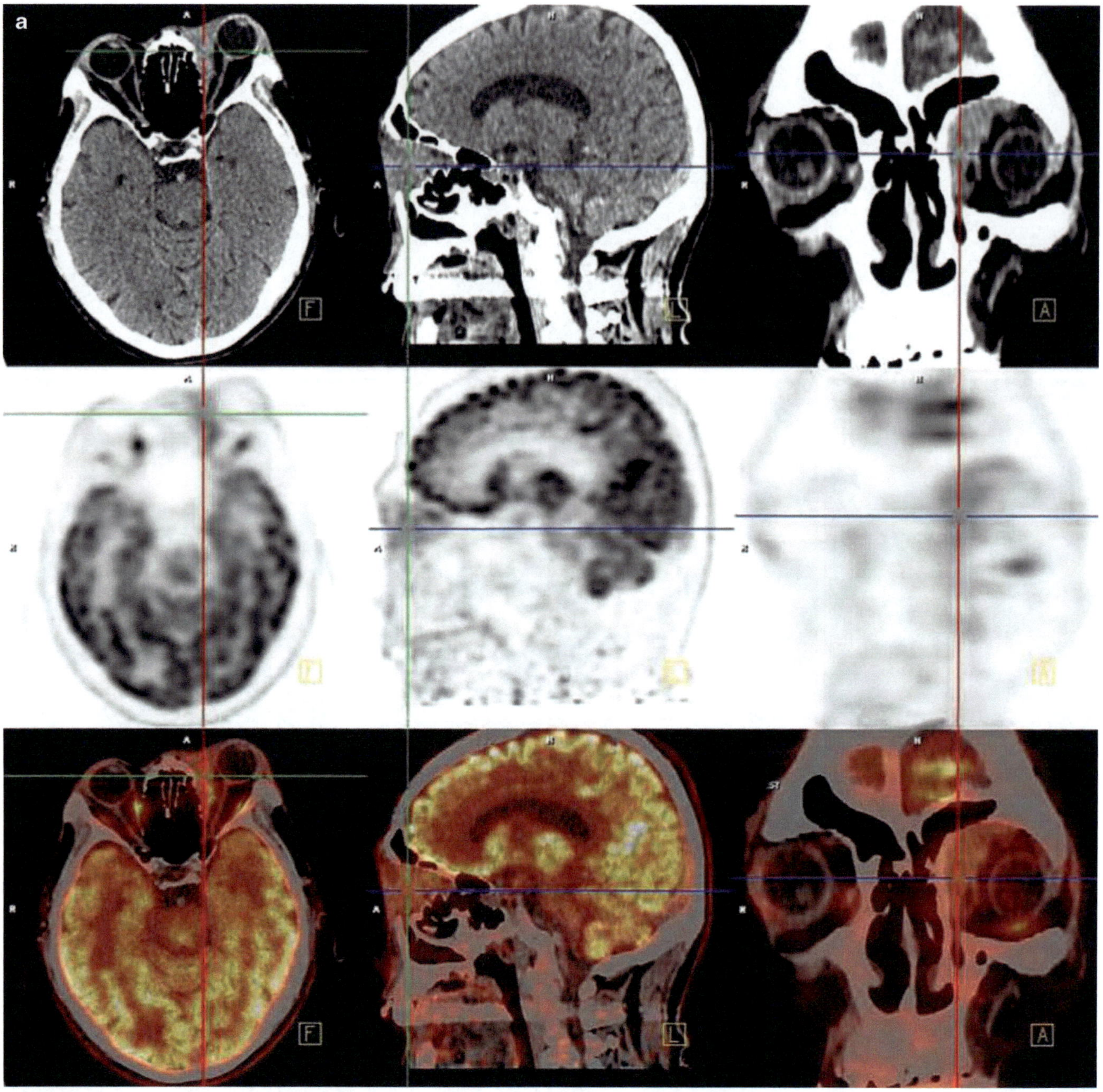

Fig. 14.4 FDG PET/CT images of diffuse large B-cell lymphoma of the left orbit. (**a**) Cross section, sagittal plane, and coronal plane of PET, CT, and fusion images from top to bottom. (**b**) CT, PET, and fusion images of cross sections. The lower right image was the coronal plane of PET. The left eyeball was prominent, and there was a soft tissue mass (criss-cross) in the external intervertebral space of the left medial orbital muscle, with a maximum cross section of about 3.3 cm × 1.1 cm. The metabolic activity of the mass was significantly increased, with SUVmax of 16.7 (this case was provided by Dr. Xiuling Shen and Dr. Zhiming Yao from Beijing Hospital)

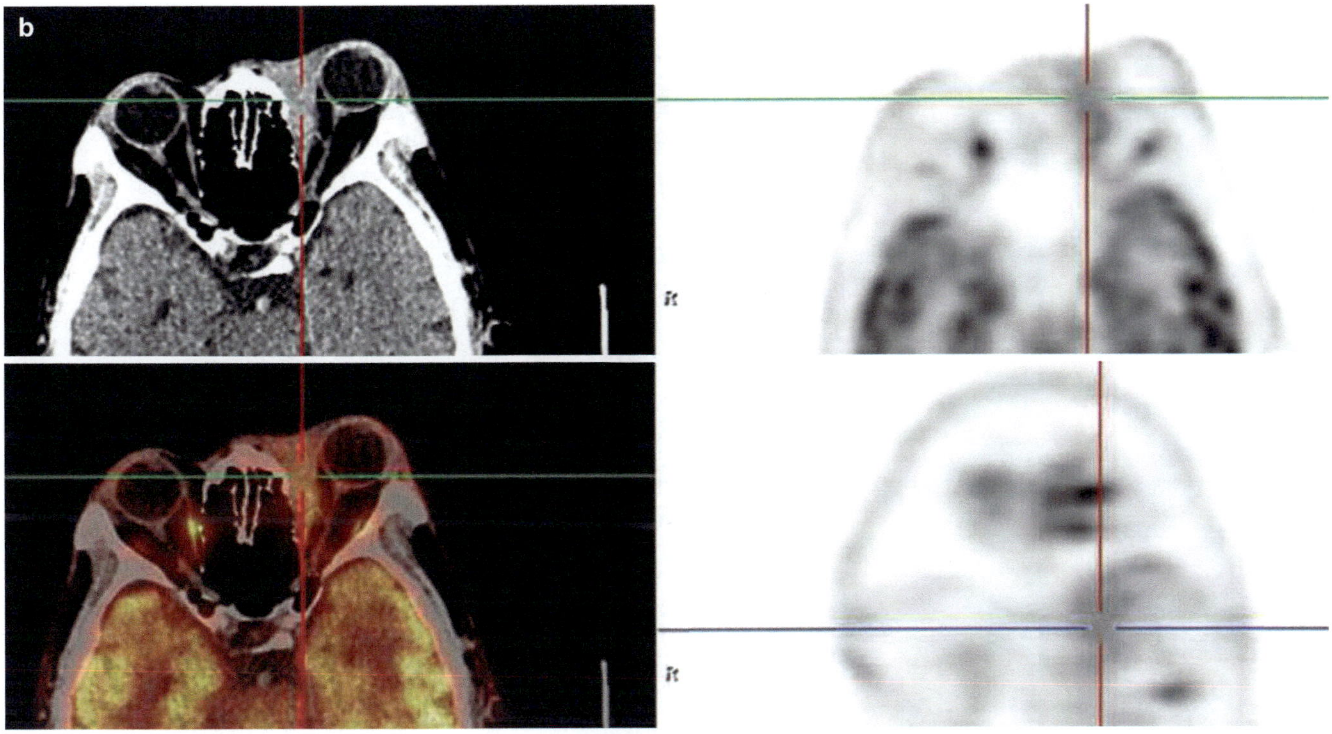

Fig. 14.4 (continued)

1.4 Differential Diagnosis

1.4.1 Inflammatory Pseudotumor

1. Similarities
   (a) Patients often present with proptosis.
   (b) Most of them are unilateral, and orbital space occupation is more common.
   (c) Increased uptake FDG in ocular lesions.
2. Key points for identification
   (a) Inflammatory pseudotumors often invade orbital adipose tissue and can form typical "mold" changes.
   (b) Ocular lymphoma usually shows as isolated soft tissue density nodules in the orbit that can invade surrounding tissues, but peripheral bone changes are relatively rare, and some patients with ocular lymphoma can be identified with involvement of other parts of the body (Fig. 14.5).

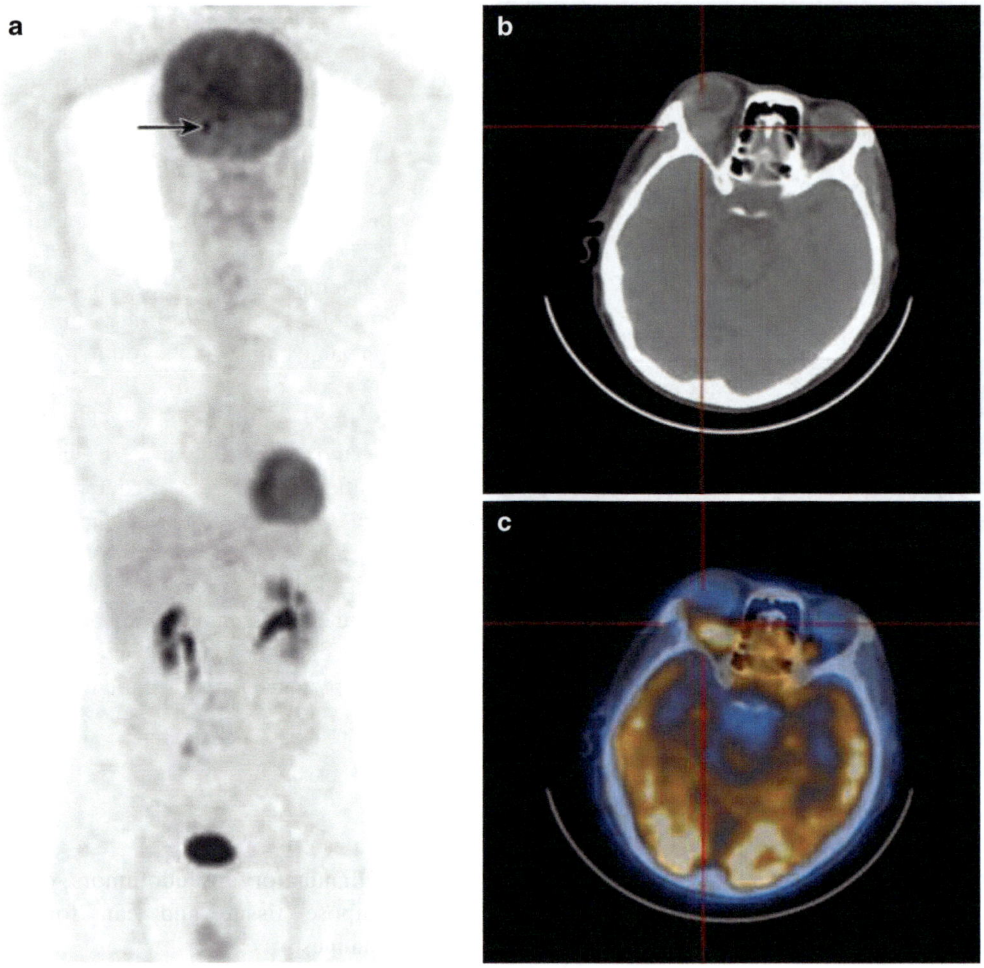

Fig. 14.5 PET/CT images of inflammatory pseudotumor of the right orbit. The patient was a 54-year-old male with right eye swelling for more than half a month: (**a**) FDG PET MIP image showed hypermetabolic nodules (black arrow) of the patient's right eye. (**b**) Cross-sectional CT image showed that the right eyeball was slightly protruding; soft tissue density nodules were visible behind the right eyeball, involving the right lacrimal gland; the adjacent eye muscle thickened; the right eye thimble was intact; and no obvious abnormalities were observed in the adjacent bone (criss-cross). (**c**) Cross-sectional PET/CT fusion images showed intense FDG uptake in nodules, with SUVmax of 12.8 (criss-cross). Inflammatory pseudotumor mostly occurs in one eye, and patients may present with proptosis, and some patients may have typical "mold" changes. The differential diagnosis between inflammatory pseudotumor and ocular lymphoma needs to be combined with the patient's clinical examination and laboratory results, and biopsy is still needed to confirm the diagnosis

1.4.2 Ocular Metastatic Tumor

1. Similarities
   (a) Most of them are isolated soft tissue density nodules in the eye.
   (b) Multiple lesions in the whole body.
2. Key points for identification
   (a) Choroid involvement is more common in metastatic tumors of the eye, while in lymphoma of the eye, intraocular involvement is less common, and orbital tissue involvement is often.
   (b) Primary tumor from the esophagus, lung, breast, etc. found during systemic imaging can provide evidence for the differential diagnosis of ocular lymphoma and metastatic tumor.
   (c) Tumor markers, bone biopsy, and other clinical test results will be helpful to the diagnosis (Fig. 14.6).

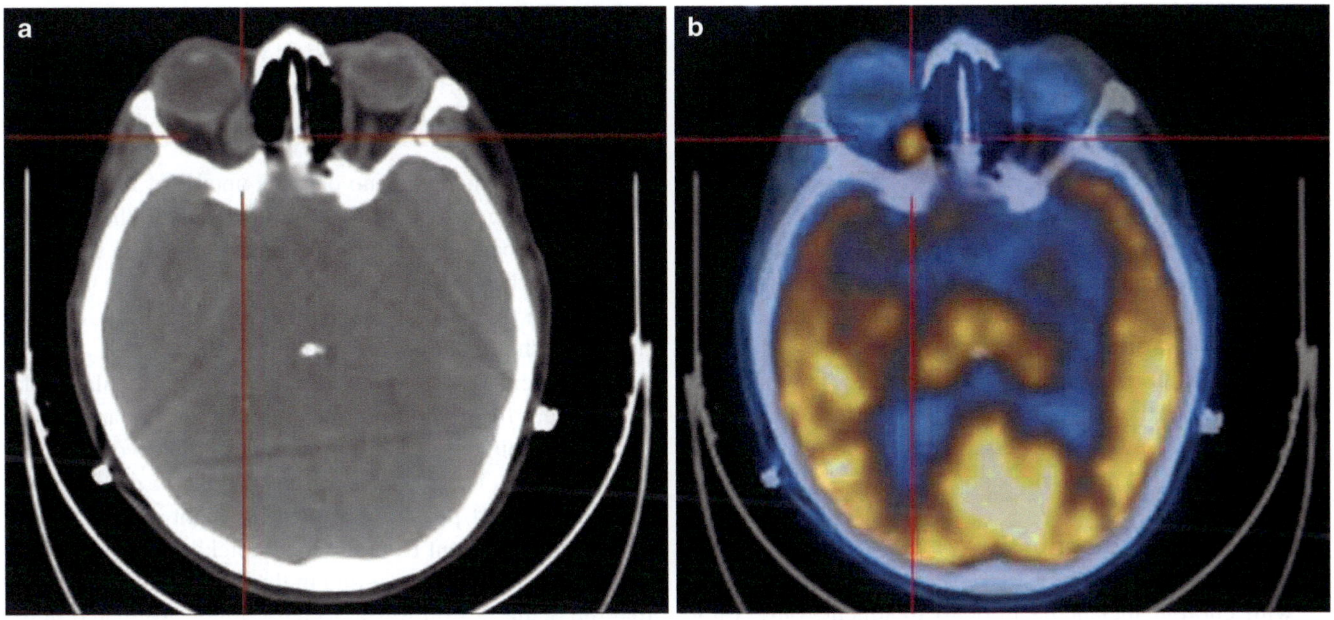

Fig. 14.6 PET/CT images of metastatic tumor of the right orbit. The patient was a 56-year-old female with biopsy of cervical lymph node showing metastatic carcinoma: (**a**) Cross-sectional CT image showing soft tissue density nodule in the right medial orbital wall. (**b**) Cross-sectional PET/CT fusion image showed increased FDG uptake and SUVmax was 6.9 in the nodule (criss-cross). PET/CT also showed mass with increased FDG uptake in the right lower lobe and focal increased FDG uptake in the lymph nodes, bone, lungs, liver, and other parts of the whole body, which was considered to be right lung cancer with multiple metastasis in the above sites. Results of immunohistochemistry later confirmed that it was a poorly differentiated adenocarcinoma deriving from lung tissue, indicating that PET/CT could be used to search for the primary site and stage of tumor

1.5 Summary

Ocular lymphoma is one of the most common malignant neoplastic lesions in the orbit, which tends to occur in middle-aged and elderly patients. The clinical manifestations of patients are associated with infiltration of the structure with lymphoma. Patients often present with orbital soft tissue mass; the degree of increased FDG uptake in the ocular lymphoma lesion depends on the pathological type of lymphoma. It is necessary to distinguish ocular lymphoma from inflammatory pseudotumor or metastatic tumor of the eye.

2 Choroidal Melanoma

2.1 Clinical Overview

Choroidal melanoma is the most common intraocular malignant tumor in adults, mostly occurring in middle-aged and elderly people, accounting for about 5% of all melanomas. There are no obvious gender difference and no obvious heritability, and it is more common in Caucasians. Choroidal melanoma is more common in one eye, while it is less common in both eyes. According to the 1980 WHO standard, choroidal melanoma can be classified into four types – spindle cell type (A, B), epithelioid cell type, mixed type, and other types. Clinically, spindle cell type is more common.

Common clinical symptoms include visual loss, pain, photopsia, floaters, etc. Some patients have no obvious symptoms. The treatment of choroidal melanoma is based on tumor location, extent of involvement, size, and systemic status. Pupillary thermotherapy is usually applied to the treatment of small choroidal melanoma. For small tumors without melanin, photodynamic therapy is often used. For medium-size tumors, radiotherapy, local tumor resection, or enucleation of the eyeball can be selected. Large choroidal melanoma is often treated through enucleation of the eyeball. However, the mortality rate of the disease is high, even if the patients are excised without definite metastasis, with 5-year mortality rate as high as 17–53%. It is easy for tumors to metastasize to the whole body through blood flow, and liver metastasis is relatively common. The metastasis rate of 5-year and 10-year survival rate is 25% and 35%.

2.2 PET/CT Diagnostic Points

2.2.1 General Diagnosis

1. It tends to occur in the population aged from 40 to 50 years old and rarely in children or elderly people over 70 years old.
2. The disease mostly occurs in one single eye.
3. It usually occurs in the posterior pole of the eyeball.
4. It is usually manifested by gradual decrease in vision.

2.2.2 CT Diagnostic Points

1. Slightly higher-density protuberance of the posterior extremity of the eyeball in mushroom form.
2. There is a semi-circular detachment of the retina on one or both sides of a partial lesion.

2.2.3 FDG PET Diagnostic Points

1. Reedy et al. performed FDG PET/CT scan in patients with choroid melanoma prior to treatment; only 14/50 patients' PET showed increased FDG uptake in tumors (SUVmax $\geq$ 2. 5). The tumor detection rates by FDG PET were 33.3% and 75.0% in the tumors with stage T_2 and in tumor with stage T_3 by AJCC, respectively, and that is 0% in the tumors with stage T_1.
2. A research on 14 cases of choroidal melanoma conducted by Faia et al. indicated that the mean SUVmax of lesions was 3.7 and the SUVmax of tumors was positively correlated with the thickness and the maximum base diameter of tumors. The SUVmax was higher in focal necrosis and mixed cell melanoma.

2.3 Typical Cases

Case 1: A 40-year-old male patient presented with blindness in his right eye for 1 week. Pathology: Choroid melanoma (Fig. 14.7)

Reminder: There was no obvious uptake of FDG in choroidal melanoma, so attention should be paid to the differentiation from benign lesions, and MRI examination should be combined when necessary.

Case 2: A 53-year-old patient presented with vision decline in the right eye for 2 months (Fig. 14.8).

Reminder: This is another type of typical ocular melanoma, i.e., focal intense FDG uptake in the melanoma lesions, although this manifestation is similar to ocular metastatic tumor. The mushroom-like nodule of ocular melanoma in the left posterior wall of the right eyeball of this patient was different from the focal thick lesion of metastasis. No other lesion was found in the body, which supported that the ocular lesion was a primary tumor originated in the right eye.

Case 3: A 68-year-old male patient presented with progressive vision decline in the left eye for more than 4 months (Fig. 14.9).

Reminder: This case was not easy to be distinguished from metastatic tumor, but there was no previous history of tumor, and no signs of tumor outside the eye could be seen by PET systemic imaging in this case, which did not support the diagnosis of metastasis.

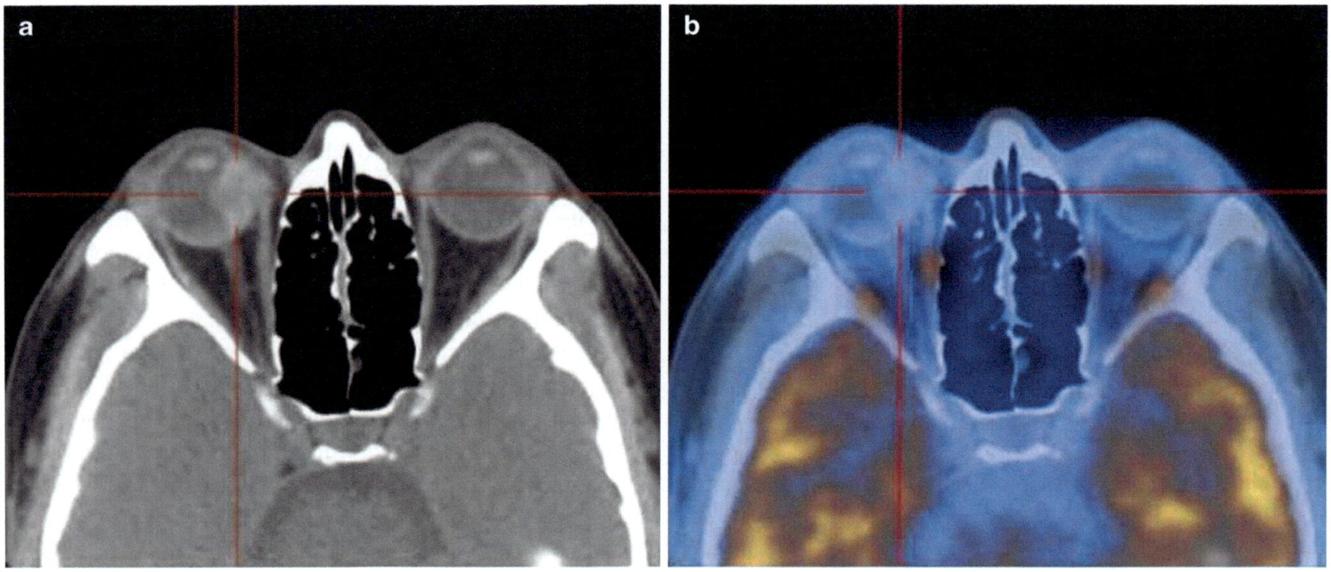

Fig. 14.7 PET/CT images of choroidal melanoma on the right side. (**a**) CT image showed a slightly denser nodule in the left posterior wall of the right eyeball protruding toward the eyeball. (**b**) PET/CT fusion image showed no increased FDG uptake in the lesion (criss-cross)

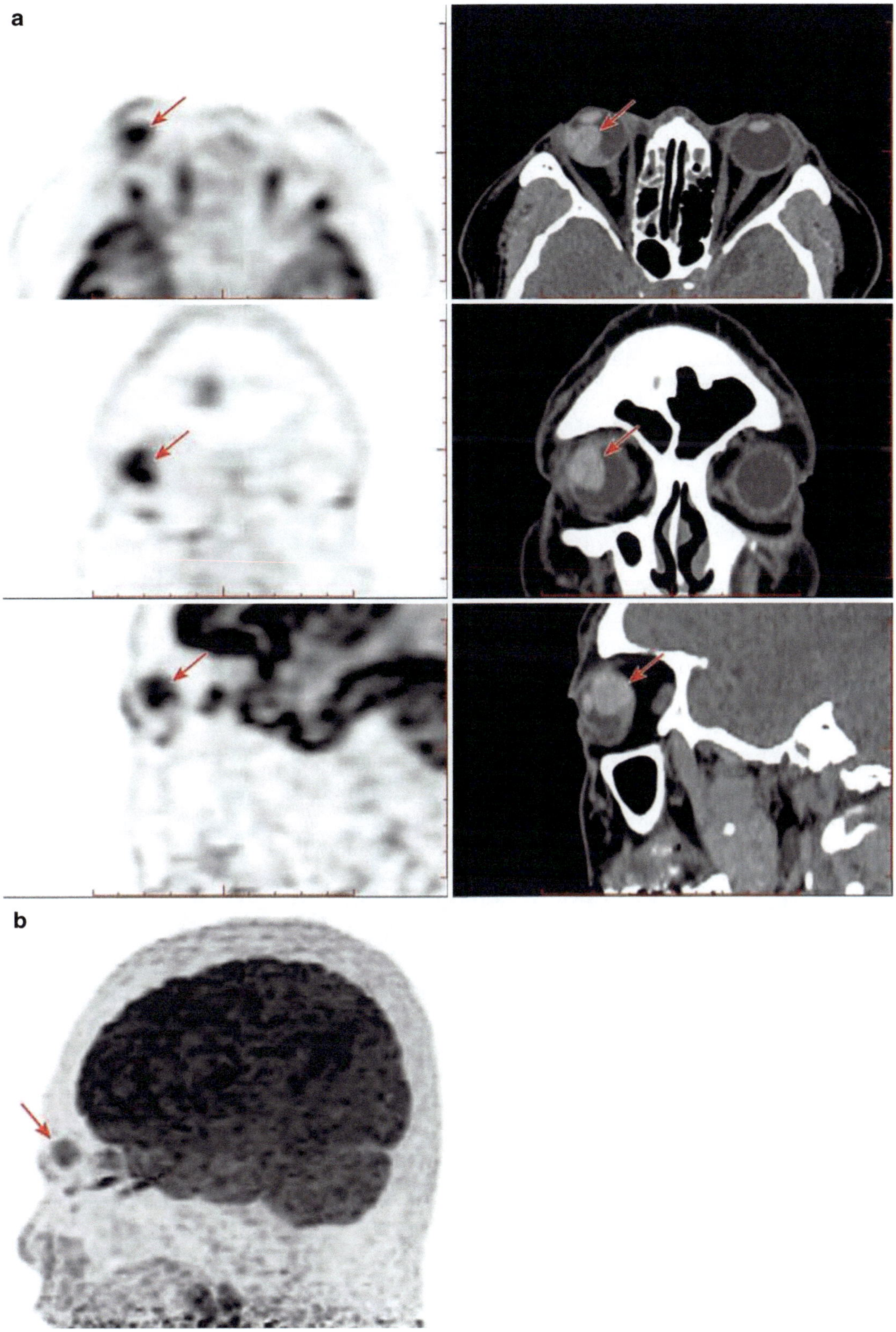

Fig. 14.8 FDG PET/CT images of melanoma of the right eye. (**a**) CT and PET cross-sectional images were presented in the upper row, CT and PET coronal plane images in the middle row, and CT and PET sagittal plane images in the lower row. The melanoma of the posterior wall of the left eyeball at the temporal side of the eye showed a mushroom shape mass with a high density and clear boundaries; PET showed increased FDG uptake in the mass (red arrow), with SUVmax of 11.1. (**b**) PET MIP lateral image of the brain (Provided by Dr. Congxia Chen and Dr. Zhiming Yao from Beijing Hospital)

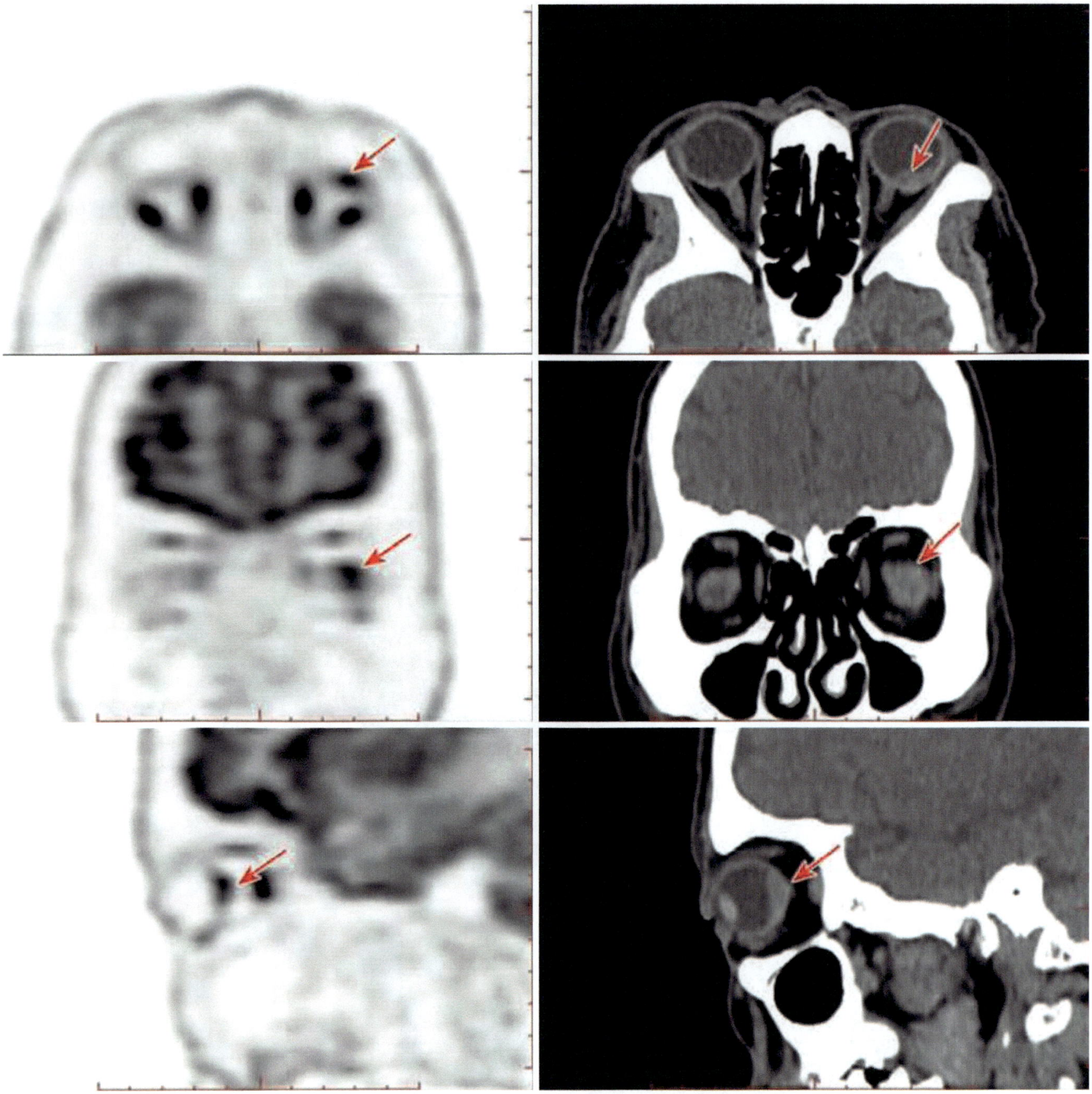

Fig. 14.9 FDG PET/CT images of melanoma of the left eye. CT and PET cross-sectional images were presented in the upper row, CT and PET coronal plane images in the middle row, and CT and PET sagittal plane images in the lower row. A nodule with slightly high density and clear boundaries was seen in the posterior wall of the left eyeball at the temporal side, with intense FDG uptake and SUVmax of 9.2 (red arrow) (Provided by Dr. Congxia Chen and Dr. Zhiming Yao from Beijing Hospital)

2.4 Rare Cases

The patient, a 65-year-old woman, presented with progressive vision decline in her right eye. Pathology: Right breast cancer with ipsilateral axillary lymph node metastasis and right eye choroid melanoma (Fig. 14.10)

Reminder: Patients with dual cancer are relatively rare. In these patients, attention should be paid to distinguish whether the eye lesions are metastatic tumors or other types of primary tumors. FDG uptake of choroidal metastatic tumors is often higher than that of melanoma, which can be helpful for diagnosis.

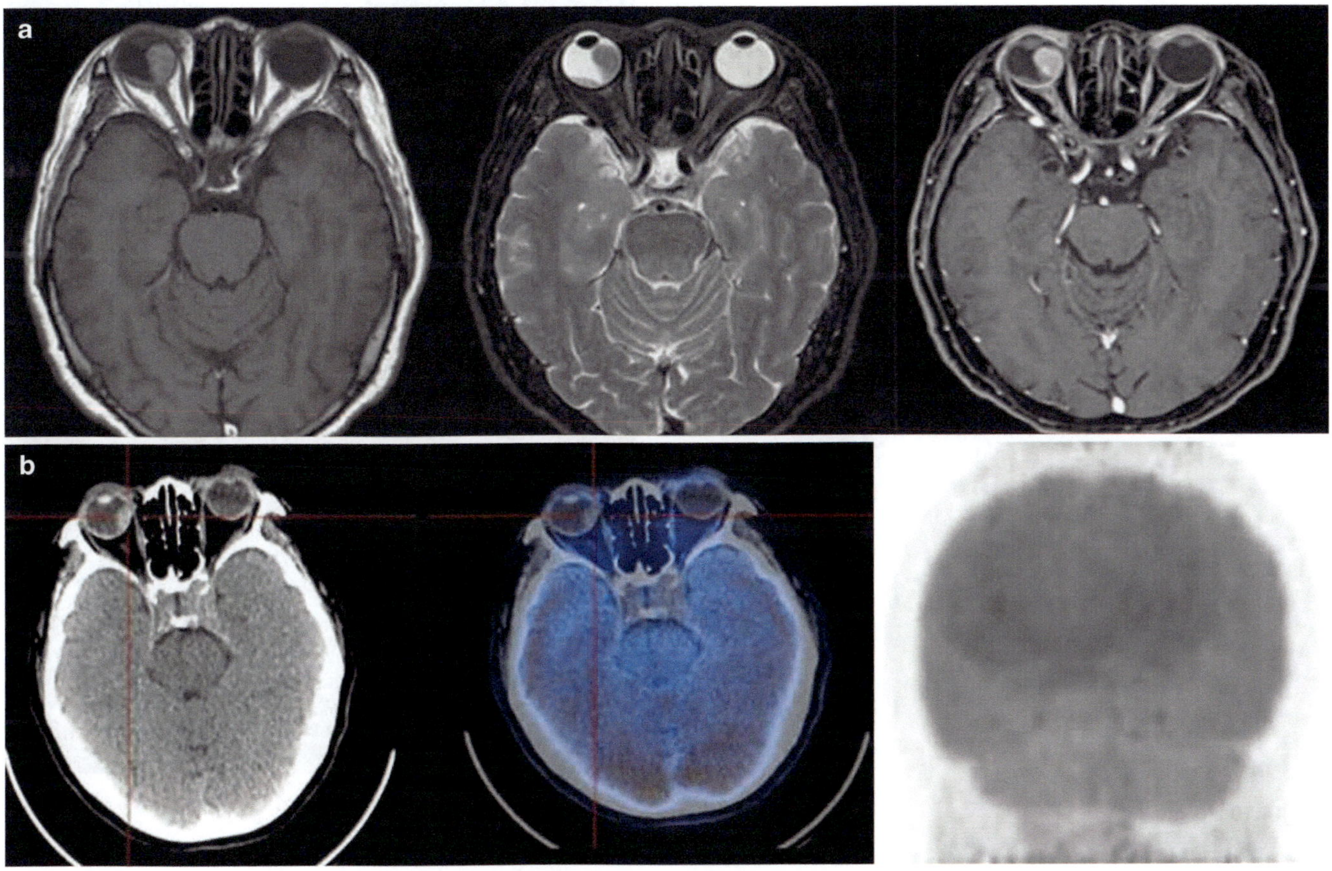

Fig. 14.10 PET/CT images of choroidal melanoma on the right side. (**a**) Cross-sectional MR image. T_1 and T_2 MRI slight short signal nodules in the left posterior wall of the right eyeball, which protruded into the vitreous body, and the enhanced MRI showed uneven and obvious enhancement in the nodule. (**b**) PET/CT image in cross section of the eyeball and PET MIP image of the head. No increased FDG uptake in slightly high-density nodules (criss-cross) in the left posterior wall of the right eyeball. (**c**) PET/CT images of the breast cross section and PET MIP images of the body. Intense FDG uptake in soft tissue density nodules in the outer upper quadrant of the right breast (black long arrow and criss-cross on MIP figure), with its SUVmax being 20.7; the nodule was confirmed breast cancer. Increased FDG uptake in multiple lymph nodes in the right axillary (black short arrow) with SUVmax being 5.7–11.4, which was considered as lymph node metastasis from breast cancer

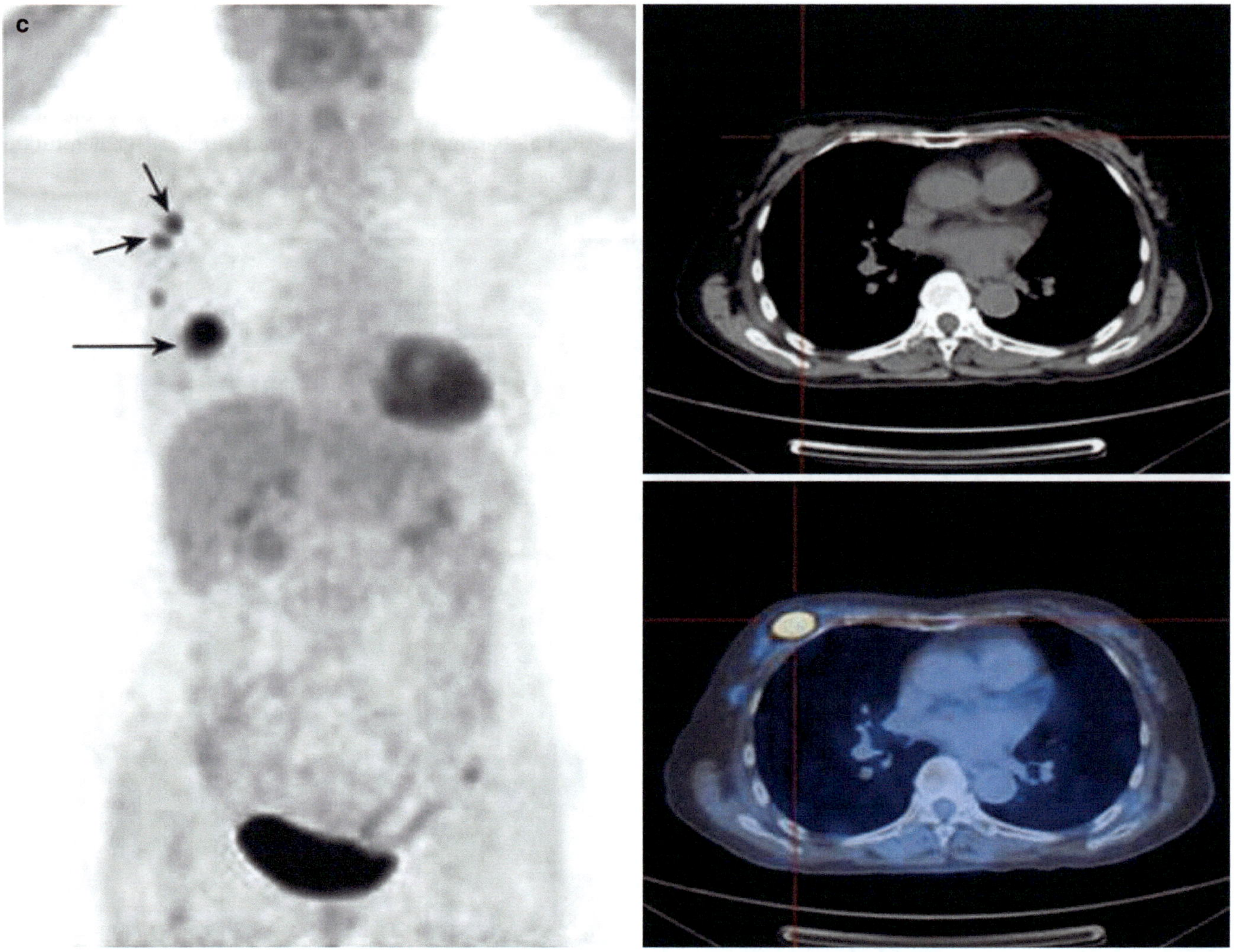

Fig. 14.10 (continued)

2.5 Differential Diagnosis

Choroidal metastatic tumor:

1. Similarities
   (a) The patient may present with progressive vision decline.
   (b) Most cases are unilateral.
2. Key points for identification
   (a) Choroidal melanoma is often manifested as slightly high-density nodules in the posterior pole of the eyeball, and usually there is no obviously increased FDG uptake in small lesions of melanoma. However, it is difficult to distinguish choroidal melanoma with increased FDG uptake from metastatic tumor with increased FDG uptake by PET alone.
   (b) Choroidal metastatic tumor often presents as soft tissue density protuberance in the posterior wall of the eyeball, accompanied by obviously increased FDG uptake. FDG PET/CT is a good tool to detect both primary tumor and metastasis out of the eye; this is very helpful for differential diagnosis (Fig. 14.11).
   (c) Reminder: Ocular metastatic tumors often metastasize to choroid through blood circulation, and about 50% of patients with choroid metastatic tumors cannot be identified for the primary lesions. However, the application of PET/CT can improve the diagnosis rate of the primary lesion of choroid metastatic tumors and help in making the early diagnosis of the patients.

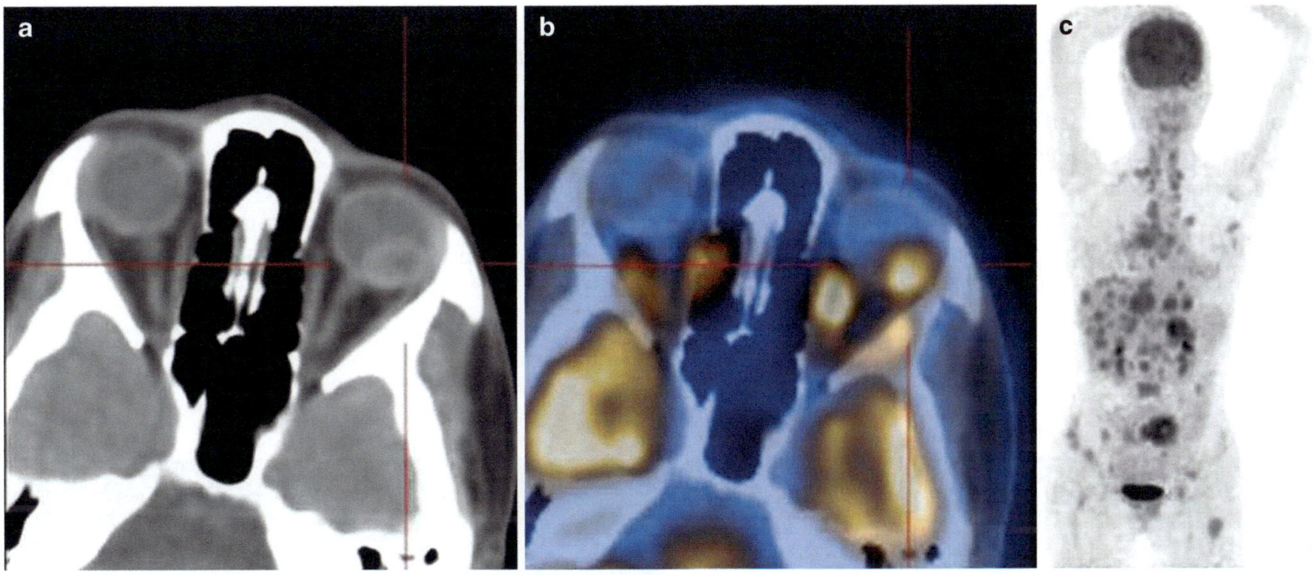

Fig. 14.11 PET/CT images of the left choroid metastatic tumor. The patient was a 31-year-old female who developed cough and phlegm white with occasional bright red blood and fever at night after catching cold half a month ago: (**a**) Cross section of CT image showed annular soft tissue density nodules in the left eye. (**b**) Cross section of PET/CT fusion image showed annular increase of FDG uptake in the lesion, with SUVmax of 8.4, and the central density of the annular lesion was low, and there was no obvious uptake of FDG, suggesting that liquefactive necrosis might occur in the center of the ocular lesion. (**c**) FDG PET MIP image also found multiple hypermetabolic lesions in the right hilum of the lung and other parts of the body, suggesting right lung cancer with multiple metastases. Histopathological examination confirmed lung adenocarcinoma. Choroidal metastatic tumors are often associated with significant uptake of FDG (criss-cross) and can be distinguished from choroidal melanoma

2.6 Summary

Choroidal melanoma is the most common intraocular malignant neoplastic lesion in adults. It tends to occur in middle-aged and elderly people, mostly in a single eye, and often shows slightly high-density nodules in the posterior pole of the eyeball. The FDG uptake of lesions may be associated with the size and pathological type of lesions. Attention should be paid to the differentiation with choroid metastatic tumor during diagnosis and to the presence of liver metastasis.

3 Retinoblastoma

3.1 Clinical Overview

Retinoblastoma is the most common intraocular malignant tumor among infants and young children, with no significant gender difference. Its incidence decreases with age, and most children are diagnosed before the age of 4. Forty percent of retinoblastomas are of genotype and autosomal dominant inheritance. The onset of this kind of children is early, and both eyes are involved for most of them. Sixty percent of retinoblastomas are non-genetic, and the onset is late, and the onset is mainly in one eye. A very small number of children with pineal tumors may be associated with trilateral retinoblastoma.

Based on the growth mode of the tumor, retinoblastoma can be classified into endophytic type, exogenous type, mixed type, diffuse type, and mossy type, among which mixed type is the most common type clinically. Enucleation was the only and standard treatment for retinoblastoma in the nineteenth and twentieth century. There are many current therapeutic alternatives, including radiotherapy, chemotherapy, enucleation, cryotherapy, laser therapy, thermotherapy, sclera application therapy, etc. In recent years, new therapies such as immunotherapy and gene therapy have also been emerging. Through early diagnosis and comprehensive treatment, the survival rate of children can reach 90–95%.

3.2 PET/CT Diagnostic Points

3.2.1 General Diagnosis

1. Patients are mainly infants and children.
2. It can be unilateral or bilateral, and very few patients can have pineal region involved.
3. Patients may have "white pupils."

3.2.2 CT Diagnostic Points

1. Retinoblastoma usually presents as a mass protrusion from the posterior of the eye into the vitreous body, which can be in plaque or half-moon shape.
2. Flake necrosis or plaque and speckle calcification can be seen in the lesion.

3.2.3 FDG PET Diagnostic Points

FDG uptake occurs in ocular lesions of most IRRS stage III patients. Studies have shown that PET has limited diagnostic value for retinoblastoma, but can reduce the missed diagnosis of metastases outside the head.

3.3 Typical Cases

The female patient was 6 years old and presented with gradual vision decline in the right eye for more than half a year (Fig. 14.12).

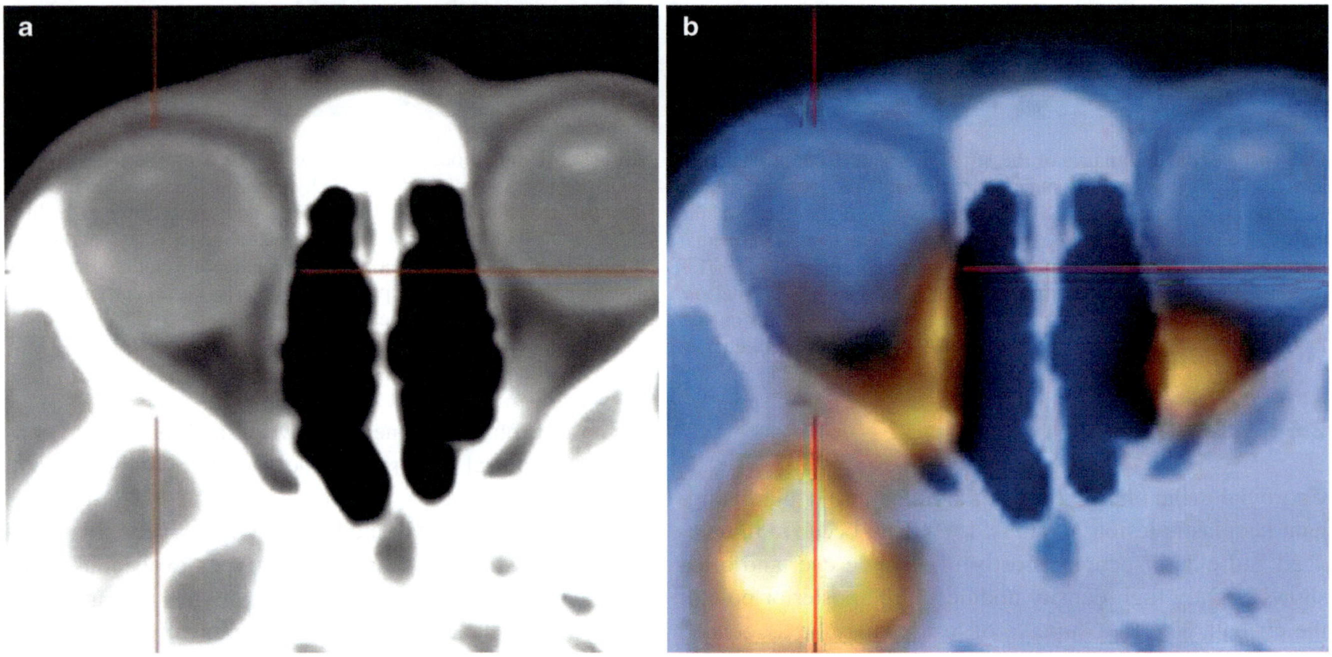

Fig. 14.12 PET/CT images of the right retinoblastoma. (**a**) The cross-sectional CT image showed heterogeneous nodules in the right eyeball, which were dominated by soft tissue density and speckled calcification. (**b**) Cross-sectional PET/CT fusion images showed mild FDG uptake in the edges of the above lesions (criss-cross), with SUVmax of 1.6–1.9

Reminder: the age of the patient and the typical calcification in the lesion can help the diagnosis and differential diagnosis.

3.4 Differential Diagnosis

Persistent hyperplastic primary vitreous (PHPV):

1. Similarities
   (a) It tends to occur among infants and young children.
   (b) Children may present with "white pupils."
2. Key points for identification
   (a) PHPV usually occurs in one eye, but retinoblastoma can be monocular or binocular.
   (b) PHPV can be manifested as reduced eyeball, and the mixed type of anterior and posterior eyeball is more common. However, retinoblastoma is usually manifested as enlargement of the eyeball, often occurring in the posterior part of the eyeball, and calcification lesions can be observed in some lesions.

3.5 Summary

Retinoblastoma is the most common malignant tumor in the eyes of infants and young children. It is usually diagnosed before the age of 4 and usually occurs in the posterior of the eye. It can be accompanied by plaque and speck-like calcification, and most IRSS stage III patients have FDG uptake in ocular lesions. Retinoblastoma should be distinguished from the persistent hyperplastic primary vitreous which often occurs in infants and young children and often presents as "white pupil."

4 Intraocular Tuberculosis

4.1 Clinical Overview

Intraocular uvea is rich in blood vessels with slow blood flow, and mycobacterium tuberculosis is easy to be retained in this area and produce infection. After mycobacterium tuberculosis invades the eye tissue, it can directly invade the uvea or cause uveitis and other ocular lesions through the immune response. It can also invade the eye tissue through blood transmission in the primary or secondary infection stage and induce hypersensitive ocular inflammation. Clinical manifestations are low fever, night sweats, fatigue, weight loss, and other symptoms. The disease is chronic and latent, which can invade any tissues in the eye. The most common clinical diseases are uveitis, retinitis, and so on.

4.2 PET/CT Diagnostic Points

1. CT and MRI diagnostic points Tuberculosis in different parts of the eye is mostly manifested as local inflammatory infiltration, and pathological changes of tuberculosis are found in tissue biopsy. CT lesions also resemble tumors in morphology. The diagnosis of intraocular tuberculosis should be closely combined with clinical symptoms, chest imaging manifestations, and tuberculin test.
2. PET/CT diagnostic points Increased FDG uptake is observed in active tuberculosis lesion, and a systemic PET/CT examination of tuberculosis lesion in the lungs or elsewhere is helpful in the diagnosis.

4.3 Typical Cases

Case 1: A 22-year-old male patient presented with progressive vision decline in the left eye for 4 months and no other symptoms (Fig. 14.13).

Reminder: It was difficult to distinguish this case from malignant lesions, sarcoidosis, etc. Finally, mycobacterium tuberculosis was found in sputum examination and confirmed, and the symptoms were relieved after anti-tuberculosis treatment.

Case 2: A 17-year-old female patient presented with swelling of the left eyelid 2 months ago without obvious cause, without red eye pain and photophobia tearing. Pathology: Tuberculous granulomatous lesions (Fig. 14.14)

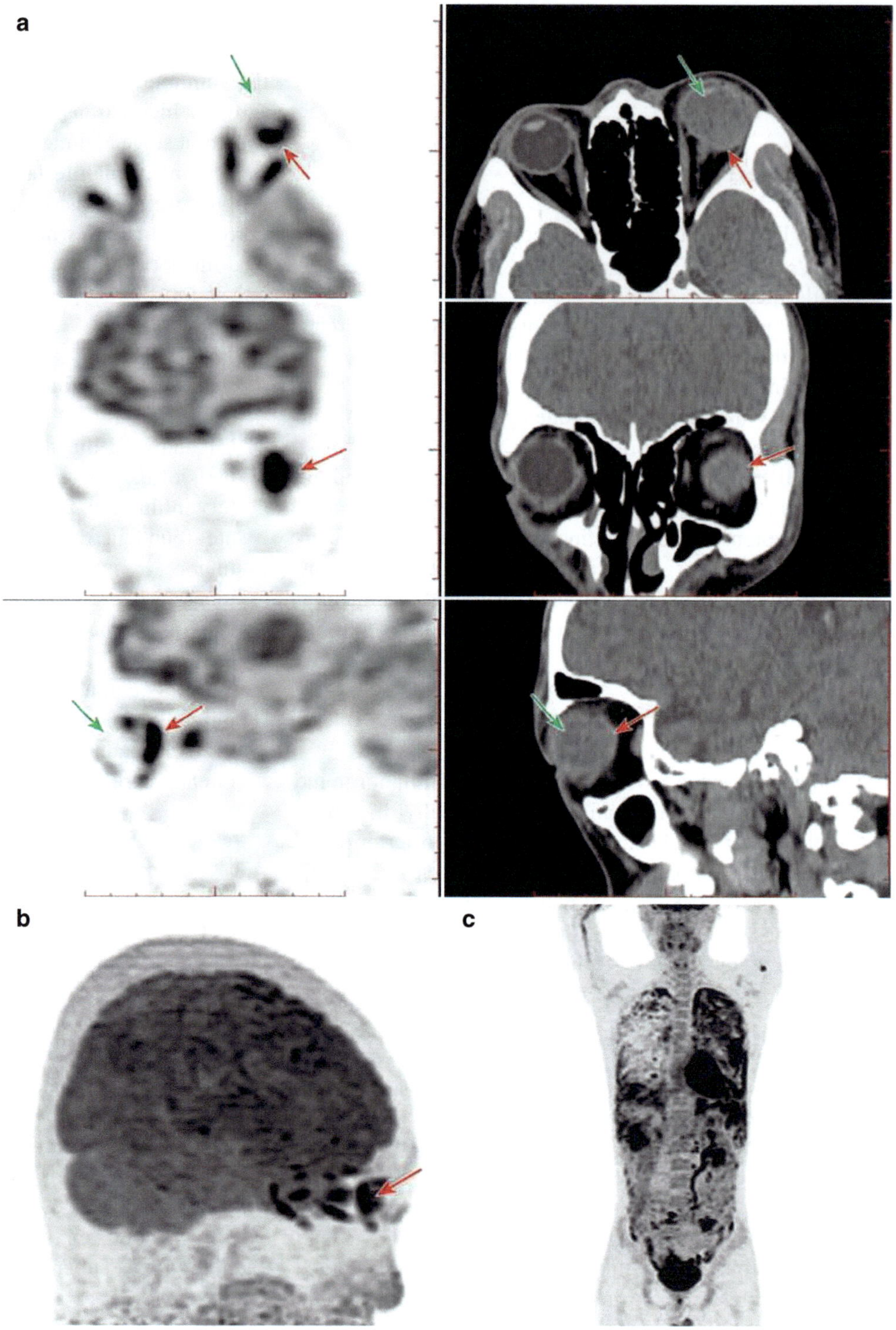

Fig. 14.13 FDG PET/CT images in a patient with tuberculosis in the left eye, brain, lymph node, lung, pleura and peritoneum, kidney and bone. (**a**) CT and PET cross-sectional images were presented in the upper row, CT and PET coronal plane images in the middle row, and CT and PET sagittal plane images in the lower row: the vitreous opacity in the right eye sphere was seen with increased density and unclear boundary. The annular inhomogeneous FDG uptake in the posterior wall was significantly increased (red arrow), SUVmax was 19.5, and FDG uptake in the anterior opaque vitreous body was not abnormal (green arrow). (**b**) FDG PET MIP lateral image of the head: inhomogeneous increased FDG uptake in lesion in the left eye (red arrow). (**c**) Anterior PET MIP images of the whole body: multiple lesions with intense FDG uptake in many organs were shown, pleura and peritoneum lesions was especially numerous (provided by Dr. Congxia Chen and Dr. Zhiming Yao from Beijing Hospital)

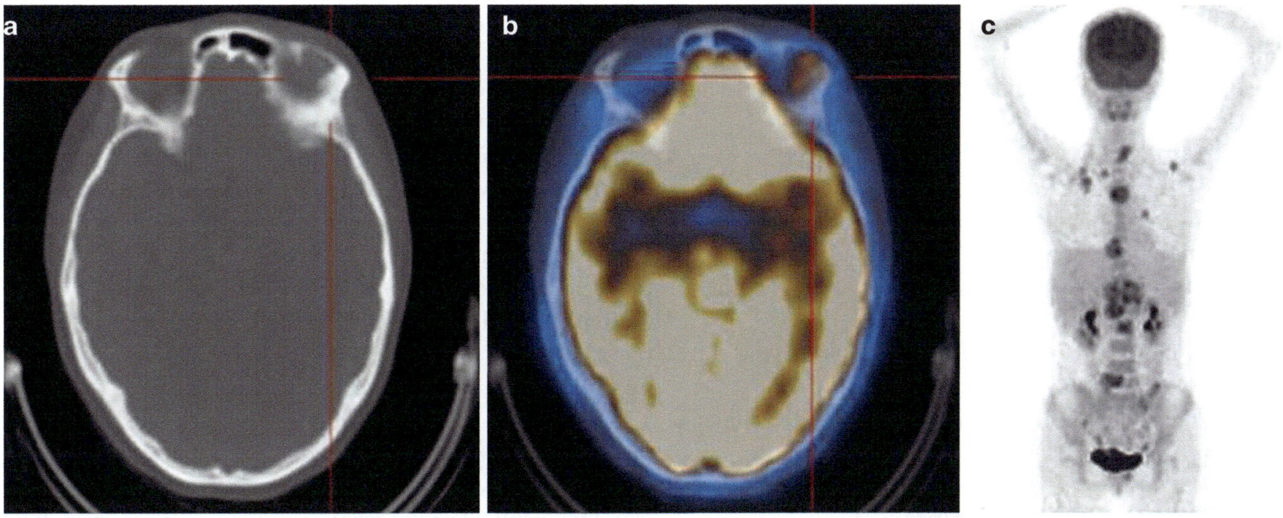

Fig. 14.14 PET/CT images of tuberculosis granulomatous lesions. (**a**) CT image. (**b**) PET/CT fusion image. (**c**) PET MIP image. Soft tissue density shadow in the left lateral orbit, with increased FDG uptake and SUVmax 5.5–5.9 and 2.2 cm × 1.7 cm in size (criss-cross). Multiple small nodules were seen in both lungs with low metabolism and multiple bone destruction throughout the body with high metabolism. PET was misdiagnosed as left orbital malignancy (lacrymal gland origin) with lung and multiple bone metastases

4.4 Summary

Intraocular tuberculosis is relatively rare, and diagnosis of tuberculosis by PET/CT alone is difficult. Diagnosis should be made after understanding well whole body PET/CT signs and clinical manifestations.

5 Intraocular Metastatic Tumors

5.1 Clinical Overview

Intraocular metastatic tumor is the most common malignant tumor of the eye, which refers to the metastasis and growth of malignant tumors originating in other parts of the body. Almost all malignant tumors in the human body may have intraocular metastasis, but due to the lack of lymphatic vessels in the orbit and ocular tissues, tumors mainly metastasize to the orbital soft tissue and uvea through blood. Moreover, as the ophthalmic artery branches at right angles with the internal carotid artery, the probability of metastasis of cancer embolus with blood flowing into the skull is higher than that of the intraocular artery. Therefore, it is generally believed that the incidence of intraocular metastatic tumor is very low, which has been reported abroad as 1/150000–1/130000. Clinical findings showed that about 2.3% of patients with cancer had intraocular metastasis, among which choroid was the most common site of metastasis, and its incidence was reported to be 0.01–12.00%. Clinical reports show that choroid metastatic tumor accounts for only 1% of intraocular tumors, but 81–88% of intraocular metastatic tumors.

Intraocular metastatic tumor is more common in lung cancer and breast cancer. As for the primary tumor lesion of eye metastases, breast cancer has been the most reported type in foreign countries, while lung cancer has been the most reported type in China. The patients are mostly 40–70 years old, and there is no significant difference in the ratio of male to female. About 1/3 of patients with intraocular metastatic tumor have no history of primary cancer when they visit the ophthalmology department. Therefore, if the relevant examination results do not match the characteristics of the primary tumor in the eye, metastatic tumor should be highly suspected, and lung and breast screening should be given emphasis.

Therapies of intraocular metastatic tumor include enucleation, radiotherapy, chemotherapy, endocrine therapy, etc., most of which tend to adopt conservative individual multidisciplinary comprehensive treatment. After treatment, the short-term visual acuity prognosis is better, but the life prognosis is very poor. The treatment is intended to improve the quality of life of patients with advanced cancer. The overall prognosis is associated with age, primary lesion, and metastasis of other organs in the body.

5.2 PET/CT Diagnostic Points

5.2.1 General Diagnostic Points

1. The patient has a history of cancer or primary tumor lesions found on PET/CT; most of the primary tumors are lung cancer, followed by breast cancer.
2. Most are accompanied by multiple metastatic tumors in other sites and/or lymph node metastases.

3. Intraocular metastases are more common in the posterior wall of the eyeball.
4. It can be binocular involvement and also can be single eye multi-focal distribution.

5.2.2 CT Diagnostic Points

1. Localized thickening of the wall of the eyeball (mostly seen in the posterior wall), which is flat or nodular in shape, with clear boundaries and uniform or slightly high density.
2. The larger metastatic tumor presents as a mass in the ocular wall.
3. Some patients are accompanied with retinal detachment and hemorrhage.

5.2.3 FDG PET Diagnostic Points

1. Corresponding to the same CT metastatic tumor, the local nodular metabolic activity of the eyeball is increased.
2. Due to partial volume effect, thin and small eye metastases show slightly higher local metabolic activity in fine strip and flake shape, which should be carefully compared with the contralateral healthy eyeball.
3. The FDG activity of the detached retina and the site of hemorrhage is usually normal.
4. Due to the fact that the high radiation uptake of brain tissue can cover the lesion, the lesion should be observed after the eyeball is placed in an appropriate position and the color level of the image is carefully adjusted.

5.3 Typical Cases

Case 1: A male patient, 32-year-old, blurred vision in his right eye for 1 month (Fig. 14.15)

Reminder: Whole body PET supported the hypothesis that the lesion with increased FDG uptake in the right eyeball is caused by lung cancer metastasis.

Case 2: Female patient, 50-year-old, a water-like shadow in her left eye for 3 months (Fig. 14.16)

Reminder: The whole body PET results supported the hypothesis that the increased metabolic activity of the left eyeball is caused by lung cancer metastasis.

Case 3: A 41-year-old female patient presented with blurred vision in her left eye for half a month (Fig. 14.17).

Reminder: Whole body PET results supported the hypothesis that ocular lesions were metastatic tumors from lung cancer.

Case 4: A 60-year-old male patient presented with left eye tearing and swelling for more than 1 month (Fig. 14.18).

Reminder: Body PET results supported the hypothesis that ocular lesions were metastatic tumors from esophageal cancer.

Case 5: A 50-year-old female patient presented with vision decline in the left eye for more than 1 month (Fig. 14.19).

Reminder: Body PET results supported the hypothesis that ocular lesions were metastatic tumors from breast cancer.

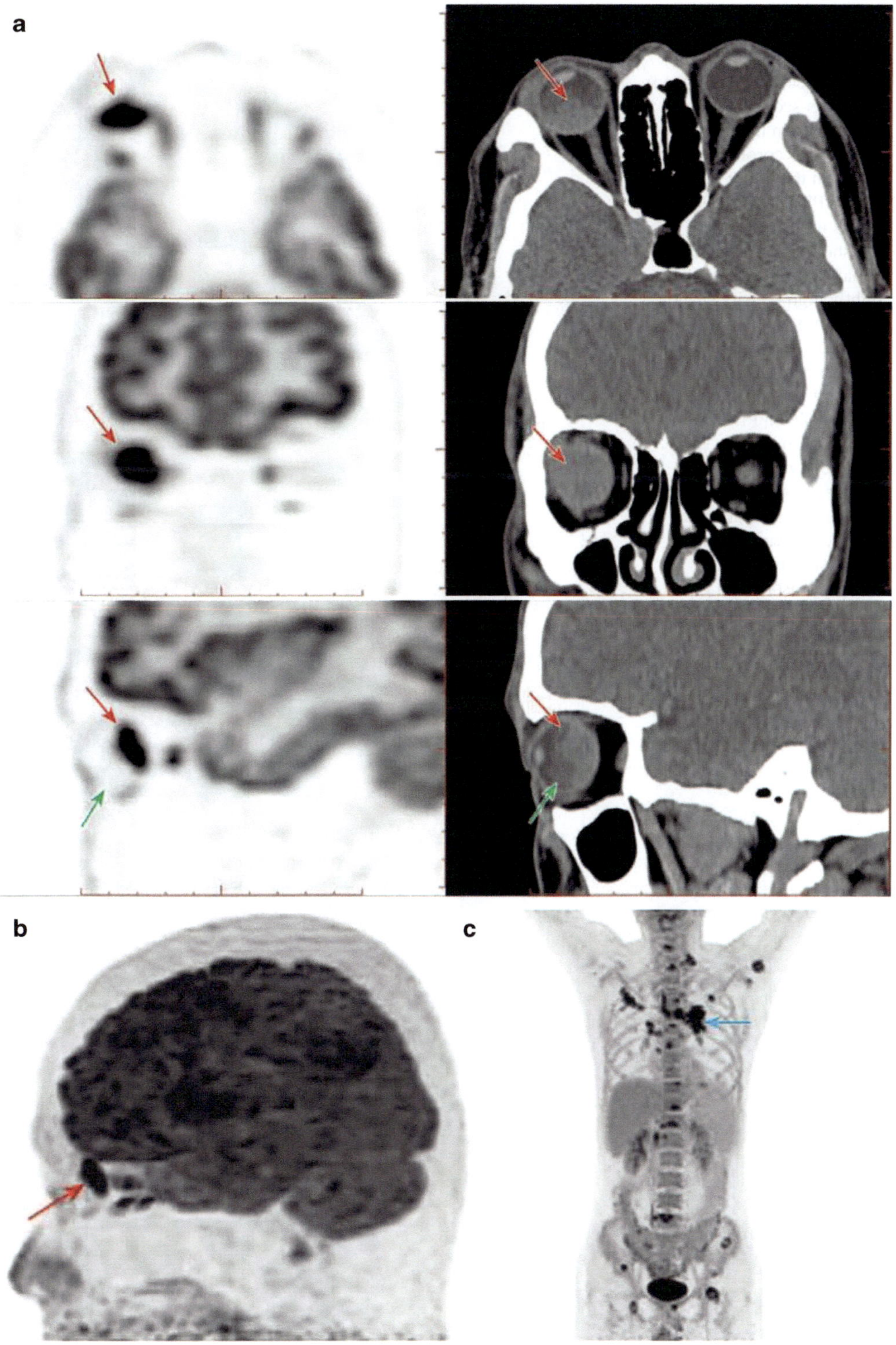

Fig. 14.15 FDG PET/CT images of metastatic tumor of the right eye of the patient with left lung cancer. (**a**) CT and PET cross-sectional images were shown in the upper row, CT and PET coronal plane images in the middle row, and CT and PET sagittal plane images in the lower row: Increased FDG uptake in irregular nodules with slightly high-density shadows on the posterior wall of the right eyeball with clear boundaries (red arrow); its SUVmax was 28.1. Vitreous opacity around the posterior wall of the right eye was seen without abnormal metabolic activity (green arrow). (**b**) FDG PET MIP lateral image of the head: A mass lesion with increased metabolic activity was seen in the right eyeball (red arrow). (**c**) Whole body PET MIP anterior image: PET MIP imaging showed typical left lung cancer (blue arrow), hilar mediastinal lymph node metastasis, and multiple distal metastasis; FDG uptakes in these malignant lesions were increased or intense

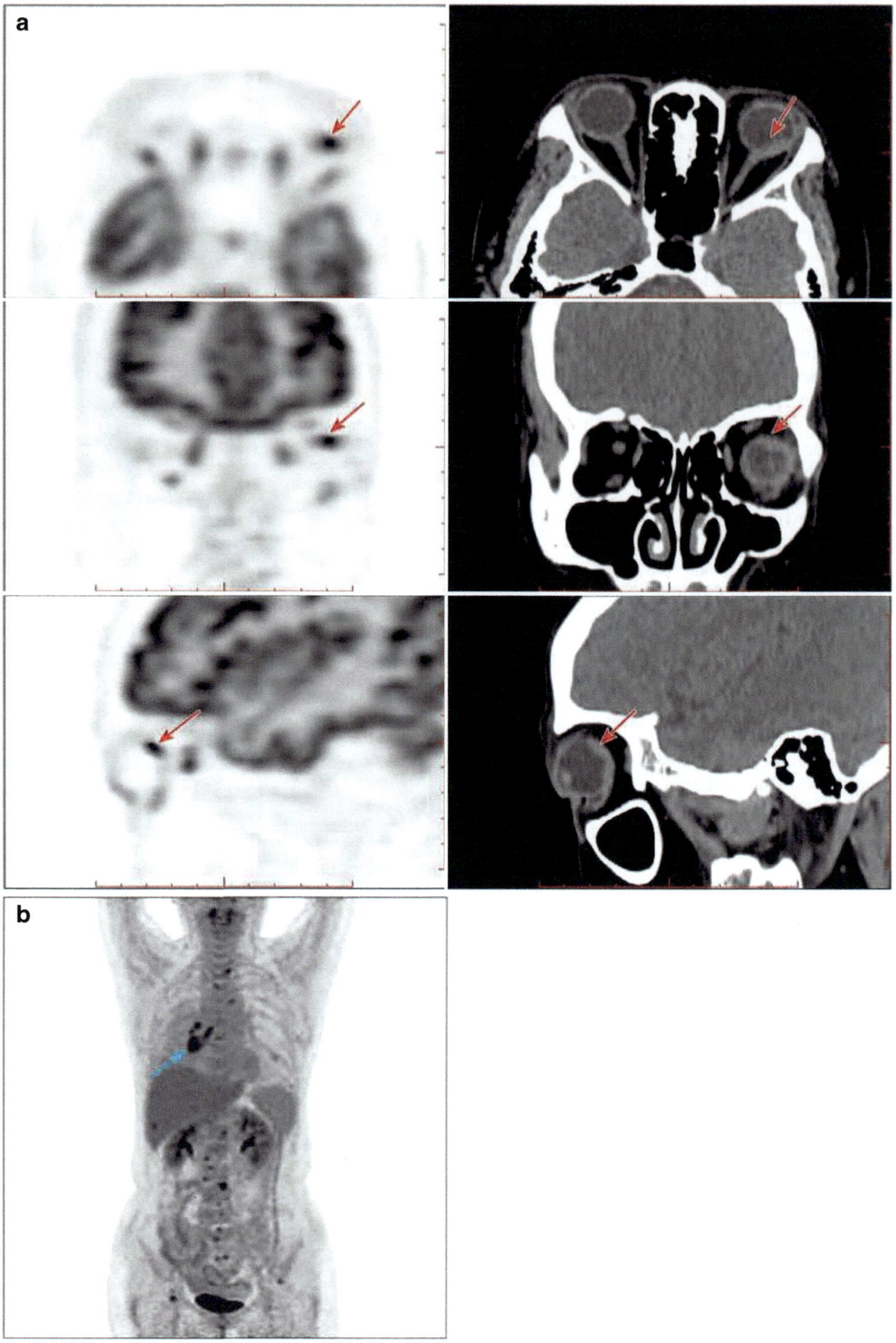

Fig. 14.16 FDG PET/CT images of metastasis in the left eye of the patient with right lung cancer. (**a**) CT and PET cross-sectional images were shown in the upper row, CT and PET coronal plane images in the middle row, and CT and PET sagittal plane images in the lower row: The metastatic tumor of the left eyeball showed a flattened, slightly high-density shadow (red arrow) on the posterior wall of the left eyeball in the lateral temporal with a clear boundary and focal increased FDG uptake on PET (red arrow, SUVmax 9.9). (**b**) Whole body PET MIP anterior image: typical right lung cancer (blue arrow), mediastinal lymph node metastasis, and multiple distant metastases on PET

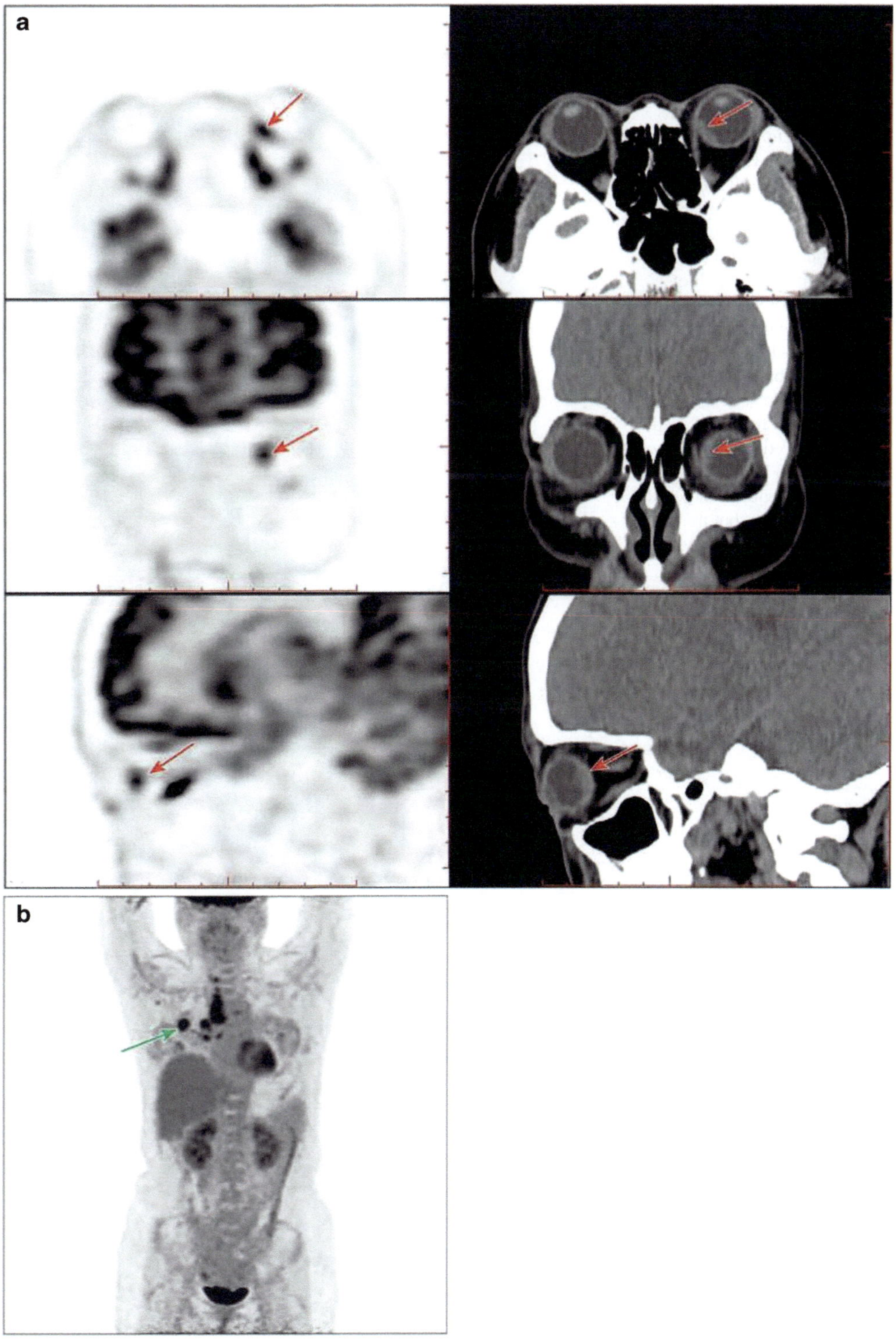

Fig. 14.17 FDG PET/CT images of metastases in the left eye of the patient with lung cancer and multiple lymph node metastasis. (**a**) CT and PET cross-sectional images were shown in the upper row, CT and PET coronal plane images in the middle row, and CT and PET sagittal plane images in the lower row: The posterior wall of the left eyeball was thickened with intense FDG uptake (red arrow, SUVmax 9.3). The lesion had a clear boundary. (**b**) Body PET MIP anterior images: right lung cancer was identified with intense FDG uptake (green arrow); metastatic tumor of the right lung and hilar mediastinal lymph node metastasis were easily observed in PET MIP image

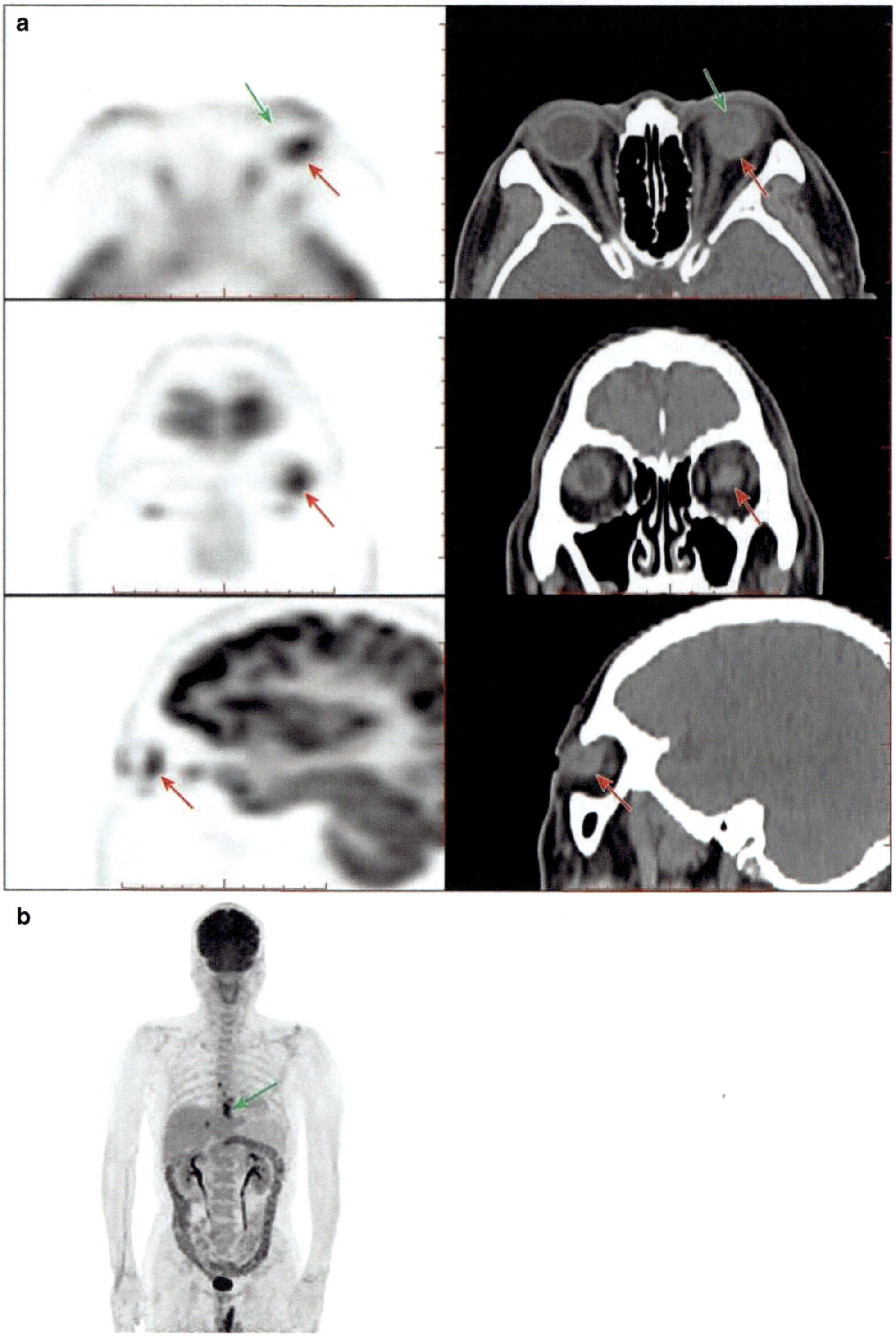

Fig. 14.18 FDG PET/CT images of esophageal carcinoma metastasizing to the left eye. (**a**) CT and PET cross-sectional images were shown in the upper row, CT and PET coronal plane images in the middle row, and CT and PET sagittal plane images in the lower row: Metastatic tumor of the left eye in the posterior wall of the left eyeball was manifested as flake-like slightly high-density shadow with unclear boundary and hypermetabolic activity on PET with SUVmax 10.0 (red arrow). The retinal detachment in front of the lesion had an equidensity with unclear boundary, but no abnormal metabolic activity was observed (green arrow). (**b**) Anterior image of whole body PET MIP: primary esophageal cancer presented with intense hypermetabolic activity (green arrow) and paraphrenic and mediastinal lymph node metastasis

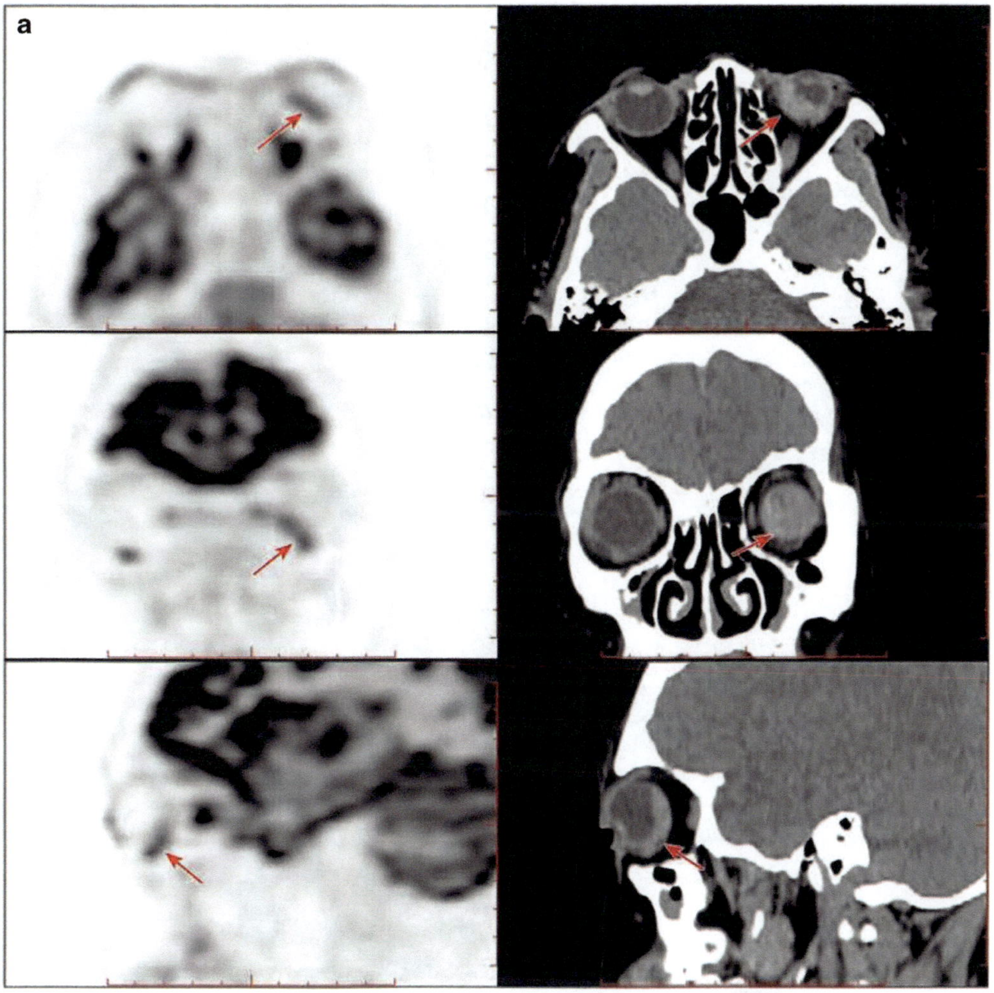

Fig. 14.19 FDG PET/CT images of metastatic breast cancer to the left eye. (**a**) CT and PET cross-sectional images were shown in the upper row, CT and PET coronal plane images in the middle row, and CT and PET sagittal plane images in the lower row: Metastatic tumor of the left eye showed a flat, slightly high-density shadow in the posterior wall of the left eyeball with clear boundaries and uneven and patchy increase in the metabolic activity of PET corresponding parts (red arrow), with SUVmax of 7.8. (**b**) CT and PET cross-sectional images were shown in the upper row, CT and PET coronal plane images in the middle row, and CT and PET sagittal plane images in the lower row: The upper part of the metastatic tumor of the left eye was detached from the retina, presenting a slightly high-density shadow, but no abnormal metabolic activity was observed (red arrow). Although the manifestations on CT images of eyeball metastatic tumor and retinal detachment were similar, the differences in metabolic activity on PET image between the two were helpful for the identification. (**c**) Anterior image of whole body PET MIP: breast cancer presented with significantly increased metabolic activity (green arrow) and multiple distal metastases

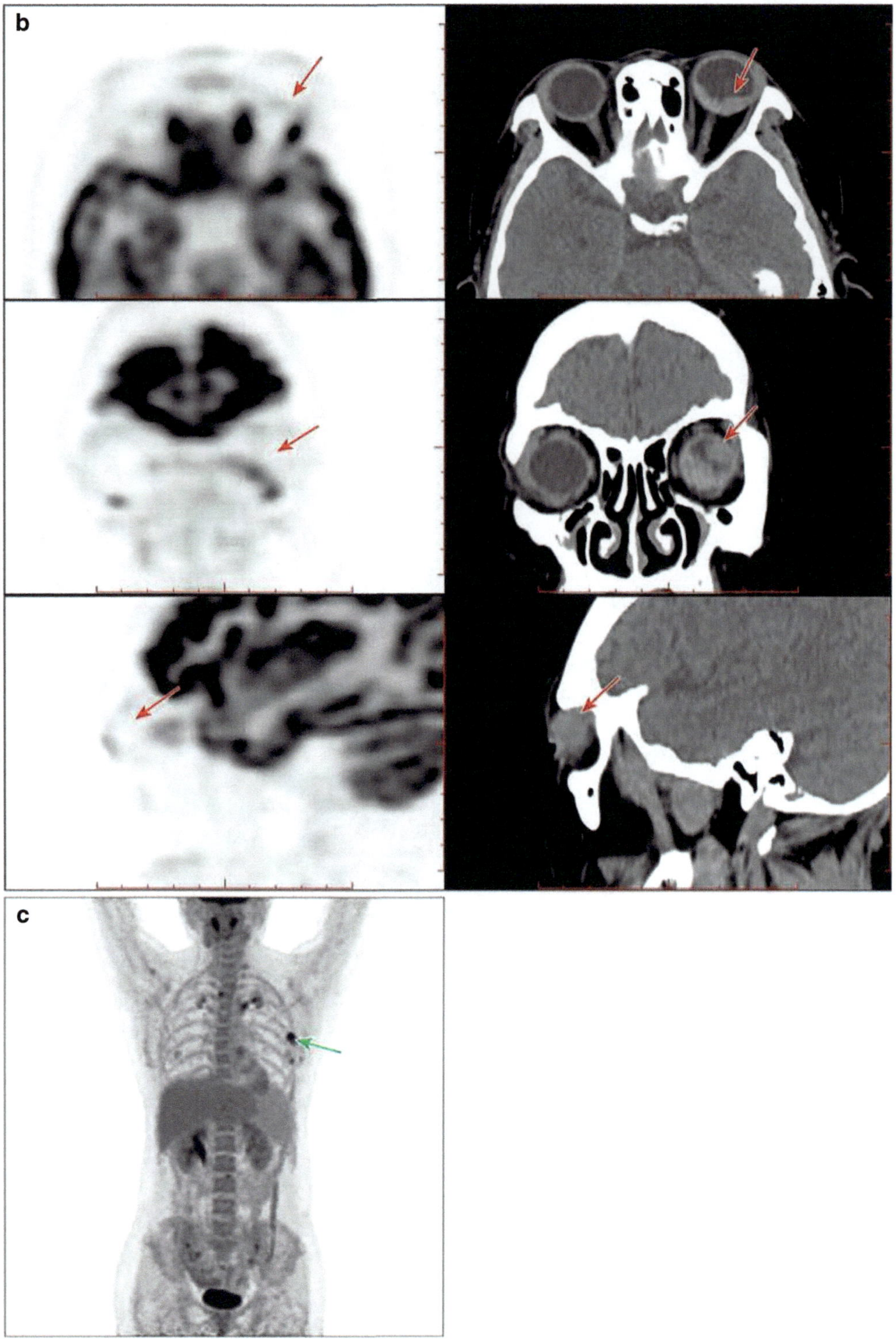

Fig. 14.19 (continued)

5.4 Rare Cases

The patient, a 68-year-old male, underwent a reduction operation owing to retinal detachment of his right eye and was found to have an intraoperative space at the bottom of his right eye (Fig. 14.20).

Reminder: What is rare in this case is that the ocular wall thickening is not obvious and the lesion area is slightly lower density due to the high density of surgical silicone oil. PET showed its advantage in this case, showing the location of the ocular metastasis. Whole body PET imaging in this case revealed a primary lung cancer with intense FDG uptake (green arrow) and lymph node and distal metastases, supporting the ocular lesions as metastatic tumors of lung cancer.

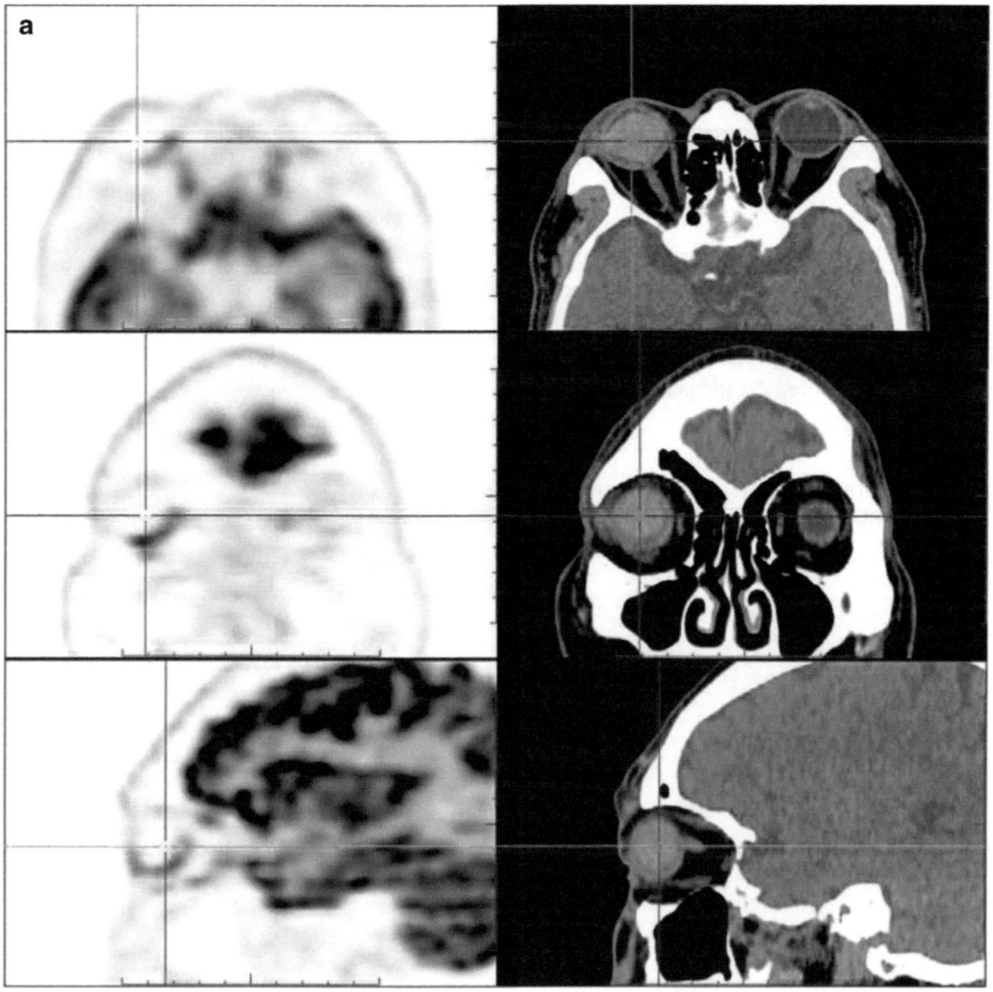

Fig. 14.20 FDG PET/CT images of metastatic left lung cancer to the right eye. (**a**) CT and PET cross-sectional images were shown in the upper row, CT and PET coronal plane images in the middle row, and CT and PET sagittal plane images in the lower row: There was a diffuse high-density shadow in the left eyeball without abnormal metabolic activity (criss-cross), which was considered to be caused by the surgical injection of silicone oil. (**b**) CT and PET cross-sectional images were shown in the upper row, CT and PET coronal plane images in the middle row, and CT and PET sagittal plane images in the lower row: The semi-circular shadow between the posterior wall of the eyeball and the high-density shadow in the eyeball was slightly lower with a clear boundary, but no obvious thickening of the ocular wall was observed. The non-uniform metabolic activity of the semi-circular shadow in the posterior wall of the PET eyeball was observed with increased localized lesions (red arrow), with SUVmax of 7.9. (**c**) The anterior image of body PET MIP showed multiple lesions with increased metabolic activity

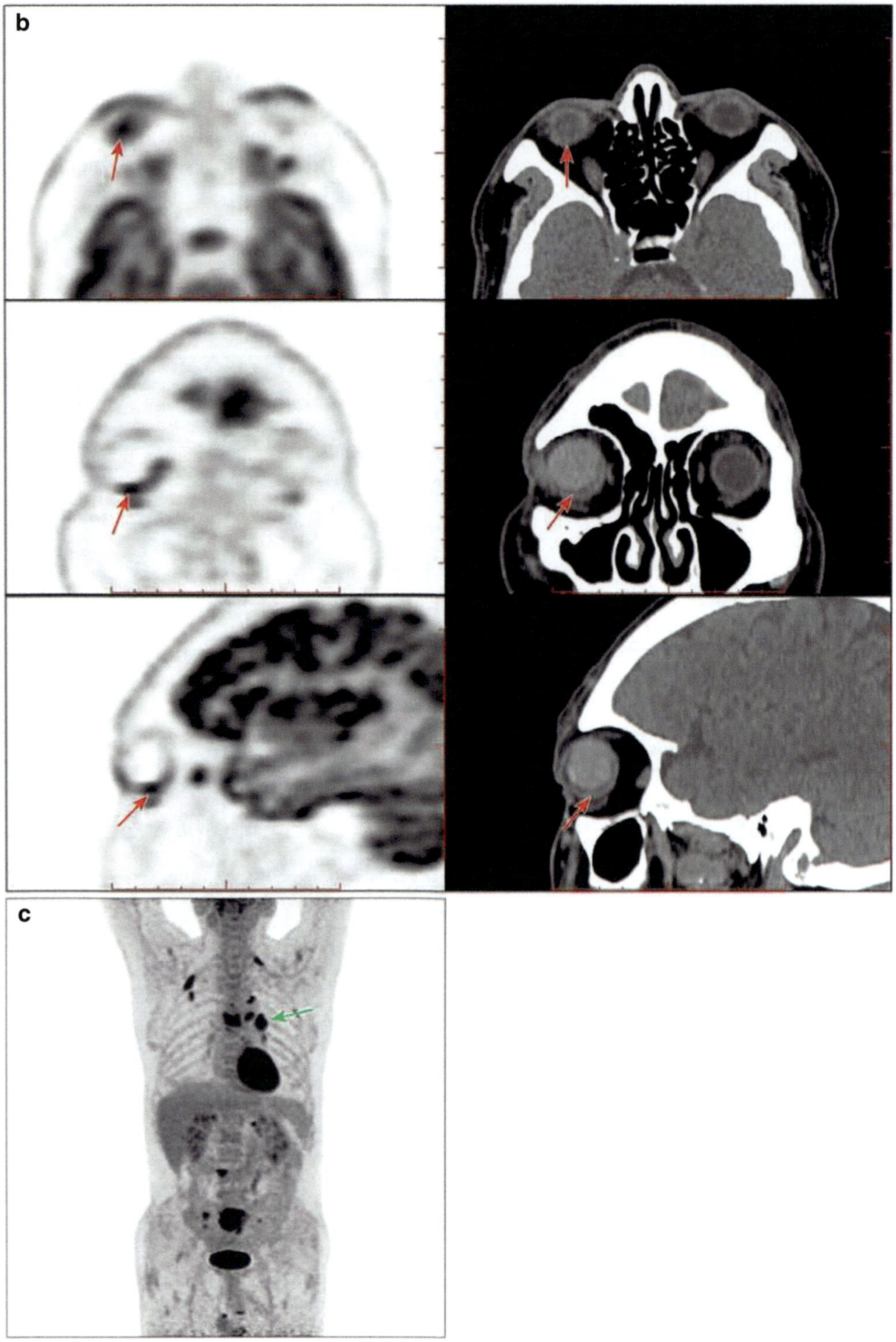

Fig. 14.20 (continued)

5.5 Differential Diagnosis

Nonspecific intraocular inflammatory granuloma is extremely rare and easy to be confused with neoplastic lesions if they do not spread out of the eye. The intraocular inflammatory granuloma also has increased FDG uptake on PET, and the lesion usually has more extensive involvement than tumors. Clinical symptoms such as fever and pain and laboratory examination results such as elevated white blood cells support the differential diagnosis. The diagnosis of this disease should be carried out in close combination with the clinical situation.

A 61-year-old male had fever with body muscle pain and without known cause for 10 days and had right eye pain and redness and blurred vision for 5 days (Fig. 14.21).

Reminder: In this case, the involvement of the right eye is extensive, and the thickening of the ocular wall is mainly out-

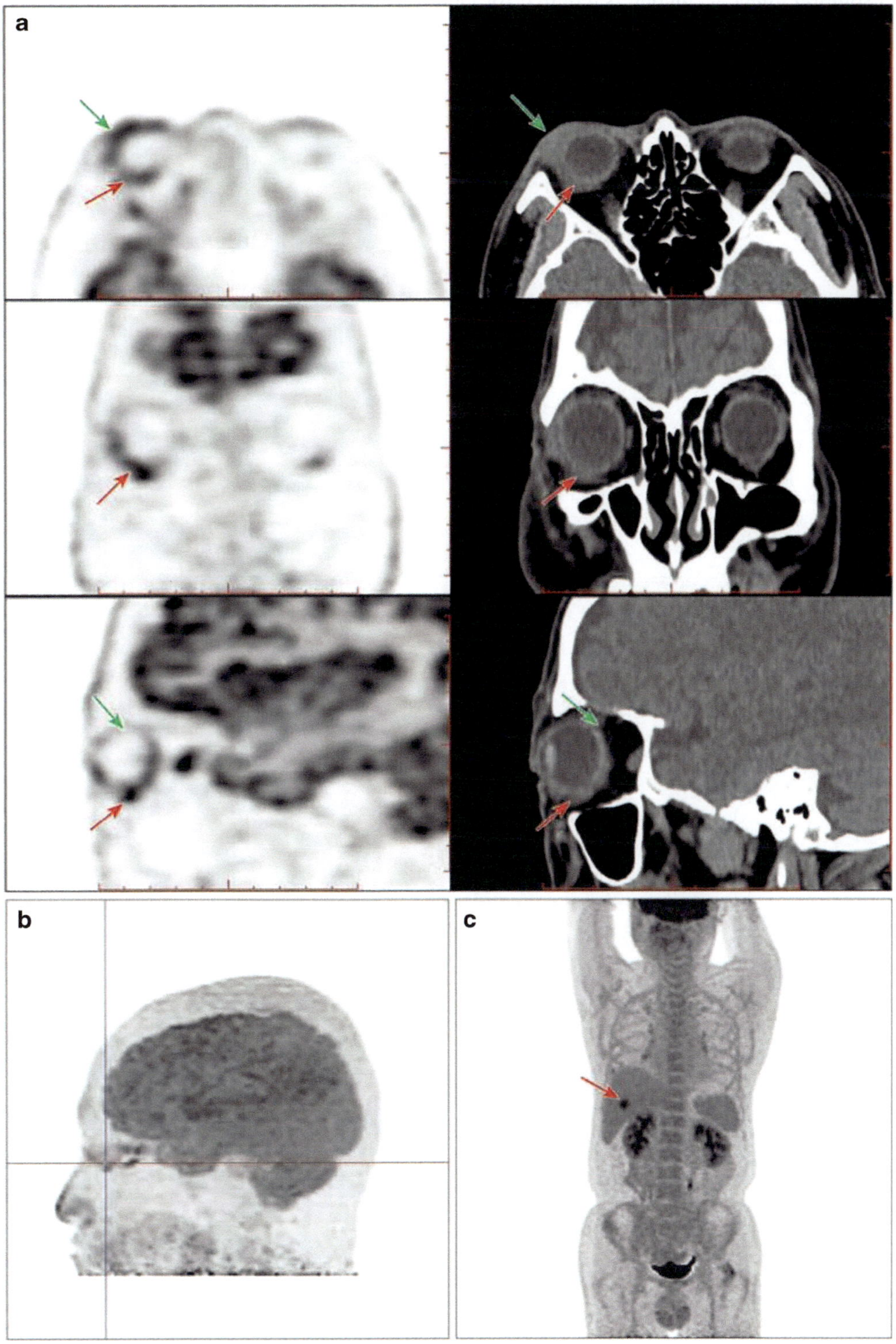

Fig. 14.21 FDG PET/CT images of infectious endophthalmitis in the right eye in patient with liver abscess. (**a**) CT and PET cross-sectional images were shown in the upper row, CT and PET coronal plane images in the middle row, and CT and PET sagittal plane images in the lower row: The anterior, lateral, and posterior walls of the right ocular bulb were inhomogeneously thickened and protruded (red arrow), accompanied by swelling of the right eyelid and lacrimal gland (green arrow), and the FDG uptake of PET in corresponding parts was inhomogeneously increased, with SUVmax of 9.4. (**b**) Later images of head FDG PET MIP: Non-uniform increased metabolic activity of the right eye (criss-cross). (**c**) Anterior image of body PET MIP: Focal intense metabolic activity in hepatic abscess (red arrow)

ward protruded with diffusely increased FDG uptake. After the right eye surgery and systemic plus local anti-infection treatment, the symptoms were relieved. The biopsy of liver lesion proved to be liver abscess.

5.6 Summary

Owing to the fine and complex ocular structure, high-resolution image technique is required for identification and diagnosis. MRI examination has become a common method since it can provide accurate positioning and abundant morphological information. But FDG PET/CT is capable of not only detecting the metabolic activity in the lesions but also showing lesion's morphological structure; in addition, "one-time whole body scan" of PET/CT lets it to be superior to other imaging examination in search of the primary lesions and metastasis, and PET/CT also can be performed in patients contraindicated for MRI. Therefore, PET/CT is very helpful in patients suspected with intraocular metastatic tumors.

Part IV

PET/CT of Tumors of Ear and Temporal Bone

General Introduction of PET/CT of Tumors of the Ear and Temporal Bone

15

Guoren Yang, Zhenguang Wang, and Tingting Lu

The structure of the ear and temporal bone is subtle and complex, and except for the auricle and cartilage of the external auditory canal, other parts are all irregular cavities in the temporal bone. Therefore, special imaging techniques and post-processing methods are required to show the anatomical structures and lesions in this area. Clinical ear and temporal bone tumors are rare. According to reports, temporal bone malignant tumors account for only 1/180 of head and neck malignant tumors and 1/1100 of systemic tumors. At present, there have been few reports on the application of PET/CT in ear and temporal bone lesions. In this chapter, the anatomical structure of the ear is summarized so that readers can have a primary understanding of the structure and adjacent relationship of the ear. Besides, the advantages, disadvantages, and possible gain value of PET/CT in ear and temporal bone tumors are introduced based on the conventional imaging including high-resolution CT.

1 Normal Anatomy

1.1 Temporal Bone

The temporal bone is of irregular shape, one on each side, which is involved in the formation of the skull base and lateral wall of the skull cavity. The temporal bone is divided into squamous, petrous, tympanic, and mastoid parts and styloid process with the external auricle as the center.

The squamous part is located above the anterior door of the outer ear and involved in forming the lateral wall of the skull cavity. The tympanic part and the petrous part constitute part of the skull base; the tympanic part surrounds the external auditory canal in the front, the bottom, and the back; and most of the bony part of the external auditory is composed of the tympanic part. The petrous part is tapered and contains the internal ear structure. The mastoid part includes the internal ear, the middle ear mastoid process, and part of the osseous external auditory canal.

In anatomy, the petrous apex is the temporal bone cone in front of the labyrinth of the internal ear. The structure around the temporal petrous apex is complex, so it is helpful for image diagnosis to be familiar with the adjacent relation of this area. In front of the petrous apex is the infratemporal fossa and pterygopalatine fossa, with the foramen lacerum and sphenoid pterygium process. Posterior lies the nasopharyngeal anterior lateral wall, connecting the nasopharyngeal Eustachian tube; the medial side is close to the clivus, and there are foramen ovale, foramen spinosum, external opening of carotid artery, and foramen jugular from the front to the back in the lateral side. The surrounding structural lesions can invade the petrous part.

1.2 External Ear

The external ear includes the auricle, the external auditory canal, and the tympanic membrane, which is a channel for conducting sound waves. 1/3 of the outer is cartilage and 2/3 of the inner is bone.

1.3 Middle Ear

It includes the tympanic cavity, pharyngotympanic tube, mastoid sinus, and mastoid cells.

1. Tympanic cavity: The tympanic cavity is an irregular air space in the petrous part of the temporal bone, containing three auditory ossicles – malleus, incus, and stapes. The three auditory ossicles are connected to form an ossicular chain, and the two ends are, respectively, connected to the

G. Yang (✉) · T. Lu
Shandong Cancer Hospital, Jinan, Shandong, China

Z. Wang
The Affiliated Hospital of Qingdao University, Qingdao, Shandong, China

Z. Yao, S. Li (eds.), *Atlas of PET/CT in Oncology - Volume 1*, https://doi.org/10.1007/978-981-99-1172-1_15

tympanic membrane and vestibular window. There are six walls around the tympanum:

(a) Upper wall: tympanic cavity cover, which is a thin bony plate separating the tympanic cavity from the middle cranial fossae. Lesions in the middle ear can invade this wall and enter the intracranial cavity upward, causing intracranial complications of otogenic origin.
(b) Inferior wall: the jugular fossa, which is separated from the initial part of the jugular vein by a thin bony plate.
(c) External wall: the majority is the tympanic membrane, above which lies the external wall of the tympanic cavity.
(d) Inner wall: it is the external wall of the internal ear, also known as the labyrinth wall.
(e) Anterior wall: the posterior wall of the internal carotid artery, above which lies the pharyngotympanic tube.
(f) Posterior wall: it is the mastoid wall, above which there is the entrance of the mastoid sinus, connected to the tympanic cavity and mastoid sinus.

2. The tympanic cavity is divided into three parts according to the upper and lower margin of the pars tensa of the tympanic membrane: the upper tympanic cavity is located above the upper margin of the pars tensa of the tympanic membrane; the lower tympanic cavity is located below the lower margin of the pars tensa of the tympanic membrane. The middle part is the middle tympanic cavity. Malignant tumors in the tympanic cavity are mostly located in the middle and lower tympanic cavity.
3. Pharyngotympanic tube: The pharyngotympanic tube is a channel connecting the nasopharyngeal cavity and tympanic cavity, which opens inward to the nasopharyngeal cavity, with the opening at the Eustachian orifice, and opens outward to the anterior wall of the tympanic cavity with the opening at the pharyngotympanic tube. The nasopharyngeal cancer can invade the middle ear through the pharyngotympanic tube.
4. Mastoid sinus: The mastoid sinus connects forward the upper tympanic cavity through the mastoid entry and connects backward the mastoid cells, and lesions in the middle ear may invade the mastoid cells through the mastoid sinus.

1.4 Internal Ear

The internal ear is a labyrinthine structure in the petrous part of the temporal bone, with irregular shape and complex structure. The main function is to receive acoustic wave and sensory stimulation. The labyrinth consists of the outer osseous labyrinth and the inner membranous labyrinth.

1. Osseous labyrinth: The osseous labyrinth is an irregular bone tunnel located in the petrous part, including the cochlea, vestibule, and osseous semicircular canals, three of which are arranged along the long axis of the petrous part of the temporal bone in order from the anteromedial side to posterolateral side, and they are connected with each other. The vestibule is located in the middle of the osseous labyrinth, connected with the cochlea in the front and three semicircular canals in the back. The semicircular canal consists of three small tubes arranged at right angles to each other, namely, the anterior osseous semicircular canal, the posterior osseous semicircular canal, and the external osseous semicircular canal. The anterior osseous semicircular canal is perpendicular to the long axis of the petrous part of the temporal bone, while the posterior osseous semicircular canal is parallel to the long axis of the petrous part of the temporal bone.
2. Membranous labyrinth: The membranous labyrinth is a membranous sac enclosed within the osseous labyrinth, including the elliptic sac, the balloon, the membranous semicircular canal, and the cochlea canal. Between the membranous labyrinth and the osseous labyrinth, there is filled with endolymph fluid, but the endolymph fluid and the perilymphatic fluid are not connected.
3. Internal auditory canal: The internal auditory canal begins at the internal acoustic pore behind the petrous part of the temporal bone and passes laterally into the temporal bone. The internal auditory canal contains the facial nerve, the vestibular cochlea nerve, and the labyrinth artery.

2 Imageological Examination Techniques

1. X-ray radiography: According to the different projection positions, X-ray radiography includes the lateral projection of the temporal bone (including Schuller's view and Runstrom's view), the axial projection of the temporal bone (namely, Mayer's), the transorbital position of the internal auditory canal, the posterior and anterior oblique projection (namely, Stenvers view) of the temporal bone, etc. Because of the imaging mode of X-ray radiography, there are two disadvantages: (1) two-dimensional projection imaging with overlapping anterior and posterior structures, while the temporal bone shape is irregular and the acoustic meatus is subtle and complex in structure, which makes most of the lesions difficult to show; and (2) lower-resolution, suboptimal display of fine structures. This examination has been replaced by CT and MRI.
2. Conventional CT: Conventional CT is usually adopted with an axial scanning thickness of 2 ~ 5 mm. The scanning plane passes through the external auricle and

the upper orbital margin, namely, the upper auditory orbit line. This plane is applicable to displaying most structures of the external, middle, and internal ear. Soft tissue algorithm is adopted for images. Conventional CT is mainly used to evaluate the relationship between ear lesions and surrounding structures. Contrast-enhanced scan can be adopted to further determine the blood supply characteristics of lesions and the relationship between lesions and blood vessels.

3. High-resolution CT (HRCT): High-resolution CT (HRCT) is the preferred method for the examination of lesions in the ears and temporal bone. It can be used for coronal and sagittal reconstruction to comprehensively display the fine structure of the ears and temporal bone.

   HRCT is performed using a slice thickness of <2 mm for thin slice scanning. The baseline is parallel to the supraorbital line, and the entire temporal bone is scanned using an axial scan to cover the entire structure of the middle ear and internal ear. Because it is volumetric scanning and has isotropic characteristics, it can be reconstructed at any orientation by post-processing, avoiding the disadvantages such as inconvenient position and high radiation of direct coronal and sagittal scanning. Coronal reconstruction can be used to determine the reconstruction plane on the lateral cranial positioning image. Most of them are adopted with the long axis parallel to the occipital clivus, which is equivalent to the scanning plane of 70° (the inferior orbital line is 0°).

   The volume data obtained by spiral CT can be used for a variety of computer post-processing, including multiplanar reformation technique (MPR), maximum intensity projection (MIP), shaded surface display (SSD), CT virtual endoscopy technology (CTVE), volume reconstruction technology (VR), etc., to achieve a comprehensive observation of the structure of interest.

4. Magnetic resonance imaging (MRI): MRI has diagnostic value for tumors of the internal auditory meatus, especially small acoustic neuroma. MRI should be performed on the basis of HRCT in the temporal bone for suspected ear tumors invading the labyrinth, nerves, and blood vessels or invading the skull. If acoustic neuroma is suspected, a MRI should be performed first.
5. PET/CT examination technique: PET/CT is rarely used in ear and temporal bone tumors and is generally not taken as the preferred method. It has clinical application value or gain value mainly in the following aspects: (1) to judge the invasion of ear tumors to surrounding structures, especially when the range of CT and MRI is ambiguous; (2) to guide the site of biopsy when the tumor coexists with inflammation; (3) to determine whether there is residual or recurrence of malignant tumors of the ear after surgery and radiotherapy; (4) to find out the primary lesion if the ear and temporal bone lesions are suspected to be metastatic tumors; and (5) to understand whether there is a distant metastasis and determine the postoperative comprehensive therapeutic regimen.

16 PET/CT of Tumors of the Ear and Temporal Bone

Guoren Yang, Zhenguang Wang, Dacheng Li, and Tingting Lu

1 Overview

Ear tumors can be classified into tumors of the external ear and external auditory canal, middle ear, and internal ear.

Tumors of the external ear and external auditory canal may originate from various tissues including the bone, cartilage, blood vessels, skin, glands, etc., most of which are benign. Common tumors include osteomas, papillomas, fibromas, ceruminous adenomas, hemangiomas, etc. Clinical symptoms are generally not obvious, and when the tumor is large and exerts compression or obstruction on the external auditory canal, the affected side is inflicted with hearing loss, infection in the external auditory canal, and other manifestations. Malignant tumors are rare, most of which are metastatic. The primary malignant tumors are squamous cell carcinoma, and other types of tumors include basal cell carcinoma, adenoid cystic carcinoma, ceruminous gland adenocarcinoma, etc. Clinical manifestations include earache, hearing loss, discharge of pus and bleeding, facial paralysis, etc. The external ear and external auditory canal are shallow and exposed, and polypoid or cauliflower-like masses of the external auditory canal can be easily found by physical examination. Obtaining pathological diagnosis is the main means of diagnosis, and imaging including PET/CT examination is mainly intended to determine the range and understanding whether there is metastasis.

Tumors of the middle ear are rare, and the middle ear is deep and hidden, so it is difficult to obtain pathological diagnosis. Most malignancies of the middle ear are secondary to or associated with inflammation and are often diagnosed late because of the confusion between the two. Common benign tumors of the middle ear include facial neuroma and glomus tumors of the tympanic cavity. Carcinoma of the middle ear accounts for 1.5% of the tumors of the ear, of which squamous cell carcinoma is the most common type with high degree of malignancy, followed by basal cell carcinoma, adenocarcinoma, and metastatic tumor which are rare. Primary tumors of the external ear, nasopharynx, and so on can invade the middle ear, and it is often difficult to determine the primary site on imaging.

The vast majority of ear tumors occur in the external and middle ear, but very few occur in the internal ear. The overwhelming majority of tumors in the labyrinth and internal auditory canal are schwannomas, which can originate from the vestibular nerve, cochlear nerve, and facial nerve, most of which originate from the vestibular nerve. Schwannomas in the internal auditory canal are more common than those in the labyrinth. Most of them are unilateral, while a few can be bilateral, which is called type II neurofibromatosis.

2 Osteoma of the Ear

2.1 Clinical Overview

Osteoma is a benign bone tumor originating from the periosteum tissue, which usually occurs on the bone wall of the skull, maxilla, mandible, and sinuses and is rarely seen in the ear. Auricular osteoma can be seen in the external auditory

G. Yang (✉) · T. Lu
Shandong Cancer Hospital, Jinan, Shandong, China

Z. Wang · D. Li
The Affiliated Hospital of Qingdao University, Qingdao, Shandong, China

Z. Yao, S. Li (eds.), *Atlas of PET/CT in Oncology - Volume 1*, https://doi.org/10.1007/978-981-99-1172-1_16

canal, mastoid process, tympanic cavity, squamous part of the temporal bone, etc., among which the external auditory canal and mastoid process are more inflicted. Osteomas can be classified into dense type and loose type. Osteomas of the external auditory canal are of mostly dense type, which are usually unilateral and single, and grow slowly.

2.2 PET/CT Diagnostic Points

CT images show spherical or hemispherical bone density nodules and masses in the osseous parts of the external auditory canal, with prominent protruding toward inside the external auditory canal cavity, characterized with regular and smooth surfaces. It has pedicle and is connected with the bone wall of the external auditory canal, and a few are with broad base. They are mostly unilateral occurrence and grow singly.

^{18}F-FDG PET image showed no metabolic activity in lesions.

2.3 Typical Cases

The patient, a 45-year-old male, was present due to "occupancy of the external auditory canal found by this examination" (Fig. 16.1).

2.4 Summary

Since there was no abnormal metabolic activity of ear osteoma, this disease was not an indication of FDG PET/CT and was usually diagnosed by CT.

3 Malignant Tumor of the External Auditory Canal

3.1 Clinical Overview

The reason of malignant tumor of the external auditory canal is not known, and it is mostly related to injury, chronic inflammation, and fungal infection of the external auditory canal. Squamous cell carcinoma is the most common pathological type, followed by adenoid cystic carcinoma. Early carcinoma of the external auditory canal often does not have subjective symptom, can show only for slight pruritus or ache, and is not easy to discover. The lesion progression may involve cartilage or bone, with persistent severe earache and radiating to the ipsilateral temporal, shoulder, and occipital regions. When accompanied with infection, it can be inflicted with discharge of pus and stream fluid in the ear, and advanced tumor can invade the middle ear and parotid gland and even invade into the skull upward.

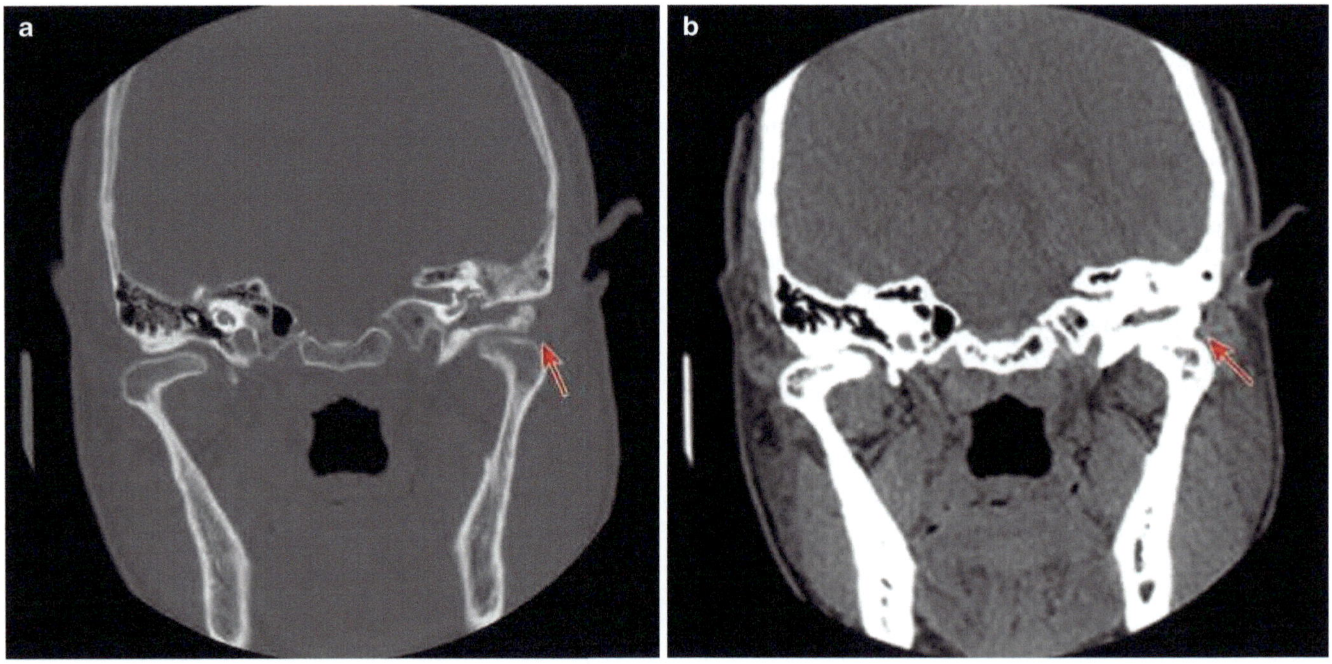

Fig. 16.1 CT images of osteoma in the external auditory canal. (**a**) Coronal CT bone window image. (**b**) Coronal CT soft tissue window image. The arrow in the figure shows the bone density nodules of the left external auditory canal, protruding into the cavity of the external auditory canal, with a slightly wider base connected to the bone wall of the external auditory canal, with neat and smooth edges

Tumors of the external auditory canal are easily pathologically diagnosed. Imaging methods, including PET/CT, are mainly used to determine the primary site and lesion invasion scope and to understand the metastasis, which are of reference value for guiding biopsy, surgical selection, and postoperative comprehensive treatment. The imaging findings of malignant tumors of the external auditory canal of different pathological types are not specific.

3.2 PET/CT Diagnostic Points

1. The external auditory canal is filled with density shadow of soft tissue, and the external auditory canal is damaged by bone. Bone destruction, invasion of surrounding structures, and edema of surrounding soft tissues are the main bases for CT to judge malignant lesions of the external auditory canal.
2. The lesion progresses and invades in all directions; the lesion can invade the middle ear and mastoid process to the medial side, the skull base, and the skull and invade the parotid gland outward.
3. ^{18}F-FDG PET shows increased metabolism of tumors in the external auditory canal, which helps to determine the extent of invasion of surrounding structures, cervical lymph node metastasis, and distant metastasis.

3.3 Typical Cases

The patient was a 49-year-old female with left ear discomfort for 1 month (Fig. 16.2).

Follow-up ^{18}F-FDG PET/CT after surgical operation 6 months for a poorly differentiated nonspecific adenocarcinoma of the left external auditory canal (Fig. 16.3)

Follow-up ^{18}F-FDG PET/CT after surgical operation 8 months for squamous carcinoma of the left external auditory canal; she was reexamined with ^{18}F-FDG PET/CT (Fig. 16.4).

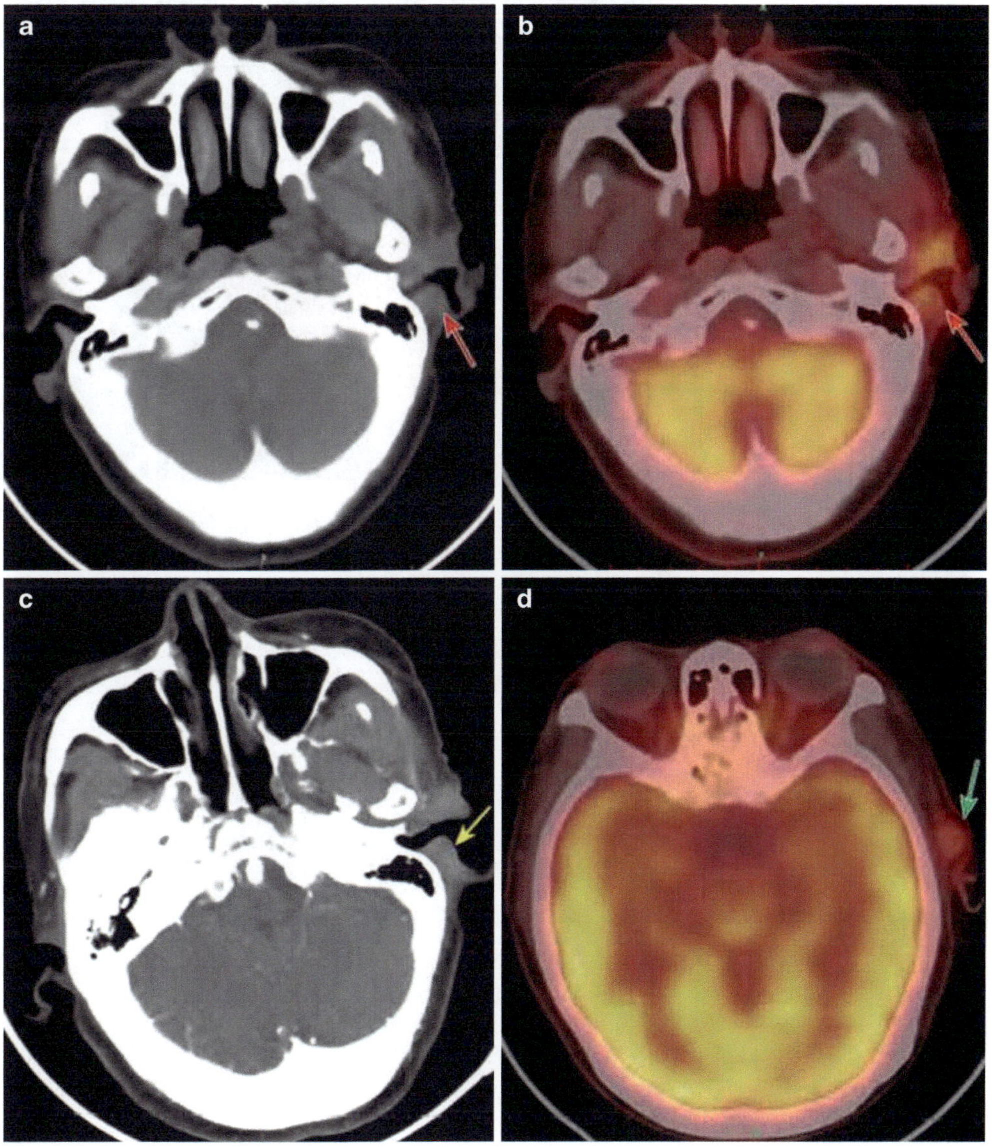

Fig. 16.2 ^{18}F-FDG PET/CT and enhanced CT images of basal cell carcinoma of the external auditory canal. (**a**) CT image. (**b**) ^{18}F-FDG PET/CT fusion image showed the soft tissue of the left external auditory canal was significantly thickened and hypermetabolic (red arrow) with SUVmax 7.1. (**c**) Enhanced CT images showed obvious enhancement of soft tissue lesions in the left external auditory canal (yellow arrow). (**d**) ^{18}F-FDG PET/CT fusion image showed enlarged lymph nodes in front of the left ear with increased metabolism and SUVmax of about 3.8, which was considered as lymph node metastasis (green arrow). It was confirmed through pathology with basal cell carcinoma of the left external auditory canal

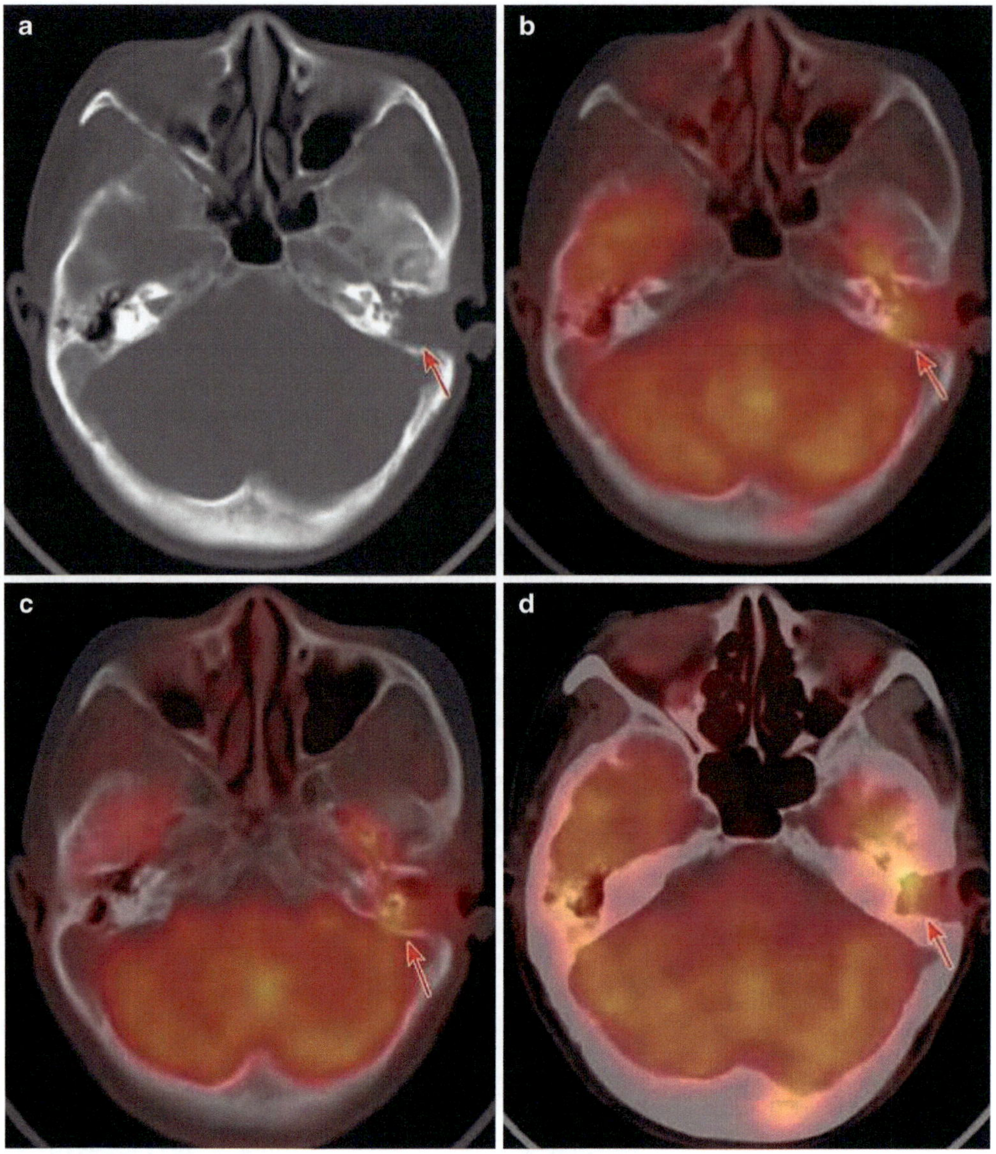

Fig. 16.3 ^{18}F-FDG PET/CT images of recurrent adenocarcinoma of the external auditory canal after resection. (**a**) CT bone window image, bone absence in the left posterior wall of the external auditory canal and the left mastoid part of the temporal bone; soft tissue density lesions were seen in the left external and middle ear canal, and the surrounding bone showed bone destruction like worm erosion, with lesions invading the petrous part of the temporal bone. (**b, c**) Bone window fusion images. (**d**) Window fusion image of soft tissue showed significantly increased metabolism in soft tissue lesion and surrounding bone destruction area, with SUVmax 8.7, and lesions invading the skull base in front and above. Pathology confirmed recurrence

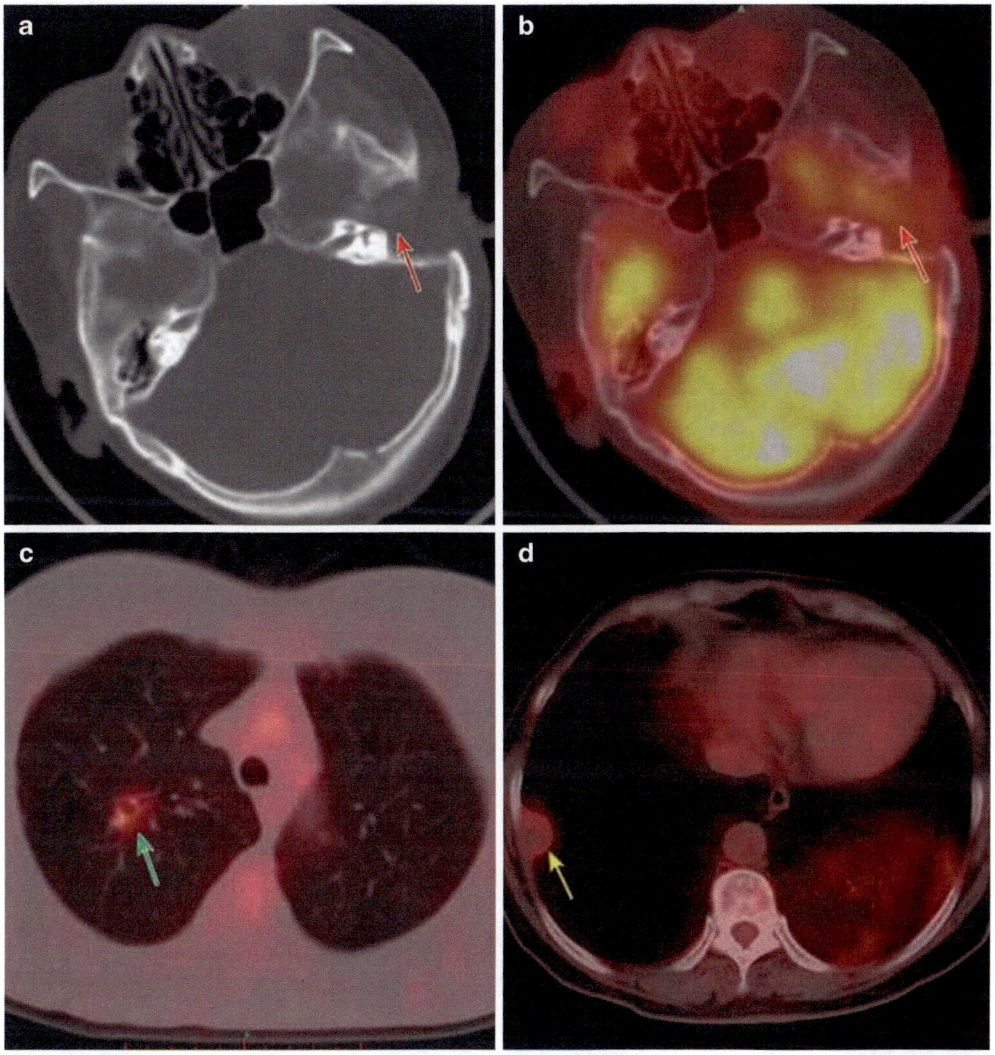

Fig. 16.4 ^{18}F-FDG PET/CT images of recurrence and metastasis occurred after resection of squamous cell carcinoma of the external auditory canal. (**a**) CT image of bone window of the left external auditory canal: bone of the left posterior wall of the external auditory canal and the left mastoid part of the left temporal bone was absent, and the anterior bone of the operative area was seen with destruction like worm-eaten shape. (**b**) PET/CT fusion image of the left external auditory canal: the lesions in the above left external auditory canal showed increased metabolism, with SUVmax 4.3 (red arrow). (**c**) Lung PET/CT fusion image: increased metabolism (SUVmax 3.2) in the cavitary nodules in the upper lobe of the right lung. (**d**) Chest PET/CT fusion image: right pleural nodules with increased metabolism and SUVmax 2.7. The diagnosis with ^{18}F-FDG PET/CT image showed recurrence with pulmonary metastasis (green arrow) and right pleural metastasis (yellow arrow). A puncture biopsy of the right pleural nodule showed infiltration of highly differentiated squamous cell carcinoma in the proliferative fibrous adipose tissue, which was considered to be metastatic based on the medical history

3.4 Differential Diagnosis

Granulation tissue: Granulation tissue is usually secondary to other diseases such as inflammation, trauma, surgery, etc. In most cases, there is no peripheral bone damage, or the damage is mild. Inflammation of the external auditory canal is easy to be diagnosed. There is no soft tissue mass formation (Figs. 16.5 and 16.6).

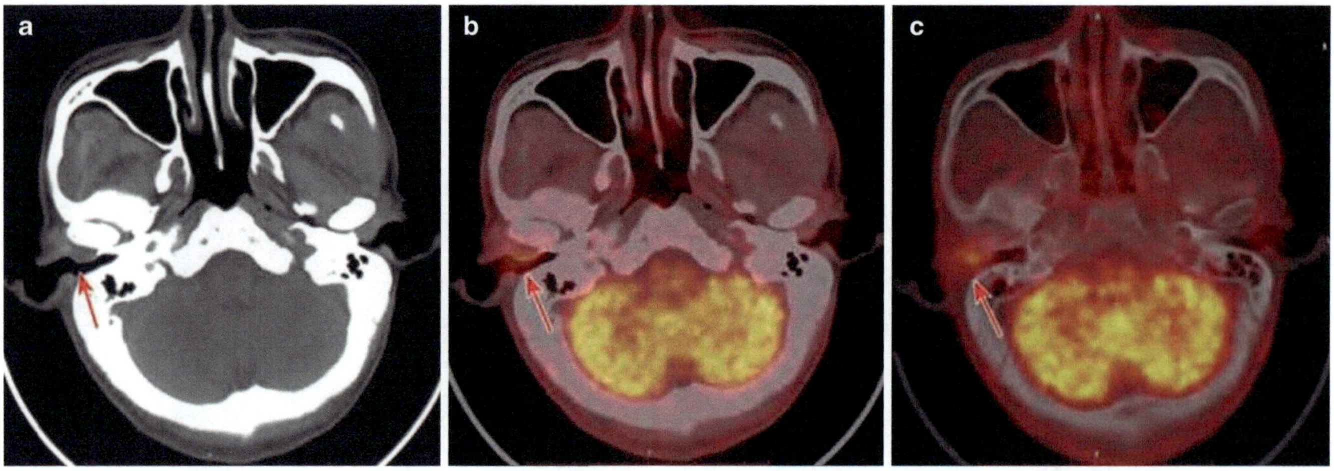

Fig. 16.5 ^{18}F-FDG PET/CT images of otitis externa. (**a**) CT image (soft tissue window) showed slight thickening of soft tissue in the anterior wall of the right external auditory canal with smooth edges. (**b**) PET/CT fusion image (soft tissue window) showed mild increased local metabolism, with SUVmax of 4.4. (**c**) PET/CT fusion image (bone window) showed no adjacent bone destruction and erosion. The patient was effectively treated with antibiotics

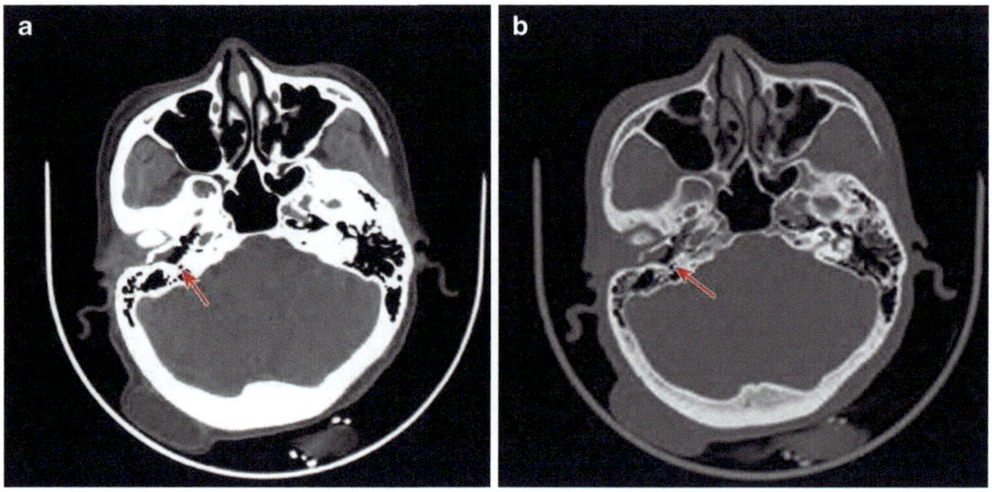

Fig. 16.6 CT images of fungal infection of the external auditory canal and middle ear. (**a**) CT soft tissue window image. (**b**) CT bone window image. The arrow in the figure showed the right external auditory meatus—tympanic cavity had soft striate tissue density shadow with smooth edges and without adjacent bone erosion. Pathology: There was a little keratinized substance under the microscope (in the right external auditory canal tissue), and the fungal spore-like structure was found inside, which was consistent with fungal infection. Hexamine silver (+)

3.5 Summary

The external auditory canal tumors with hypermetabolic activity are easily confused with infectious diseases of the external auditory canal.

4 Carcinoma of the Middle Ear

4.1 Clinical Overview

Carcinoma of the middle ear is more common in middle-aged and elderly patients. The majority of the cases were pathologically squamous cell carcinomas arising from the mucosae epithelium of the middle ear cavity. Due to the inter-connection of the tympanic cavity, tympanic sinus, mastoid air chamber, pharyngotympanic tube, and other parts, malignant tumors of the middle ear are easy to spread to the inferior tympanic cavity, perilabyrinth, and mastoid air chamber, and often have obvious damage to the adjacent bone, and can also invade the petrous apex, parotid gland, and temporomandibular joint. Next is sarcoma, which is associated with local radiation exposure, trauma, viral infection, and malignant transformation of some benign tumors, and it develops rapidly and may have early distant metastases. Adenocarcinoma of the middle ear is rare and originates from the mucous gland of the mucosa of the tympanic membrane, which grows slowly and can have local invasion and exert damage.

About 80%–85% of patients with carcinoma of the middle ear have a history of chronic suppurative otitis media, so there are no characteristic clinical symptoms, and in addition to long-term chronic mastoiditis manifestations of the middle ear, the patient may suffer from bleeding, pus, and severe pain in the auditory canal, facial paralysis, etc.

4.2 PET/CT Diagnostic Points

1. Soft tissue density mass in the middle ear cavity, invading the surrounding tissues with the tympanic cavity as the center, can invade the external auditory canal, pharyngotympanic tube, internal ear, mastoid sinus, mastoid process, etc. and even invade the parotid gland, inferior temporal fossa, and intracranial part.
2. There is extensive and obvious bone damage; the edge of the damaged lesion is of worm-eaten shape and irregular; the ossicle is damaged; moderate or significant enhancement is seen.
3. ^{18}F-FDG PET shows increased metabolism in the lesion. PET/CT can be used to determine the lesion invasion scope, metastasis of cervical lymph node, and distant metastasis and is also of help to determine whether it is a direct invasion to the middle ear, such as nasopharyngeal carcinoma.

4.3 Typical Cases

The patient, a 41-year old male, was present 3 months after surgery for adenoid cystic carcinoma of the right tympanic cavity, with right earache for 1 month and with drooping of the angle of the mouth over 1 week (Fig. 16.7).

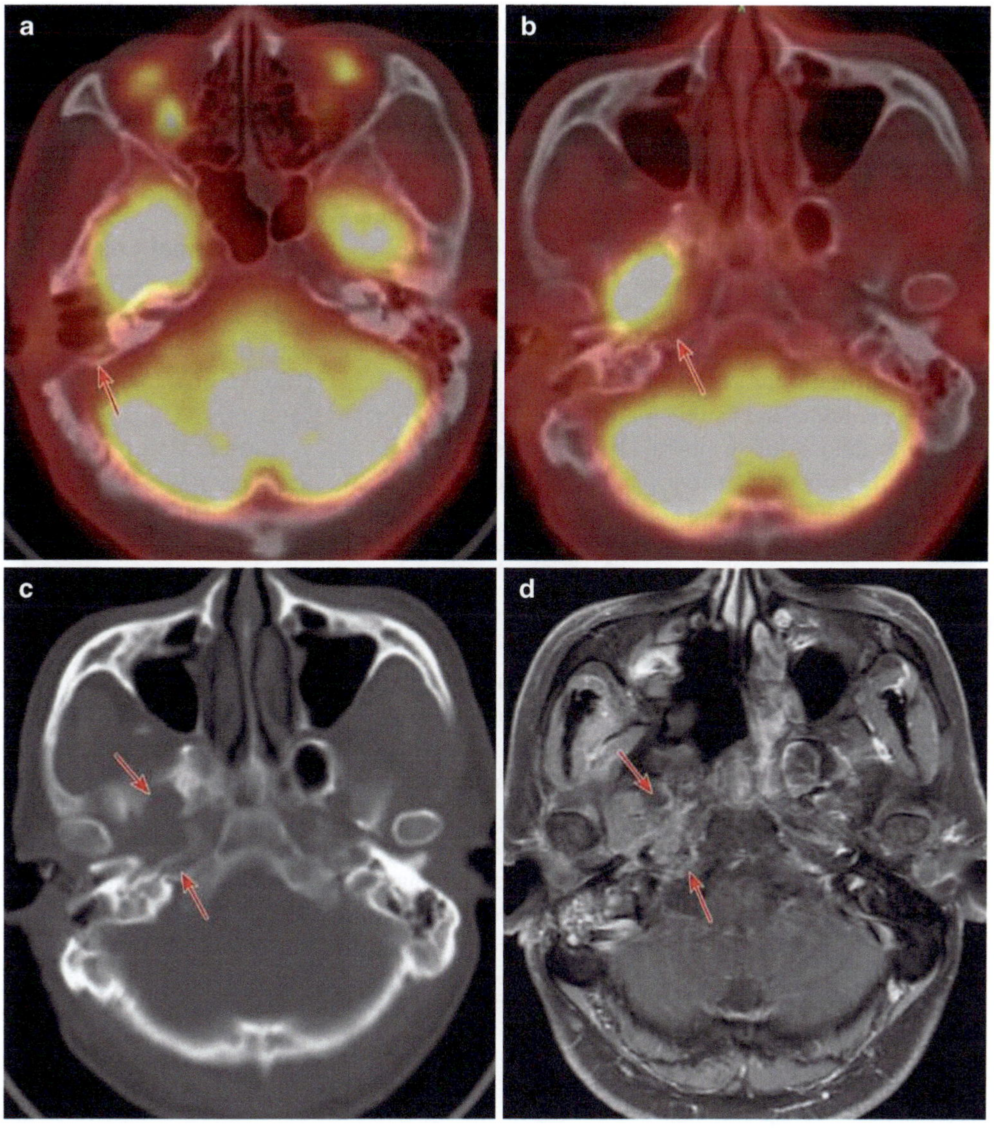

Fig. 16.7 ^{18}F-FDG PET/CT images showing local invasion after surgery for adenoid cystic carcinoma of the tympanic cavity of the middle ear. (**a**) PET/CT cross section of fusion image at the level of the right tympanic cavity: Bone loss was found in the bone wall around the right tympanic cavity and in the right mastoid part, and no abnormal increase in metabolism was observed locally. (**b, c**) PET/CT fusion image and CT window image of the right temporal bone, respectively: osteolytic bone destruction was observed in the petrous apex of the right temporal bone, the pterygoid process and the greater wing of sphenoid bone. A soft tissue mass was noted with increased metabolism (SUVmax12.2). (**d**) Enhanced MR image of the right temporal bone: irregular morphology of the damaged area showed moderate heterogeneous enhancement. The patient had a local invasion after middle ear carcinoma

4.4 Differential Diagnosis

1. Congenital cholesteatoma It more commonly occurs in the superior tympanic cavity, with regular margins and clear masses, which may be accompanied by erosion of the middle ear wall or loss of the ossicle.
2. Glomus tympanicum tumor There are density nodes in the promontory and the surrounding soft tissues, mostly without obvious bone destruction.

5 Metastatic Tumor of the Temporal Bone

5.1 Clinical Overview

Metastatic tumors of the temporal bone are rare and most common in the elderly. There are three main routes:

1. Hematogenous metastasis: The temporal bone is rich in bone marrow and blood supply, and primary tumors in other areas can be transferred to the temporal bone through blood flow, among which breast cancer is the most common, followed by lung cancer, kidney cancer, prostate cancer, melanoma, etc.
2. Lymphatic metastasis: Upper respiratory tract and digestive tract tumors have been reported to invade the temporal bone through the retropharyngeal lymph nodes.
3. Direct invasion: The adjacent relationship around the temporal bone is complicated, and tumors with multiple channels communicating with adjacent structures can directly invade the temporal bone, such as nasopharyngeal carcinoma and parotid malignant tumor. The clinical manifestations of temporal bone metastases include headache, abducent nerve paralysis, hearing loss, etc., and imaging findings are not specific.

5.2 PET/CT Diagnostic Points

1. CT findings are varied and associated with the biological behavior and pathological type of primary cancer. The metastatic tumors to the nose are mainly osteolytic bone destruction and rarely osteogenic one. Bone metastasis of breast cancer is mostly osteolytic, mainly manifested as worm-biting-like or rat-biting-like irregular bone destruction, with or without soft tissue density mass. In lung cancer, bone metastasis usually occurs in adenocarcinoma, mainly with osteolytic bone destruction. Small cell undifferentiated carcinoma and a few adenocarcinoma can present osteoblastic metastasis. The majority of renal carcinoma is osteolytic metastasis. Osteoblastic metastases may resemble benign fibrous bone disease.
2. ^{18}F-FDG PET/CT findings of bone metastases mostly show increased metabolic manifestations, and the degree of metabolism increase depends on the pathological type and metabolic level of primary tumor and the type of local bone destruction. The metabolic activity of osteolytic bone metastasis was increased significantly, while that of osteogenic bone metastasis was slightly higher or even without increase. The osteogenic changes of the temporal bone can be detected by CT, and the osteogenic metastasis of the temporal bone can be diagnosed by combining with lesion's metabolic activity.
3. Single bone metastasis in patient is rare; most are multiple bone metastases. ^{18}F-FDG PET/CT is a systemic examination, which is of great value in the detection of the metastasis in the whole body and understanding well the primary lesion. The discovery of bone metastases in other locations of body is very helpful in improving the diagnostic confidence of bone metastases in the temporal bone.

5.3 Typical Cases

Case 1: A 55-year-old female patient with a right breast mass for 10 months and a headache for 2 months. Pathology: (Biopsy of the right breast) Poorly differentiated invasive carcinoma (Fig. 16.8)

Case 2: Male patient, 66 years old. Due to headache, bone destruction was found in the petrous part of the left temporal bone. PET/CT examination was requested to find out the primary lesion. Pathology: Medium differentiation adenocarcinoma in the upper lobe of the right lung with metastasis to the petrous part of the left temporal bone and sacrum (Fig. 16.9)

Case 3: Male patient, 52 years old. 7 years after surgery for atypical carcinoid tumors of the thymus. Bone metastasis was found for 1 year, and octreotide was used for treatment for 1 year. PET/CT examination was applied to understand the recurrence and metastasis (Fig. 16.10).

Case 4: A typical case photo of poorly differentiated squamous cell carcinoma of the left pharyngeal recess (Fig. 16.11)

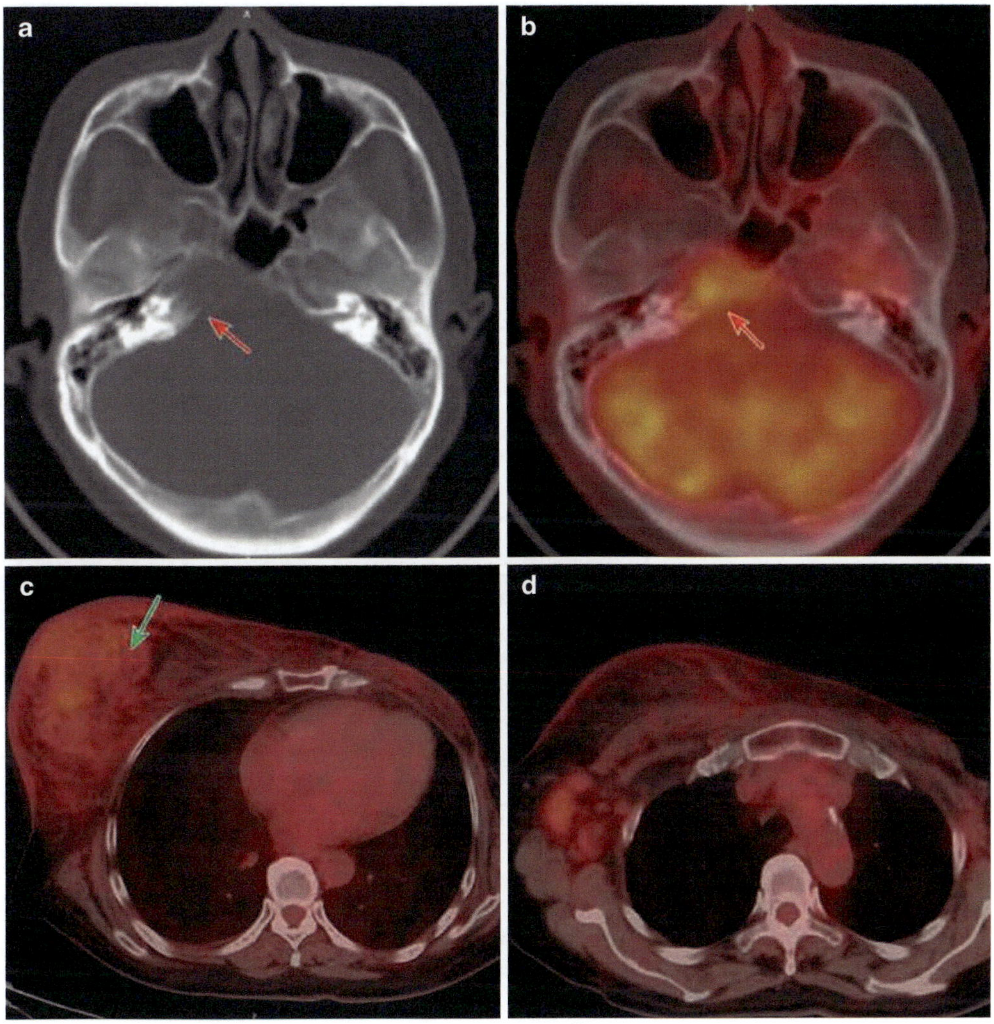

Fig. 16.8 ^{18}F-FDG PET/CT image of metastases of the petrous apex of the temporal bone. (**a** and **b**) CT bone window image and cross section of PET/CT fusion image of the temporal bone, respectively: CT showed osteolysis bone destruction at the petrous apex of the right temporal bone, with irregular edges of the lesion destroyed; PET/CT fusion image showed increased metabolism in bone destruction lesion, with SUVmax of about 5.0. (**c**) Breast PET/CT fusion image: The right breast was seen with enlargement, there were multiple soft tissue density masses (green arrow), and there was skin thickening of the right breast with increased metabolism and SUVmax being 3.9. (**d**) Axillary PET/CT fusion image: Multiple enlarged lymph nodes were seen in the right axilla with increased metabolism, which was considered as lymph node metastasis

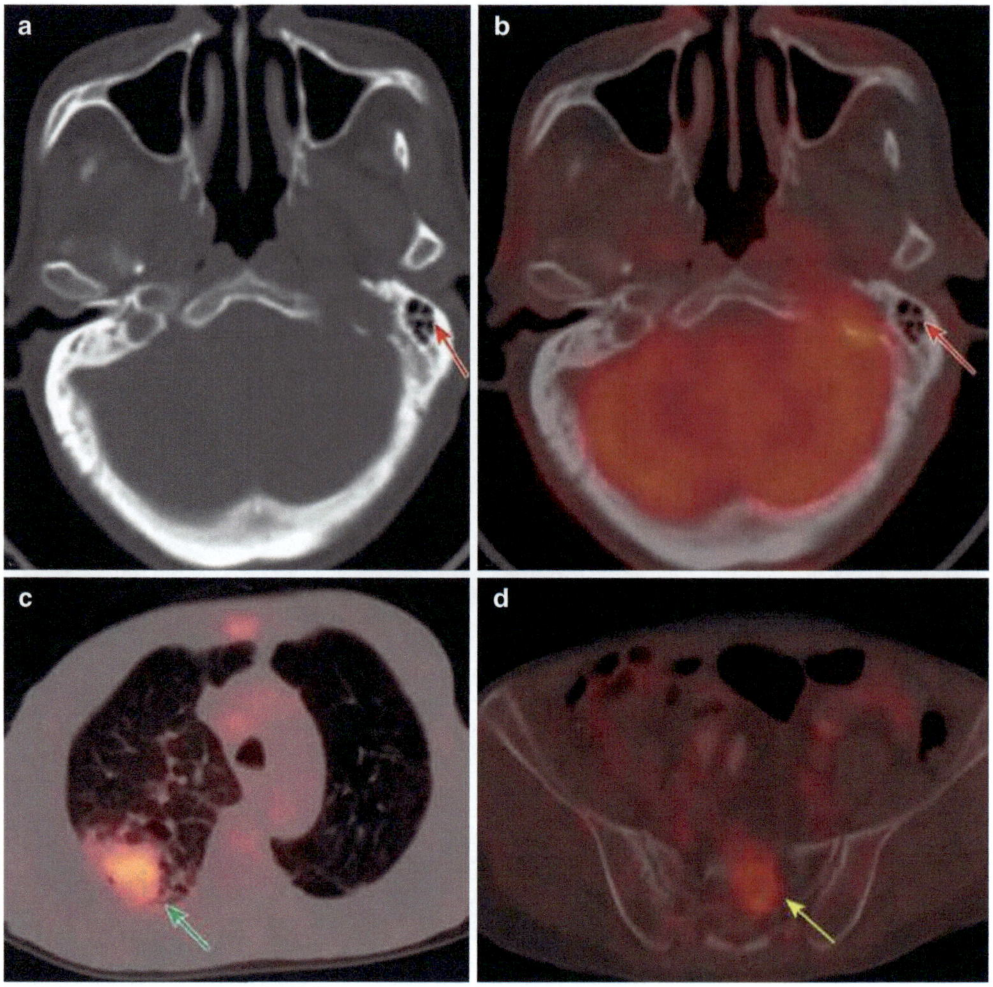

Fig. 16.9 ^{18}F-FDG PET/CT images of petrous metastasis of the temporal bone of lung cancer. (**a** and **b**) CT bone window image and cross section of PET/CT fusion image of the temporal bone, respectively: CT showed osteolysis bone destruction at the petrous part of the left temporal bone (red arrow), which damaged the edge of the lesion in an irregular, worm-biting-like appearance and invaded the jugular vein foramen; PET/CT fusion image showed increased metabolism in the bone destruction lesion, with SUVmax of 3.6. (**c**) Lung PET/CT fusion image: Subpleural differentiation of lobar soft tissue density masses in the upper lobe of the right lung (green arrow), with increased metabolism and SUVmax of about 3.9. (**d**) Sacral PET/CT fusion image: Sacral osteolytic bone destruction with increased metabolism (yellow arrow)

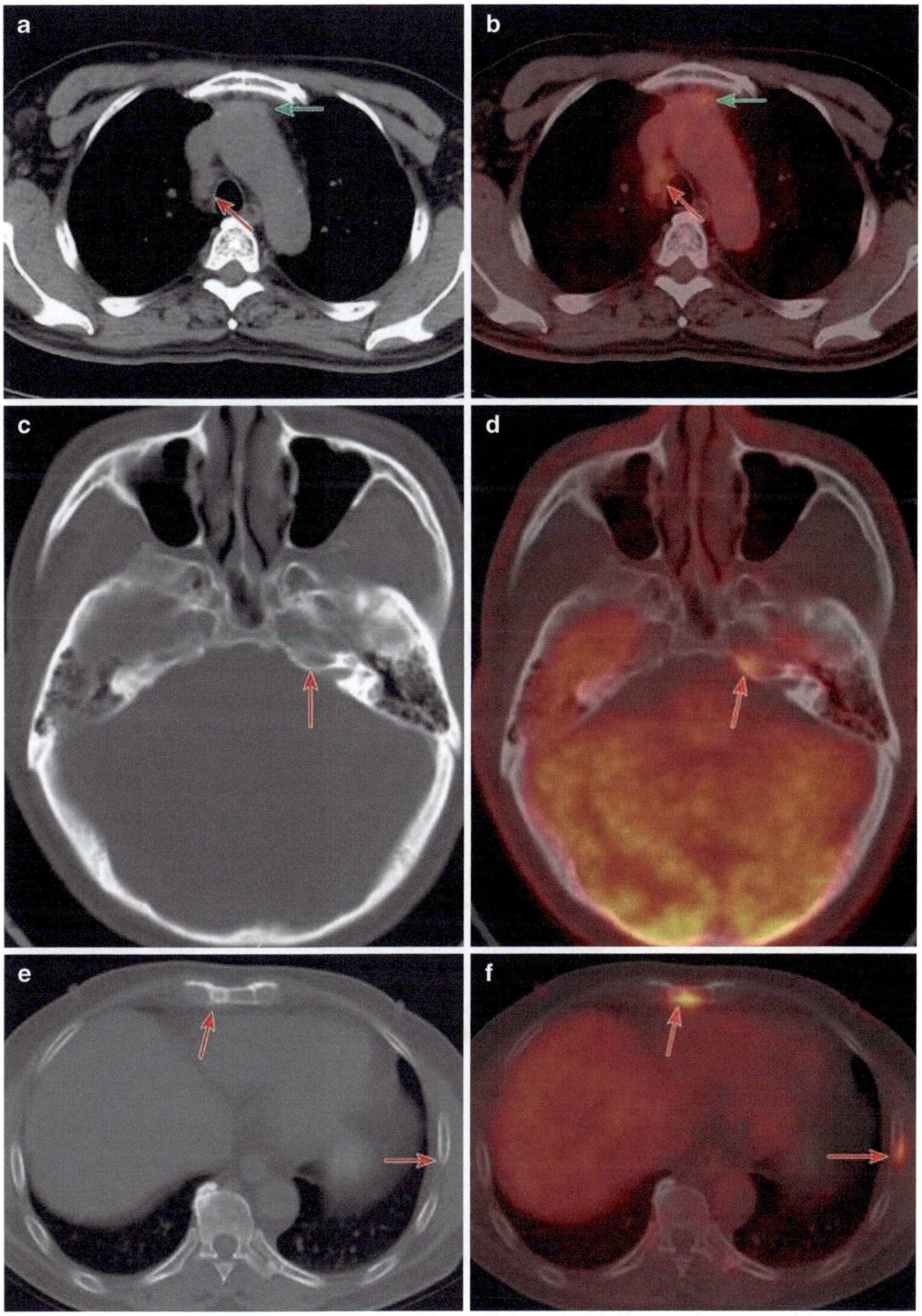

Fig. 16.10 ^{18}F-FDG PET/CT images of postoperative recurrence after surgery for atypical carcinoid tumors of the thymus and metastasis to the petrous part of the temporal bone. Figures **a**, **c**, and **d** were CT images, while Figures **b**, **d**, and **f** were PET/CT fusion images. (**a** and **b**) After thymus operation, local region was seen with irregular soft tissue density lesion (green arrow) and increased metabolism, with SUVmax being about 3.7. Enlarged lymph nodes were discovered (red arrows) in the mediastinum near the right lower trachea with increased metabolism. (**c** and **d**) Focal increased metabolism in the petrous apex of the left temporal bone, with SUVmax 4.3, and no definite bone destruction was found on CT. (**e** and **f**) Sternum osteogenic destruction with increased metabolism and SUVmax 4.9; a focal metabolic increase in the left rib with no confirmable bone destruction. The diagnosis based on PET/CT was recurrence with mediastinal lymph node metastasis and multiple bone metastases. Although lesions with focal increased FDG uptake in the petrous apex of the left temporal bone and left rib showed no definite bone destruction on CT, there were other metastatic lesions out of the head (such as sternal bone metastasis) detected by PET/CT, so it had adequate confidence to identify the focus with increased FDG uptake in the petrous apex of the left temporal bone as a metastatic tumor

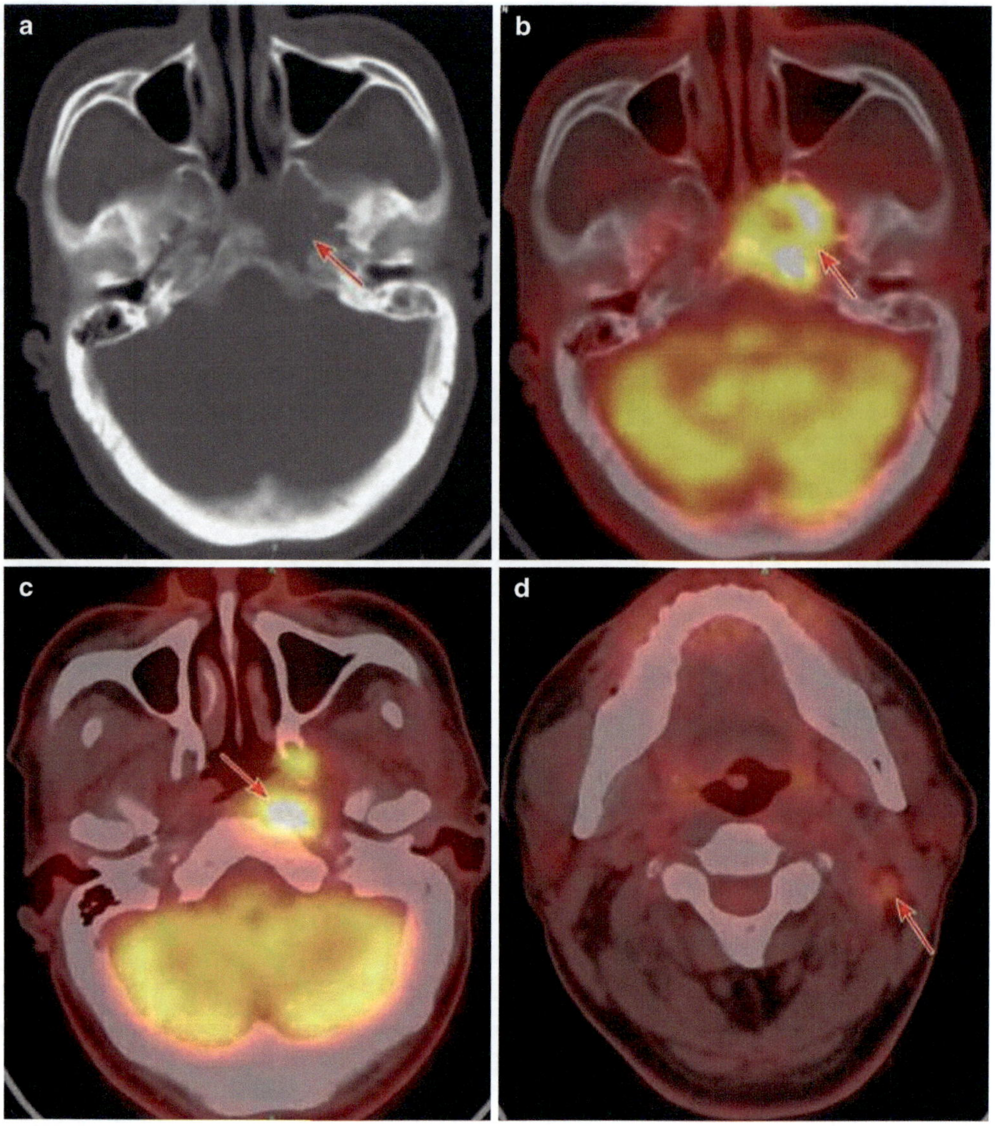

Fig. 16.11 ^{18}F-FDG PET/CT images of nasopharyngeal carcinoma directly invading the petrous apex of the temporal bone. (**a** and **b**) CT bone window image and cross section of PET/CT fusion image of the temporal bone, respectively: CT showed osteolysis bone destruction at the petrous apex of the left temporal bone, basal part of the occipital bone, and greater wing of the left sphenoid bone, soft tissue density lesion was observed, the edge of the destruction area was irregular, and the part was in worm-eaten shape. PET/CT fusion images showed increased focal metabolism in the bone destruction area, and SUVmax was about 11.2. (**c**) PET/CT fusion image at the lower level of Fig. **b**: the left pharyngeal recess became shallow and disappeared, local soft tissue thickened and metabolism increased, SUVmax was about 12.3, and the medial muscle of left wing was invaded. (**d**) Submaxillary plane PET/CT fusion image: lymph node metastasis was seen in the left cervical II region

5.4 Differential Diagnosis

Langerhans cell histiocytosis (LCH):

1. Clinical overview: LCH is a group of tissue-cell proliferative diseases with unknown causes; it is a group of heterogeneous diseases clinically. The pathology is characterized with proliferation of mature eosinophilic cells and Langerhans cells, of which eosinophilic granulomas are the most common. CT image shows osteolytic bone destruction accompanied by soft tissue mass formation, with clear and sharp margins of the destruction lesion, and soft tissue mass shows no invasion to the surrounding bone. In the repair stage, the margin of the damaged lesion may show osteosclerosis, and the range of the late stage sclerosis expands. Osteolytic lesions may contain residual bone fragments, known as "buttonlike dead bones."
2. PET/CT diagnostic points: Most of them are highly metabolized and difficult to distinguish from osteolytic bone metastases. However, PET/CT is used for systemic imaging, and most of them are able to show primary body lesions, which is helpful for the diagnosis of metastatic tumors (Fig. 16.12).

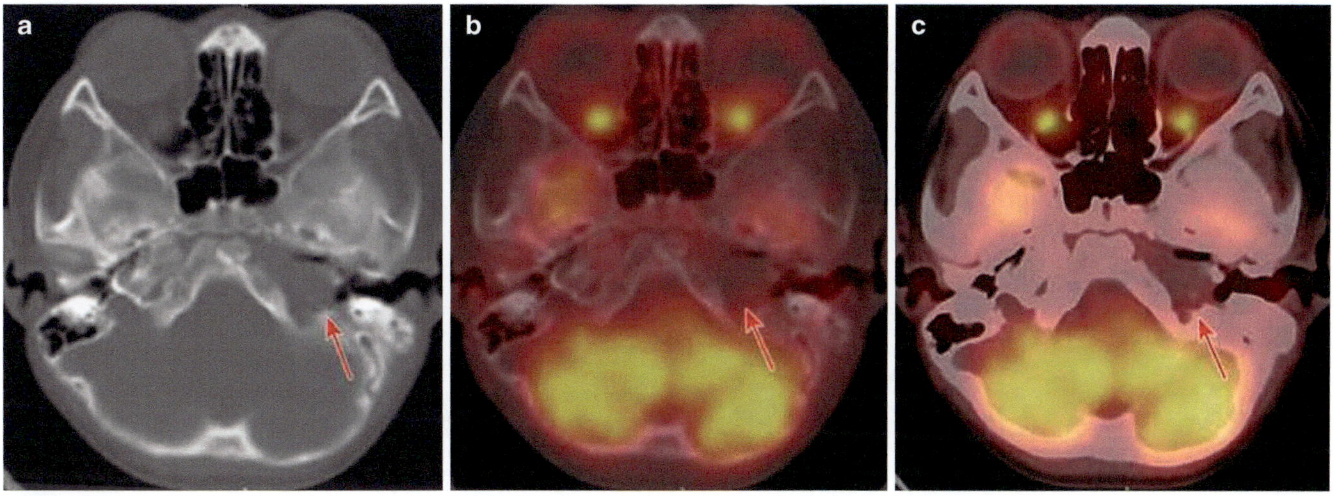

Fig. 16.12 ^{18}F-FDG PET/CT images of Langerhans cell histiocytosis. A 5-year-old child patient with Langerhans cell histiocytosis was reviewed with ^{18}F-FDG PET/CT images after six cycles of chemotherapy: (**a**) CT image (bone window) was seen with osteolytic bone destruction of the petrous part of the left temporal bone and soft tissue density lesion with smooth, sharp margins and no erosion. (**b**) PET/CT fusion image (bone window). (**c**) PET/CT fusion image (soft tissue window). Figures **b** and **c** showed no metabolism in the lesion, while Figures **a** and **c** showed small bone fragments in soft tissue lesions

5.5 Summary

The application value of ^{18}F-FDG PET/CT for temporal bone metastases is higher than that for primary tumors, which is mainly used in:

1. Searching for primary tumors: ^{18}F-FDG PET/CT is helpful for searching for primary tumors in the detection of metastatic tumors or bone destructions in the temporal bone.
2. Understanding the lesion invasion scope: For those inflicted with direct spreading and invasion to the temporal bone, such as nasopharyngeal carcinoma, ^{18}F-FDG PET/CT examination is helpful to determine the local invasion scope and know whether there is local lymph node metastasis or distant metastasis.
3. For patients with known primary lesion, ^{18}F-FDG PET/CT can be used for tumor staging.

Part V

CT of Neck Neoplasms

General Introduction of PET/CT of Neck Neoplasms

17

Yuetao Wang, Xiaoliang Shao, and Feifei Zhang

1 Overview

Head and neck tumors are common in Asian countries while relatively uncommon in Western ones. Many factors are related to the occurrence of head and neck tumors, including smoking, alcohol abuse, environmental pollution, viral infection, heredity, diet, and chemical contact. The pharynx, larynx, thyroid, and salivary glands are the most common sites of neck tumors which may metastasize to the cervical lymph nodes in the early stage. Most of laryngopharyngeal tumors are squamous cell carcinoma originating from epithelial tissues. See Chap. 4 of Part II for details. Thyroid cancer accounts for 0.2–1.0% of all human malignant tumors, and papillary carcinoma is the most common type. At present, thyroid cancer is the solid tumor with the fastest-growing incidence and mostly occurs in women. Salivary gland tumors account for about 3% of head and neck tumors, 80% of which are parotid gland tumors, and also include sublingual, submandibular, and minor salivary gland tumors. Lymphomas often involve cervical lymph nodes and Waldeyer's ring and occasionally originate from the thyroid gland, parotid gland, and throat. Rare cervical tumors include rhabdomyosarcoma and fibrosarcoma. Pathologically, tumor differentiation and infiltration depth are related to the prognosis.

Painless cervical lymph node enlargement is often the first clinical manifestation of either head and neck neoplasms or metastases from other sites. Some patients with neck tumors may present with hoarseness, dysphagia, etc. Besides palpation, B-ultrasonography is the most widely used method to detect and evaluate lesions. Owing to the superficial location of neck tumors, invasive endoscopic examination such as laryngoscopy and ultrasound-guided aspiration is easy to be performed. Accordingly, histopathological specimens can be obtained to make a definite diagnosis. SPECT/CT has an auxiliary value for qualitatively diagnosing thyroid tumors and salivary gland tumors. CT, MRI, and PET/CT can be used to evaluate the lesion range, relationship with adjacent anatomical structures, lymph node metastasis, etc. Also, PET/CT can accurately evaluate the distant metastasis, hence further assisting the clinical staging of the tumors.

1.1 Applied Anatomy of the Neck

The neck is located between the head and the shoulders and superior to the chest. The neck area is small. The upper boundary is a line connecting the inferior border of the mandible, angle of the mandible, mastoidale, superior nuchal line, and external occipital protuberance. The lower boundary is a line connecting the jugular notch, sternoclavicular joint, supraclavicular border, scapula, and acromion to the spinous process of the seventh cervical vertebra. The neck is divided into the anterior portion of the neck, including the anterior cervical region, sternocleidomastoid region, and lateral cervical region and the posterior nape. The neck is supported by the cervical spine. The infrahyoid region of the anterior neck contains thyroid glands and parathyroid glands, with the cervical respiratory tract and the cervical digestive tract behind as well as great vessels and nerves arranged longitudinally on both sides. The root of the neck contains the cupula of the pleura and apex of the lung, as well as oblique blood vessels and nerves.

Y. Wang (✉)
Changzhou Key Laboratory of Molecular Imaging, The First People's Hospital of Changzhou, The Third Affiliated Hospital of Soochow University, Changzhou, Jiangsu, China

X. Shao · F. Zhang
The First People's Hospital of Changzhou, Changzhou, Jiangsu, China

Z. Yao, S. Li (eds.), *Atlas of PET/CT in Oncology - Volume 1*, https://doi.org/10.1007/978-981-99-1172-1_17

The neck is divided into four regions: anterior cervical region, mainly including the hypopharynx, larynx, esophagus, thyroid glands, and parathyroid glands; two lateral cervical regions, including the sternocleidomastoid and carotid sheath vessels; and posterior cervical region, mainly including the cervical spine and its surrounding muscles.

The imaging diagnosis of neck neoplasm is closely related to the tumor location. In surgery, superficial muscles are used as landmarks, and the neck is divided into anterior triangles (submental, submandibular, carotid, and muscular), posterior triangle (occipital), and subclavian triangle. In imaging studies, the neck is divided into various spaces according to the cervical fascia, and intrinsic organs are located within the spaces.

1.2 Neck Lymph Node Levels

Lymph nodes belong to lymphatic organs and they are round or oval gray-red bodies of different sizes. One side of the lymph nodes is convex and distributed by afferent lymphatic vessels. The other side is concave, centered by the hilum of the lymph node, and distributed by nerves, blood vessels, and efferent lymphatic vessels. Lymph nodes are usually distributed in groups, arranged along blood vessels, and inconstant in numbers. The primary function of the lymph nodes is to filter lymph, produce lymphocytes, and initiate immune response. The sentinel lymph node (SLN) is the first lymph node or group of nodes draining the lymph from an organ or site. When a lesion such as a tumor starts there, SLN can intercept or eliminate tumor cells and prevent the cancerous dissemination. At this point, the lymph nodes undergo pathological changes such as cell proliferation and result in lymph node enlargement. If regional lymph nodes cannot prevent the cancerous dissemination, the lesion may spread far away along the lymphatics. Hence, a regional lymph node enlargement often indicates a lesion in its drainage area.

Lymph nodes in the head and neck are arranged in an annular pattern at the head and neck junction and longitudinally along the veins at the neck, and few are located around the digestive tract and the respiratory tract, including the submental, submandibular, anterior cervical, superficial cervical, and deep cervical lymph nodes. In addition to lymphatic drainage from the head and neck, cervical lymph nodes receive some lymphatic drainage from the chest and upper limbs. The lymph then travels from efferent lymph vessels downward and directly or indirectly into the deep lateral cervical lymph nodes. Currently, the cervical lymph nodes are widely divided into seven levels (Table 17.1). Among them, levels II–IV make up the internal jugular chain which receives drainage from the parotid, submandibular, submental, retropharyngeal, and anterior cervical lymph nodes and hence is a key area for neck dissection.

Table 17.1 Neck lymph node levels

Level	Sublevel	Lymph node group	Boundary	Features
I	IA (submental) IB (submandibular) Bounded by the digastric muscles	Submental and submandibular lymph node groups	Bounded above by the mandible and below by the digastric muscle and the hyoid bone	Level I lymph nodes receive lymphatic drainage from the chin, lips, cheek, floor of the mouth, anterior oral tongue, palate, sublingual gland, and submandibular gland
II	IIA (anterior- inferior) IIB (posterior-superior) Separated by the vertical plane defined by the spinal accessory nerve	Upper jugular group	The anterior boundary is the stylohyoid muscle, and the posterior boundary is the upper third of the posterior border of the sternocleidomastoid muscle. The upper jugular nodes extend from the level of the skull base (above) to the level of the inferior border of the hyoid bone (below)	Primary sites of laryngeal cancer metastases
III		Middle jugular group	The anterior boundary is the lateral border of the sternohyoid muscle, and the posterior boundary is the middle third of the posterior border of the sternocleidomastoid muscle. The middle jugular nodes extend from the inferior border of the hyoid bone (above) to the junction between the superior belly of the omohyoid muscle and the internal jugular vein or the inferior border of the cricoid cartilage (below)	Progresses superiorly from level II and inferiorly to level IV
IV		Lower jugular lymph group	The lower jugular nodes extend from the inferior border of the cricoid cartilage (above) to the superior border of the clavicle (below). The anterior boundary is the lateral border of the sternohyoid muscle, and the posterior boundary is the lower third of the posterior border of the sternocleidomastoid muscle	An extension down of level III
V	VA (posterior triangle level) VB (supraclavicular level) Bounded by the lower border of the cricoid cartilage	Posterior triangle and supraclavicular lymph groups	The anterior boundary is adjacent to the posterior boundary of levels I, III, and IV or the posterior border of the sternocleidomastoid muscle. The posterior boundary is the anterior border of the trapezius muscle, and the inferior boundary is the clavicle	
VI		Central compartment nodes (including prelaryngeal, paratracheal, perithyroidal, and retropharyngeal nodes)	Level VI is defined by the infrahyoid (strap) muscles. The superior boundary is the lower border of the hyoid bone, the inferior boundary is the suprasternal notch, and the lateral boundaries are the common carotid arteries. The anterior boundary is the superficial layer of the deep fascia, and the posterior boundary is the deep layer of the deep fascia	The prelaryngeal lymph nodes receive lymphatic drainage from the subglottic region
VII		Superior mediastinal nodes	Located between the common carotid arteries from the superior border of the manubrium to the innominate vein	Closely related to the thyroid, hypopharyngeal, and cervical esophageal cancer

2 Essentials for PET/CT Image Acquisition

2.1 Normal Physiological Distribution of ^{18}F-FDG in the Neck

^{18}F-FDG can be absorbed by normal tissues of the neck, such as the muscle, gland, lymphoid tissue, fat, and mucous membrane. The physiological ^{18}F-FDG uptake is usually symmetrical on both sides, and the symmetry is one of the features for identifying a physiological or pathological uptake. Nevertheless, the pathological uptake may also show bilateral symmetry, and due to the position, the physiological uptake may also show bilateral asymmetry. Especially, the postoperative image is acquired under more complex situations, and a diagnosis should be made closely combined with clinical conditions.

The parotid gland and the submandibular gland usually show mild to moderate homogeneous FDG uptake, and some of them show no FDG uptake. The thyroid usually shows unremarkable FDG uptake. The ^{18}F-FDG uptake is relatively low in the tongue muscle and is noted in the cervical cord of some individuals. Cervical lymph nodes often show different degrees of physiological uptake, mainly due to the ^{18}F-FDG uptake by some lymphocytes and macrophages. The pharyngeal lymphoid ring (inner ring: Waldeyer's tonsillar ring) composed of the palatine and lingual tonsils can be clearly shown in the coronal plane. The mucosa of the oropharynx and nasopharynx usually shows physiological FDG uptake, which is more obvious in the presence of non-specific inflammation, manifesting as strip uptake distributed along the mucosal surface. The FDG uptake is usually unremarkable in the cervical bone and none in each sinus cavity (Figs. 17.1, 17.2, 17.3, 17.4, 17.5, 17.6, 17.7, 17.8, and 17.9).

There is usually unremarkable uptake in the muscle of the neck. When the uptake appears in the muscle, it is often associated with muscular tension of the neck and often shows homogeneously increased uptake in the whole muscle on both sides or on one side. The condition can be judged by observing anatomical structures and medical history taking. For example, a patient who recently underwent an operation is prone to an increased uptake in unilateral muscle. The uptake in some muscle tendons may be localized and should

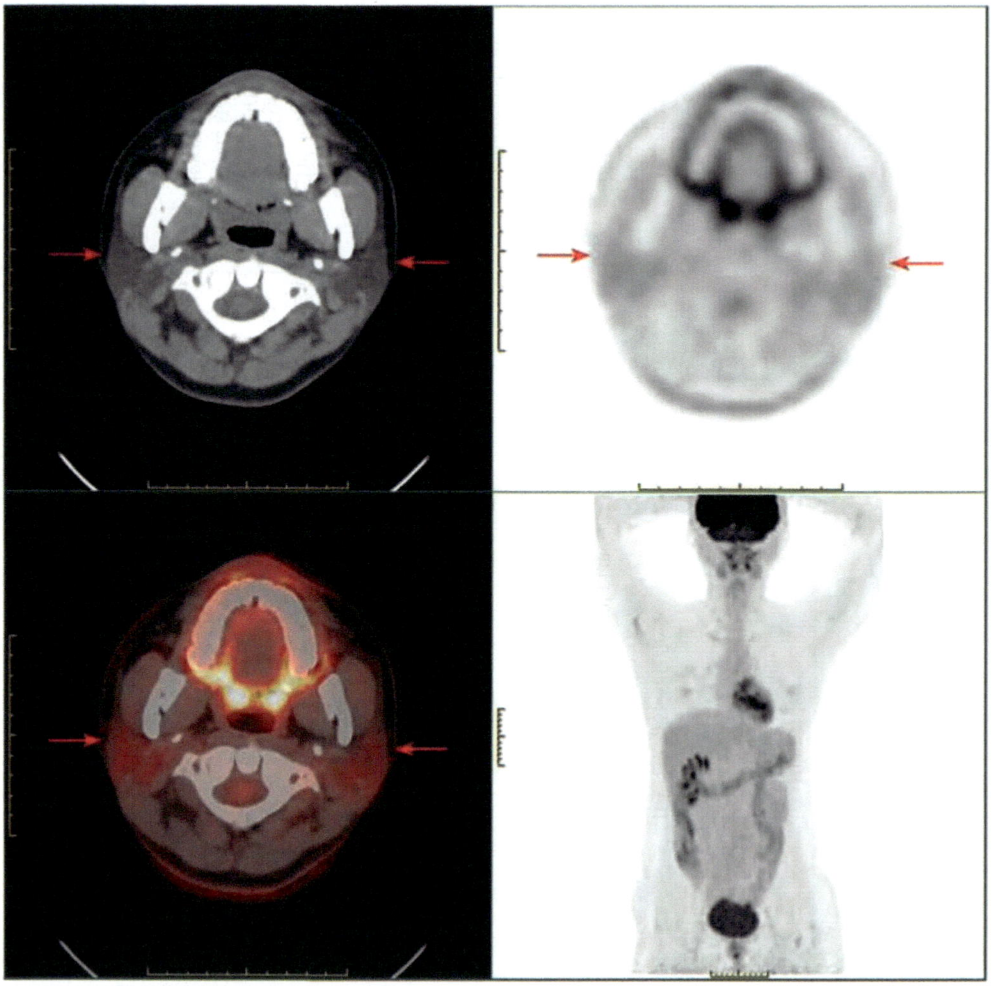

Fig. 17.1 Physiological ^{18}F-FDG uptake in the bilateral parotid glands. A 19-year-old female presented with imaging findings of a mild diffuse increased FDG uptake in the bilateral parotid glands and basically symmetrical and homogeneous distribution on both sides, without significantly abnormal density (arrow)

be carefully identified in the axial, coronal, and sagittal planes (Figs. 17.10, 17.11, and 17.12).

Under cold conditions, there may be a symmetrical increased uptake in adipose tissues on both sides of the neck. This is caused by the activation of the brown adipose tissue and is more likely to occur in thinner women. The brown adipose tissue is mainly distributed in the root of the neck, bilateral clavicular regions, and both sides of the vertebral column (Figs. 17.13 and 17.14).

Surgical history and postoperative complications have a significant impact on the FDG PET/CT imaging. Hence, the medical history should be inquired carefully. The non-specific inflammation in the field of surgery can present increased FDG uptake and cause false positive findings. Surgical injury to the recurrent laryngeal nerve results in a compensatory increased FDG uptake in the contralateral vocal cords, whereas usually there is no increased FDG uptake in the diseased vocal cords (Figs. 17.15 and 17.16).

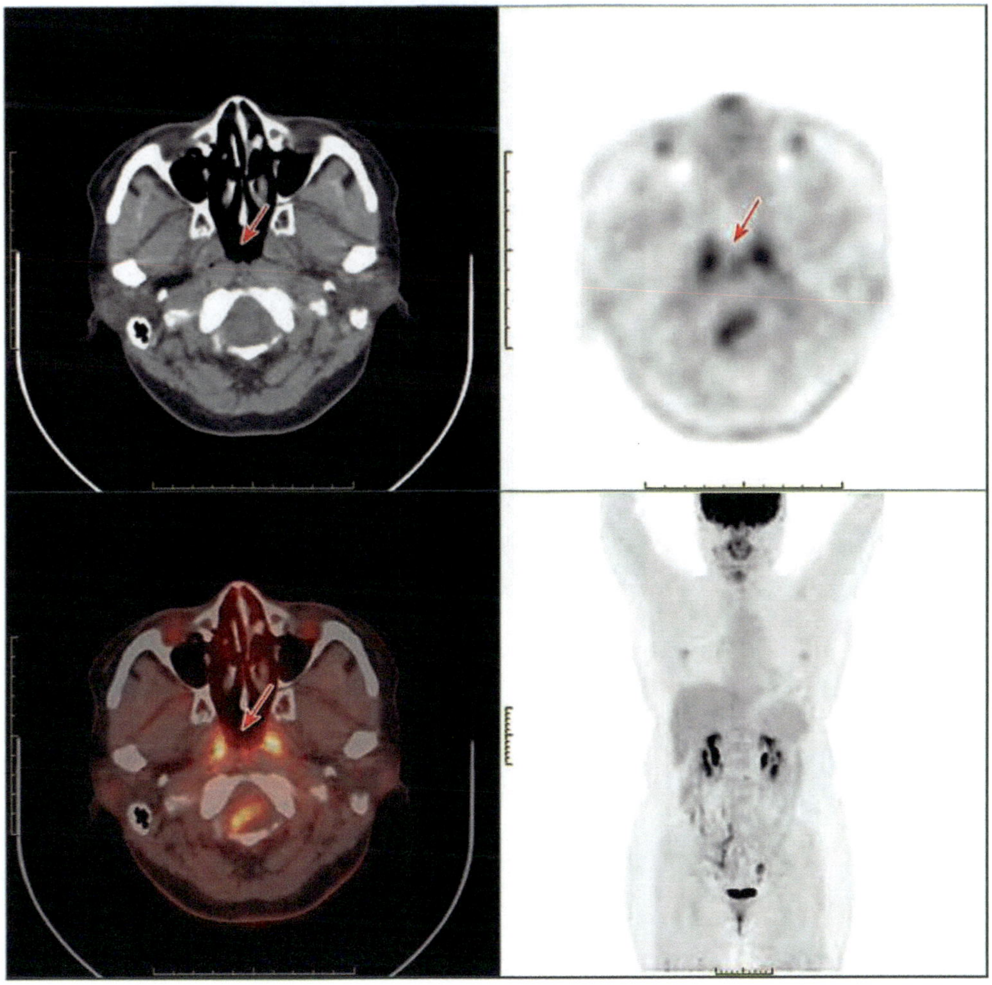

Fig. 17.2 Physiological ^{18}F-FDG uptake in the nasopharynx. A 46-year-old female presented with a symmetrical increased FDG uptake in both lateral walls of the pharynx (arrow), without significantly abnormal density. Bilateral auditory tubes are unobstructed

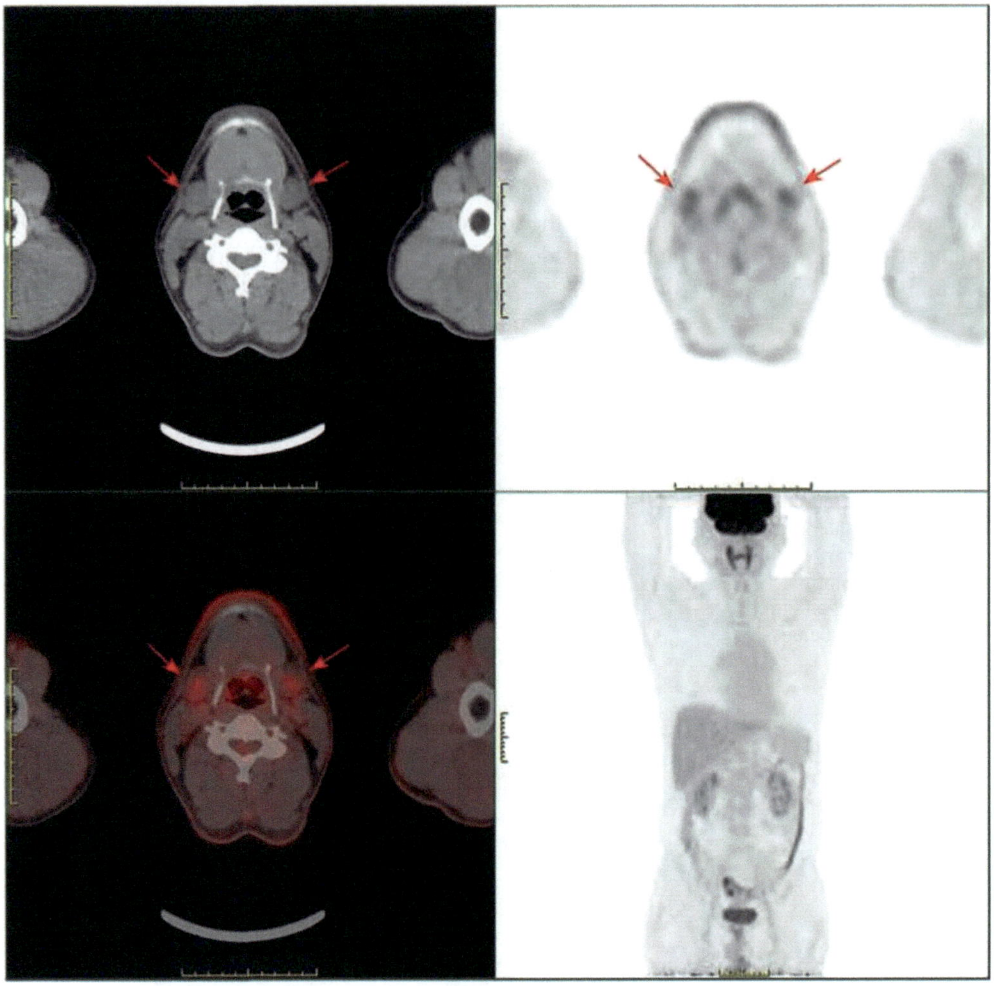

Fig. 17.3 Physiological ^{18}F-FDG uptake in the submandibular glands. A 52-year-old male presented with a diffuse FDG uptake in the bilateral submandibular glands. The distribution of FDG is less homogeneous and basically symmetrical on both sides, without significantly abnormal density (arrow)

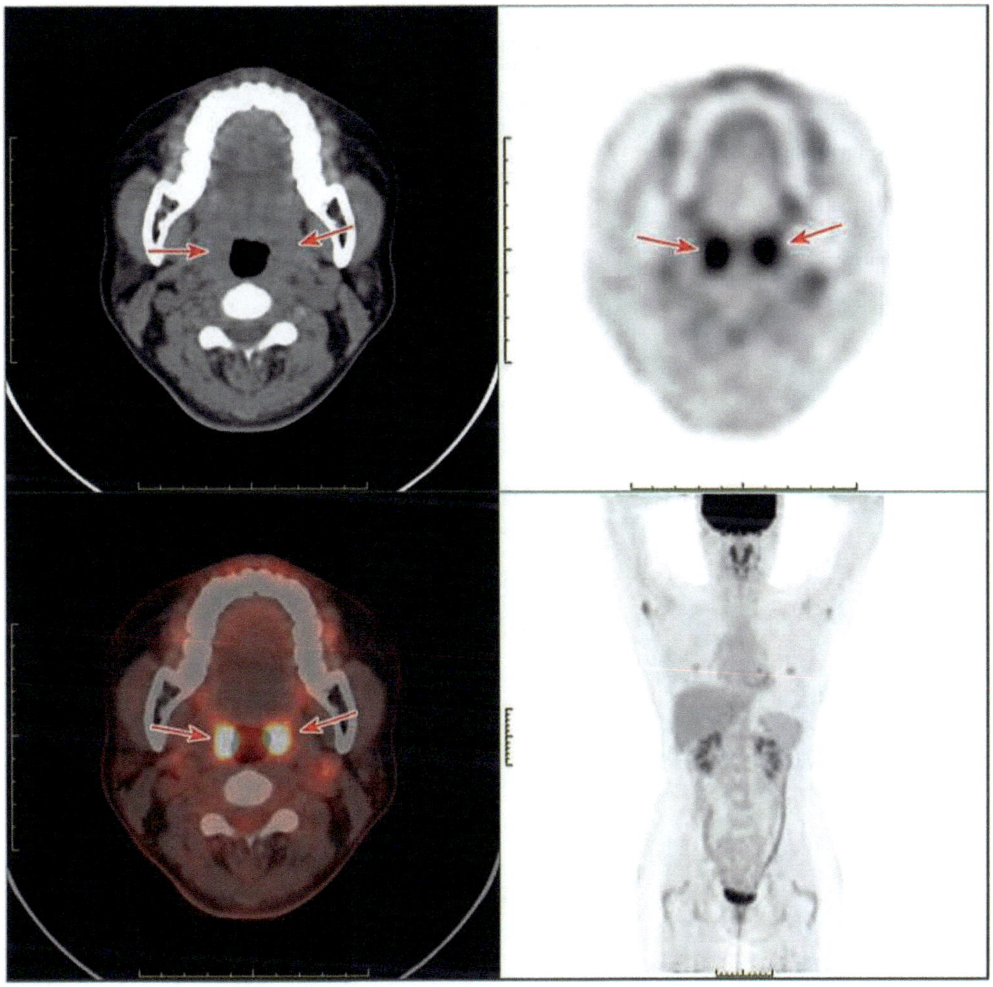

Fig. 17.4 Physiological ^{18}F-FDG uptake of in the palatine tonsils. A 43-year-old female presented with imaging findings of increased FDG uptake in the bilateral palatine tonsils as well as symmetrical and homogeneous distribution, without remarkable enlargement or abnormal density shadow (arrow)

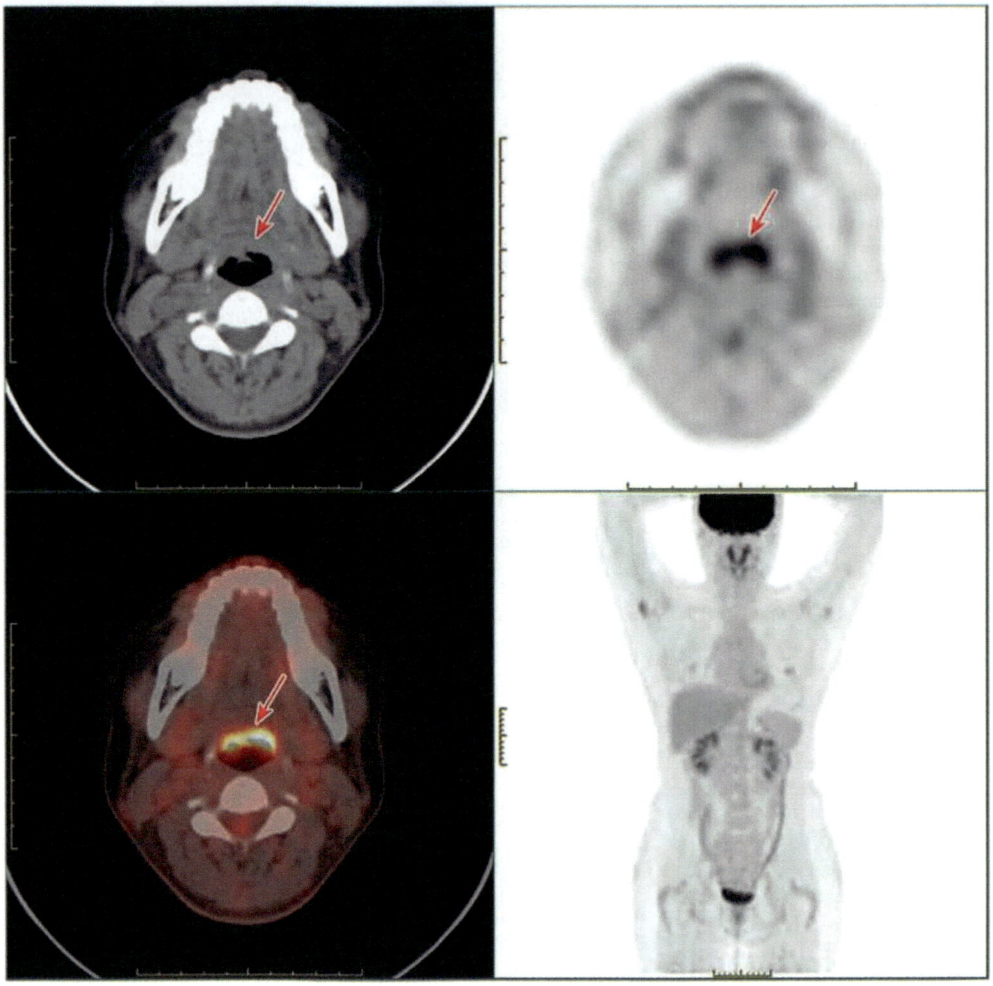

Fig. 17.5 Physiological ^{18}F-FDG uptake in the lingual tonsils. A 43-year-old female presented with imaging findings of increased FDG uptake in the lingual tonsils at the root of the tongue and a strip-like distribution, without remarkable enlargement or abnormal density (arrow)

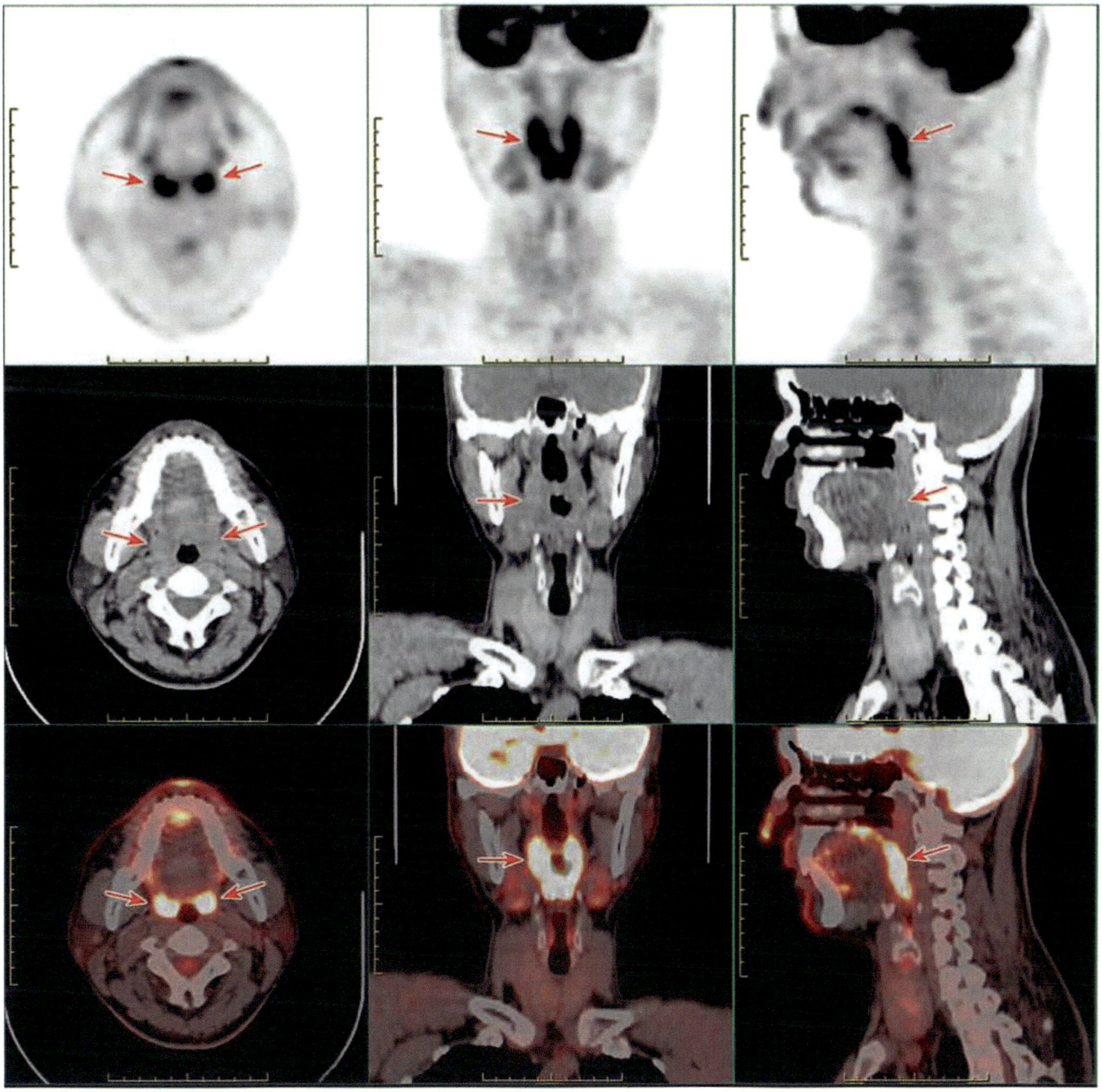

Fig. 17.6 Physiological ^{18}F-FDG uptake in the pharyngeal lymphoid ring (inner ring: Waldeyer's tonsillar ring). A 50-year-old male presented with imaging findings of a diffuse increased of FDG uptake in the tubal tonsils, palatine tonsils, and lingual tonsils as well as in the lateral pharyngeal bands and retropharyngeal lymph nodes, with an "annular" distribution in the coronal plane (arrow)

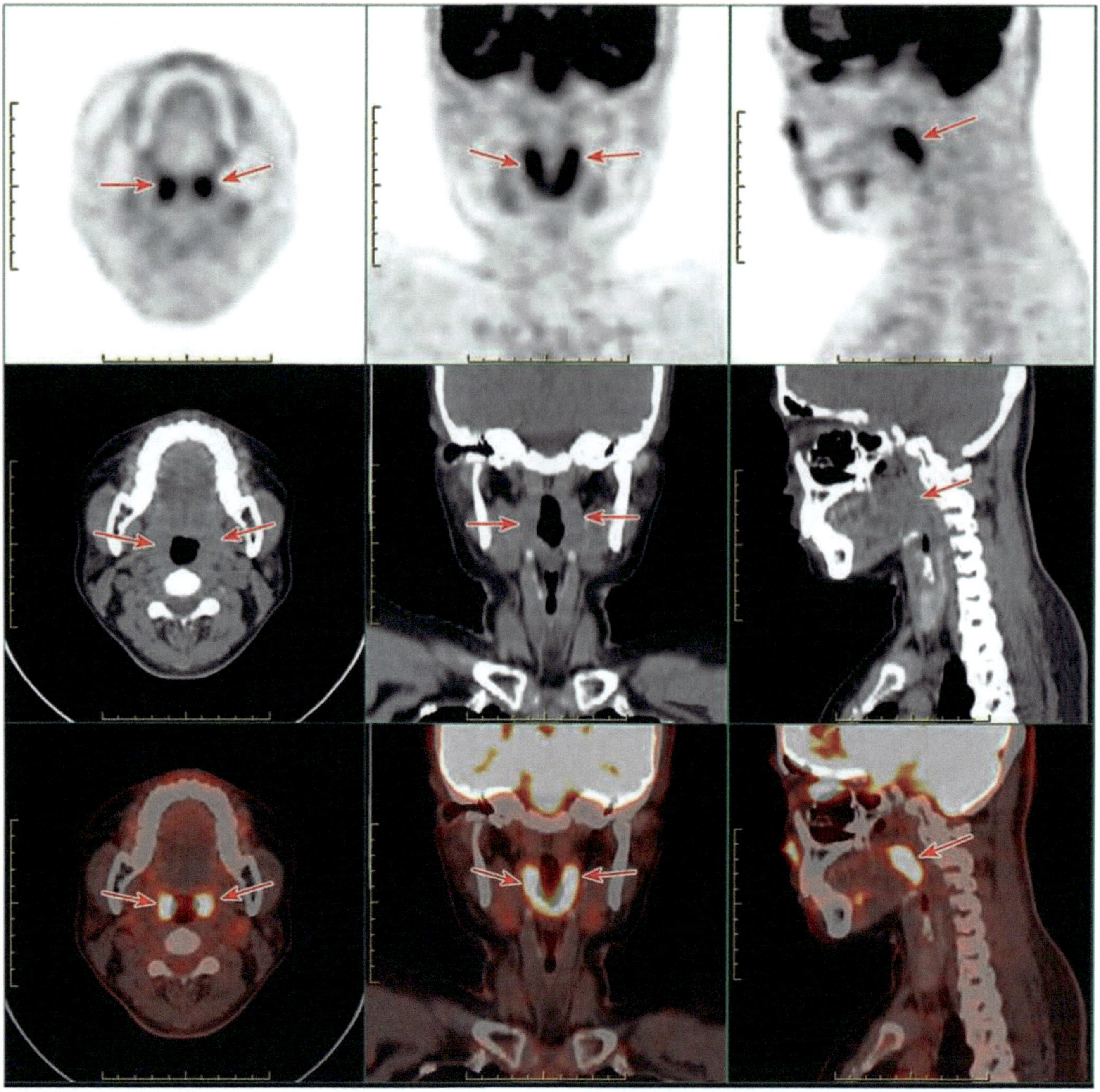

Fig. 17.7 Physiological ^{18}F-FDG uptake in the pharyngeal lymphoid ring (inner ring: Waldeyer's tonsillar ring). A 43-year-old female presented with imaging findings of a diffuse increased FDG uptake in the tubal tonsils, palatine tonsils, and lingual tonsils as well as in the lateral pharyngeal bands and retropharyngeal lymph nodes, with an "annular" distribution in the coronal plane (arrow)

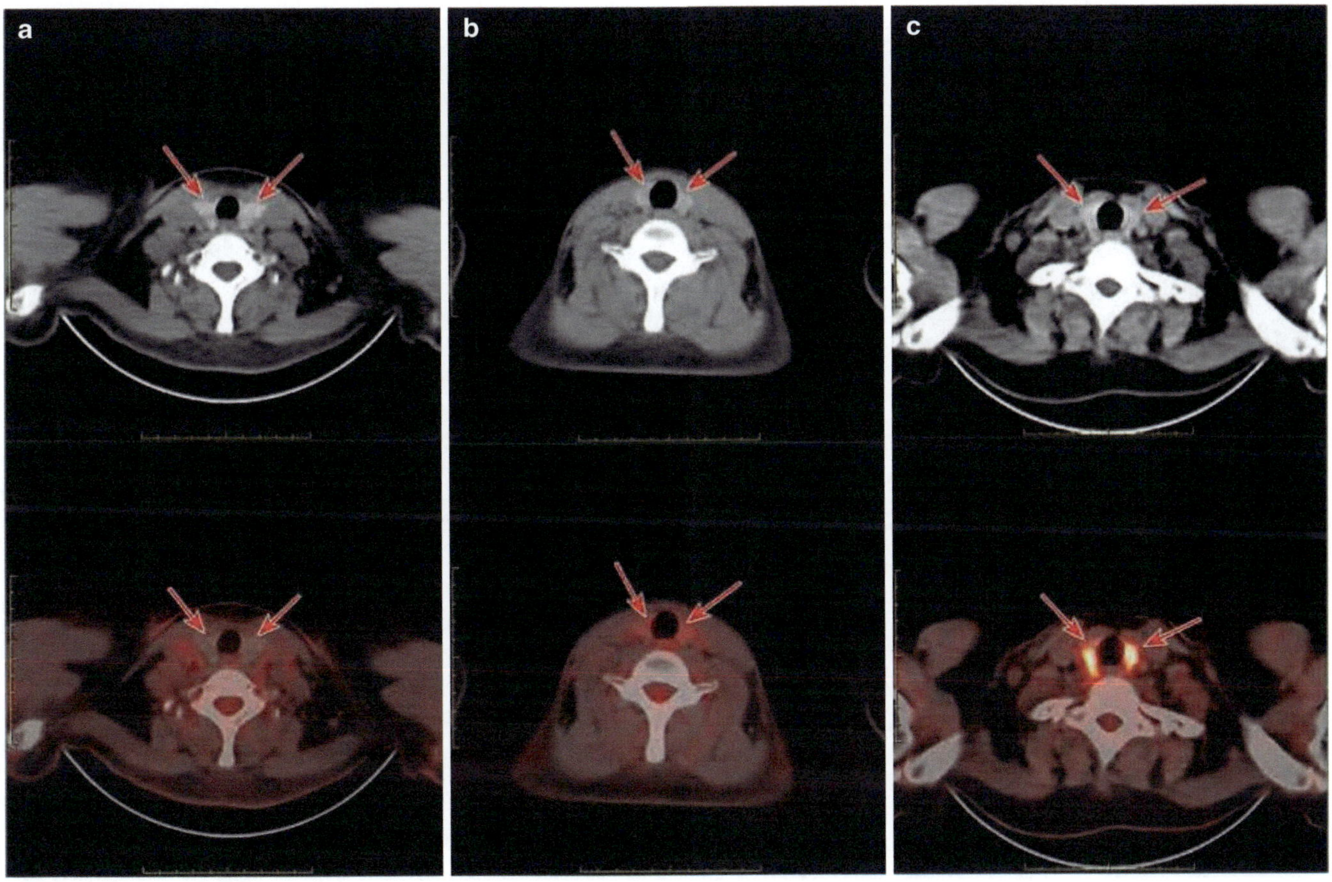

Fig. 17.8 ^{18}F-FDG PET/CT images of the thyroid glands. (**a**) A 43-year-old female presented with thyroid FDG uptake close to the background radiation. (**b**) A 19-year-old female presented with a mild increased thyroid FDG uptake. (**c**). A 59-year-old female presented with a diffuse increased thyroid FDG uptake, with basically bilateral symmetry (arrows). Unremarkable results in the above subjects were found by either thyroid function test or the B-scan ultrasonography

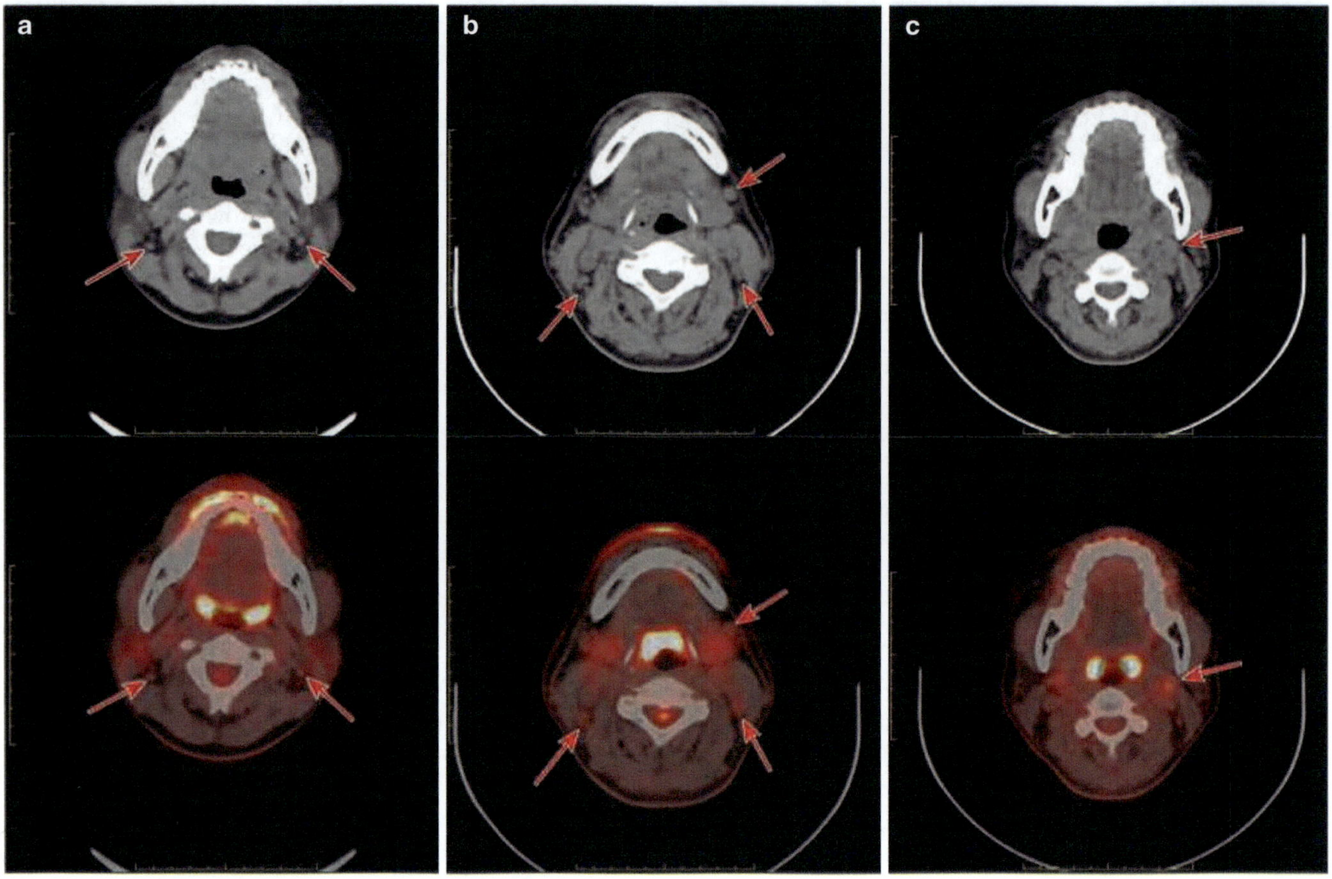

Fig. 17.9 ^{18}F-FDG PET/CT images of the cervical lymph nodes. (**a**) A 19-year-old female. The FDG uptake in level II lymph nodes in both sides of the neck, being close to that in the background. (**b**) A 50-year-old male presented with a mild increased FDG uptake in the scattered lymph nodes of level I in the left neck and level III in both sides of the neck. (**c**) A 43-year-old female presented with increased FDG uptake in the level II lymph node in the left neck. Arrows indicate lymph nodes with increased FDG uptake

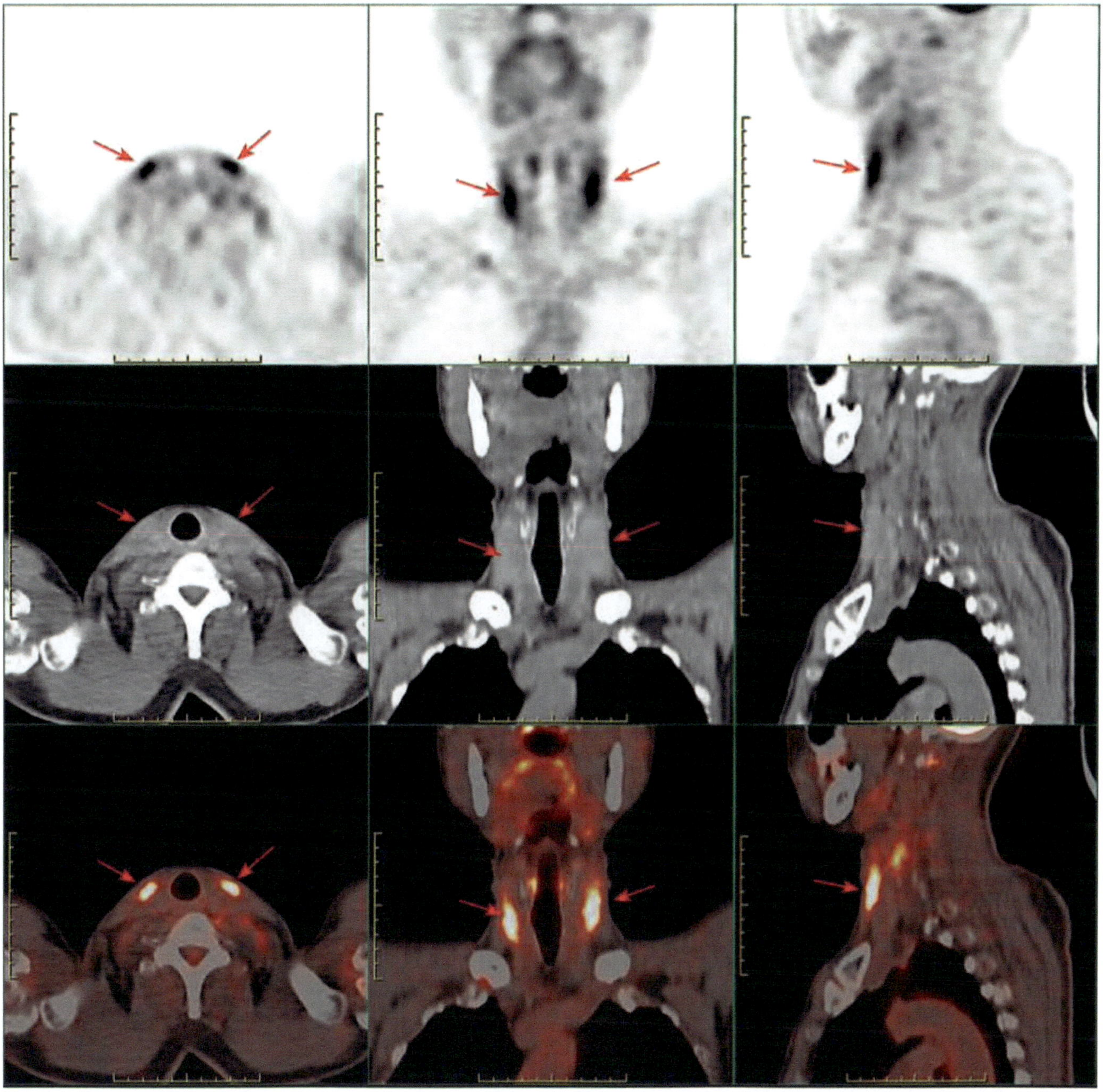

Fig. 17.10 Physiological ^{18}F-FDG uptake in the bilateral sternocleidomastoid muscles. A 5-year-old male presented with imaging findings of a symmetrical increased FDG uptake in the bilateral sternocleidomastoid muscles, without significantly abnormal density (arrow)

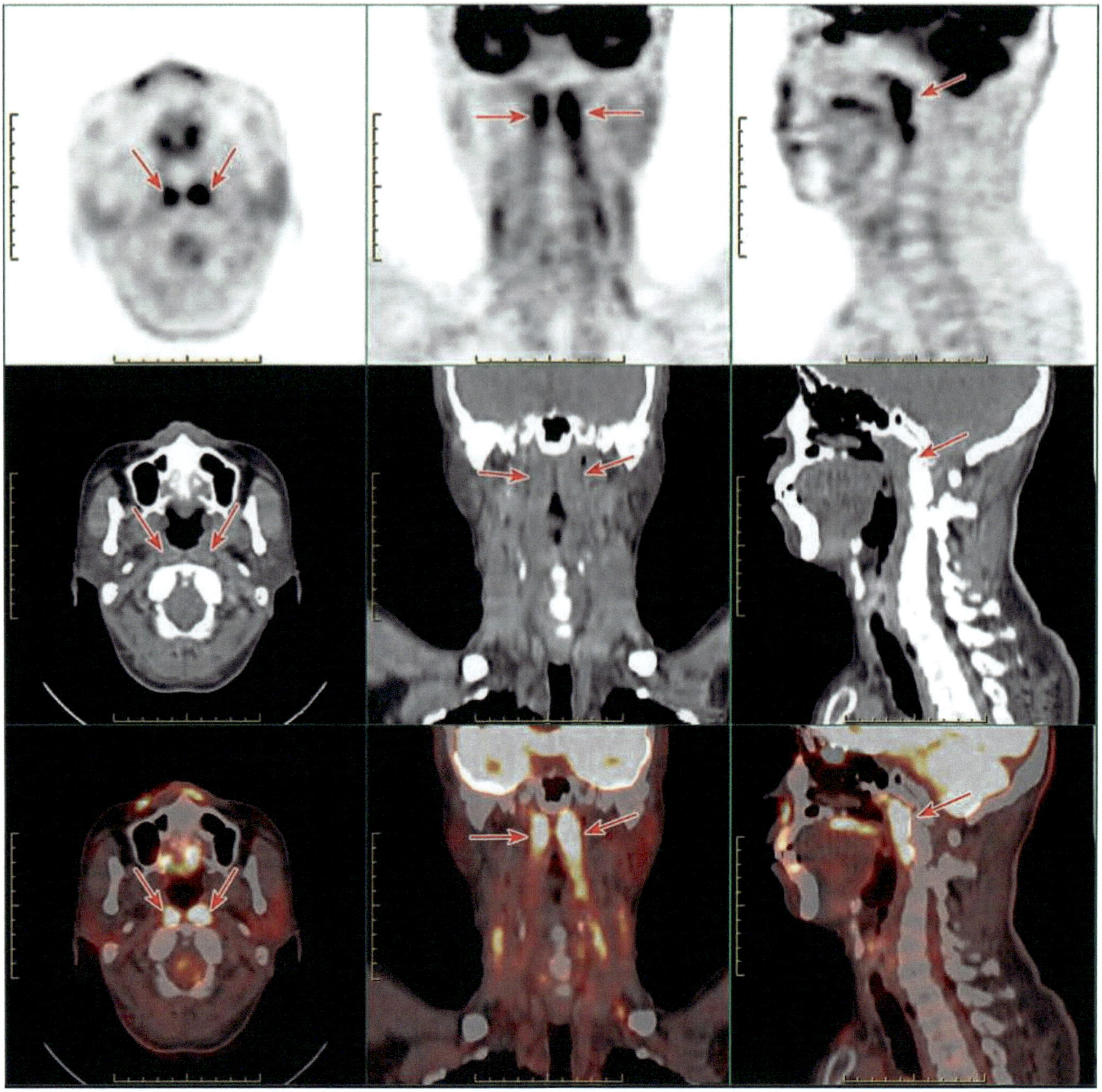

Fig. 17.11 Physiological ^{18}F-FDG uptake in the bilateral longus colli muscles. A 65-year-old male presented with a symmetrical increased FDG uptake in the bilateral longus colli muscles, without significantly abnormal density (arrow)

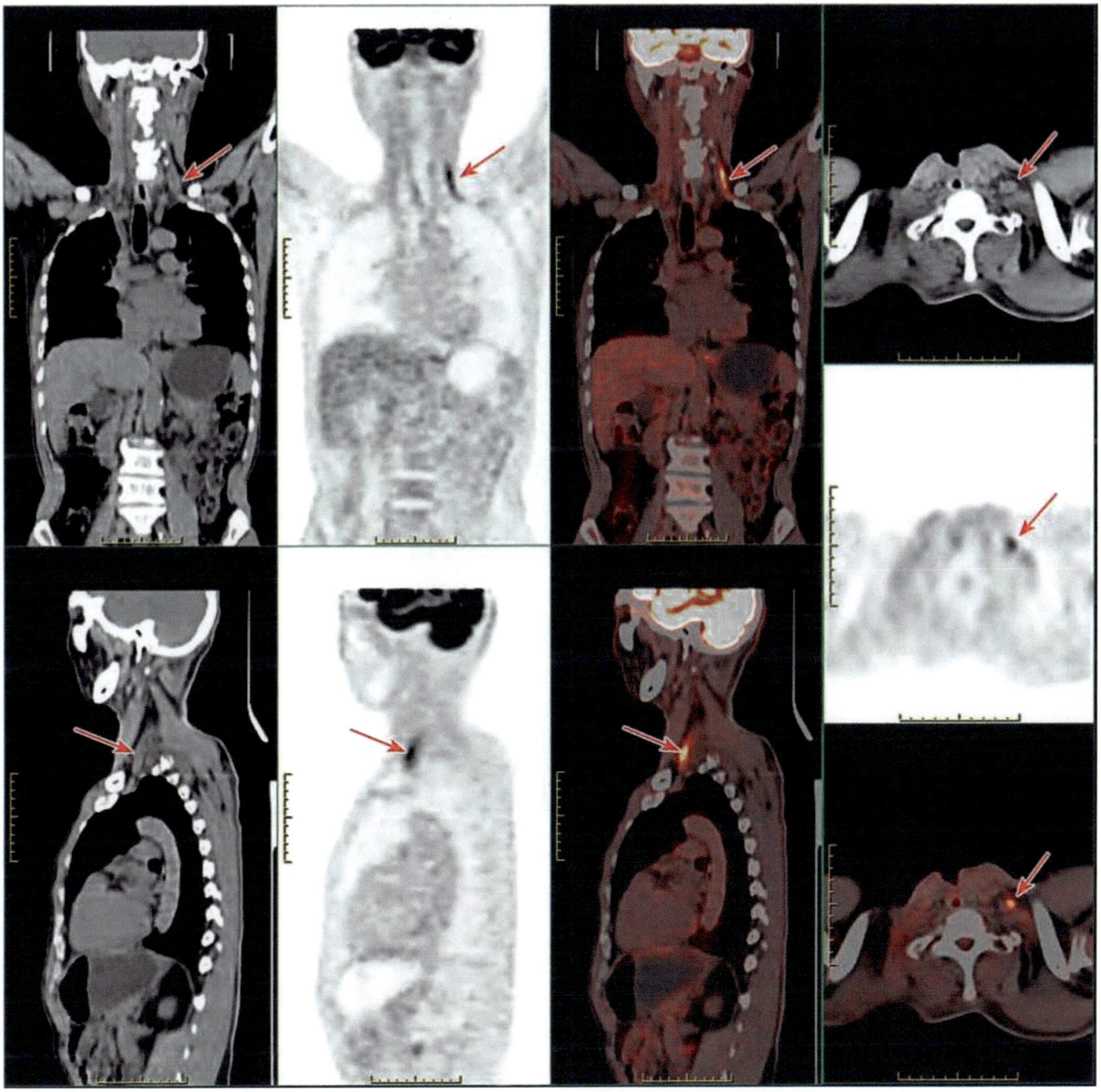

Fig. 17.12 Physiological ^{18}F-FDG uptake in the left musculi subclavius. A 59-year-old male presented with status post-tracheotomy for laryngeal cancer. PET/CT shows a diffuse increased FDG uptake in the left musculi subclavius without significantly abnormal density (arrow)

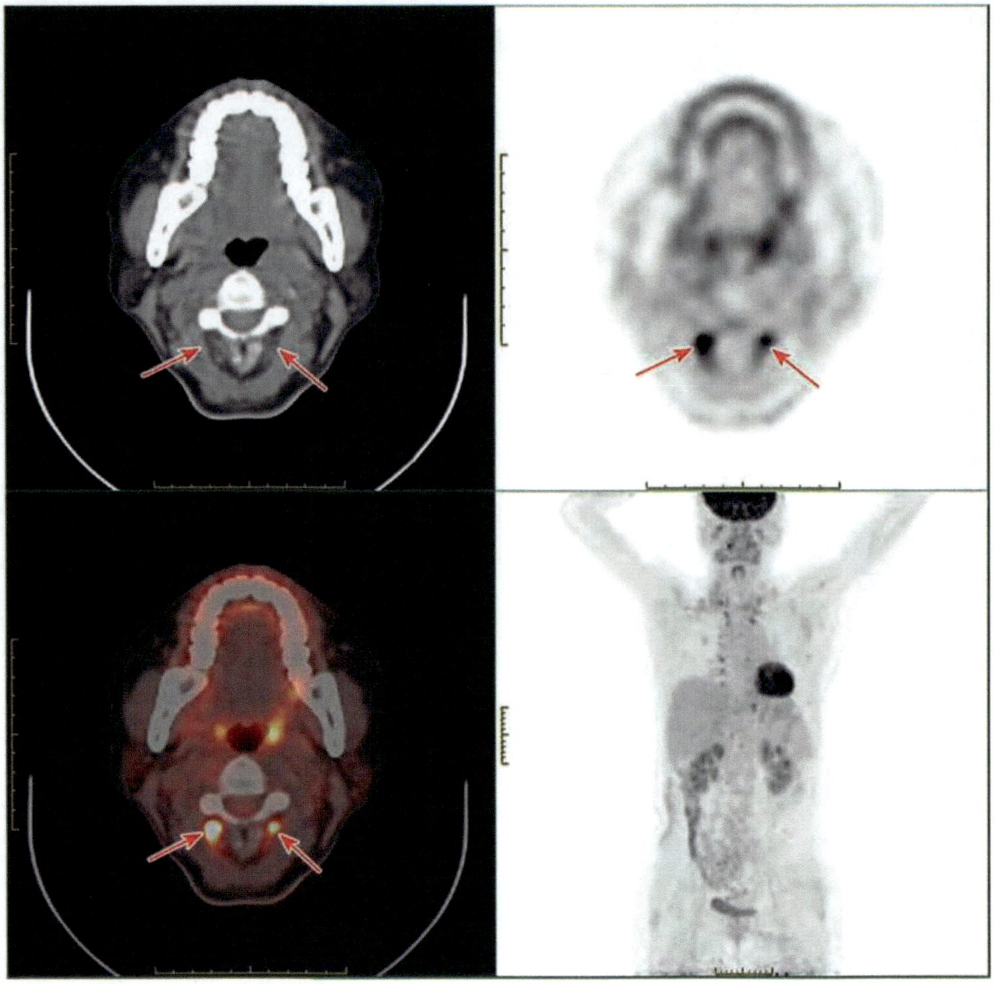

Fig. 17.13 Physiological ^{18}F-FDG uptake in the brown adipose tissue in both sides of the neck. A 54-year-old female presented with a symmetrical increased FDG uptake in adipose tissues between the semispinalis capitis and the obliquus capitis inferior of both sides of the neck (arrow)

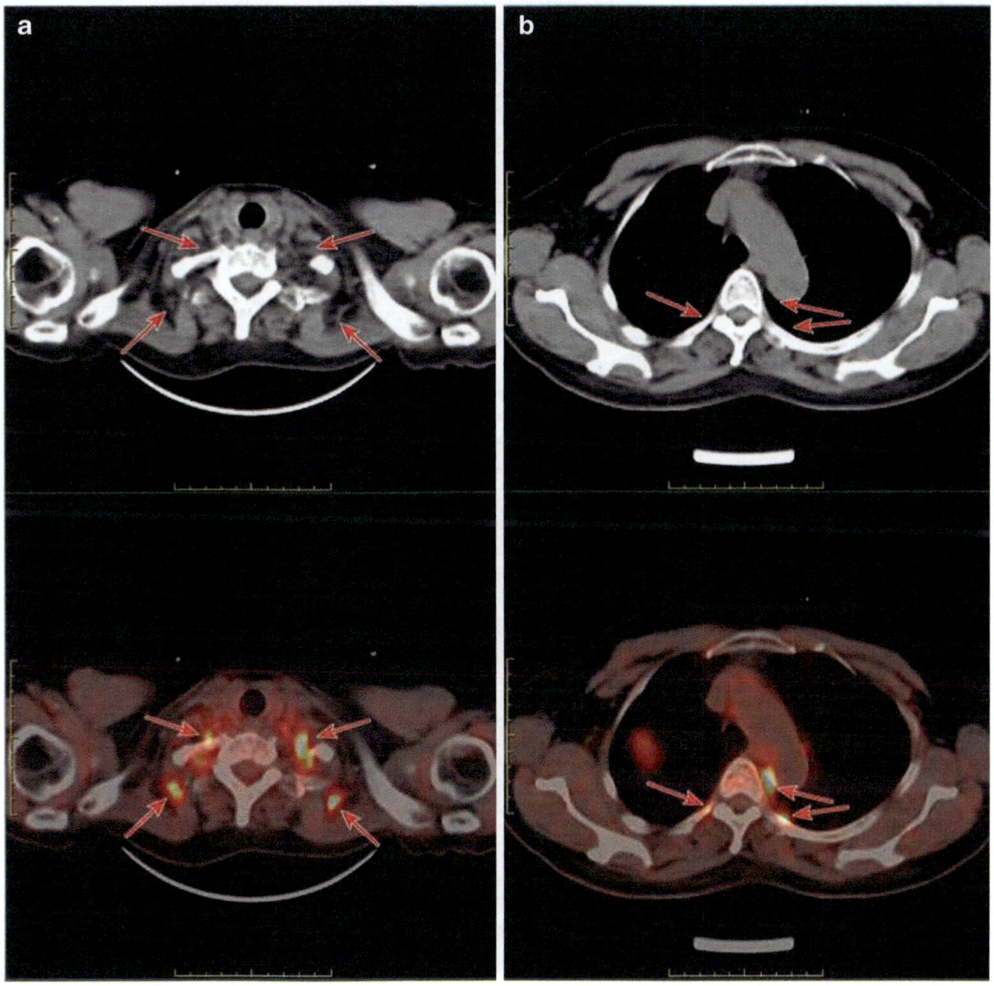

Fig. 17.14 Physiological ^{18}F-FDG uptake in the brown adipose tissue in the bilateral neck, mediastinum, and paraspinal tissues. A 57-year-old female presented with imaging findings: (**a**) A symmetrical increased FDG uptake in both sides of the neck and in the adipose tissue of the bilateral clavicular spaces. (**b**) Increased FDG uptake in the inside of the descending aorta and in the adipose tissue of the bilateral paraspinal tissues. Arrows indicate increased metabolic activity in the brown adipose tissue

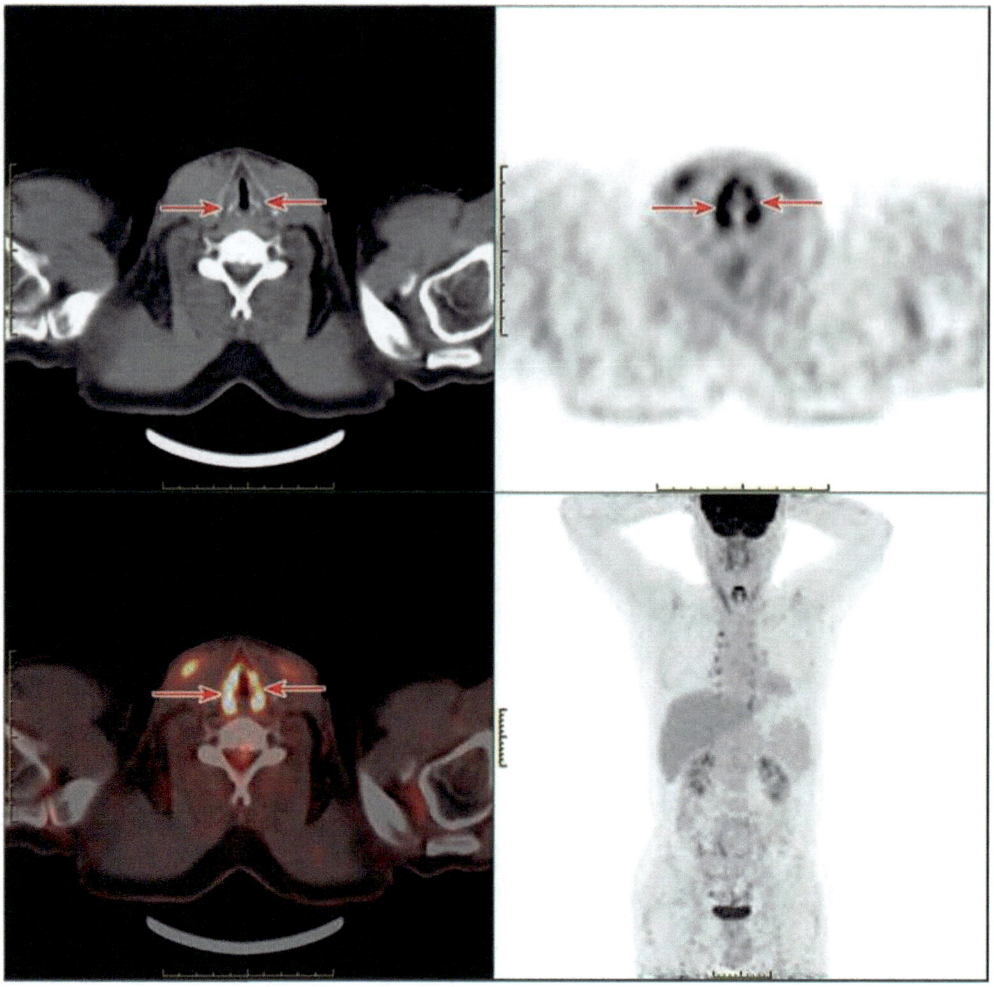

Fig. 17.15 Physiological ^{18}F-FDG uptake in the vocal cords. A 48-year-old male presented with imaging findings of a diffuse increase in FDG uptake in the bilateral vocal cords and basically symmetrical distribution on both sides, without swelling or abnormal density (arrow)

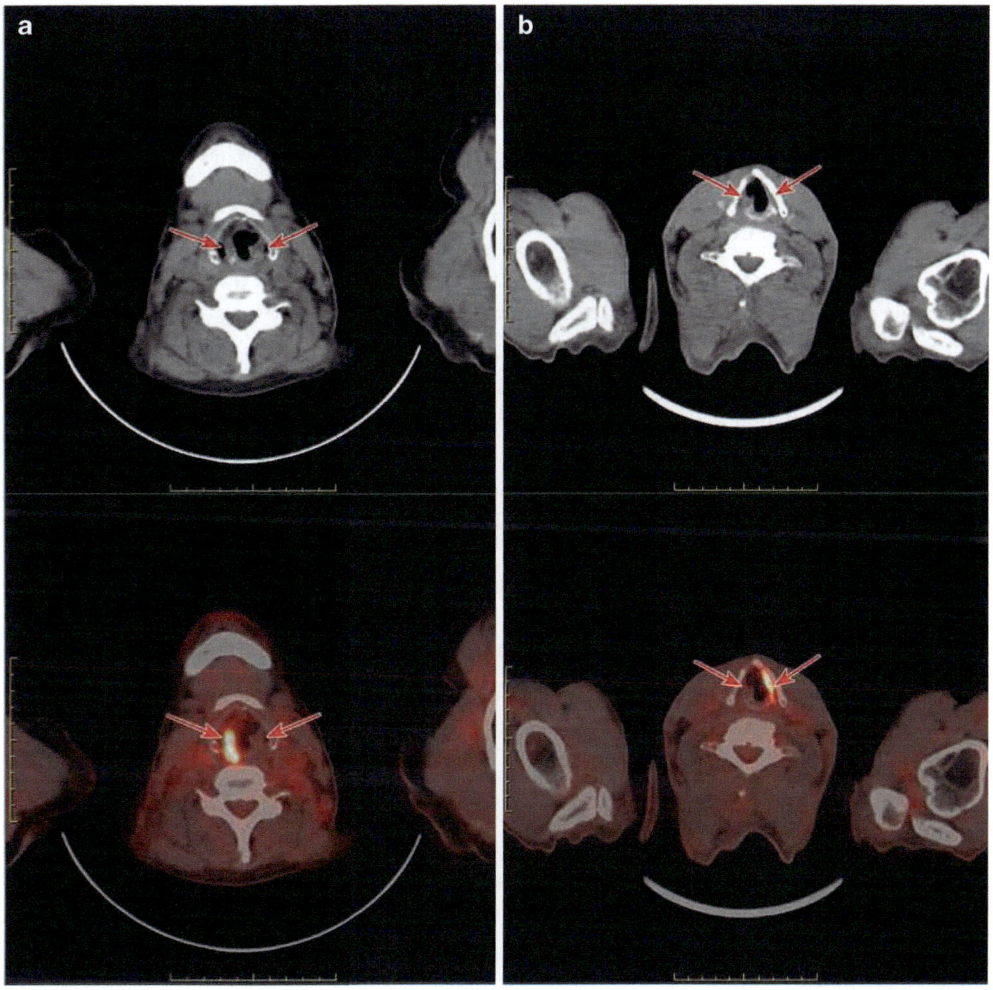

Fig. 17.16 ^{18}F-FDG PET/CT images of vocal cord paralysis. (**a**) A 70-year-old female. Post the surgery for invasive ductal carcinoma of the left breast for 13 years and post the chemotherapy for multiple metastases. The laryngoscopy showed left vocal cord paralysis. PET/CT shows the FDG uptake in the left vocal cord is close to the background and increased FDG uptake in the right vocal cord (functional compensation), without significantly abnormal density. (**b**) A 66-year-old male presented with status post the esophageal cancer surgery for more than 1 year and the anastomotic recurrence. The laryngoscopy showed the right vocal cord paralysis. The FDG uptake in the right vocal cord is close to background and increased in the left one (functional compensation), without significantly abnormal density. Arrows indicate the vocal cords

2.2 Preparation for the Examination

Before the examination of ^{18}F-FDG PET/CT imaging for neck tumor, fasting for more than 6 hours is required, and blood glucose should be routinely tested before injection of ^{18}F-FDG to ensure that fasting blood glucose is below 11 mmol/L. The blood glucose of diabetic patients should reach the above level without hypoglycemic drugs and insulin intervention on the same day. For patients evaluated before treatment, it is necessary to inquire whether the aspiration biopsy has been performed and the specific time. The local increased ^{18}F-FDG uptake caused by the above invasive examination can last for 1 week or longer. After treatment, medical histories of previous operation, radiotherapy, and chemotherapy should be inquired. Non-specific inflammatory response 4 weeks after radiotherapy and 2 weeks after chemotherapy can lead to increased ^{18}F-FDG uptake, while decreased FDG uptake in the bone marrow within the radiotherapy target area will exist for a long time (Figs. 17.17 and 17.18).

About 1 h before and after the injection of ^{18}F-FDG, the patient should be asked to rest quietly, in order to avoid the physiological uptake of vocal cords caused by speaking. During the examination, the patient should be asked to keep as relaxed as possible to avoid the increased ^{18}F-FDG uptake caused by neck muscle tension.

In order to avoid the effect of increased FDG uptake of the activated brown adipose tissue on its surrounding organs, especially lymph nodes, it is necessary to keep the patient warm before and during examination.

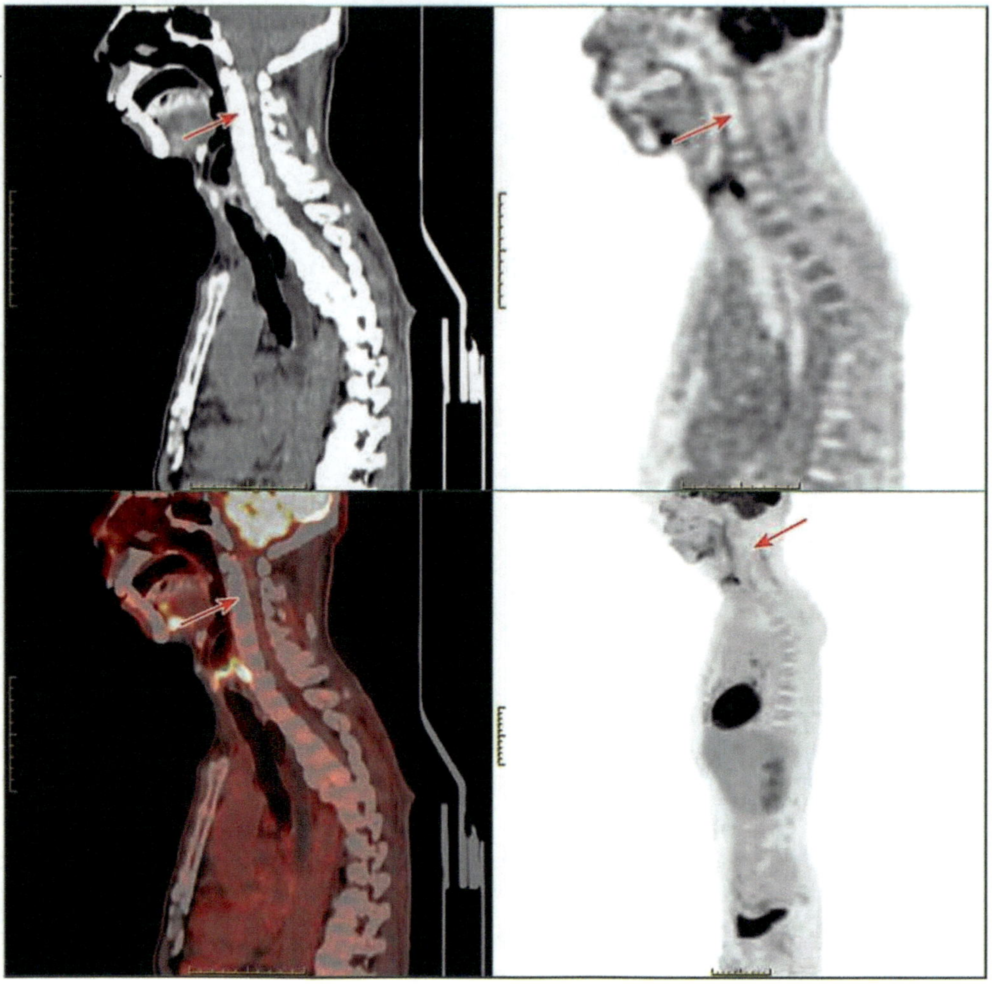

Fig. 17.17 Decreased ^{18}F-FDG uptake in the local cervical vertebra after the radiotherapy for nasopharyngeal cancer. A 56-year-old male presented with status post the radiotherapy for nasopharyngeal cancer. PET/CT shows a diffuse decreased ^{18}F-FDG uptake in the radiotherapy area of the cervical vertebra (arrow)

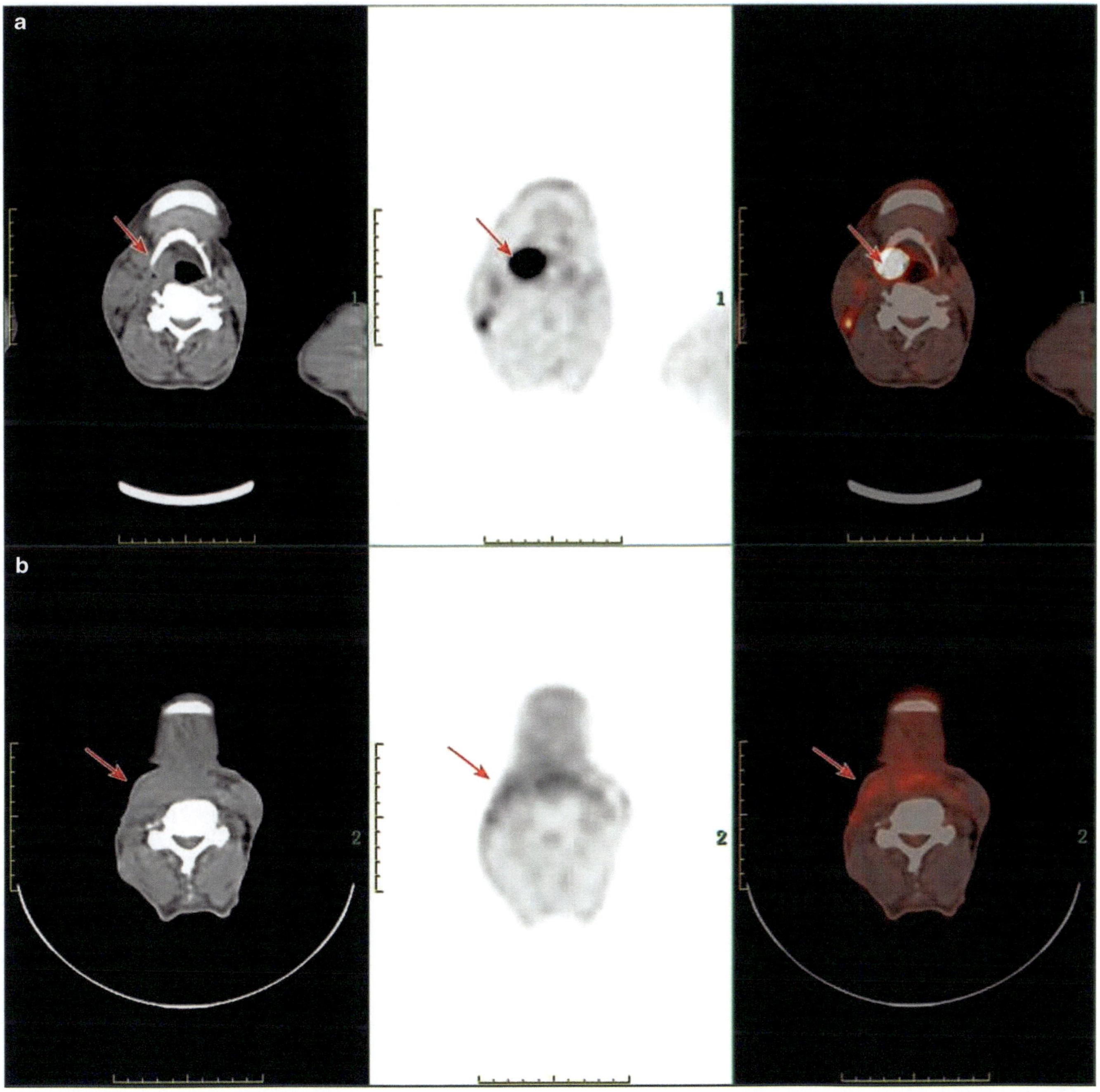

Fig. 17.18 Series of ^{18}F-FDG PET/CT images before and after the surgery as well as after the radiotherapy in a patient with hypopharyngeal cancer. A 59-year-old male presented with hypopharyngeal squamous cell carcinoma: (**a**). PET/CT images before the surgery for nasopharyngeal cancer; increased FDG uptake in the right pyriform sinus soft tissue mass, with a long diameter of 2.7 cm and SUVmax of 18.7. Hypopharyngeal cancer was considered. (**b**). PET/CT images 20 days after the resection of hypopharyngeal cancer; mild swelling of soft tissues in the field of operation, with a mild increased FDG uptake, SUVmax of 3.6, and strip-like and heterogeneous distribution. (**c**). PET/CT images 11 months after the resection of hypopharyngeal cancer. (**d**). PET/CT images 8 months after the resection and the radiotherapy for hypopharyngeal cancer: a mild increased FDG uptake in the soft tissues in the field of operation, with a reduction of SUVmax to 2.2, narrowing of the scope, and heterogeneous distribution. Postoperative changes were considered

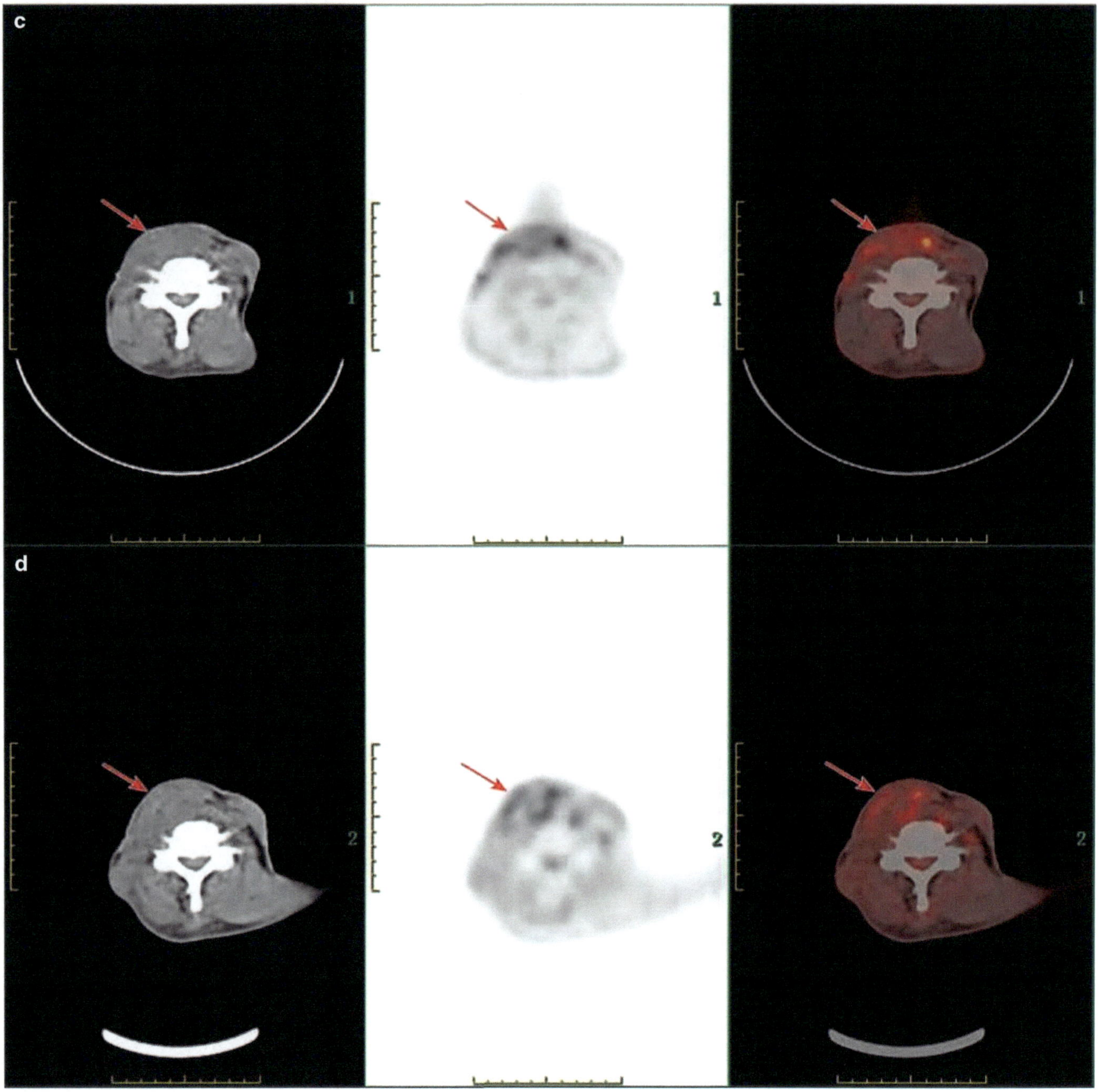

Fig. 17.18 (continued)

2.3 The Artifacts That May Affect Diagnosis and the Associated Treatment Strategies

A routine whole-body PET/CT scan usually requires the patient to maintain arms raising overhead. When the arm is close to the head and neck, artifacts will be generated on the neck image.

Therefore, in order to show the neck structure more clearly with perfect whole-body image quality, a neck PET/CT scan should be performed after completing the whole-body PET/CT scan with the patient placing the arms on both sides of the body during neck scan (Figs. 17.19 and 17.20).

PET/CT imaging uses CT without contrast to correct attenuation and simultaneously obtain the diagnostic information from CT. However, during the attenuation correction, CT artifacts may result in an overestimate to the standardized uptake value (SUV) of a lesion. The increased ^{18}F-FDG uptake around metallic objects, such as earrings, necklace, and dentures, is the artifact caused by over-attenuation correction. At this time, images without CT attenuation correction should be reviewed for the differentiation, and patients should be asked to remove the removable metal objects before examination. Oral CT contrast agent is beneficial to improving the diagnostic efficiency of CT; however, high concentration of contrast agent will lead to the false appearance of increased ^{18}F-FDG uptake. Therefore, PET/CT scans should use a lower concentration of oral contrast agent than CT scan does.

Since CT images and PET images are not acquired simultaneously, the movement of patients during the examination will produce artifacts. The common artifacts are the poor image registration and information fusion between CT and PET, among which the head and neck movement artifacts are more common, mainly due to the longtime of PET/CT examination and the involuntary head movement of patients. At the same time, the cervical organs have a certain range of motion, and the position of the neck during movement may change. Therefore, when performing PET/CT scan, the head should be fixed (special head support), and the central axis of the neck should be aligned with that of the trunk as far as possible. For patients who cannot maintain the above posture, the possible anatomical positioning changes caused by changes in the neck position should be considered in the image analysis (Figs. 17.21 and 17.22).

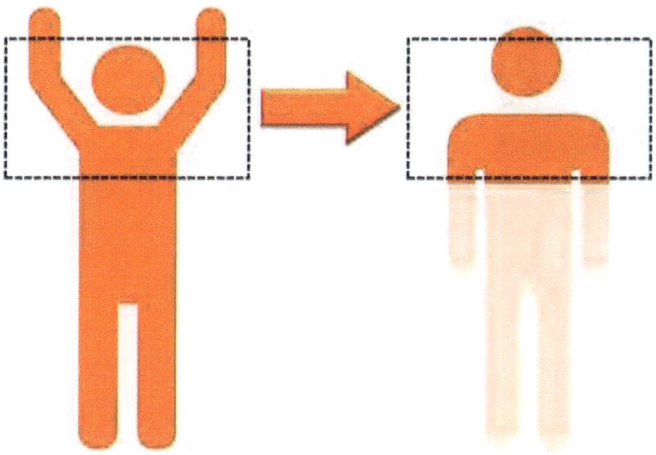

Fig. 17.19 PET/CT image acquisition techniques for the assessment of neck tumors. In order to avoid the neck artifacts caused by the upper limbs, the PET/CT image acquisition of neck tumors should adopt a two-step method: (1) step 1, whole-body PET/CT scan with raising upper limbs overhead; and (2) step 2, neck PET/CT scan with placing upper limbs by the sides of the body

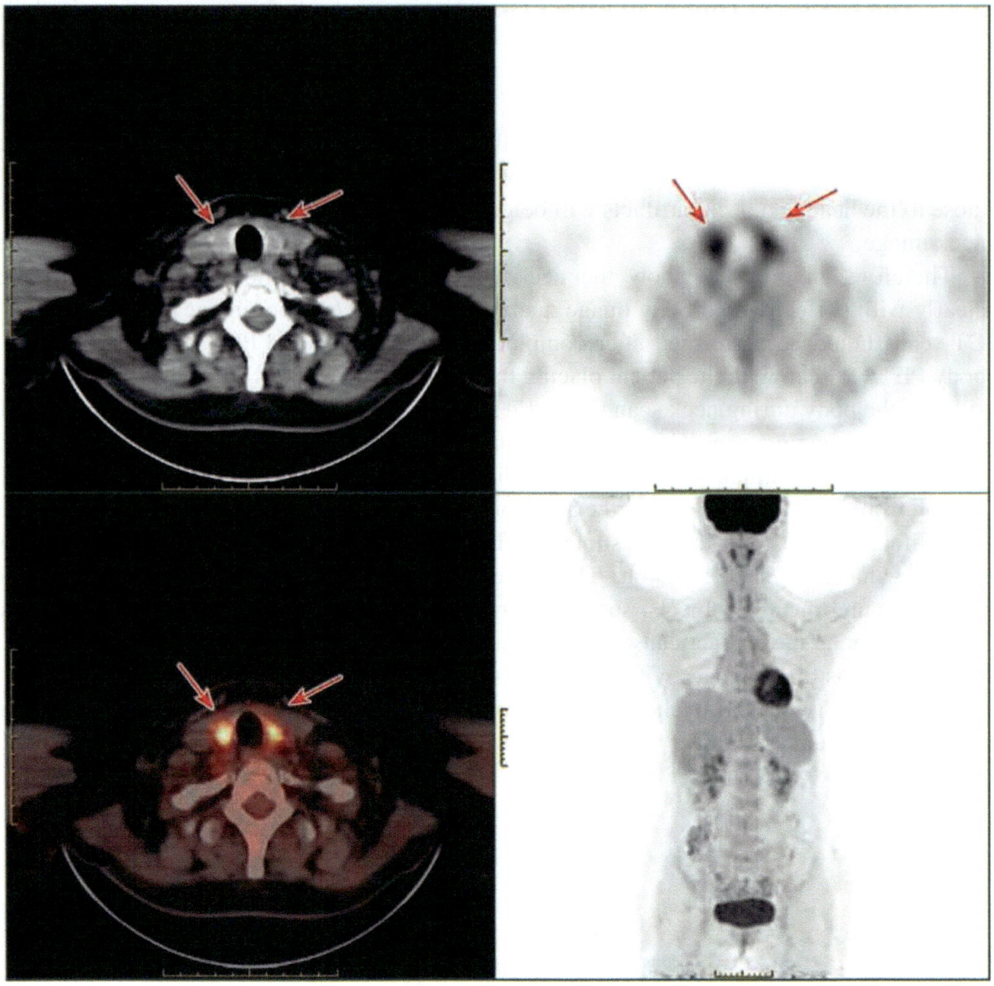

Fig. 17.20 Neck artifacts caused by raising upper limbs overhead. A 58-year-old female raising her upper limbs overhead. The CT imaging shows axial artifacts of the neck (arrow)

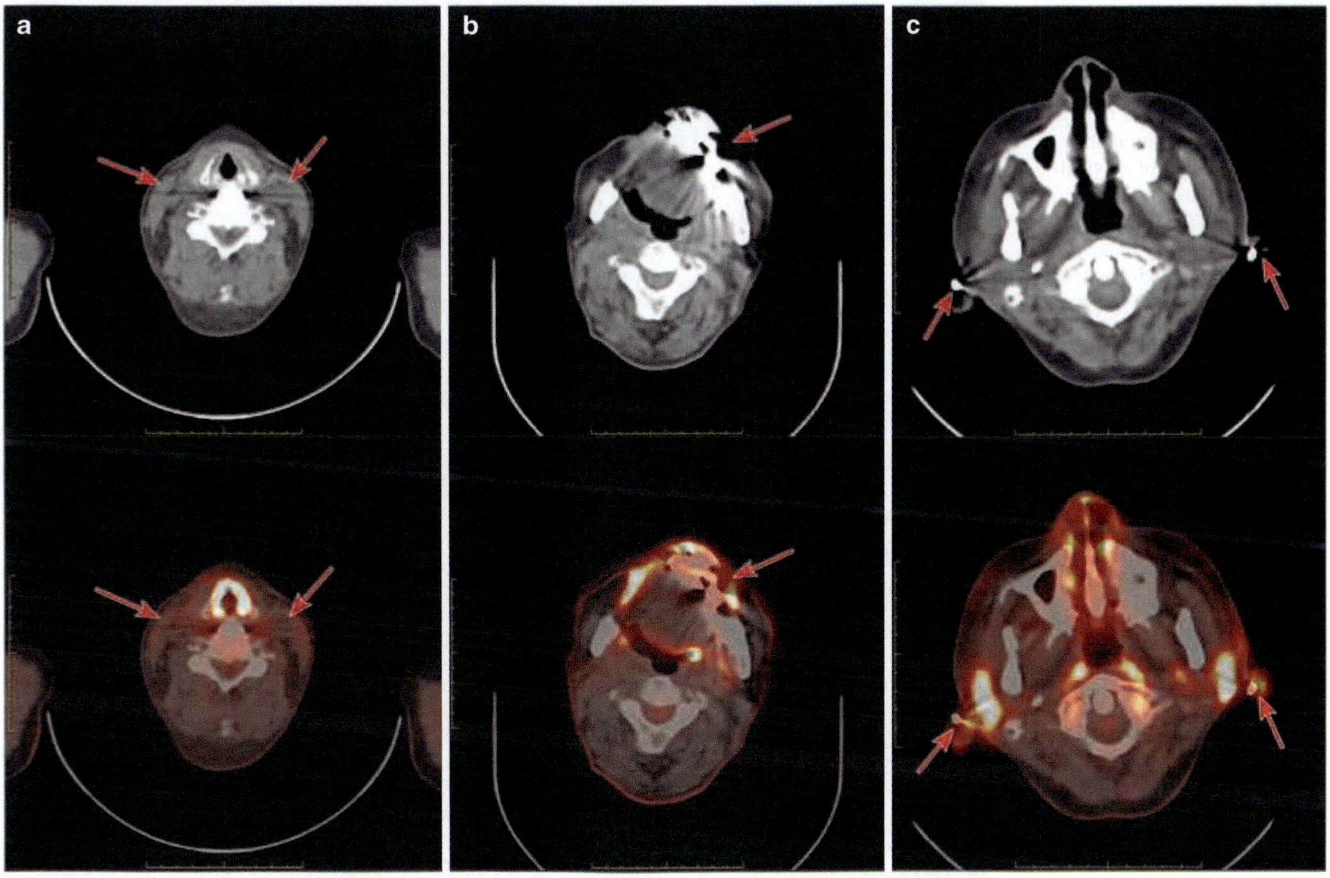

Fig. 17.21 PET/CT images of common metal artifacts in the neck. (**a**) A 52-year-old female, post-cervical internal fixation surgery. Imaging findings of axial radial artifacts on both sides of the internal fixation shadow. (**b**) A 71-year-old male, post the surgery for the recurrence of right gingival squamous cell carcinoma, partial absence of the (right) mandible, and radial artifacts around the left denture. (**c**) A 27-year-old female presented with radial artifacts around bilateral earrings. Arrows indicate artifacts

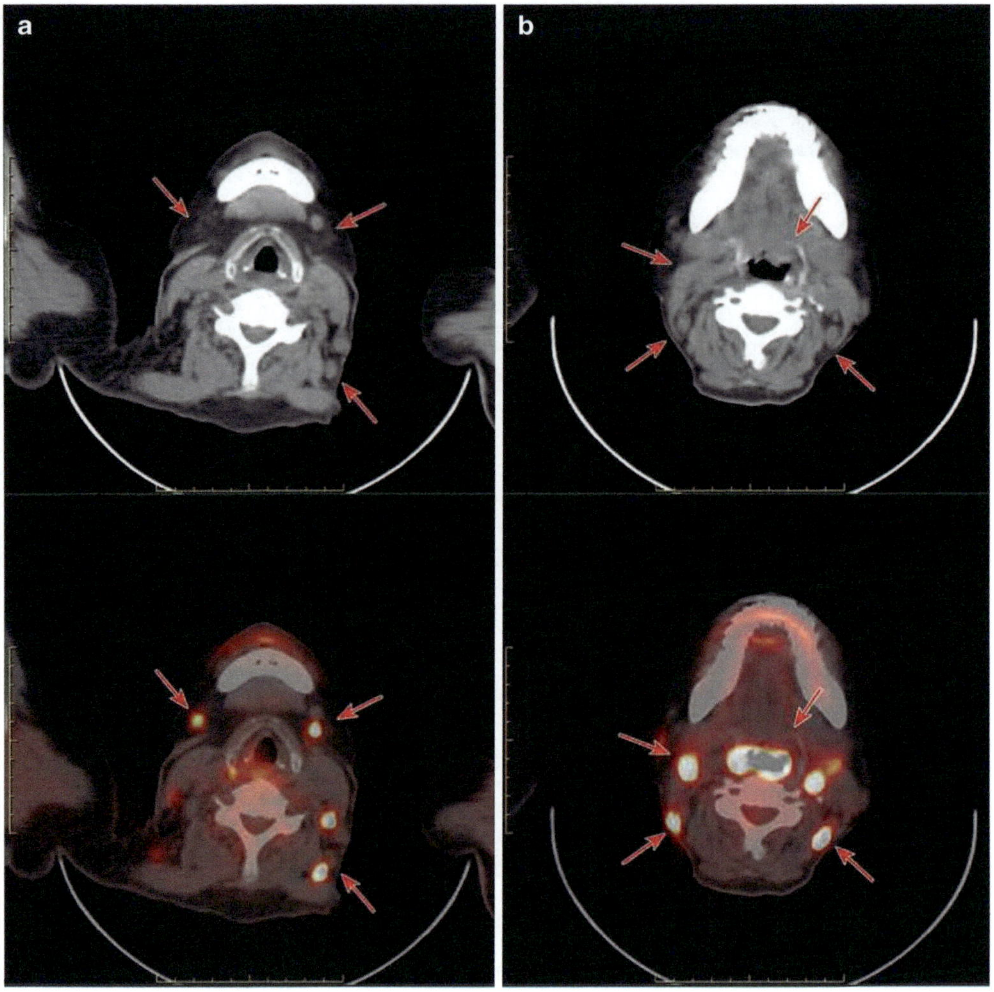

Fig. 17.22 Poor image registration and fusion of PET/CT due to neck movement. A 63-year-old female: (**a**) Due to her motion during the examination, the CT fusion images of cervical lymph nodes are not well matched with the lesions of increased FDG uptake. (**b**) Due to her cough, the CT findings are not clear in the oropharynx, and the fusion images of cervical lymph nodes are not well matched

3 Overview of the Diagnosis of Cervical Cancer by PET/CT

^{18}F-FDG PET/CT is mainly used to evaluate the infiltration range, adjacent relationship, lymph node metastasis, distant metastasis, and other conditions of neck tumors, so as to further assist clinical staging and guide the treatment plan, but it has limited value in differentiating the benign or malignant primary tumors.

1. Diagnosis of primary tumors: Head and neck tumors can be diagnosed by a variety of examination methods, and the pathological evidence is often obtained before the ^{18}F-FDG PET/CT examination. Hence, the application value of PET/CT for primary lesions is to evaluate the invasion to adjacent tissues and the involvement in surrounding organs by tumors. The sensitivity of PET/CT to different types of head and neck tumors is different. The sensitivity is high to nasopharyngeal cancer, oropharyngeal and lower pharyngeal tumors, laryngeal cancer, and oral squamous cell cancer, whereas it is relatively low to salivary gland tumors.
2. Clinical staging: Head and neck cancer is easy to be spread to local lymph nodes, and the presence of regional lymph node metastasis is vital to prognosis. For example, the 5-year survival rate of patients with lymph node metastasis is significantly decreased. ^{18}F-FDG PET/CT is mainly used to detect the lymph nodes with unremarkable enlargement and the metastasis lymph nodes missed by other imaging techniques, and it can further assist in making the radiotherapy plan. Blood metastasis is rare at the initial assessment of head and neck tumors, and distant metastasis may also occur when radiotherapy is ineffective and tumor progresses. The use of PET/CT as a one-stop-shop imaging protocol for staging and restaging can change the treatment regimen for 12%–34% of patients. Thus, a routine application of PET/CT is recommended for some patients in the initial staging and restaging (Fig. 17.23).
3. Efficacy evaluation: Compared with CT, MRI, and other structural imaging techniques, ^{18}F-FDG PET/CT has unique advantages in early efficacy evaluation. During the treatment, there was a linear relationship between the

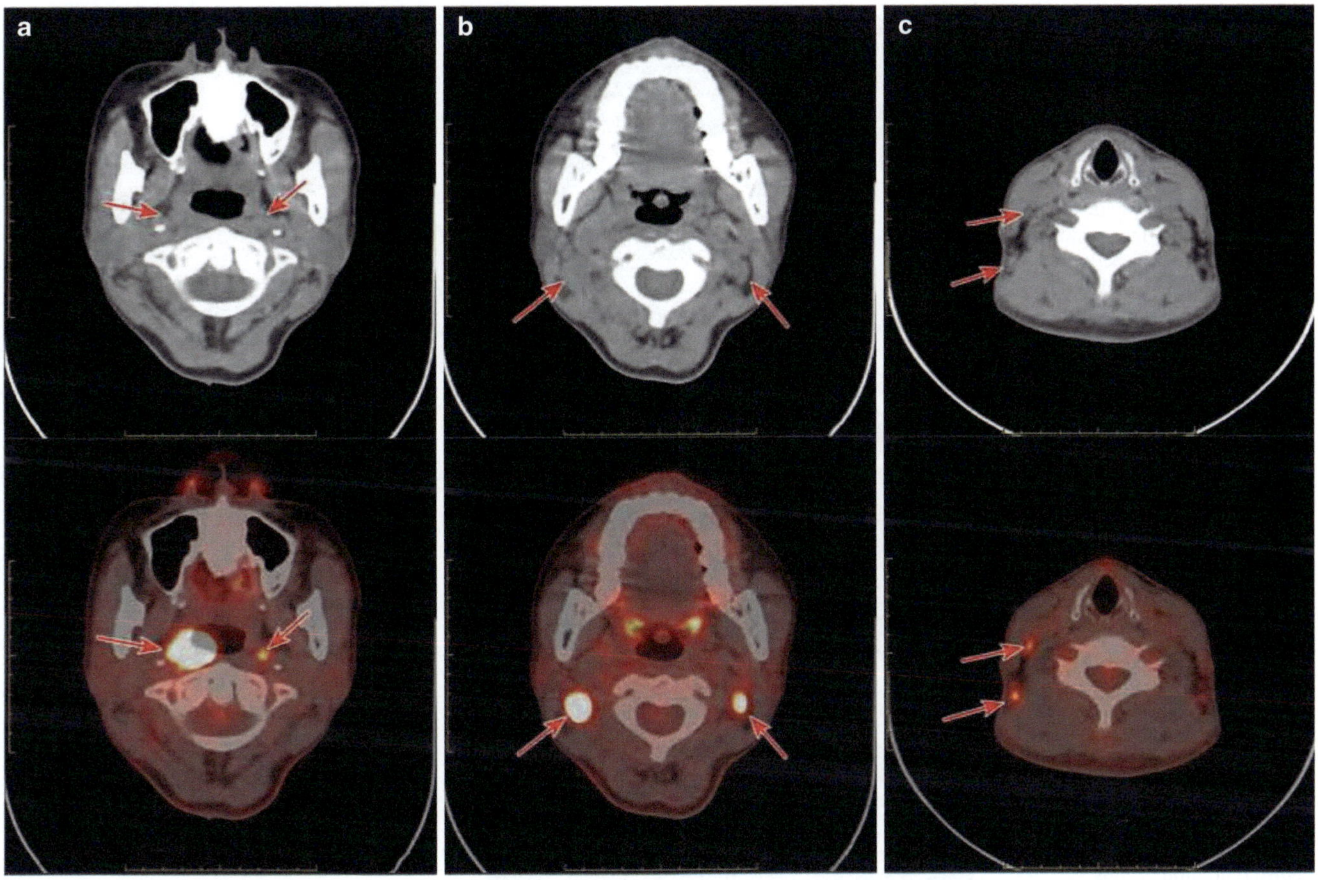

Fig. 17.23 Nasopharyngeal carcinoma with cervical lymph node metastases (pretreatment evaluation). A 37-year-old female diagnosed with squamous cell carcinoma of the posterior wall of the nasopharynx by nasopharyngoscopy underwent the PET/CT evaluation before treatment. Figs. **a–c** show the thickening of soft tissues in the right lateral wall of the nasopharynx with increased FDG uptake (SUVmax 24.6). Multiple lymph nodes of different sizes are noted in the left parapharyngeal space, levels II–IV of the right neck, and levels II and III of the left neck, with clear boundary, comparable density with the surrounding muscles, and varying degrees of increased FDG uptake. The larger node has a short diameter of 1.6 cm and SUVmax of 17.8. Hence, the nasopharyngeal carcinoma with bilateral cervical lymph node metastases was considered. Based on the findings, the clinical staging was $cT_3N_2M_0$ (stage III). Accordingly, the intensity-modulated radiation therapy was given after the neoadjuvant chemotherapy

concentration of ^{18}F-FDG of tumor and the growth rate of tumor cells, and the change of the glucose metabolism level is prior to that of the tumor volume. Thus, the increased FDG uptake in tumors indicates an ineffective treatment, while the rapidly decreased FDG uptake indicates a good therapeutic effect.

According to the above principles, early efficacy evaluation can be carried out effectively, so as to avoid ineffective treatment and change the treatment plan in time. However, the time window for PET/CT imaging after treatment has a significant influence on the outcome interpretation. It is generally believed that, for the purpose of observing the treatment response, or on the clinical situations suggesting that treatment is ineffective and the disease progresses, PET/CT examination can be performed at an early stage. For the purpose of restaging, PET/CT imaging is recommended 2 months after the end of radiotherapy and 2 weeks after the end of chemotherapy, in order to avoid an early inflammation and the interference of false-positive results resulting from radiation necrosis (Figs. 17.24 and 17.25).

4. Detect recurrence and metastasis: Head and neck tumors often have anatomical structure changes and scar formation caused by surgery and biopsy, as well as edema, necrosis, long-lasting infection, and fibrosis caused by radiotherapy, making it difficult to diagnose the local recurrence by routine examination methods. PET/CT is currently considered to be the preferred imaging technique for detecting the recurrence of head and neck tumors after treatment. Especially for patients with local swelling, cervical lymph node enlargement by palpation, and new-onset or persistent clinical symptoms, PET/CT can be used to identify the cause of these conditions. To reduce false-positive results, the evaluation with PET/CT imaging for the recurrence and metastasis is recommended 3–4 months after treatment (Figs. 17.24, 17.25, and 17.26).

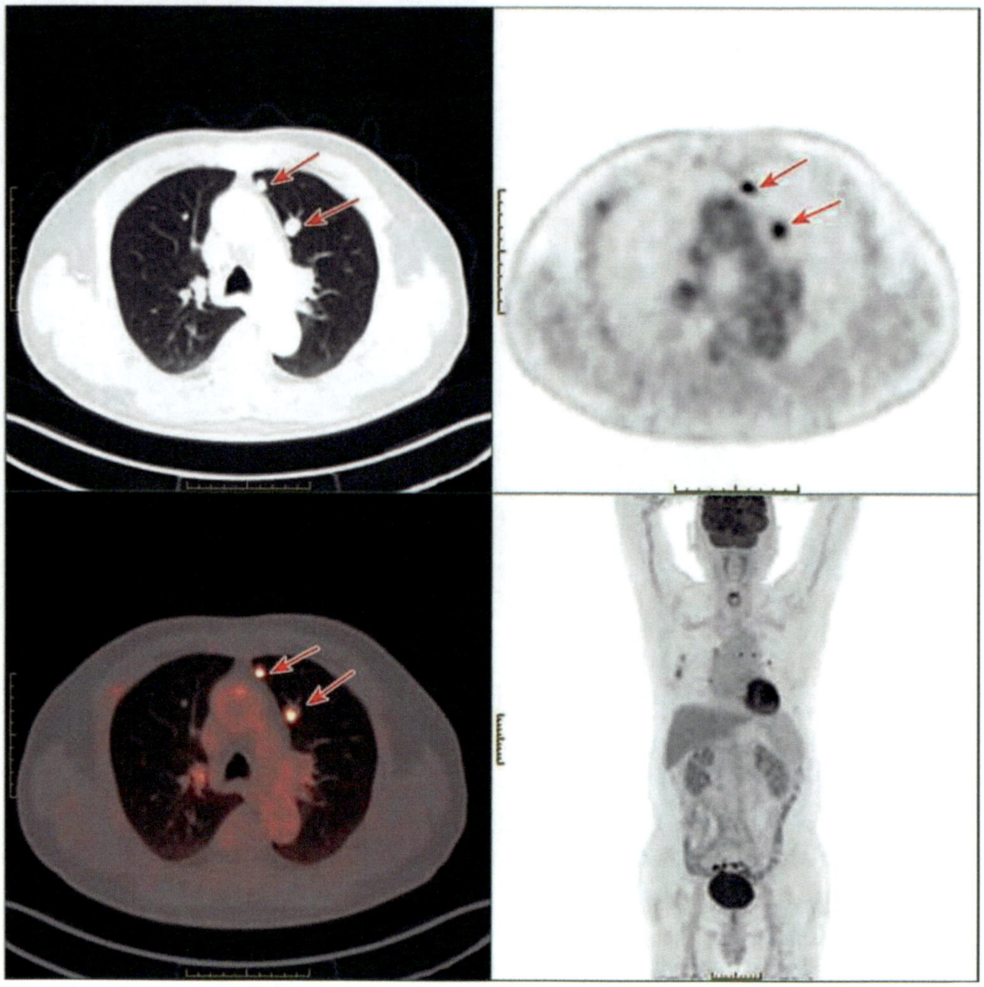

Fig. 17.24 Bilateral lung metastases (dedifferentiation) after the surgery for papillary thyroid carcinoma. A 73-year-old male presented with status post the operations for papillary thyroid carcinoma and lymphatic metastasis of the right neck. The enlargement of the lymph nodes in the left neck was found, and the serum thyroglobulin was determined to be 207.1 ng/mL. PET/CT shows increased FDG uptake in multiple nodules of both lungs. The larger one is about 1.5 cm in diameter and 7.9 in SUVmax. Accordingly, the condition was considered as bilateral lung metastases. Subsequently, the metastasis of papillary thyroid carcinoma to a half of the left central lymph node was confirmed by the surgery. An oral administration of ^{131}I 150 mCi was given after the surgery, and whole-body ^{131}I imaging showed no iodine uptake in multiple nodules of both lungs (not shown). Hence, the dedifferentiation of lung metastases was considered

5. Guide the biopsy: Pathological diagnosis is the most reliable basis for clinical staging and treatment planning. Nevertheless, accurate results are often difficult to be obtained due to sampling failure in clinical practice. PET/CT has irreplaceable advantages in determining suitable histological biopsy sites. PET can find specific areas with high uptake of ^{18}F-FDG, while CT can further provide more accurate anatomical details, significantly increasing the positive rate of biopsy. For example, large tumors often have necrotic areas, and PET/CT can clearly distinguish necrotic areas from parenchymal tumor areas, thus effectively avoiding false negatives caused by the sampling from the necrotic areas. For tumors with heterogeneous uptake of ^{18}F-FDG, the best biopsy site should be the highest uptake area.
6. Identify primary focus: In clinical practice, some patients present with painless lymph node enlargement in the neck as the first manifestation. For those with metastatic lymph nodes confirmed by aspiration biopsy, PET/CT can be used to identify the primary focus. Most cervical lymph node metastases come from head and neck tumors, such as nasopharyngeal cancer, thyroid cancer, and laryngeal cancer. Also, a considerable number of the metastases originate from organs outside the head and neck, such as the esophagus and lung. A few primary tumors of the head and neck are small, located in the submucosa or faded away naturally, and they just show cervical lymph node enlargement.

   Therefore, it is time-consuming and laborious to screen one by one with routine examination techniques, and it is more difficult to make a diagnosis because of the complex anatomical structure. Some scholars believe that PET/CT should be performed before routine examination for patients with unknown primary foci (Figs. 17.27 and 17.28).
7. Assist the radiation treatment planning: The image fusion technique of PET/CT plays an important role in determining the target area of radiation treatment. For head and neck tumors, PET/CT can increase the radiation field according to the volume of peripheral involvement, avoid

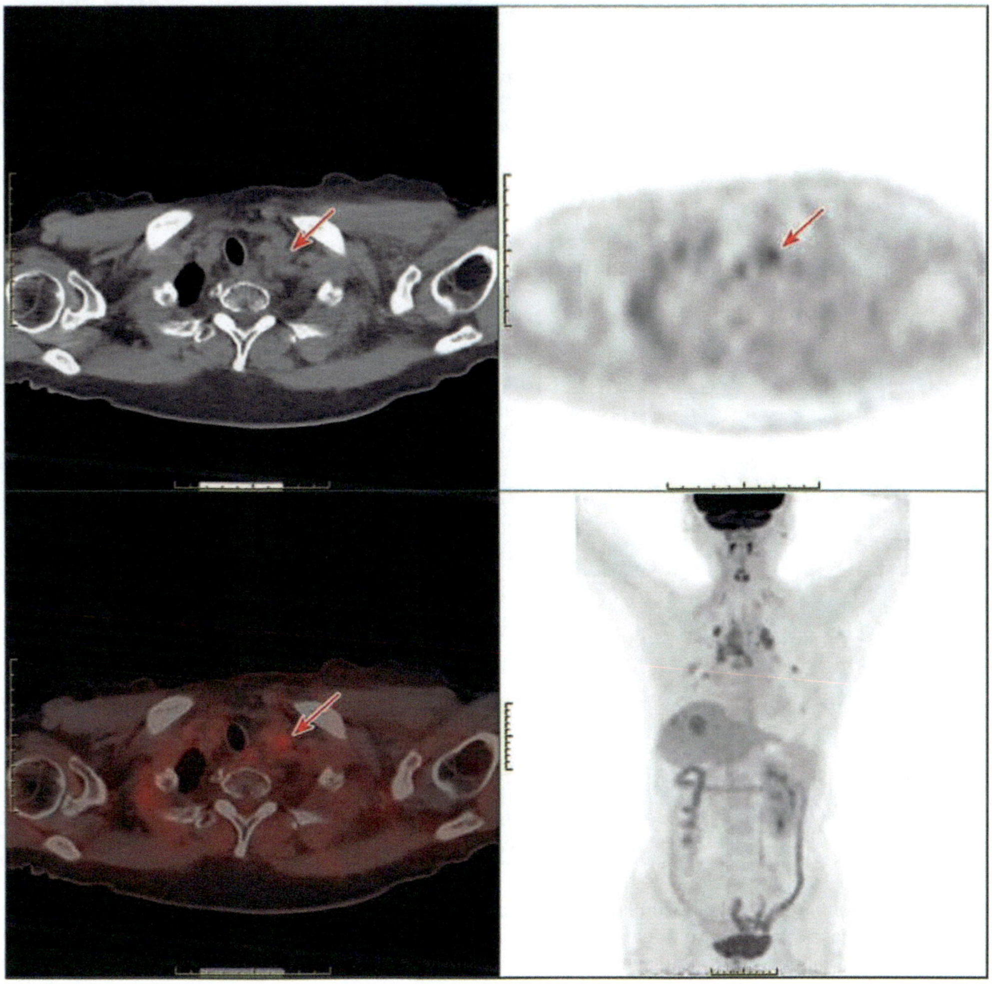

Fig. 17.25 Status post the surgery for medullary thyroid carcinoma, left cervical lymph node metastasis (extensive systemic metastasis). A 64-year-old female presented with status post the surgery for medullary thyroid carcinoma. PET/CT images show a slight increased FDG uptake in the level VB lymph node of the left neck, 1.1 cm in short diameter and 3.2 in SUVmax; metastatic lymph nodes were considered. MIP images show an abnormal increased FDG uptake in multiple foci of both lungs, mediastinum, and liver (metastasis)

normal tissues, and simultaneously increase the radiation dose of tumor target area, so as to protect organs such as the eyes, glands, and spinal cord. In addition, PET/CT can also use non-^{18}F-FDG imaging agents to delineate the unique biological targets of amino acid metabolism, angiogenesis, hypoxia, apoptosis, and other information in tumor tissues, making it an ideal tool for the conformal radiation therapy and the conformal intensity-modulated radiation therapy, but it is still in the research stage.

To sum up, PET/CT can provide "one-stop" tumor staging and therapeutic follow-up for patients with head and neck tumors. It has certain advantages in differentiating the recurrence of residual tumors from postoperative changes, and its rich diagnostic information is of great significance for making clinical treatment decisions. In this chapter, we will describe the features of ^{18}F-FDG PET/CT imaging in salivary gland tumors, thyroid tumors, and metastatic lymph nodes in the neck.

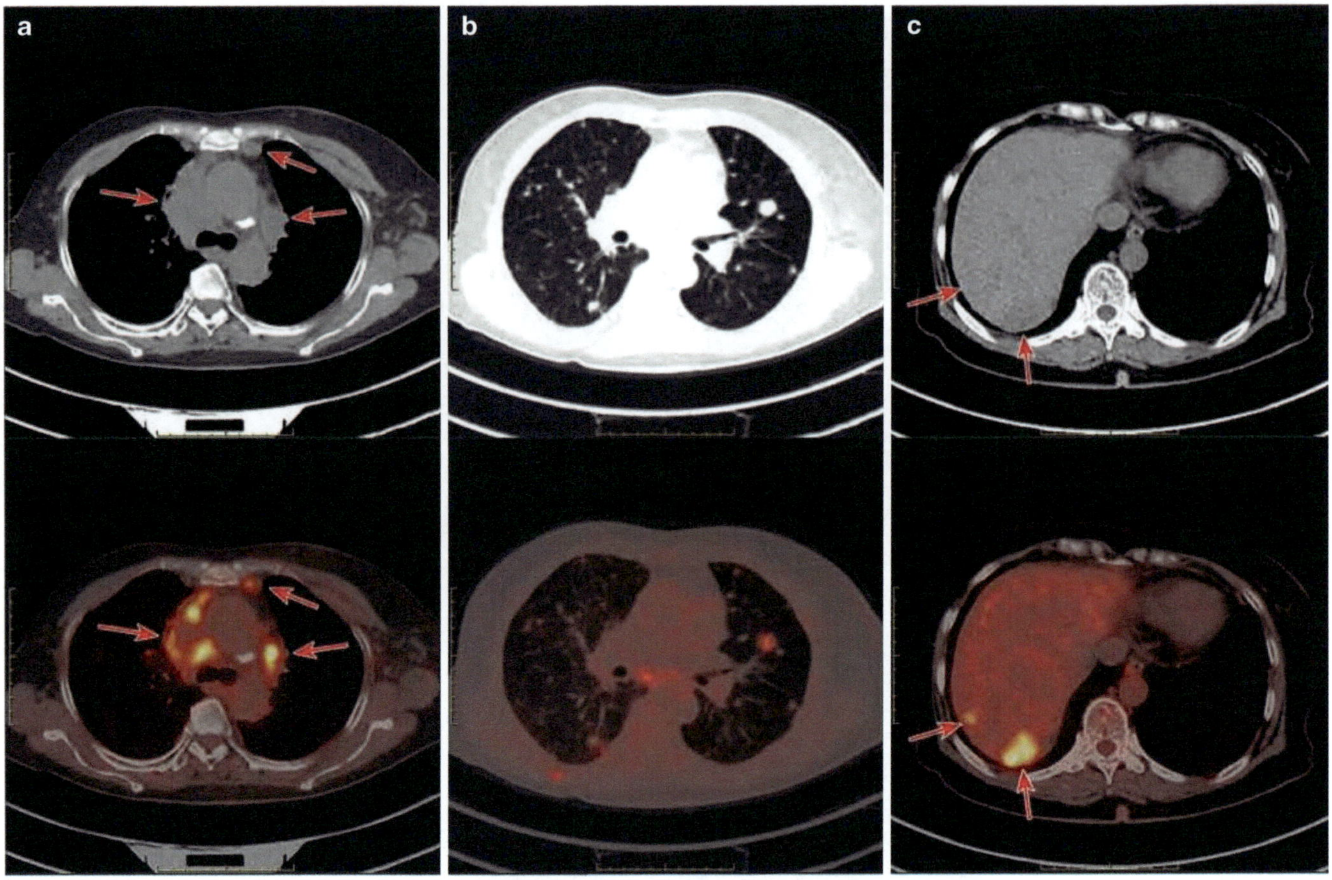

Fig. 17.26 Post the surgery for medullary thyroid carcinoma, multiple systemic metastases. A 64-year-old female, post the surgery for medullary thyroid carcinoma. PET/CT images show an abnormal increased FDG uptake in multiple enlarged lymph nodes within the mediastinum (**a**), multiple nodules in both lungs (**b**), and multiple low-density foci in the right lobe of the liver (**c**). Hence, multiple metastases of mediastinal lymph nodes, both lungs, and liver were considered

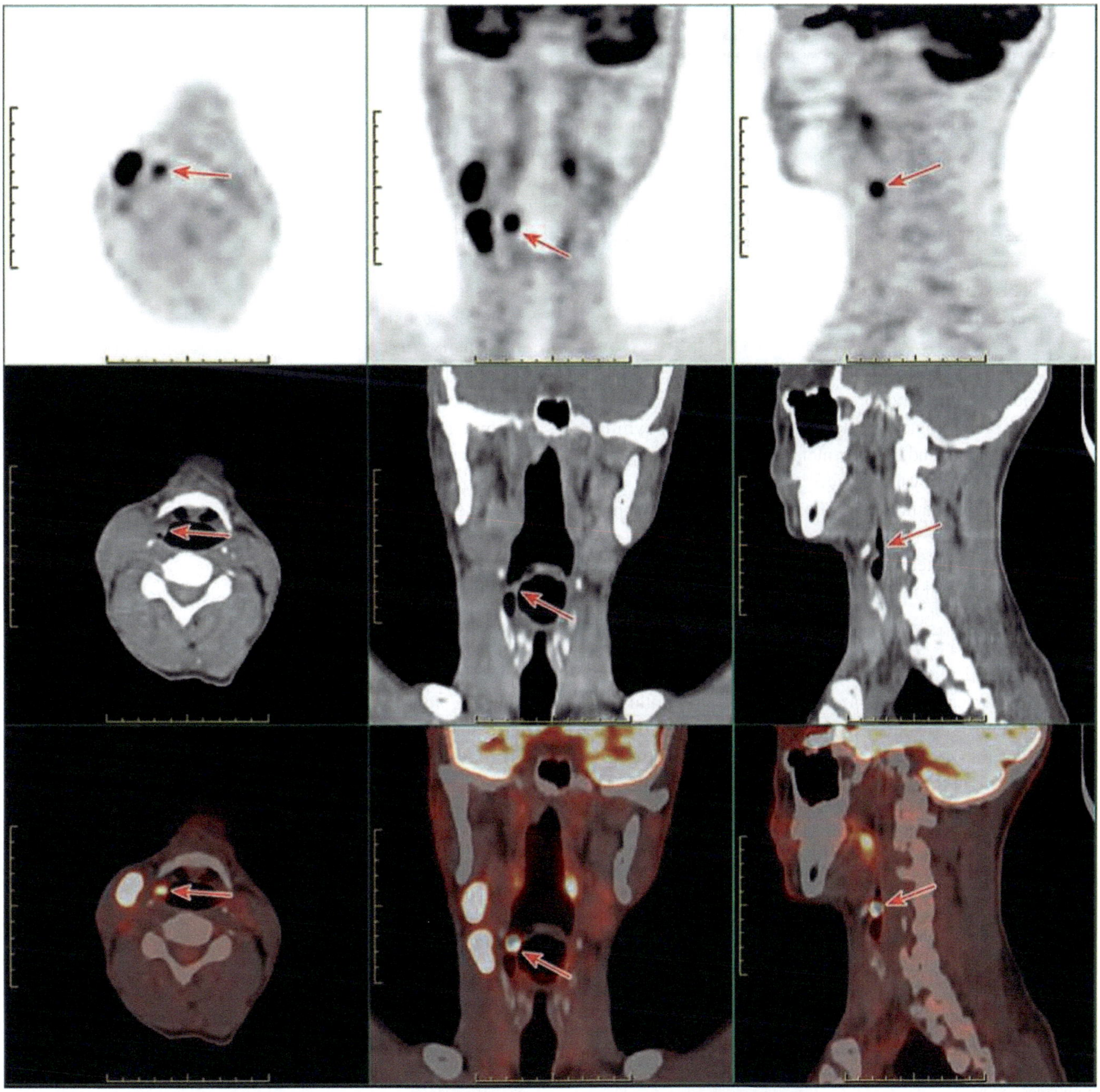

Fig. 17.27 Right cervical lymph node metastasis, with primary lesion unknown. A 53-year-old male presented with metastatic lymph nodes confirmed by the aspiration biopsy in the right neck, and the primary focus was unknown after relevant examinations. PET/CT imaging shows a focal increased FDG uptake in the right aryepiglottic fold, 1.1 cm in diameter and 12.9 in SUVmax, and CT imaging shows small nodules with the density of soft tissues; malignant lesions were considered. Increased FDG uptake is noted in multiple lymph nodes (levels II and III) in the right neck, and the larger one is 2.0 cm in short diameter and 24.7 in SUVmax. Hence, metastatic lymph nodes were considered. Accordingly, total laryngectomy plus cervical lymph node dissection was performed. The pathology showed a poorly differentiated squamous cell carcinoma at the lower right of the laryngeal epiglottis, invading the muscularis propria, about 1.2 cm × 0.9 cm in size. Metastases were noted in 4 of the 11 lymph nodes of the right neck and 2 of the 20 lymph nodes of the left neck

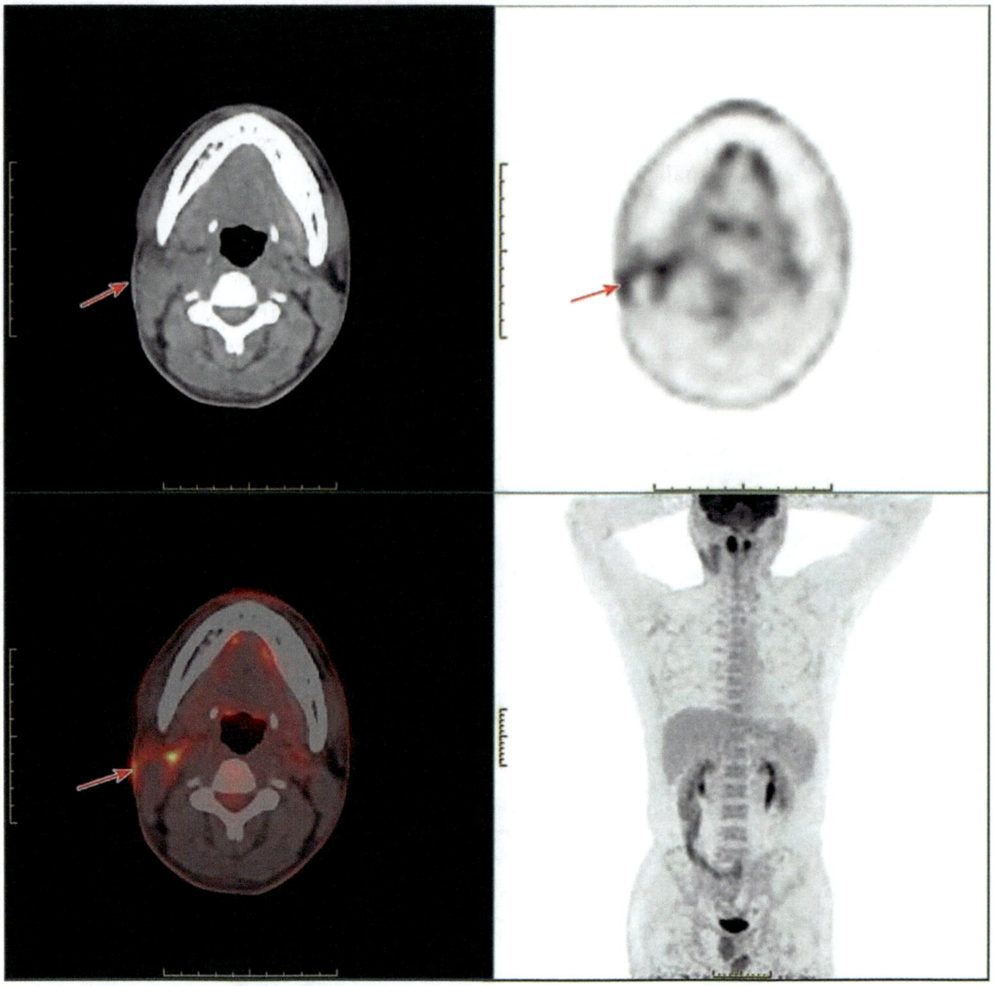

Fig. 17.28 Metastatic squamous cell carcinoma in the right cervical lymph node, with primary lesion unknown. A 26-year-old male presented with metastatic squamous cell carcinoma confirmed by the lymph node biopsy, and the primary focus was unknown after relevant examinations. PET/CT imaging shows strip-shaped FDG uptake in the biopsy area, with SUVmax of 5.0, which was considered to be postoperative changes after biopsy. There was enlargement in the right palatine tonsil, about 2.7 cm × 1.8 cm in the largest cross section, SUVmax 21.5 (arrow); whereas the left palatine tonsil showed SUVmax of 14.5. Hence, the malignant lesions of the right palatine tonsil were considered. Subsequently, low-temperature plasma radiofrequency ablation of bilateral tonsils was performed, and right tonsillar enlargement (grade III) was found. The pathology showed right tonsillar squamous cell carcinoma, 3.5 cm × 2.5 cm × 1 cm in size, and chronic tonsillitis of the left tonsil

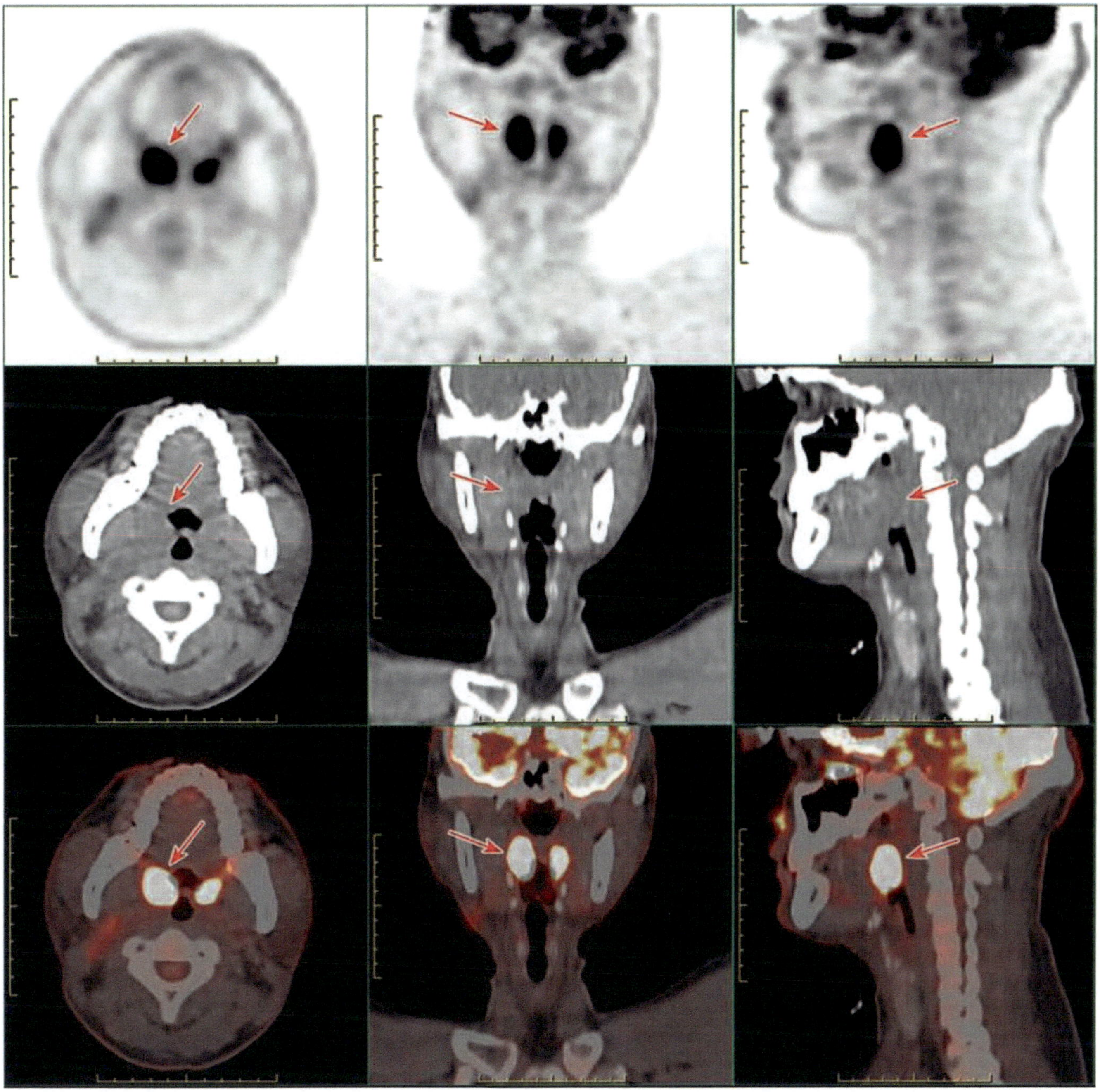

Fig. 17.28 (continued)

18 PET/CT of Thyroid Neoplasms

Linfa Li, Bin Long, and Xuemei Ye

1 Common Thyroid Malignancies

Thyroid carcinoma is one of the most common endocrine malignant tumors and usually occurs in women, and its morbidity has been on the rise in recent years. In 2015, data from the Chinese National Central Cancer Registry (NCCR) showed that the morbidity of thyroid cancer in China in 2011 was 10.32 out of 100,000 and there were 67,800 new cases of thyroid cancer (416,300 males and 189,600 females), accounting for 6.02% of the new cases of malignant tumors. In 2012, the global cancer data showed 229,900 new cases of thyroid cancer in women worldwide, ranking eighth among female cancers. A study in the United States predicted that thyroid cancer will become the third most common cancer in women by 2019. In the past few decades, the overall incidence rate of thyroid cancer in either males or females has been increasing and shows a trend of continuous increase. The trend of increase is seen mainly in papillary thyroid carcinoma but rarely in undifferentiated cancers. In contrast, the overall disease-specific mortality remained unchanged or even decreased, indicating an increase in the proportion of low-invasive subtypes and improved medical care that allows tumors to be detected early.

Thyroid carcinoma often has no clinical symptoms. With the popularity and attention given to physical examination, more and more thyroid cancer has been found by B-mode ultrasonography. A simple nodule in the thyroid is the main manifestation in 40% of patients with thyroid carcinoma, and cervical lymph node enlargement is more common in men than in women. The incidence of lymph node enlargement in patients of age less than 40 years is generally three times than that in those of age more than 50 years. Advanced cancer (T_3 and T_4) is more common in patients over 60 years of age than in those under 40 years. Regarding hoarseness due to vocal cord paralysis as the first symptom, the probability is only about 0.6%. Distant metastasis-related symptoms as the first symptom are seen in about 0.8% of patients with thyroid carcinoma. In general, common features of all types of the thyroid carcinoma include a mass noted in the thyroid gland, hard and fixed in consistency, with inhomogeneous surface and the ability to move up and down during swallowing. Patients with advanced thyroid carcinoma may develop compression symptoms. For example, a large tumor which compresses the trachea will cause the tracheal displacement and varying degrees of respiratory symptoms. When invading the trachea, the tumor may cause dyspnea or hemoptysis; when compressing the esophagus, the tumor may cause dysphagia; when invading the recurrent laryngeal nerve, the tumor may cause hoarseness; when compressing the sympathetic nerve, the tumor may cause Horner syndrome; when invading the cervical plexus, the tumor may cause pain in the ear, occipital region, shoulder, etc. Also, there are tumor-related manifestations such as metastasis to the local lymph nodes and distant organs. Undifferentiated carcinomas may show rapid nodular enlargement in a short time and feature invasion into surrounding tissues.

There are four types of thyroid carcinoma in clinicopathology: (1) papillary carcinoma, (2) follicular carcinoma, (3) medullary carcinoma, and (4) undifferentiated carcinomas. Both papillary and follicular carcinomas are differentiated thyroid carcinomas.

1.1 Differentiated Thyroid Carcinomas

1.1.1 Clinical Overview

Papillary carcinoma is the most common type of thyroid carcinoma, which originates from thyroid follicular cells and accounts for 60–70% of all thyroid carcinomas. It is more common in women and patients under 40 years of age, with low malignancy and slow growth. From finding a mass to visiting a doctor, the time interval of more than 5 years

L. Li (✉)
Cancer Hospital of the University of Chinese Academy of Sciences, Hangzhou, Zhejiang, China

B. Long · X. Ye
Zhejiang Cancer Hospital, Hangzhou, Zhejiang, China

Z. Yao, S. Li (eds.), *Atlas of PET/CT in Oncology - Volume 1*, https://doi.org/10.1007/978-981-99-1172-1_18

accounts for one third of all the intervals, and it may be more than 20 years in patients with a long course of disease. Most papillary tumors are unilateral, and a few are bilateral or located at the isthmus. Most of the lesions are simple and a few are multiple. Cervical lymph node metastasis is characterized by high incidence, early occurrence, extensive spread, slow development, cystic changes, etc., but the prognosis is good. Papillary thyroid carcinoma has variant subtypes, including tall cell variant, diffuse sclerosing variant, follicular variant, encapsulated variant, and oncocytic variant. These subtypes grow aggressively and are more prone to metastasis, with a poor prognosis compared with simple papillary carcinoma. The pathological diagnosis of papillary thyroid carcinoma is usually not difficult. The typical findings are lamellated structures formed by abundant thyroid cells and papillary in shape, showing psammoma bodies, enlarged nuclei, visible chromatin with ground-glass appearance, prominent and irregular nucleoli, and visible nuclear grooves and cell contents.

Follicular carcinoma accounts for 15–20% of thyroid carcinoma, generally occurs in patients with a higher mean age than those with follicular adenoma, and is more common in middle-aged women. It has a high degree of malignancy, is prone to distant metastasis, and spreads predominantly by bloodstream, 33% of which can spread to the lungs, bone, liver, and brain. The tumors are generally large, mostly unilateral. Hürthle cell carcinoma, also known as eosinophilic cell carcinoma, is a variant of follicular thyroid cancer and has a similar prognosis to follicular carcinoma. The treatment of Hürthle cell carcinoma is basically the same as that of follicular carcinoma, except that regional lymph node metastasis is frequent and the iodine concentration is rarely noted in the metastatic foci.

In clinical practice, ultrasonography is the most commonly used thyroid imaging technique. It is relatively cheap, easy and quick to operate, and not associated with ionizing radiation exposure. Hypoechoic solid nodules are typical of more than 90% of thyroid malignant tumors. In contrast, isoechoic or hyperechoic lesions are rarely malignant. In nuclear medicine, ^{131}I-NaI cannot only be used to perform whole-body imaging, but also has therapeutic effects, and can often be used to detect local or distant metastatic lesions that cannot be found by other imaging techniques. During the follow-up after the surgery for differentiated thyroid cancer (DTC) and/or after the radioiodine therapy, the effect of using ^{201}TI, ^{9m}Tc-MIBI, or tetrofosmin in the whole-body scintigraphy has been clear, especially for DTC without the uptake of radioactive iodine. Recently, ^{18}F-FDG PET/CT has become an ideal technique in examining patients with negative findings of radioiodine scan.

The abovementioned methods are just used to make an imaging diagnosis. Nevertheless, cytological or histopathological examinations should be adopted to confirm DTC. In recent years, fine needle aspiration (FNA) has become increasingly important in differentiating benign from malignant thyroid nodules, especially the microcarcinomas. The sensitivity and specificity of ultrasound-guided FNA are 97% and 83%, respectively.

Surgery is the main treatment, and postoperative AJCC TNM staging and a recurrence risk stratification should be performed for all DTC patients, in order to predict the prognosis and guide the individualized plans for postoperative treatment and follow-up. The internal radiation therapy with ^{131}I is required for some middle- and high-risk patients after total resection. Given a high long-term survival rate of DTC, the postoperative risk stratification focuses more on predicting the recurrence of disease rather than the risk of death. A high level of stimulated serum thyroglobulin (Tg) before ^{131}I treatment has an important predictive value for the postoperative distant metastasis of papillary carcinoma before the ^{131}I treatment. When the critical value of stimulated Tg is 52.75 μg/L, the corresponding sensitivity and specificity are 78.9% and 91.7%, respectively. BRAF mutation is associated with the recurrence-related clinicopathologic features, including lymph node metastasis, staging, local progression, tumor size, and multiple foci.

Radionuclide ^{131}I therapy is one of the important methods of the standardized treatment for DTC after surgery. Its clinical applications are as follows. First is the thyroid gland removal: removing residual thyroid tissues from the operation, so as to monitor the progress of the disease through the serum Tg level or ^{131}I whole-body imaging during the follow-up, aiding in the restaging of DTC. Second is adjuvant therapy: detecting and removing the potential tiny residual cancer foci after surgery, so as to reduce the risk of recurrence and tumor-related death. Third is the focus removal: for local or distant metastatic lesions that cannot be removed surgically, so as to improve disease-related and disease-free survival rates. In clinical practice before treatment initiation, it is sometimes difficult to clearly define the thyroid gland removal or adjuvant therapy.

Postoperative endocrine therapy for DTC – TSH-suppressive therapy. The TSH level is an independent predictor of both recurrence and mortality of thyroid carcinoma, with a positive correlation. TSH-suppressive therapy can significantly reduce the postoperative recurrence rate of DTC and prolong the survival time of patients. The level of TSH inhibition is closely associated with the DTC recurrence, metastasis, and relevant death, especially in high-risk DTC patients. TSH-suppressive therapy refers to the use of thyroid hormone after the surgery or the thyroid gland removal to inhibit TSH at or below the normal low limit or even to an undetectable level, on the one hand, to supplement the thyroid hormone lacking in DTC patients and, on the other hand, to inhibit the growth of DTC cells. This therapy can significantly reduce the risk of thyroid cancer recurrence and death, increase the survival rate of patients, and improve the quality of life of patients. TSH-suppressive therapy is not a simple thyroid hormone replacement therapy, but a new therapeutic concept. Principles of postoperative endocrine therapy for DTC are as follows: (1) All patients should receive TSH-suppressive therapy timely, in a long term, and adequately. (2) L-T_4 oral preparation is the first choice for drug therapy. The objective of TSH-suppressive therapy is to reduce tumor recurrence, metastasis, and disease-related mortality, reduce adverse reactions caused by exogenous subclinical hyperthyroidism, and improve the quality of life of patients. Therefore, the dual-risk assessment model, combining the risk stratification for the DTC recurrence and the adverse reaction of TSH-suppressive therapy, can provide a reference for guiding clinicians to adjust the dosage and course of individualized drug therapy.

The sensitivity of external radiotherapy is low in DTC patients and is not recommended for routine use. It can be used as an adjuvant for the locally advanced DTC patients who cannot receive surgery. Similarly, the efficacy of chemotherapy in DTC patients is limited.

1.1.2 PET/CT Diagnostic Points

In clinical practice, the differentiation of benign and malignant thyroid nodules mainly depends on B-mode ultrasonography, and PET/CT imaging has diagnostic value under certain conditions. PET/CT imaging is easy to operate and review results, and its sensitivity and specificity are higher than those of color Doppler ultrasonography and CT imaging, hence having greater advantages in diagnosing cervical lymph node metastasis. Meanwhile, the minimum diameter of the metastatic lesions detected by PET/CT is 0.5 cm, and the diameter of multiple metastatic lymph nodes detected by PET/CT is less than 1.0 cm. PET/CT can detect cervical lymph node metastasis earlier than color Doppler ultrasonography and CT imaging.

1. CT: Due to high iodine content in the thyroid gland, the CT value of the thyroid is significantly higher than that of the surrounding soft tissues such as cervical blood vessels and muscles. CT scan can clearly show the anatomical structure of the thyroid gland and the relationship with the surrounding tissues and organs. CT has advantage over other imaging techniques in assessing the trachea and esophagus compressed by the thyroid gland, the grade of the thyroid extension posterior to the sternum, and the enlargement of cervical lymph nodes. Also, it can be used to identify the relationship between tumors and cervical blood vessels. Therefore, CT imaging is an important technique for diagnosing thyroid carcinoma.

   Most of the thyroid papillary carcinomas have no capsule, but the surrounding tissues may undergo reactive fibrous hyperplasia due to continuous stimulation by the tumor growth, thus forming false capsule. Part of the false capsule is invaded or destroyed by tumors, and the resulting peritumoral incomplete capsular low-attenuation lesion is a typical feature of CT imaging for the diagnosis of thyroid cancer. A "residual ring-enhancing lesion" may be formed on CT scan with contrast. Other typical features for the diagnosis of malignant thyroid carcinoma are irregular or lobulated tumors of soft tissue density, with heterogeneous intensity, ill-defined margins, and peritumoral "peninsula-like" nodules. Fine sandy calcification is the other typical feature of thyroid carcinoma. It is believed that fine sandy calcification is commonly seen in malignant tumors, especially papillary carcinoma, and thyroid cancer should be considered first when finding fine sandy calcification on CT scan. The essentials for diagnosing primary lesions of follicular thyroid carcinoma are basically the same as those for papillary thyroid carcinoma. Nevertheless, the follicular thyroid carcinoma is prone to invading blood vessels, spreads by bloodstream, generally has complete capsule, and is moderately malignant. Although lymph node metastasis is rarely seen in thyroid follicular carcinoma, hematogenous spread is relatively frequent, mainly spreading to the lungs and bone. Some patients visit a doctor due to bone pain or pathological fracture, and then the bone metastasis of thyroid cancer is found. PET/CT imaging has great value in assessing systemic metastasis in patients with follicular thyroid carcinoma at middle and advanced stages.

   Since most of the DTC patients are complicated with cervical lymph node metastasis, CT findings of lymph node enlargement are also important references for differentiating benign and malignant thyroid nodules. In addition, CT imaging should be performed when the thyroid gland metastasis of the lung cancer is suspected or the thyroid metastasis of esophageal cancer needs to be differentiated.

   Also, CT imaging has some limits of examination. For example, it cannot clearly show lesions less than 1.0 cm, and the microstructure of soft tissues around lesions is not as clear as shown on MRI. For patients with thyroid neoplasms complicated with hyperthyroidism because the iodine-containing agents are not available, the contrast-enhanced scans cannot be performed, thus limiting the characterization of lesions. When diagnosing thyroid carcinoma, it is necessary to combine ultrasonography and other examinations for a comprehensive assessment.
2. PET: Due to a low metabolic activity of glucose in DTC lesions, especially those with the function of radioactive iodine uptake, ^{18}F-FDG PET/CT imaging gains limited value and is not clinically recommended. For DTC patients with dedifferentiation, there may be no radioactive iodine uptake in the metastatic foci, but meanwhile,

the glucose metabolism in the tumors usually increases. Hence, ^{18}F-FDG PET/CT imaging has a high sensitivity to detect these tumors. For patients with elevated levels of serum Tg but negative findings of ^{131}I whole-body imaging, if their metastatic lesions still cannot be identified by routine techniques, such as neck ultrasound and chest CT, ^{18}F-FDG PET/CT imaging can be used for further assessment of the lesions. Studies have shown that the sensitivity of ^{18}F-FDG PET/CT is as high as 85% in patients with negative findings of radioactive iodine imaging, but about 75% in DTC patients. The sensitivity of PET/CT can be up to 93% when combined with radioactive iodine imaging.

The metabolic activity of benign and malignant thyroid lesions can be higher than that of normal thyroid tissues. The standardized uptake value (SUV) of malignant thyroid lesions is significantly higher than that of benign lesions. Thus, ^{18}F-FDG PET/CT imaging can be used for the diagnosis of thyroid carcinoma. The SUV of primary lesions is not significantly correlated with that of metastatic lesions of thyroid carcinoma, whereas the primary lesion volume has a significant positive correlation with the SUV of the lesion of thyroid carcinoma. The SUV of thyroid carcinoma on delayed imaging is significantly higher than that on routine imaging, while this characteristic is not shown in benign lesions, hence being helpful in differentiating benign and malignant thyroid lesions.

1.1.3 Typical Cases

Case 1: A 48-year-old female presented with nodules beneath the middle lobe of the right thyroid by B-mode ultrasonography. PET/CT showed a low-density nodular lesion in the right thyroid lobe, with CTavg 21HU, size 1.1 cm × 1.0 cm, and poorly defined margins, breaking through the thyroid capsule, spotty calcification within, and abnormal intense FDG uptake SUVmax 27.4 (cross). The left thyroid lobe showed normal size and shape, with patchy calcification in foci, without significantly abnormal FDG uptake (cross). The lymph node was noted in front of the trachea, 0.7 cm in diameter, with abnormal increased FDG uptake and SUVmax 11.9 (cross). CT imaging showed the nodules in the right thyroid lobe with the characteristics of malignant tumors: low-density nodules, poorly defined margins, and breaking through the capsule, accompanied by fine calcification. PET imaging showed abnormal increased FDG uptake in nodules of the right thyroid lobe and lymph nodes in front of the trachea, indicating a possibility of malignancy as well. The density of nodules in the left lobe was slightly higher than those in the right lobe, with coarse calcification and unremarkable increased FDG uptake, suggesting a probability of benign tumors. Postoperative pathology: (1) (right) papillary thyroid carcinoma, 1.8 cm in diameter of the tumor, with collagenization of the stroma, involvement of the capsule, and metastasis to 1/1 lymph node (beside the right recurrent laryngeal nerve), and (2) (left) nodular goiter with, focal collagenization and calcification (Fig. 18.1)

Case 2: A 55-year-old female presented with thyroid nodules found by B-mode ultrasonography during physical examination. PET/CT imaging showed a low-density nodule in the left thyroid lobe, 0.7 cm × 0.9 cm in size, with poorly defined margins, breaking through the thyroid envelope, and fine calcification within (cross) and focal intense FDG uptake with SUVmax 17.0 on early PET imaging (Fig. 18.2a, cross) and SUVmax 21.4 on the delayed PET imaging (Fig. 18.2b, cross). Although no remarkable enlargement of lymph nodes was noted on CT imaging, the thyroid nodule appeared signs of thyroid carcinoma. The SUV value had increased on routine PET imaging and continued to increase significantly on the delayed imaging, suggesting a malignancy of the lesion. Postoperative pathology: (left) papillary thyroid carcinoma, 1.5 cm in the maximum diameter of the tumor, with collagenization of the stroma and involvement of the capsule, without lymph node metastasis (Fig. 18.2)

Case 3: A 30-year-old female presented with the thyroid mass accompanied by cervical lymph node enlargement for 10 days. PET/CT imaging shows a low-density tumor in the middle and lower pole of the right thyroid lobe, about 3.0 cm × 3.5 cm in size, with poorly defined margins, breaking through the thyroid envelope, incomplete capsule-lie low-density peritumoral attenuation, unclear boundary with adjacent tracheoesophageal structure, slightly compressed trachea, heterogeneous increased FDG uptake, and SUVmax 3.1 (the cross in Fig. 18.3a and the arrow in Fig. 18.3b). Multiple enlarged lymph nodes are noted in the space around the blood vessels of the right lower neck and to the right side of the suprasternal fossa, the larger one being about 1.2 cm × 1.1 cm in size, some accompanied by abnormal slightly increased FDG uptake, and SUVmax of about 2.3 (Fig. 18.3c and d, arrow). CT imaging shows typical signs of thyroid malignant tumors. Although PET imaging did not show significant FDG uptake and the SUVmax was lower than 2.5, however, differentiated thyroid cancer can present normal or slightly high glucose metabolism. Hence, it was not difficult to make a diagnosis of DTC. Given the accompanying remarkable enlargement of cervical lymph nodes, there was a probability of papillary carcinoma. The lymph node metastasis from follicular carcinoma is uncommon and often shows the distant metastasis. Postoperative pathology: right papillary thyroid carcinoma with multiple cervical lymph node metastases (Fig. 18.3)

Case 4: A 72-year-old female presented with status of postoperative radiotherapy for uterine cervical carcinoma for 9 years and found thyroid nodules for 5 days. PET/CT shows slightly low-density nodules in the left thyroid lobe, about 1.8 cm × 1.3 cm in size, with irregular shape, spotty calcification within, unsmooth and incomplete thyroid capsule, intense FDG uptake, and SUVmax of 24.1 (Fig. 18.4a, cross); in addition, multiple enlarged lymph nodes were noted within the mediastinum (stations 1R, 2R, and 4R), the largest of which being about 3.3 cm × 1.3 cm in size, with concentrated FDG uptake and SUVmax of 7.9 (Fig. 18.4b, cross). The diagnosis of these thyroid nodules was not difficult, because both CT and PET showed typical signs of malignant thyroid tumors. The key lay in the diagnosis of mediastinal lymph nodes. First, on CT imaging, these lymph nodes were low in density, plump in shape, without obvious calcification, and partially fused into bead-like shapes. On PET imaging, they showed an abnormal increased FDG uptake in massive shape. All the findings were signs of malignancy, and the metastasis was considered. Thyroid carcinoma has no cervical lymph node metastasis and rarely has skip metastasis of mediastinal lymph nodes. Combined with the history of uterine cervical carcinoma and the tumor markers, the probability of metastasis of uterine cervical carcinoma was considered. Postoperative pathology: (left) papillary thyroid carcinoma, 1.9 cm × 1.3 cm × 0.9 cm in size of the tumor, involving the fibrous tissue of the capsule and moderately differentiated metastatic squamous cell carcinoma noted in mediastinal lymph nodes. Combined with medical history, the metastasis of uterine cervical cancer was first considered (Fig. 18.4).

Case 5: A 58-year-old female presented with chest pain for 1 month. PET/CT shows homogeneous enlargement and decreased density in both lobes and isthmus of the thyroid; slightly low-density nodules in the right thyroid lobe, about 1.3 cm × 1.2 cm in size; and annular calcification, accompanied by abnormal increased FDG uptake and SUVmax of about 5.4 (Fig. 18.5a, cross); nodules with coarse calcification were noted in the left thyroid lobe, without abnormal increased FDG uptake (Fig. 18.5b, arrow). Bone destruction is noted in the upper segment of the body of the sternum, and the surrounding soft tissue is slightly swollen, accompanied by abnormally increased FDG uptake and SUVmax of about 10.8 (Fig. 18.5c, cross). For the nodule in the right thyroid

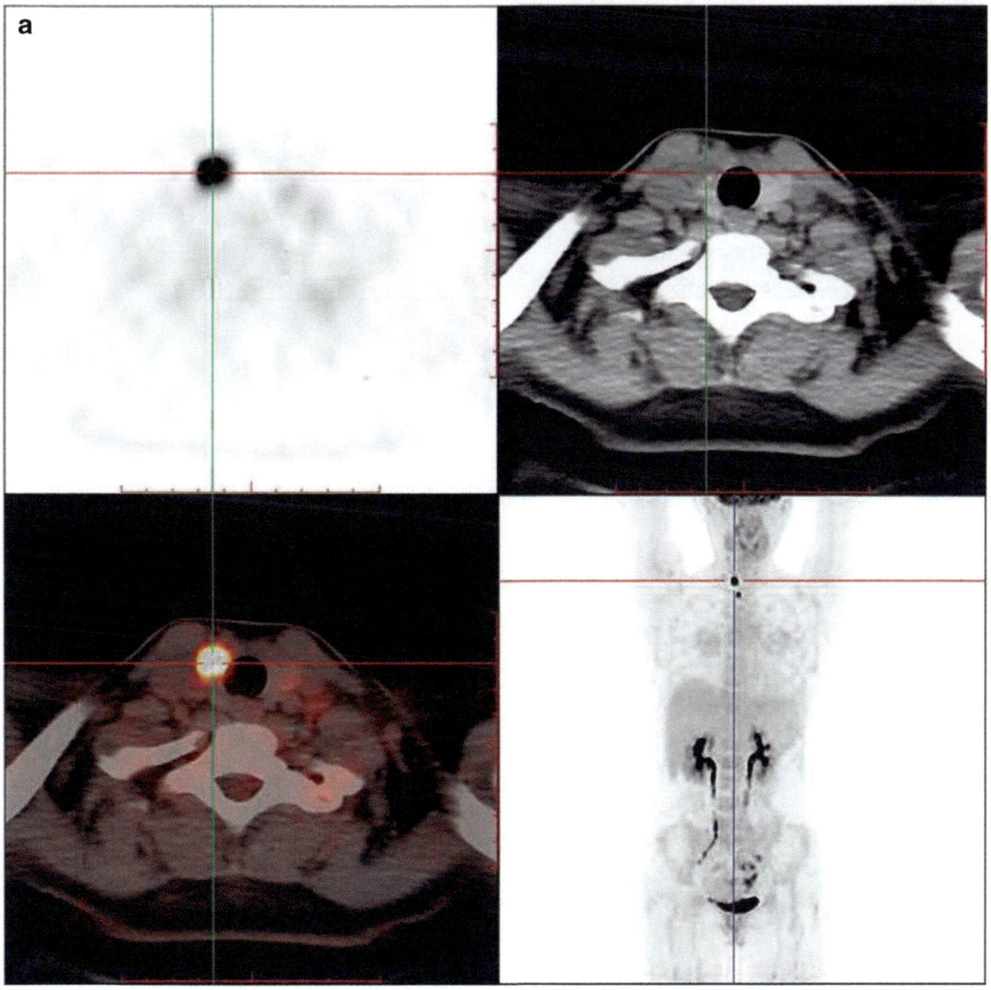

Fig. 18.1 Papillary carcinoma of the right thyroid lobe with lymph node metastasis. (**a**) PET/CT images of nodules in the right thyroid lobe. (**b**) PET/CT images of the nodules in the left thyroid lobe. (**c**) PET/CT images of cervical lymph nodes

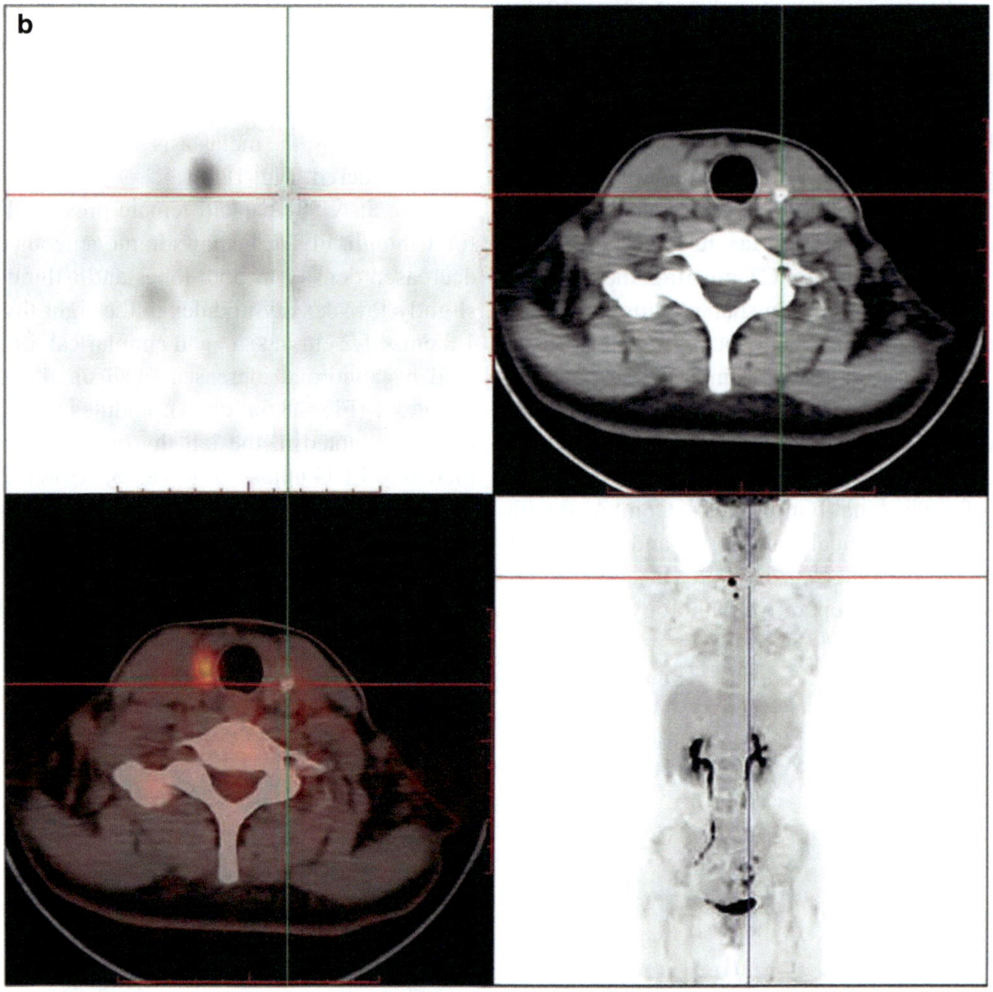

Fig. 18.1 (continued)

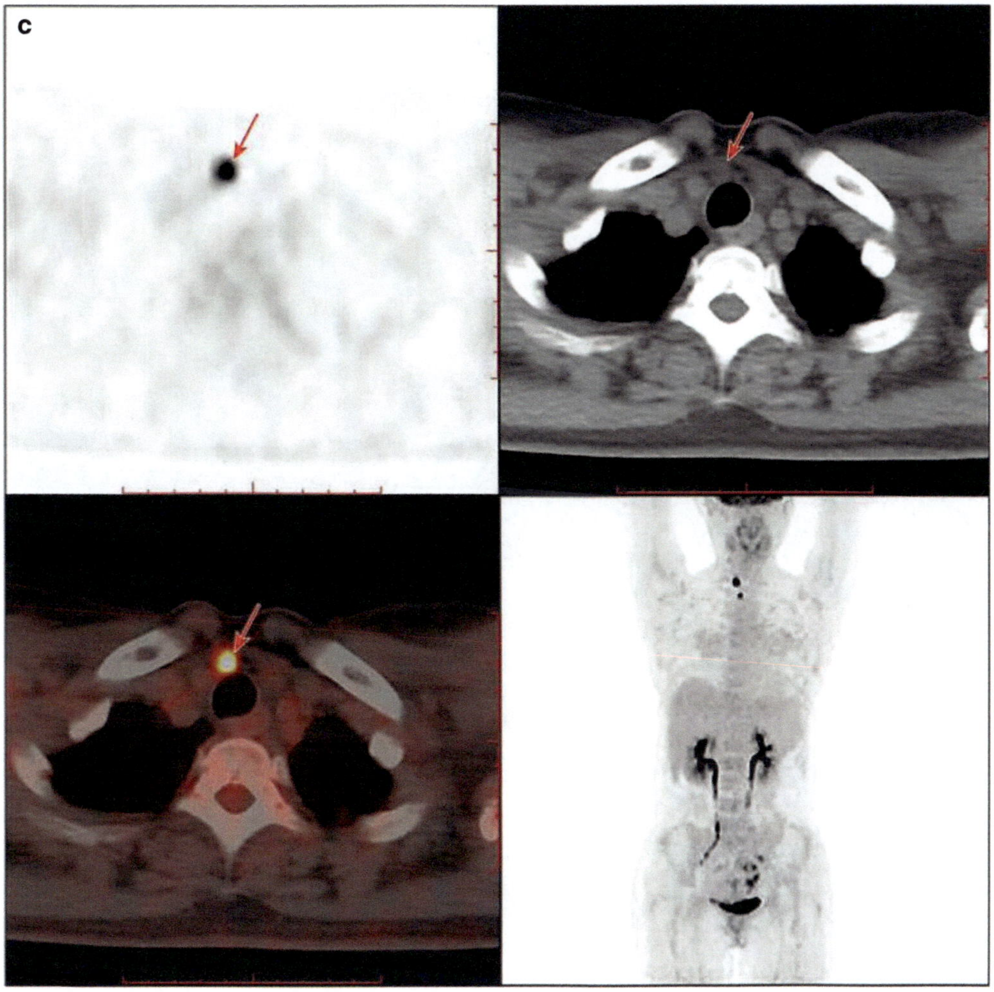

Fig. 18.1 (continued)

lobe, typical signs of malignant tumors are not shown on the CT imaging. On the contrary, the annular calcification is often a sign of benign lesions, and no lymph node with obvious enlargement or high metabolism is noted on the CT, whereas PET imaging shows a high metabolism in the nodule. Combined with the remarkable sign of sternal destruction, the bone metastasis of thyroid malignant tumors should be considered, with a probability of follicular carcinoma. Postoperative pathology: right thyroid follicular carcinoma with sternal metastasis (Fig. 18.5)

Case 6: Status post the resection of thyroid carcinoma for 2 months, with an increased thyroglobulin. On PET/CT imaging, osteolytic bone destruction is noted in the right acetabulum and pubis, accompanied by swelling of the surrounding soft tissues and intense FDG uptake (SUVmax 25.7) in the lesion (cross). If Tg increases after the surgery for thyroid follicular carcinoma, the metastatic focus in the bone should be considered. Indeed, in this case, both bone destruction and increased glucose metabolism were noted. Hence, bone metastasis of thyroid carcinoma was considered. It is worth mentioning that whole-body bone scan is not very sensitive for detecting the bone metastasis of thyroid carcinoma; on the contrary, PET/CT shows a higher sensitivity (Fig. 18.6).

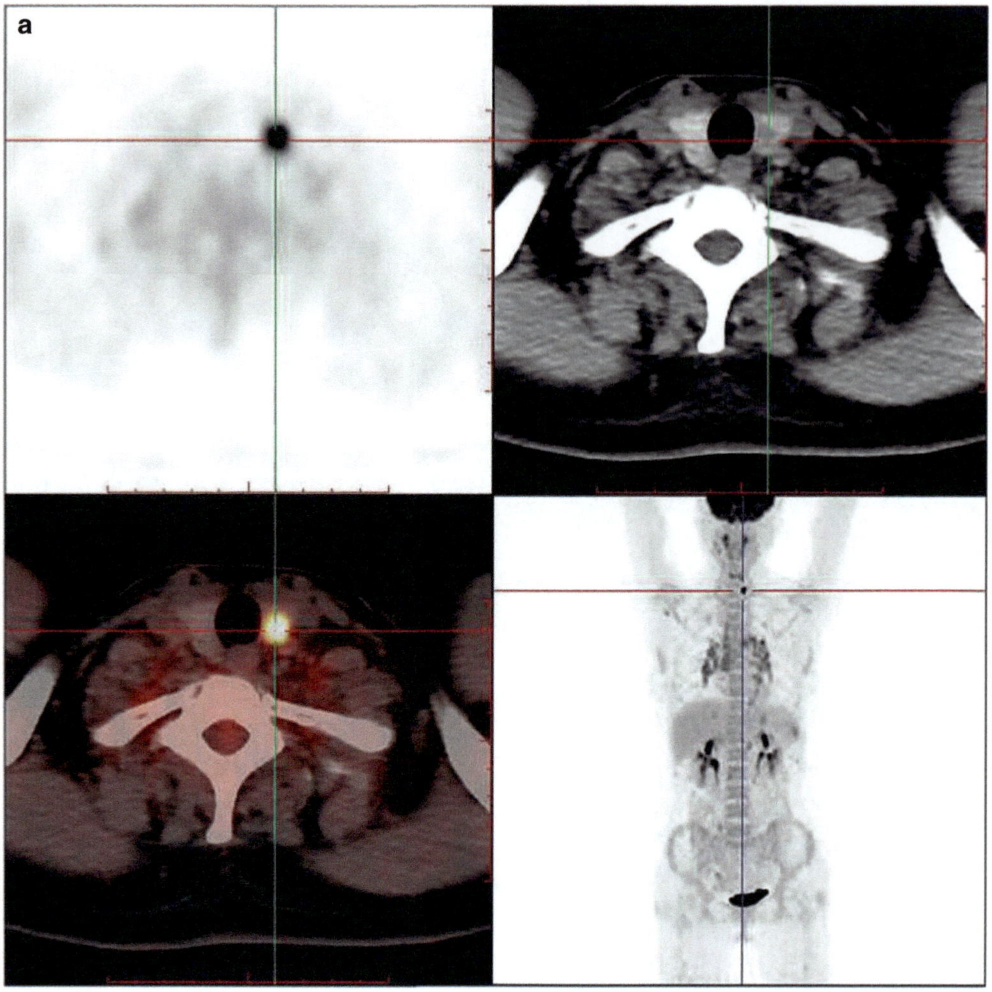

Fig. 18.2 Papillary carcinoma of the left thyroid lobe. (**a**) Routine PET/CT imaging in axial plane. (**b**) Delayed PET/CT imaging in axial plane

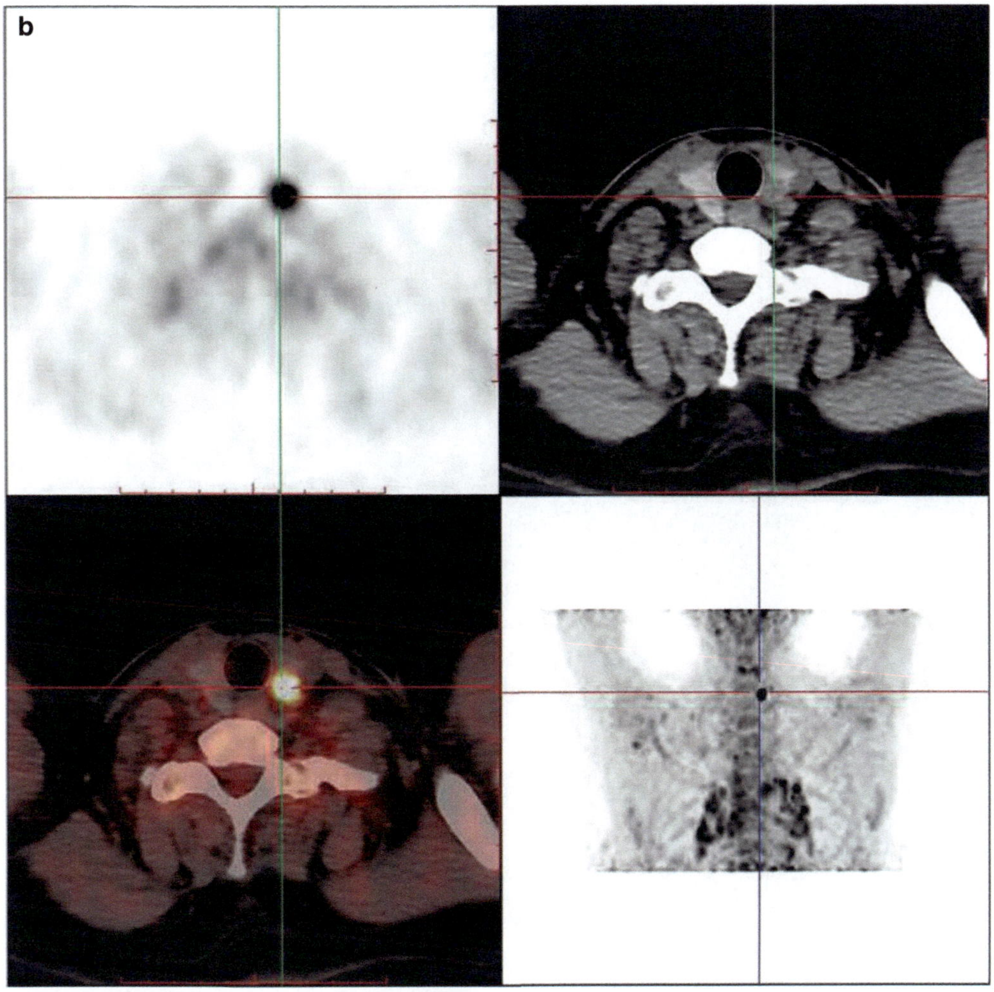

Fig. 18.2 (continued)

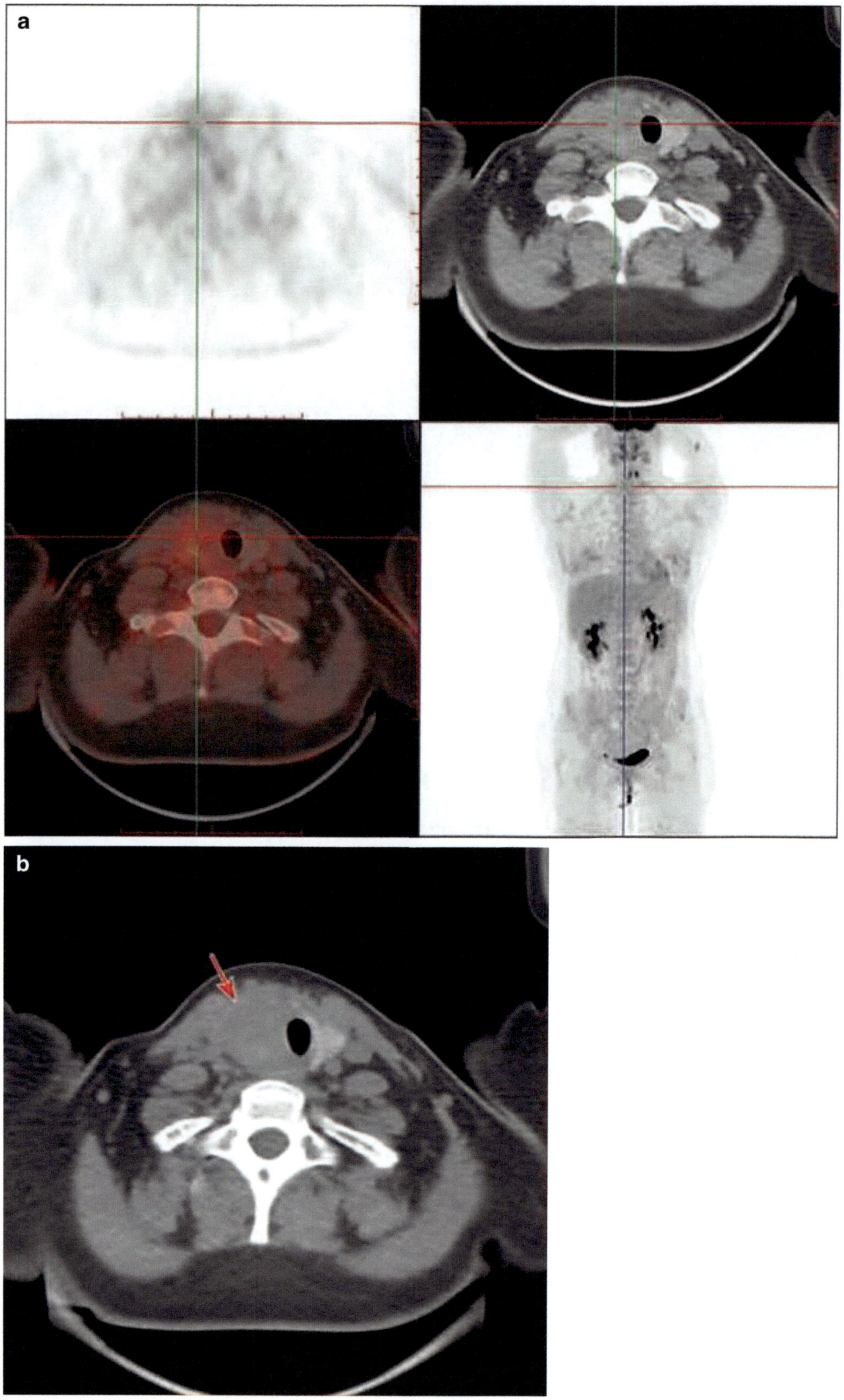

Fig. 18.3 Papillary carcinoma of the right thyroid lobe with multiple cervical lymph node metastases. (**a**) PET/CT and MIP images of nodules in the right thyroid lobe. (**b**) The CT image acquired with the same machine of PET/CT imaging. (**c**) Images of cervical lymph nodes. (**d**) Images of cervical lymph nodes

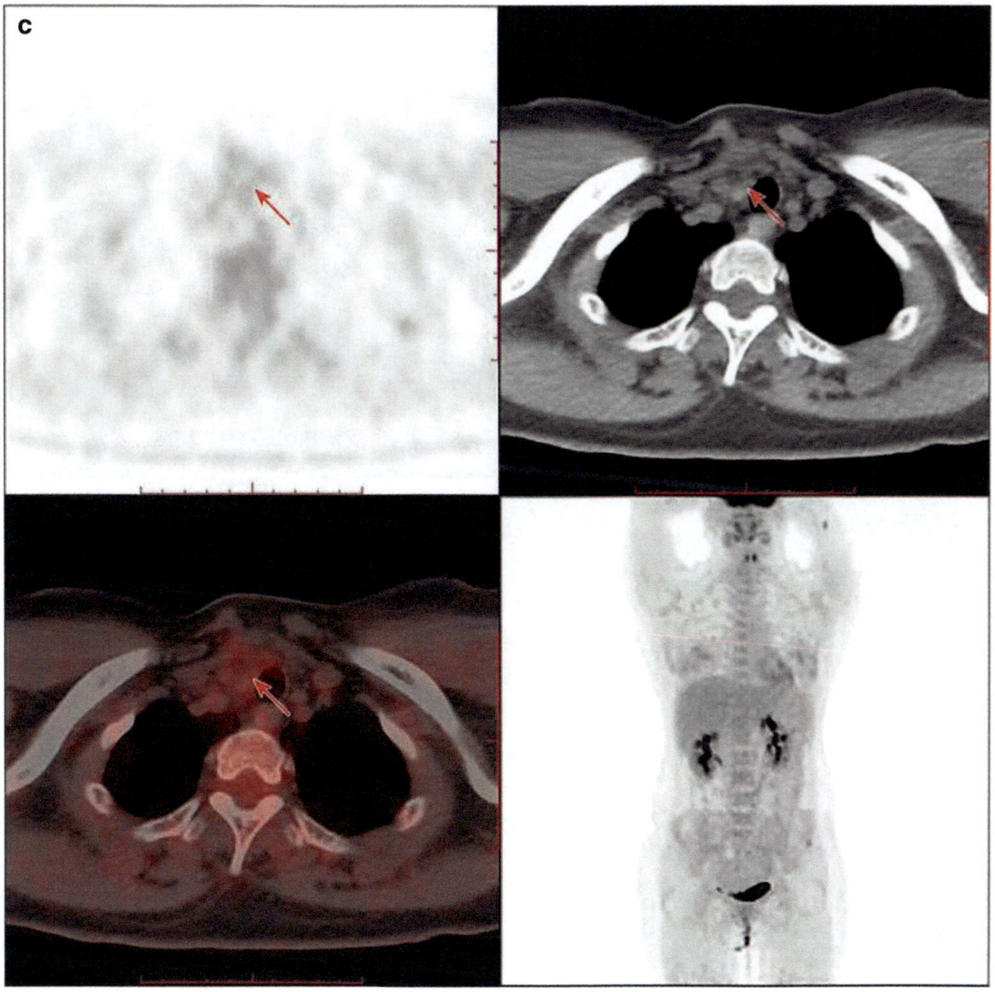

Fig. 18.3 (continued)

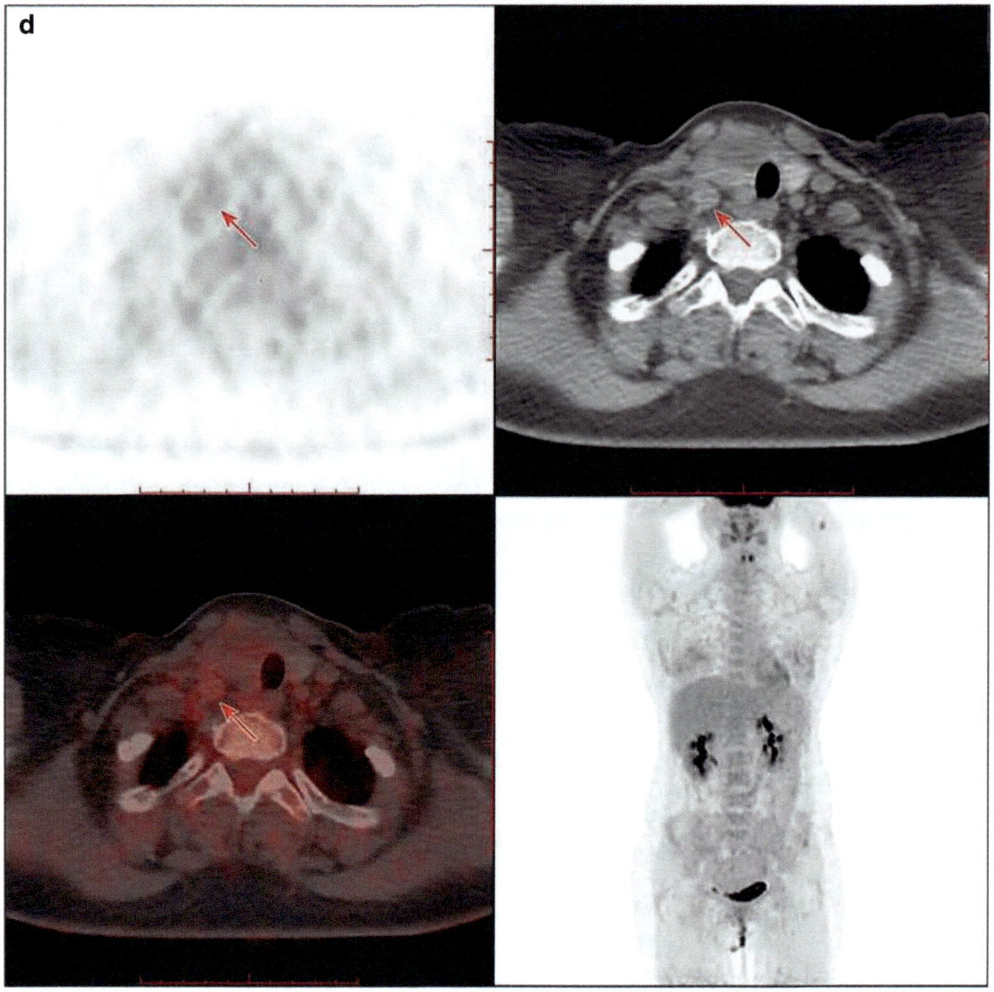

Fig. 18.3 (continued)

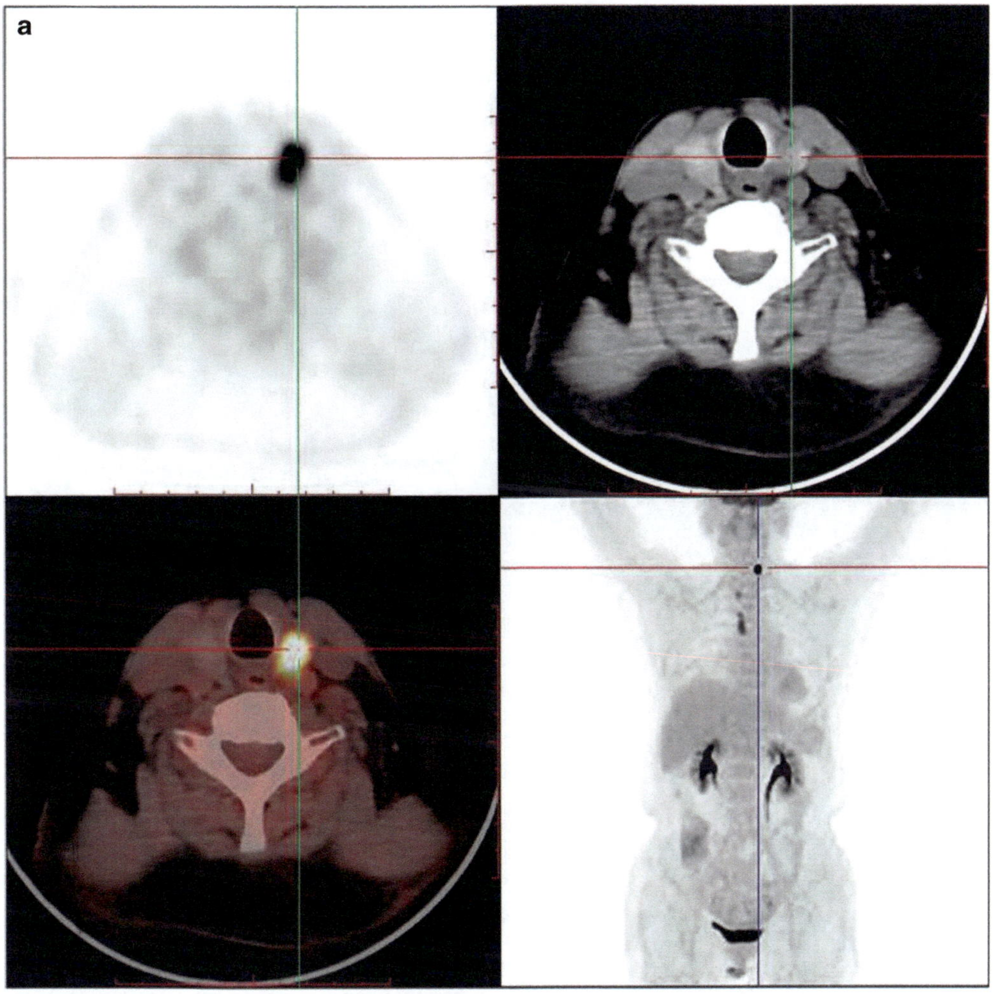

Fig. 18.4 Papillary carcinoma of the left thyroid lobe with mediastinal lymph node metastases. (**a**) Images of nodules in the left thyroid lobe; (**b**) images of mediastinal lymph nodes

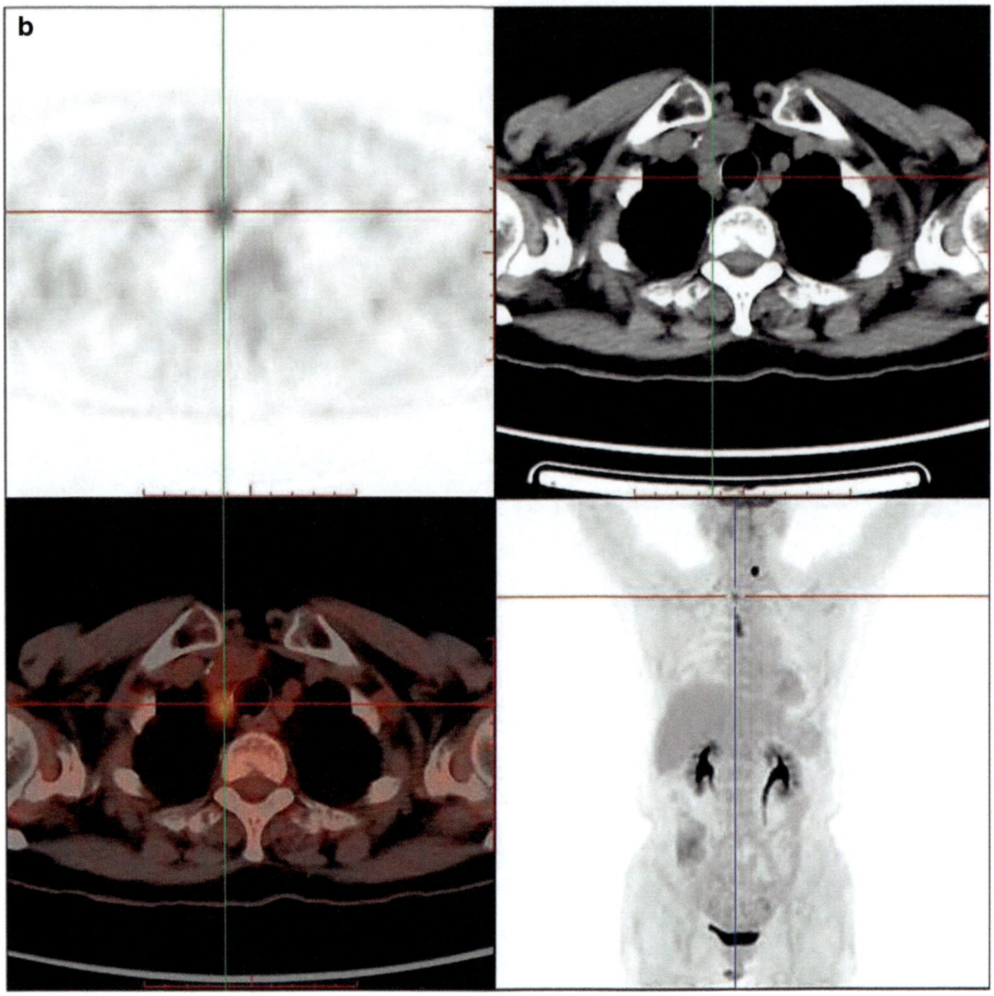

Fig. 18.4 (continued)

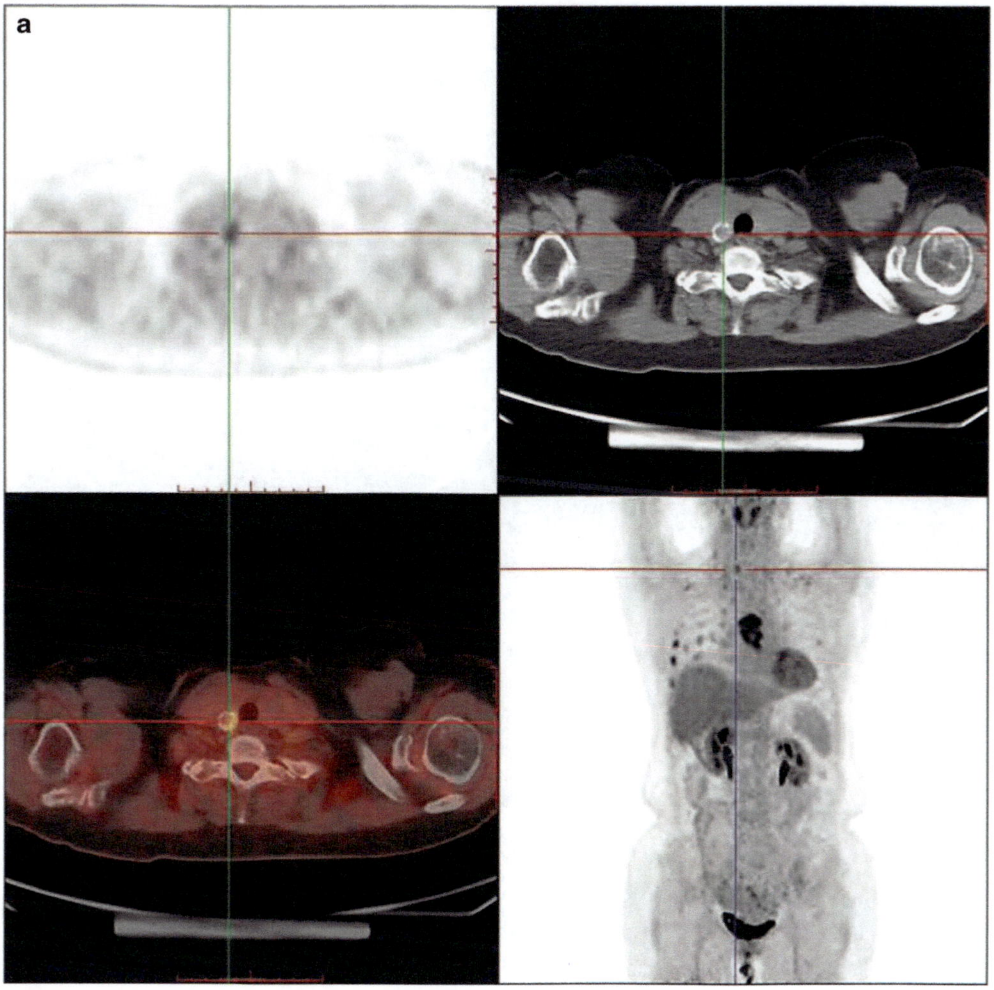

Fig. 18.5 Right thyroid follicular carcinoma with sternal metastasis. (**a**) PET/CT images of nodules in the right thyroid lobe; (**b**) PET/CT images of calcification in the left thyroid lobe; (**c**) coronal planes of the sternum

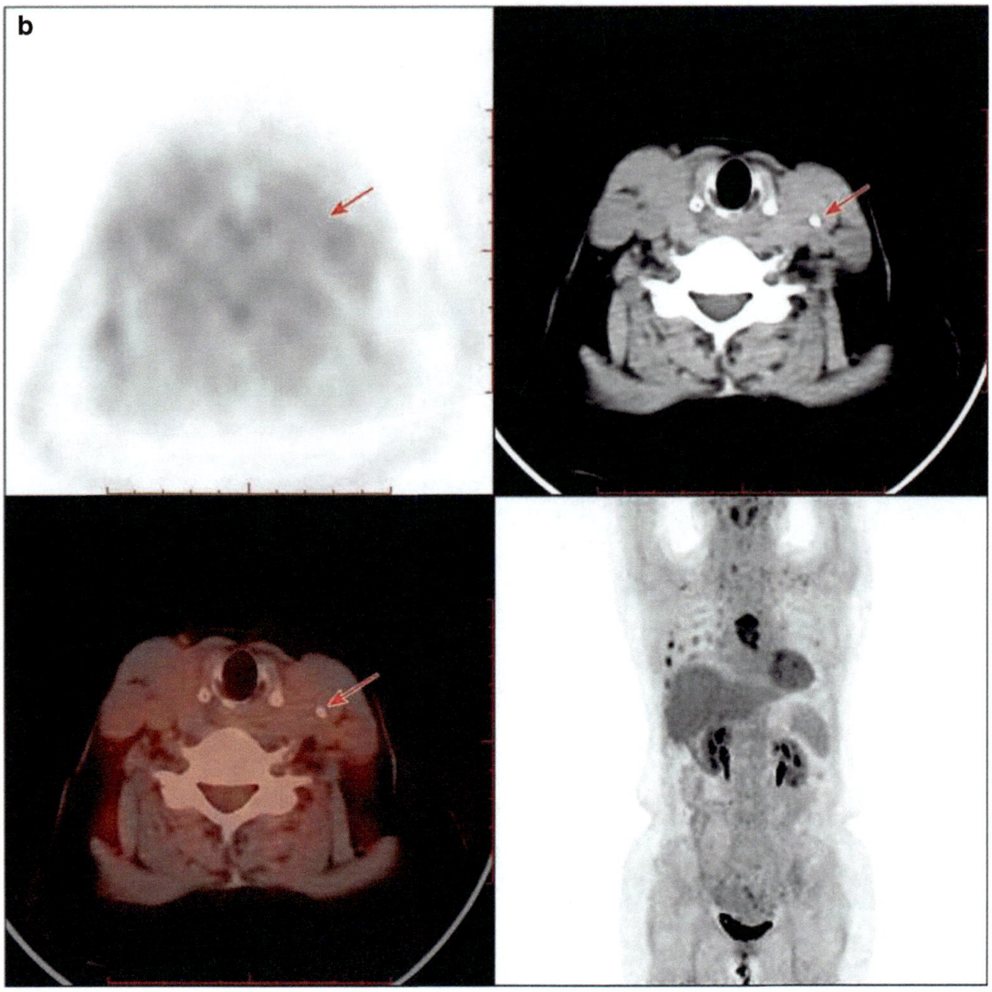

Fig. 18.5 (continued)

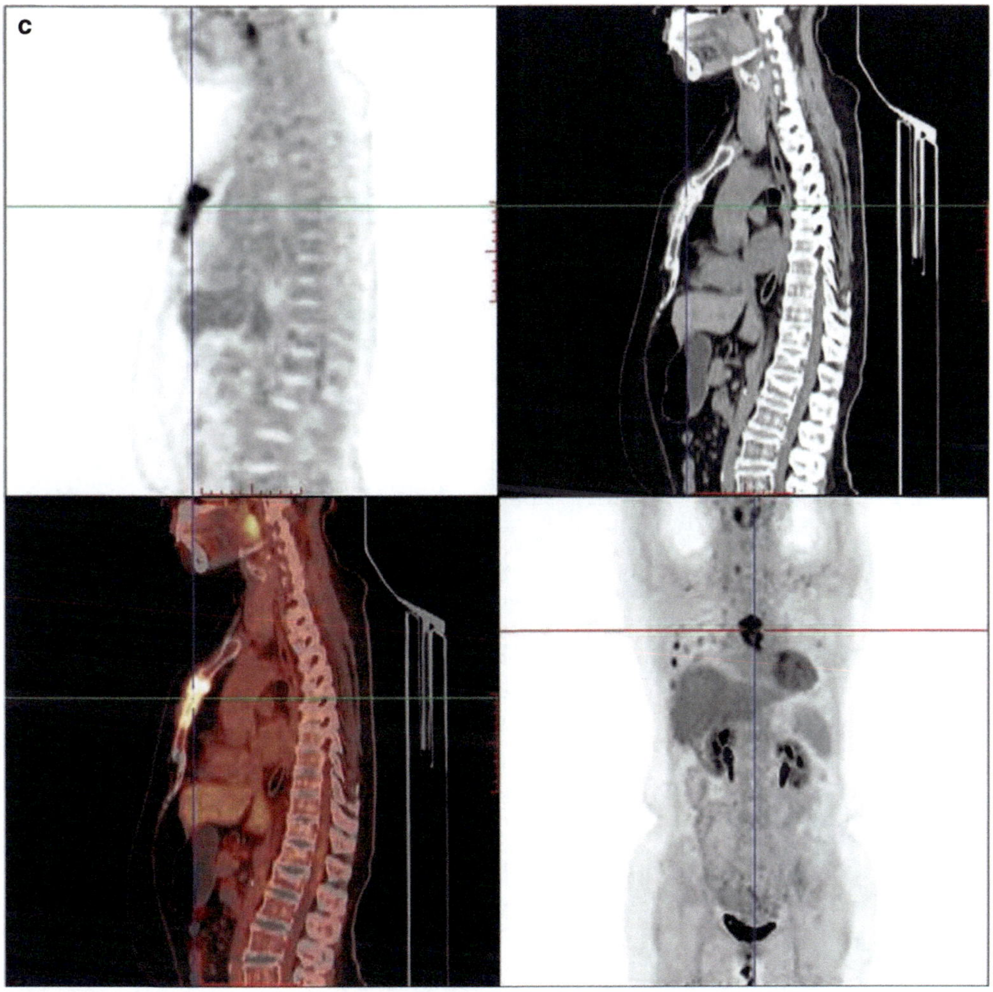

Fig. 18.5 (continued)

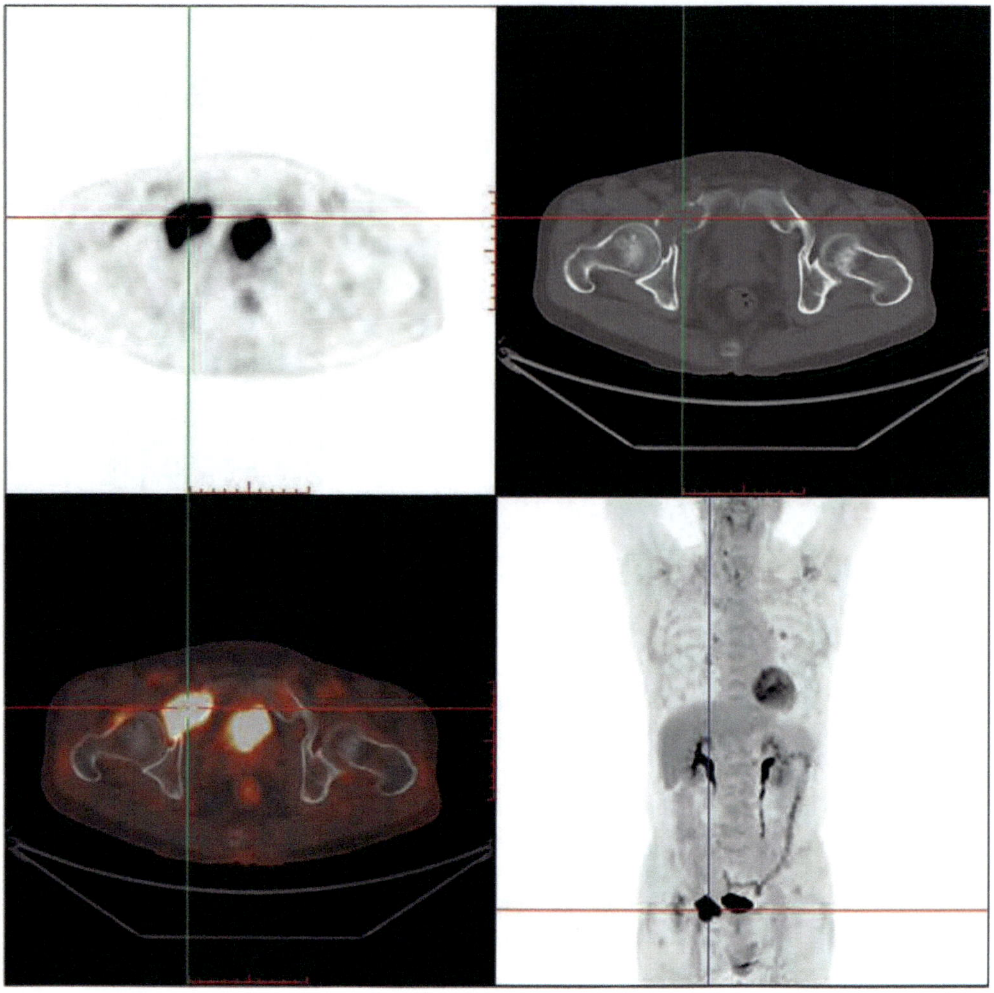

Fig. 18.6 Right hip metastasis after the surgery for follicular thyroid carcinoma

1.1.4 Summary

Differentiated thyroid carcinoma (DTC) is often referred to as a tumor with low glucose metabolism. ^{18}F-FDG PET/CT is not recommended during routine DTC follow-up; however, the results from PET/CT have a significant effect on the restaging after thyroidectomy and the patients with a high risk of poorly differentiated histological subtypes. ^{18}F-FDG PET/CT can be used in the following situations: (1) to find and locate the lesions when the serum level is increased (>10 ng/ml) and the ^{131}I whole-body scan has negative findings, (2) to assess and monitor patients whose lesions do not uptake iodine, and (3) to assess and monitor patients with invasive or metastatic DTC. Positive findings of ^{18}F-FDG PET/CT may be caused by inflammatory lymph nodes, granulomas of the wound, increased muscle activity, and other factors. Thus, for the location with positive findings of ^{18}F-FDG PET/CT imaging, it is recommended to use cytology, histology, and other examinations to further confirm whether it is a DTC lesion. Especially, these methods are often used in patients with DTC and elevated serum levels and in those with negative findings of whole-body radioactive iodine scan. The most important clinical application^{18}F-FDG PET/CT is the diagnosis, staging, and restaging as well as the treatment assessment and the prognosis estimation in patients with thyroid cancer.

However, the clinical observation shows that DTC often has a high metabolic activity of glucose on imaging studies, whereas malignant lesions may also show positive findings on ^{18}F-FDG PET/CT.

In addition, the ability of PET/CT imaging in detecting the sporadic thyroid carcinoma should not be ignored. A multicenter study showed that 1.6% of sporadic and 34% of malignant thyroid tumors were identified by PET/CT imaging. Most of the pathological types of sporadic thyroid tumors identified by PET/CT imaging were papillary carcinoma. Also, DTC with high values of both metabolic volume and total lesion glycolysis is more predisposed to lymph node metastasis.

1.2 Medullary Thyroid Carcinoma

1.2.1 Clinical Overview

Medullary thyroid carcinoma (MTC), accounting for 5–10% of thyroid cancer, is caused by parafollicular cells (also referred to as C cells) and can be classified into sporadic disorder and familial disorder, the latter being autosomal inherited endocrine syndrome. Familial medullary carcinomas involve both thyroid glands, while sporadic medullary carcinomas involve only one thyroid gland. Medullary carcinoma is highly malignant, often resulting in cervical lymphatic metastasis, with ipsilateral cervical lymphatic metastasis occurring in 53% of patients and bilateral lymphatic metastasis up to 20%. Medullary thyroid carcinoma can secrete a variety of amines and peptide hormones, inflicting on some patients with intractable diarrhea, mostly watery diarrhea, but intestinal absorption disorders are not serious, and patients can also have facial flushing and hyperhidrosis symptoms.

Medullary thyroid carcinoma can be divided into hereditary and sporadic types. The former belongs to familial autosomal dominant inheritance and is manifested as multiple endocrine adenoma type 2 (MEN 2). Currently, there are three known hereditary MTC types:

1. MEN2A type, characterized by pheochromocytoma or hyperparathyroidism, accounts for about 90% of MEN2.
2. MEN2B, accompanied with pheochromocytoma, multiple mucosal neuroma, and marfanoid type.
3. Familial medullary thyroid carcinoma (family MTC, FMTC) shows no signs of other endocrine diseases.

Clinically, there are great differences among the above-mentioned three MTC types in the incidence, gene expression, age of onset, concomitant disease, pathological changes of tumor, and prognosis. Seventy-five percent of MTC cases are sporadic, while only 25% of MTC patients are hereditary. The diagnosis of familial medullary thyroid carcinoma is based on genetic and biochemical tests instead of being on a family history of the disease. Sporadic MTC is most common in patients 50 years of age. Due to the wide application of some special examination techniques, recent years have seen dramatic improvement on the diagnosis of MTC, including CT scan for thyroid nodule and the application of molecular methods for mutation detection for sporadic MTC and MTC family people at high risk of proto-oncogenes (RET gene), so as to increase the recovery rate of the disease and greatly improve the prognosis of MTC.

FMTC differs from the usual primary tumors due to the fact that it is characterized by multicentric proliferation of C cells. Almost all MTC present bilateral proliferation as C cells as a manifestation of its initial damage. For sporadic MTC, the initial manifestation is also C-cell proliferation. The progression from C-cell proliferation to microscopically visible tumor cells may take years, but the exact duration is uncertain. Metastases may first occur in the central or peripheral areas, and at least 10% of patients with minimal MTC have cervical and mediastinal lymphatic metastases revealed intraoperatively. The incidence of cervical and mediastinal lymphatic metastasis can be as high as 90% in clinically diagnosed MTC patients. In addition, there are also cases with lung, liver, and bone metastases.

MTC initially secretes calcitonin (CT), which can be used as a tumor marker for MTC and accurately assess the prognosis of MTC. In all MTC patients, basal and stimulated calcitonin levels are increased, and basal calcitonin levels are usually closely associated with tumor size, and serum calcitonin levels are increased in the overwhelming majority of patients with clinically palpable masses, up to 100 pg/mL. In other words, basal elevation of calcitonin indicates incomplete tumor resection or tumor recurrence. Therefore, it is recommended that all patients with thyroid nodules undergo detection of serum calcitonin.

Other laboratory examination indicators include carcinoembryonic antigen (CEA), calcium aprotinin (PDN-21), chromogranin A, neuron-specific enolase (NSE), growth hormone, and adrenocorticotropic hormone (ACTH), which are secreted by MTC and can be differentiated from other types of tumors.

In terms of imaging examination, cervical ultrasound and CT examination on the neck, chest, and abdomen are mainly performed. Ultrasound plays an important role in the diagnosis of thyroid tumor, but there have been few reports on MTC ultrasound. The more consistent conclusion is that the ultrasonographic manifestations of MTC have certain characteristics, characterized with clear boundaries, regular morphology, aspect ratio ≤ 1, and more common thick calcification, but their specificity is not high enough, so that the diagnostic accuracy is low, and ultrasound is not as good as CT in the display of lymphatic metastasis and thick calcification in the central group. Increased calcitonin and CEA are found in MTC patients during postoperative follow-up, often indicating the presence of malignant C cells. The location of corresponding lesions can't be determined by conventional imaging examination. It is called occult lesion, which is mainly attributed to the small size of the tumor and diffuse metastasis to the lung, liver, or bone marrow. A single lesion is too small to be detected by conventional examination methods.

Surgery is the preferred treatment for medullary thyroid carcinoma, regardless of whether the tumor is sporadic or familial, is primary or recurrent, and is confined to the thyroid gland or invades the gland. MTC is usually manifested with multiple lesions, so total thyroidectomy is recommended for all patients with medullary thyroid carcinoma. Dissection is also necessary in the neck area where lymphatic metastases have been significant. Distant metastases of MTC are rarely treated surgically, and surgical indications are only available to prevent local complications and relieve symptoms.

Radioactive iodine is an extremely helpful tool for the diagnosis and treatment of DTC, which cannot be ingested or stored because MTC is not derived from thyroid follicular cells. External irradiation shall be avoided as much as possible, and chemotherapy has almost no efficacy. At present, more and more researches have been turned to molecular targeted drug therapy. In conclusion, the conventional non-surgical treatment of MTC is limited and less effective.

The natural course of different sporadic MTC varies greatly from one another. Long-term recessive growth may occur after surgery, and rapid invasion, spread of metastasis, and even death may also occur. The overall 10-year survival rate for all types of MTC has been 61–76%. The overall prognosis is between differentiated papillary thyroid carcinoma, follicular carcinoma, and aggressive undifferentiated thyroid carcinoma. Early diagnosis and timely operation are recommended, and the main factors that may affect the prognosis of MTC treatment include disease stage, time of diagnosis, tumor classification (sporadic or familial), gender, and age (familial MTC of stage I and female aged <40 years old are factors for good prognosis). Currently, no significant differences have been revealed between sporadic MTC and familial MTC in survival. Good prognosis mainly depends on preventive screening, early diagnosis, and timely, reasonable, and standard treatment.

1.2.2 PET/CT Diagnostic Points

MTC originates from parafollicular cells of thyroid secreting calcitonin. Therefore, as far as this type of patients is concerned, regular detection of serum calcitonin is usually adopted in prior postoperative monitoring. It is generally believed that elevated serum calcitonin levels after surgery indicate tumor recurrence or metastasis. However, many years' clinical observations have shown that although the level of calcitonin in some patients has increased in postoperative review, the recurrence and metastasis still cannot be detected by conventional imaging examination. PET/CT examination, with its unique advantages, will play a greater role in these aspects, helping to solve this problem.

Local recurrence or cervical lymphatic metastasis is usually diagnosed by ultrasound, and the CT findings are mostly manifested as single or multiple lobular nodules with irregular morphology, unclear boundaries, and inhomogeneous density reduction, accompanied with thick calcification.

Lymphatic metastasis is common, but in many cases, metastatic lymph nodes in mediastinal and hilus of the lung are difficult to distinguish from normal lymph nodes on CT, which is easy to lead to missed diagnosis or misdiagnosis. If the lesions have the above manifestations accompanied by evidently increased calcitonin, the possibility of lymph nodes metastasis from MTC should be taken into consideration. Moreover, it is necessary to combine with other examinations to improve the accuracy of preoperative diagnosis and prognosis. PET/CT, to a certain extent, can be relied on to have an overall understanding of the distribution of systemic lesions, accurate location of tumors, and its stage.

MTC has the features of neuroendocrine tumors, with diverse biological behaviors, and can be manifested as a number of types from slow-growing inert tumors to highly invasive tumors. Therefore, the SUVmax value of MTC can be high or low. PET/CT dual-phase imaging is helpful for the differentiation of benign and malignant tumors. SUVmax value in delayed imaging of malignant tumors will continue to increase, while SUVmax value in benign diseases will decrease over time.

FDG PET/CT has excellent diagnostic accuracy in the staging of non-neuroendocrine neoplasms, while its results in the diagnosis of MTC are disappointing. At present, there have been no large-scale studies to evaluate the diagnostic accuracy of FDG PET/CT in homogeneous MTC patient population, but existing data reveal that both the sensitivity and diagnostic accuracy of FDG PET/CT in MTC diagnosis are less than 60%, which is probably due to the fact that growth of MTC foci is relatively slow, with relatively rich blood vessels, so anaerobic glycolysis rate is very low, resulting in low glucose metabolism.

1.2.3 Typical Cases

Case 1: The patient, male, 5 years old, was found suffering from thyroid nodules for 1 month. On PET/CT images, there were two irregular low-density nodules in the right lobe of the thyroid, the larger one about 1.5 cm × 1.6 cm in size, with unclear boundary, which invaded into the thyroid envelope, punctiform calcification was seen inside (arrow in Fig. 18.7c), and there was increased FDG uptake (SUVmax 3.0) in the nodules (cross in Fig. 18.7a). Irregular low-density nodules were seen in the left lobe of the thyroid gland, about 2.3 cm × 0.9 cm in size, with unclear boundaries, which invaded into the thyroid envelope; its FDG uptake was increased (SUVmax 1.7) (cross in Fig. 18.7b). CT showed multiple low-density thyroid nodules on both sides, accompanied by fine calcification, unclear boundary, and incomplete capsule. Combined with high glucose metabolism on PET, it was not difficult to diagnose thyroid malignant tumor. Considering the age of the patient, the first impression might be that the patient had had differentiated thyroid carcinoma, with high possibility of papillary carcinoma. However, if combined with the levels of calcitonin and CEA tumor markers examined in the laboratory, it was not difficult to diagnose the patient with medullary thyroid carcinoma. Medullary carcinoma is often manifested as bilateral multiple lesions, easy to show with lymph node and distant viscera metastasis. However, no obvious local or distant metastases were revealed in this patient. Postoperative pathology: bilateral thyroid malignant tumor and medullary carcinoma (Fig. 18.7)

Case 2: Female patient, 22 years old. Pathology: bilateral lobar medullary thyroid carcinoma and metastasis of bilateral cervical lymphatic medullary carcinoma and bilateral pheochromocytoma of the adrenal gland (Fig. 18.8)

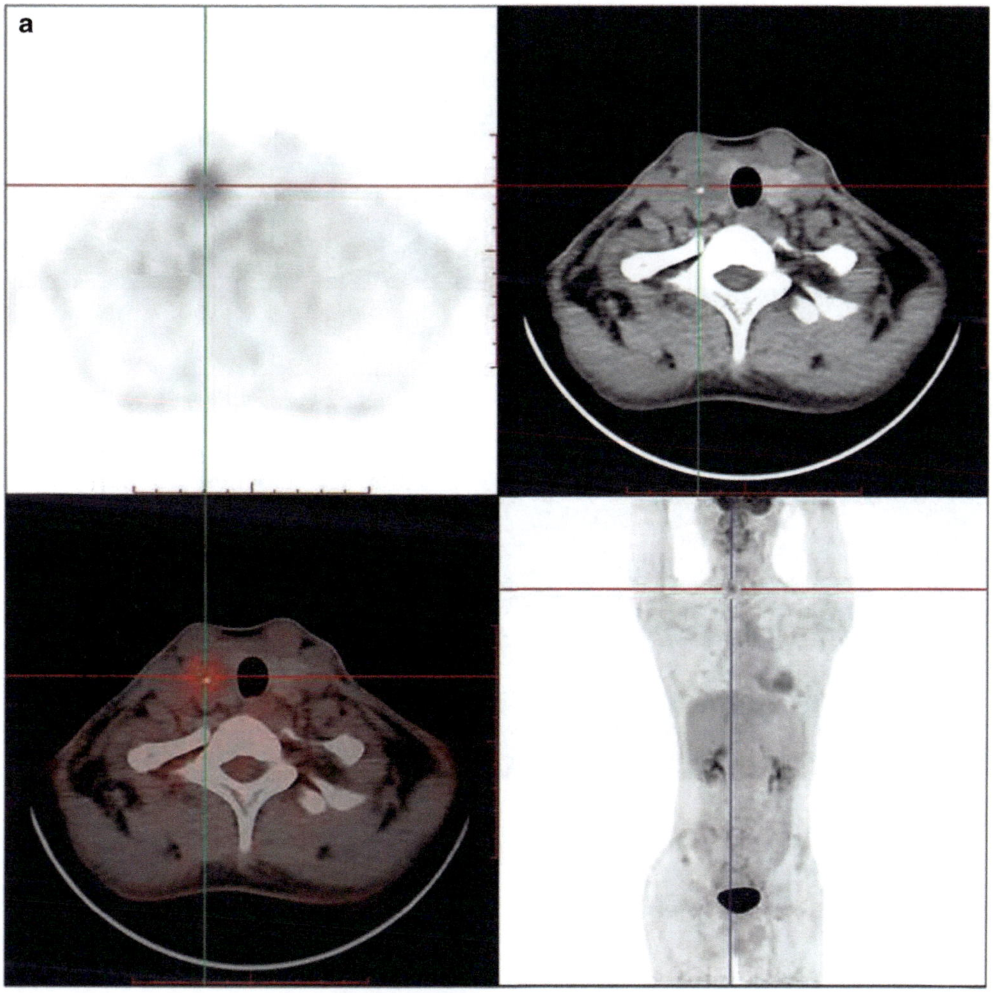

Fig. 18.7 Bilateral medullary thyroid carcinoma. (**a**) PET/CT image of thyroid nodule in the right lobe. (**b**) PET/CT image of the thyroid nodule in the left lobe. (**c**) CT image of thyroid nodule in the right lobe. (**d**) CT image of thyroid nodules in two lobes

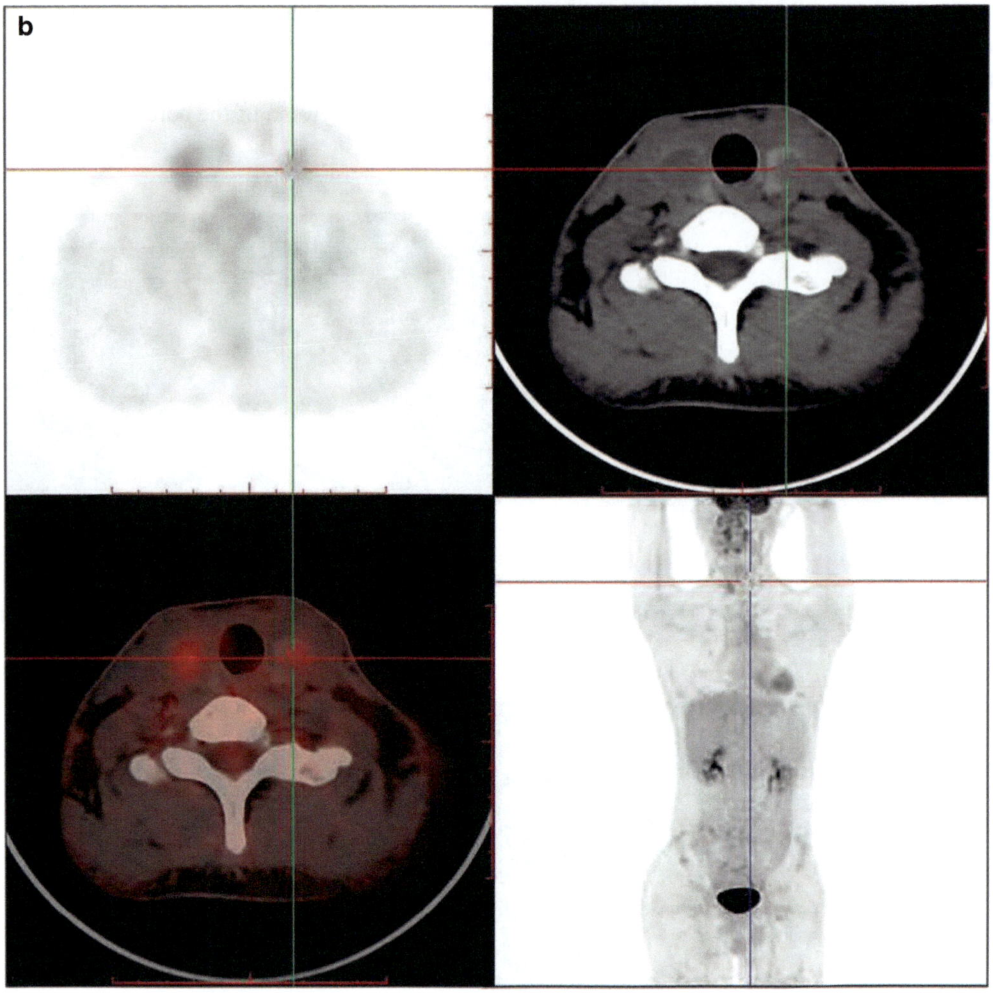

Fig. 18.7 (continued)

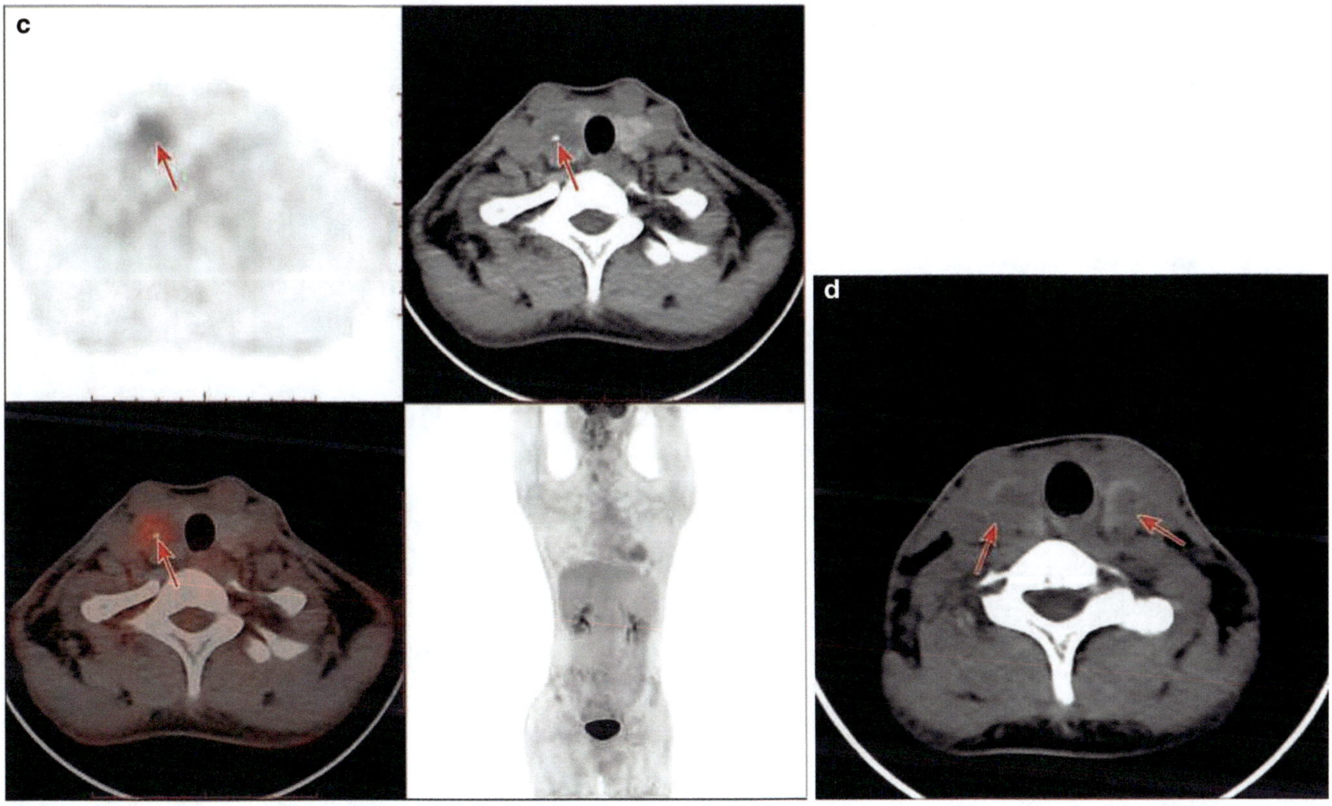

Fig. 18.7 (continued)

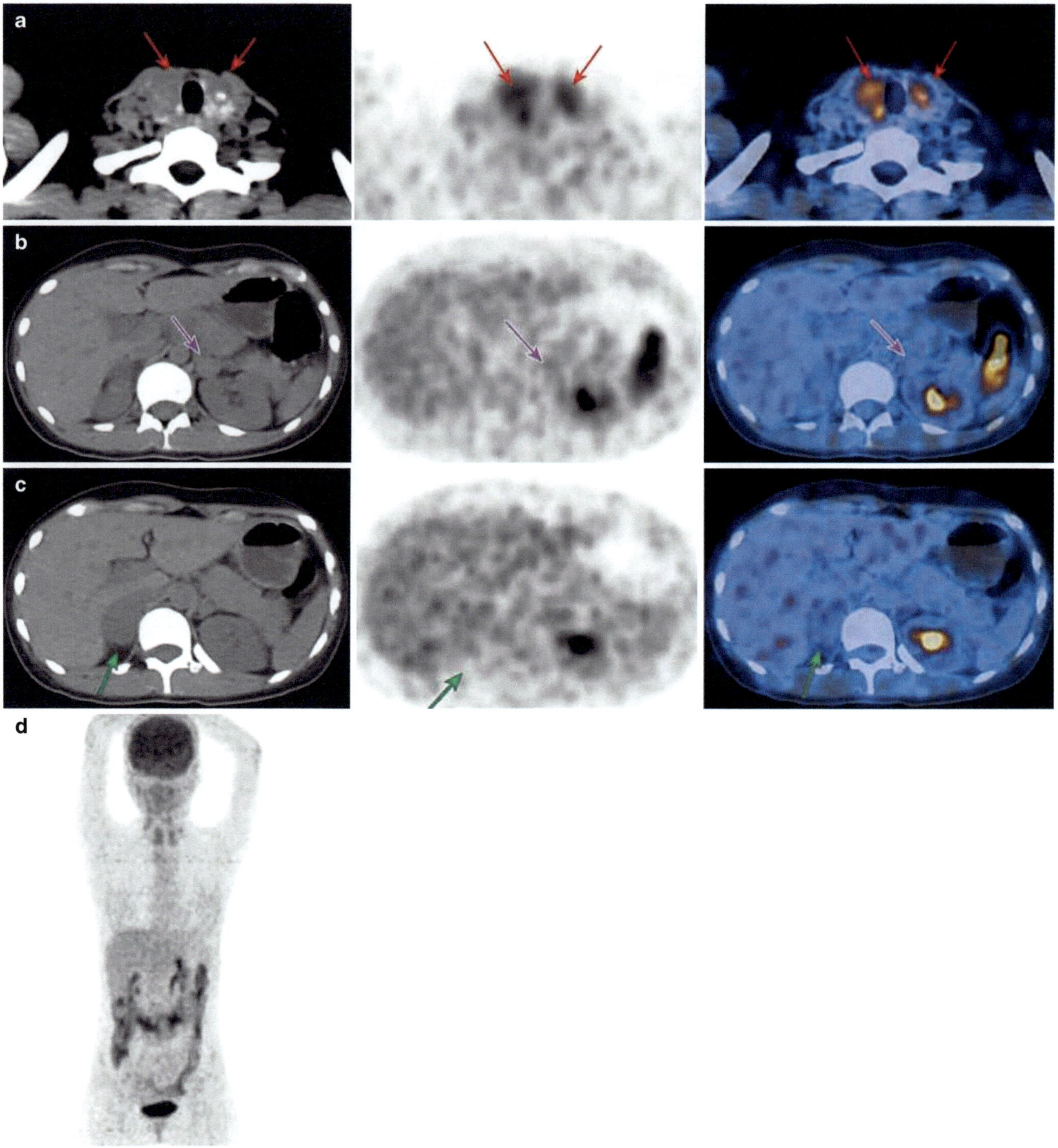

Fig. 18.8 Medullary carcinoma complicated with adrenal carcinoma (multiple endocrine tumor syndrome, MEN2 type). (**a**) Increased metabolic activity of multiple low-density nodules showed in both lobes of the thyroid (red arrow), with SUVmax of 5.4, the larger one about 1.5 cm × 1.6 cm. Nodules were with even densities, and multiple spotted calcifications were seen in the lesion, with CT value of about 583HU. (**b**) The metabolic activity of small nodules in the left adrenal area was slightly elevated (purple arrow), SUVmax was about 2.5, and its size was about 1.3 cm × 1.5 cm. (**c**) The metabolic activity of mass shadow of soft tissues in the right adrenal area was slightly higher (green arrow), SUV was about 3.0, and the size was about 2.2 cm × 3.5 cm. The adjacent posterior lobe of the liver was pressed by the mass in the adrenal area. (**d**) PET MIP image (the case was provided by Lin Xiaoping and Fan Wei, from Cancer Prevention and Treatment Center, Sun Yat-sen University)

1.2.4 Summary

PET/CT can be mainly used for the following cases where:

1. After the primary lesion is confirmed by pathological examination, the presence of potential cervical metastases in patients with early-stage thyroid cancer and retrosternal or other distant metastases in patients with middle- and advanced-stage thyroid cancer was examined.
2. Evaluation and monitoring are to be performed after MTC treatment to determine recurrence or residual lesions, such as detection of recurrence foci in patients with elevated postoperative calcitonin levels.
3. Differential diagnosis of benign and malignant thyroid neoplasms is necessary.
4. PET/CT can also be used to monitor the postoperative condition of medullary thyroid carcinoma. Although the level of calcitonin is elevated after surgery, conventional imaging may fail to detect recurrence and metastasis, and PET/CT is a useful supplement.
5. PET/CT imaging with different tracers is helpful to find rare tumors such as MTC that cause the elevation of serum CEA with and has unique advantages for the determination of the biological behavior of tumors and the overall evaluation of the metastatic lesions.

1.3 Anaplastic Thyroid Cancer

1.3.1 Clinical Overview

The prevalence of thyroid tumors has globally increased year by year, while the incidence of anaplastic thyroid cancer (ATC) with the highest degree of malignancy has decreased slightly. ATC accounts for about 1.7% of thyroid cancer in the United States and between 1.3% and 9.8% of thyroid cancer reported in other countries. The median survival time of ATC patients is 5 months, and the 1-year survival rate is 20%. This disease commonly occurs in patients over 60 years old, and the onset age is higher than other types of thyroid cancer, with a ratio between male and female about 1:2. Patients often present with rapidly increasing cervical mass or hoarseness and difficulty breathing and swallowing. Anaplastic thyroid cancer is one of the thyroid carcinomas with worst prognosis.

ATC tumors are cytologically characterized by multinucleated cells with large heteromorphic nucleus and a variety of atypical cell mitosis. Typical histopathological growth patterns are spindle-like cells, squamous cells, and giant polymorphic cells, with one manifestation or several combinations. ATC may come from the dedifferentiation of well-differentiated thyroid cancer (WDTC). Studies have shown that up to 80% of ATC patients have a history of goiter, and histological examination has shown coexistence of ATC and WDTC in 20–90% of ATC cases, or the patient has a history of surgical resection of WDTC or poorly differentiated thyroid cancer (PDTC). In the process of dedifferentiation, the accumulation of gene mutations and nuclear instability leads to the evolution of WDTC into PDTC, eventually resulting in the formation of ATC. The most common mutations in ATC were *TP53* and *β-catenin*, and mutations in these two genes are rarely seen in WDTC. *BRAF* and *RAS* mutations can be seen in WDTC and ATC, and if it occurs in the former, it indicates the potential of tumor dedifferentiation. *PIK3C* and *PTEN* mutations are also found in WDTC and ATC. *RET*/papillary carcinoma rearrangement mutations are found in papillary thyroid carcinoma and indicate the possibility of tumor dedifferentiation. *RET*/papillary carcinoma and *PAX8/PPARγ* are seen in papillary and follicular carcinoma of the thyroid, but are not detected in ATC. These molecular mutations will provide new targets for the clinical treatment of thyroid cancer and help to determine the prognosis and assist in diagnosis. However, although *BRAF* and *RAS* have high positive rate of mutation, they lack specificity. Although *RET*/papillary carcinoma and *PAX8/PPARγ* can be used to determine the thyroid-specific origin of tumors, they are rare in ATC. Mutations in *TP53* and *β-catenin* alone may suggest dedifferentiated thyroid cancers, although they are occasionally seen in poorly differentiated thyroid cancers. Therefore, molecular studies based on DNA/RNA are not currently considered necessary for the diagnosis and management of ATC patients.

Once ATC is diagnosed, tests shall be performed as soon as possible to understand the patient's basic status, assess the tumor stage, and determine the best treatment. About 10% of ATC is confined to the thyroid, 40% of which have tissue invasion outside the thyroid and/or lymph node metastasis, and the remaining 50% have extensive metastasis. The thyroid function of ATC patients is often inhibited due to large tumor volume, and some ATC patients also show significant thyrotoxicosis. However, it is worth mentioning that, unlike differentiated thyroid cancer, serum Tg cannot be used for ATC tumor monitoring. ATC tumors often invade the parathyroid glands and in rare cases present with malignant tumor-associated hypercalcemia. Imaging examinations include high-resolution ultrasound, ^{18}F-fluorodeoxyglucose positron emission tomography/computed tomography (^{18}F-FDG PET/CT), magnetic resonance imaging (MRI), or computed tomography (CT), all of which are mainly used to assess the degree of tumor invasion, whether there is distant metastasis, etc. Distant metastasis is seen in ATC patients in the lungs (37.2%), mediastinal lymph nodes (25%), liver (10.1%), bone (6.4%), kidney (5.3%), heart and adrenal glands (5.2%), and brain (4.4%). ATC tumors grow rapidly and often involve the vocal cords, resulting in vocal cord paralysis and hoarseness. All patients should be evaluated for vocal cord function. Fiberoptic laryngoscope examines the contralateral vocal cords, movement of the vocal cords, pathological changes in the larynx, and lesions in the subglottic and upper trachea.

TNM stage: All ATC are IV stage. Stage IVa: The tumor lesion is confined to the thyroid gland (T_{4a}), N_0, M_0 (no distant metastasis). Stage IVb: The primary tumor reaches T_4 invasion, N_0–N_3, M_0. Stage IVc: The tumor has distant metastasis.

Most patients with ATC have a poor prognosis, and all patients are clinically assessed for prognosis, including age, sex, tumor size, histology, and tumor stage. The 1-year survival rate was 72.7%, 24.8%, and 8.2%, respectively, in patients with IVa, IVb, and IVc stages. Patients characterized with extensive surgical excision, gender of female, and young age (<60 years old), small tumor volume (<5–7 cm), reception of high-dose radiotherapy, no distant metastasis, coexisting WDTC, and comprehensive treatment have a relatively good prognosis.

In terms of treatment, the treatment of local lesions is dominated by surgery, with total or subtotal thyroidectomy combined with central region and bilateral cervical lymph node dissection. In order to prevent airway or esophageal compression, patients with systemic metastasis should receive palliative treatment after removal of the primary tumor in time. Some patients need preoperative and postoperative adjuvant therapy and surgical resection (R0/R1) combined with chemoradiotherapy (>40Gy). Local lesion control and overall survival rate of the patients are significantly improved. As far as radiation therapy is concerned, it is recommended to use intensity-modulated radiation therapy (IMRT), which is accurately targeted and has little damage to the spinal cord and the normal tissues near the tumor. The commonly used cytotoxic chemotherapy drugs for ATC include paclitaxel analogues (paclitaxel, docetaxel), anthracycline (aclarubicin), and platinum (cisplatin, carboplatin), which are often used in combination.

The treatment of advanced metastatic ATC is mainly systemic chemotherapy, which is not responded to radioactive iodine scanning/treatment. In recent years, some new targeted therapeutic drugs have been clinically proven to have certain efficacy, such as multi-kinase inhibitor (sorafenib), tyrosine kinase inhibitor (axitinib), epidermal growth factor receptor tyrosine kinase inhibitor (gefitinib), imatinib, etc.

1.3.2 PET/CT Diagnostic Points

Undifferentiated thyroid carcinoma is usually large in size, hard in substance, and without capsule, and carcinoma tissues often invade surrounding tissues with obvious bleeding and necrosis. Its CT images are characterized with low-density or mixed density masses, irregular shape, unclear boundary, internal or marginal flocculent or patchy high-density areas, thick calcification lesion, and slight enhancement. Invasion into peripheral structure and necrosis of lymph node are common. Most of the lesions have different degrees of adhesion or invasion to the surrounding structures, mainly affecting the adjacent strap muscles, trachea, esophagus, blood vessels, larynx, and other structures, and it may be accompanied with the ipsilateral thrombus of the internal jugular vein. Additionally, a thorough examination should be conducted to exclude distant metastasis from other sites. Although the undifferentiated carcinoma originates from follicular cells, it is poorly differentiated and lacks iodine uptake ability. Moreover, it destroys the iodine uptake ability of normal thyroid follicles without obvious enhancement, which is different from that of differentiated thyroid papillary carcinoma. Different from nodular goiter, the latter is manifested as an irregular enlargement of the thyroid gland and multiple, scattered, regular low-density nodules within the gland, often characterized with patchy and mottling thick calcification. Lymphoma can invade unilateral or bilateral thyroid glands, with uniform density and no obvious enhancement. Cervical lymphatic enlargement is common, but lymph node density is uniform and necrosis is rare. If the patient is older and the mass increases rapidly in a short period of time, and if there is a large area of low-density necrosis inside, the possibility of undifferentiated cancer should be considered.

Although ATC does not take in iodine, it has a high metabolism of glucose. It is recommended that PET/CT should be used positively to evaluate ATC, especially in advanced metastatic ATC. PET/CT can be used effectively to differentiate between metastatic and non-metastatic ATC, and it is superior to CT in terms of value and sensitivity in the evaluation of resectability of tumors and follow-up.

1.3.3 Typical Cases

The patient, a 58-year-old woman, had nodules in both lungs for 1 month. PET/CT images showed irregular mass of soft tissue in the left lobe of the thyroid gland, originating from the lower margin of the thyroid cartilage to the level near the upper margin of the sternum, and low-density shadows were seen inside. The mass was about 5.5 cm × 4.3 cm in size, so that the surrounding tissues were compressed, the trachea moved to the right, and there was heterogeneously increased FDG uptake in the mass, with SUVmax about 13.2 (Fig. 18.9a, cross). Multiple swelling lymph nodes were observed in the VI region of the neck, the larger of which was about 1.1 cm in diameter and with FDG uptake increased, with SUVmax about 8.7. Multiple swelling lymph nodes were seen in the anterior superior mediastinum, the largest of which was about 3.2 cm × 2.3 cm in size, with increased inhomogeneous FDG uptake and SUVmax about 8.9 (Fig. 18.9b, cross). Quasi-circular nodules of different sizes were observed in both lungs, with clear boundaries, the larger one located in the left lower lung, with a size of about 2.9 cm × 2.4 cm, whose FDG uptake increased with SUVmax about 9.6 (arrows in Fig. 18.9c and d). CT images showed a large low-density thyroid mass with irregular morphology, unclear boundary, and invasion into surrounding tissues and blood vessels. The rapid growth in the mass led to ischemia and necrosis, accompanied by multiple enlarged lymph nodes, fusion, and necrosis and with pulmonary metastasis. PET showed increased glucose metabolism in both primary lesions and metastatic lesion, which was consistent with the manifestation of undifferentiated thyroid carcinoma. Postoperative pathology: left thyroid malignant tumor accompanied with necrosis. First consideration was taken into for undifferentiated carcinoma, involving the thyroid envelope, accompanied with vascular cancer embolus, and mediastinal lymphatic metastasis. Pathology of pulmonary nodule puncture: metastatic carcinoma was considered in combination with medical history (Fig. 18.9).

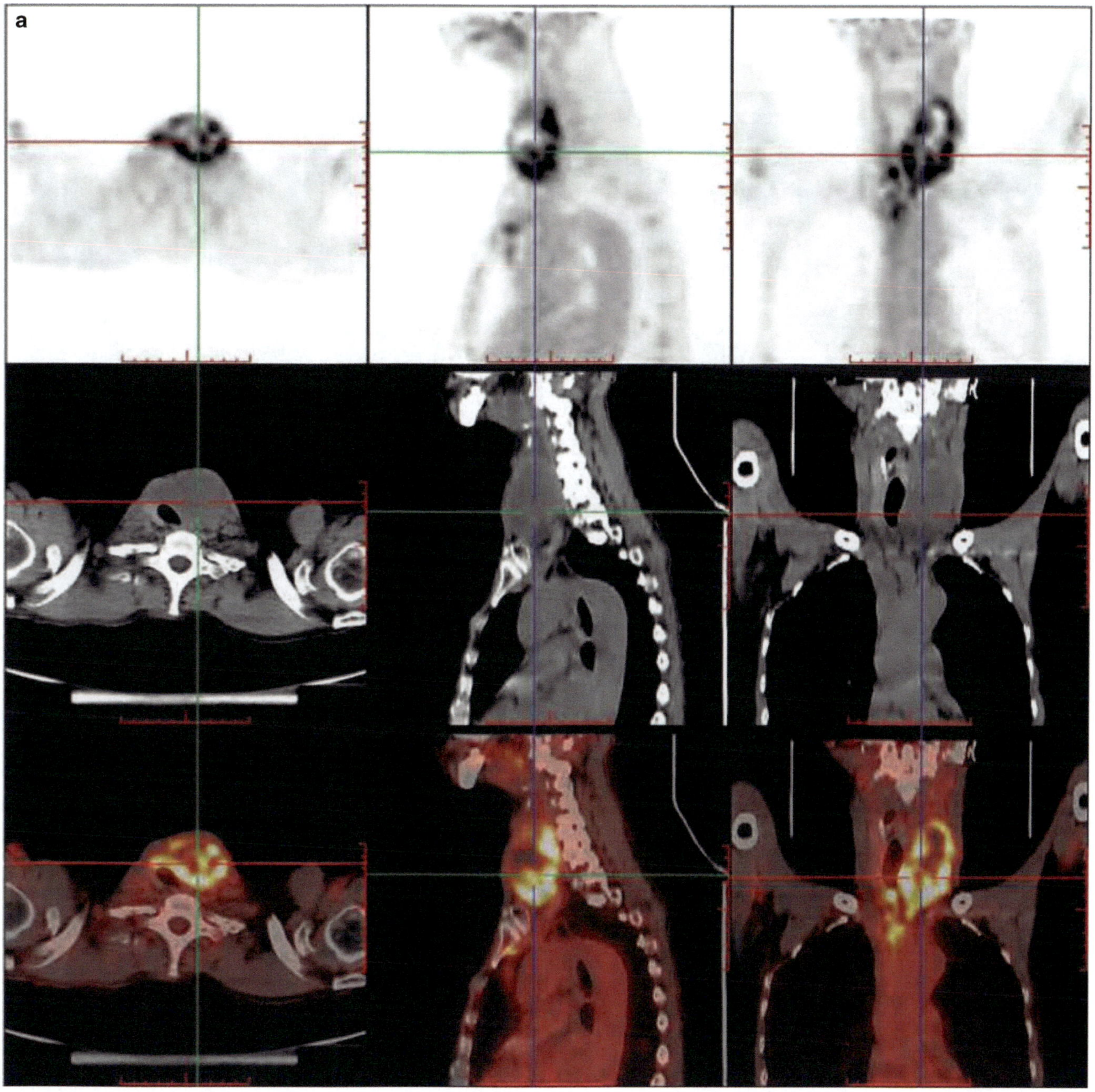

Fig. 18.9 Undifferentiated carcinoma of the left thyroid accompanied with mediastinal lymph node and pulmonary metastasis. (**a**) PET/CT images of thyroid masses. (**b**) PET/CT images of cervical and mediastinal lymph nodes. (**c**) PET/CT image of multiple pulmonary nodules. (**d**) PET/CT image of multiple pulmonary nodules

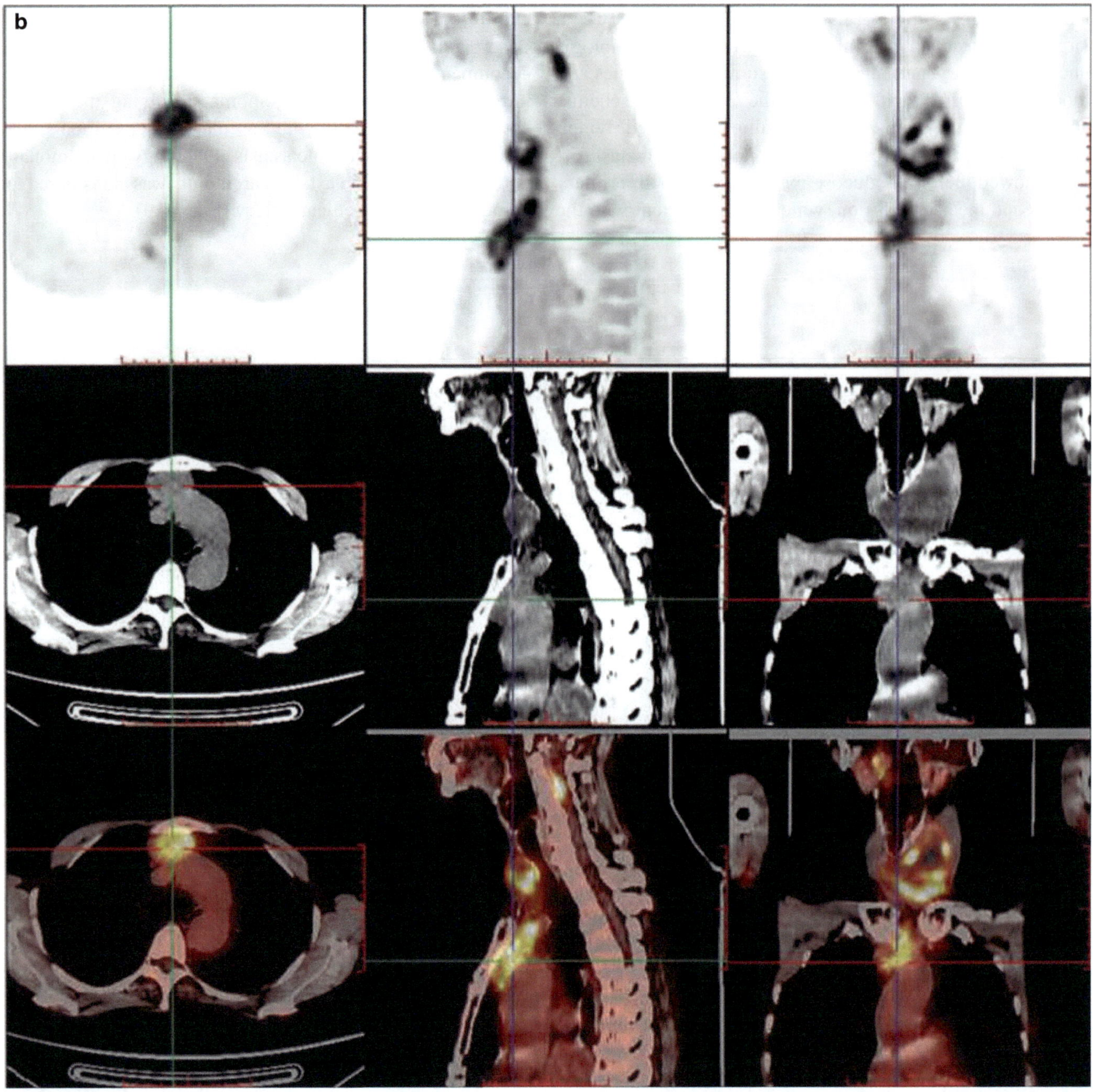

Fig. 18.9 (continued)

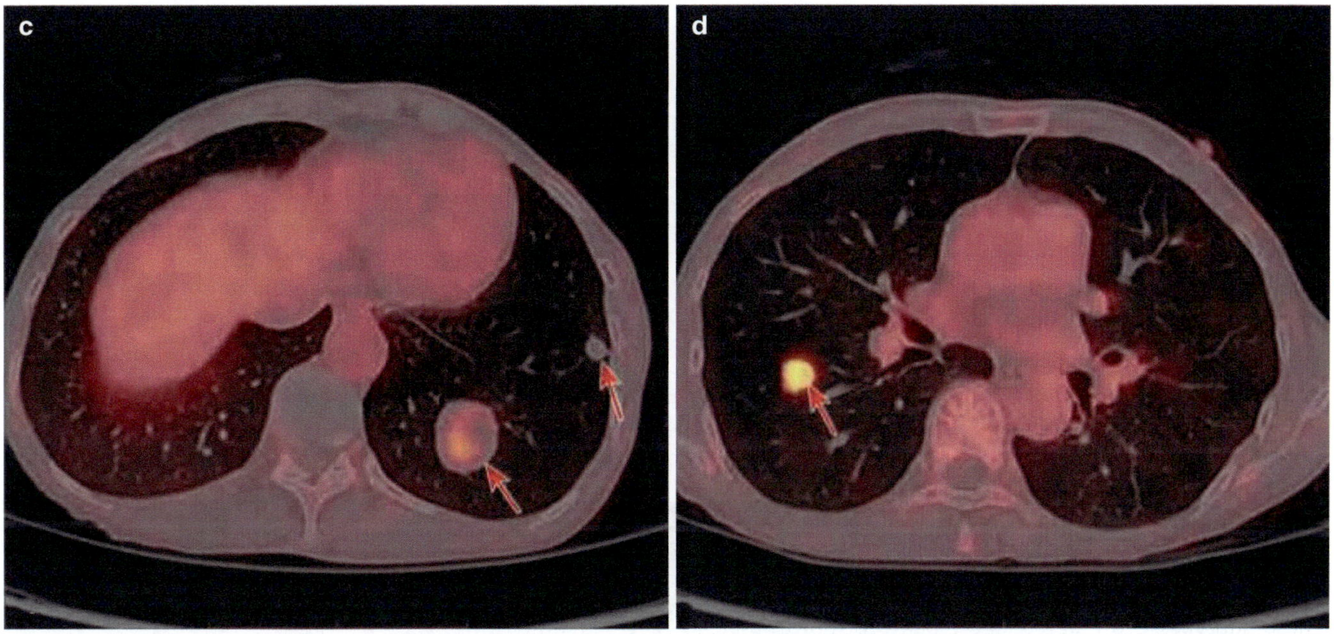

Fig. 18.9 (continued)

1.3.4 Summary

Undifferentiated thyroid cancer (ATC) is prone to being subject to lymphatic metastasis and distant metastasis. PET/CT has a high sensitivity in ATC, which can be used to have a good evaluation of the local and distant metastasis of the tumor, accurately stage ATC, and help the clinic to better evaluate the tumor and make appropriate treatment regimen. In addition, PET/CT also plays an important role in the post-operation follow-up of ATC. Therefore, it is recommended to conduct FDG PET/CT examination as early as possible in the diagnosis, staging, and restaging of ATC in order to accurately assess the disease.

2 Other Malignant Tumors of the Thyroid

2.1 Clinical Overview

There are many types of other malignant tumors of the thyroid, which are mainly divided into epithelial cells and non-epithelial cell sources. The former includes thyroid squamous cell carcinoma, mucoepidermoid carcinoma, and spindle cell tumors, and the latter includes lymphoma, sarcoma, and malignant teratoma.

Due to different tumor types, the clinical manifestations and treatment methods vary. Thyroid lymphoma is a relatively rare disease, accounting for 1% of all lymphomas. It is common in middle-aged and elderly people. There are more female patients than male patients, and the ratio of male to female is 1:2.7. It is often accompanied by Hashimoto's thyroiditis. It is unclear whether the lymphocytic infiltration of thyroid lymphoma leads to the occurrence of chronic lymphocytic thyroiditis or whether it is caused by long-term chronic stimulation of lymphocytes of thyroiditis. The clinical manifestations are rapid enlargement of the thyroid gland in one or both sides in a short time, and some of them may be accompanied by enlargement of lymph nodes, and the density of lymph node is the same as that of the primary tumor. The patients often have fever, weight loss, and other symptoms. Pathologically, B cell is the most common source, most commonly found in diffuse large B-cell and mucosa-associated lymphoma, and chemical therapy is the preferred treatment. Other malignant tumors are very rare clinically, such as thyroid squamous cell carcinoma. Before diagnosis, the metastasis of squamous cell carcinoma in other parts of the body and direct infiltration in its adjacent organs such as the larynx and trachea should be excluded. Primary thyroid squamous cell carcinoma is not sensitive to radiotherapy and chemotherapy, and the therapeutic effect and prognosis are poor.

2.2 PET/CT Diagnostic Points

The common manifestations of other malignant tumors of the thyroid in PET/CT are abnormal increased FDG uptake. For example, abnormal hypermetabolic lesions, uniform density, rare necrosis, vascular floating sign, and no obvious space-occupying effect are the main CT signs in the diagnosis of primary thyroid lymphoma. Other types of malignant tumors are mostly characterized by unclear boundary, inhomogeneous density, invasion of the surrounding tissues, and inhomogeneously increased FDG uptake. At the same time, pay attention to observe whether there are regional lymph nodes or distant metastases to assist in the diagnosis of primary diseases.

2.3 Typical Cases

Case 1: In a 53-year-old male patient, 3 years after surgery of left thyroid papillary carcinoma, a right thyroid mass was found for 1 month. Pathology: ① (right) papillary thyroid carcinoma (tumor size 3.5 cm × 3 cm × 2 cm), involving thyroid envelope and nerve, with nodal metastasis (right level II 3/7, right level III 3/5, right level IV 9/17, right level V 0/7). ② (Superior mediastinum) Papillary thyroid carcinoma and moderately to poorly differentiated squamous cell carcinoma (tumor body 4 cm × 3 cm × 2 cm, the latter accounting for about 60%) were found in the fibrous tissue, involving nerves (Fig. 18.10).

Case 2: A 52-year-old female patient who underwent surgical resection for a right thyroid mass 4 years ago. Postoperative pathology: right thyroid follicular lymphoma (grade 3A), followed by puncture of the left thyroid mass. Pathology: left thyroid mass with a cord-like diffuse hyperplastic lymphoid tissue (considered low-grade B-cell lymphoma, maybe MALT lymphoma) (Fig. 18.11)

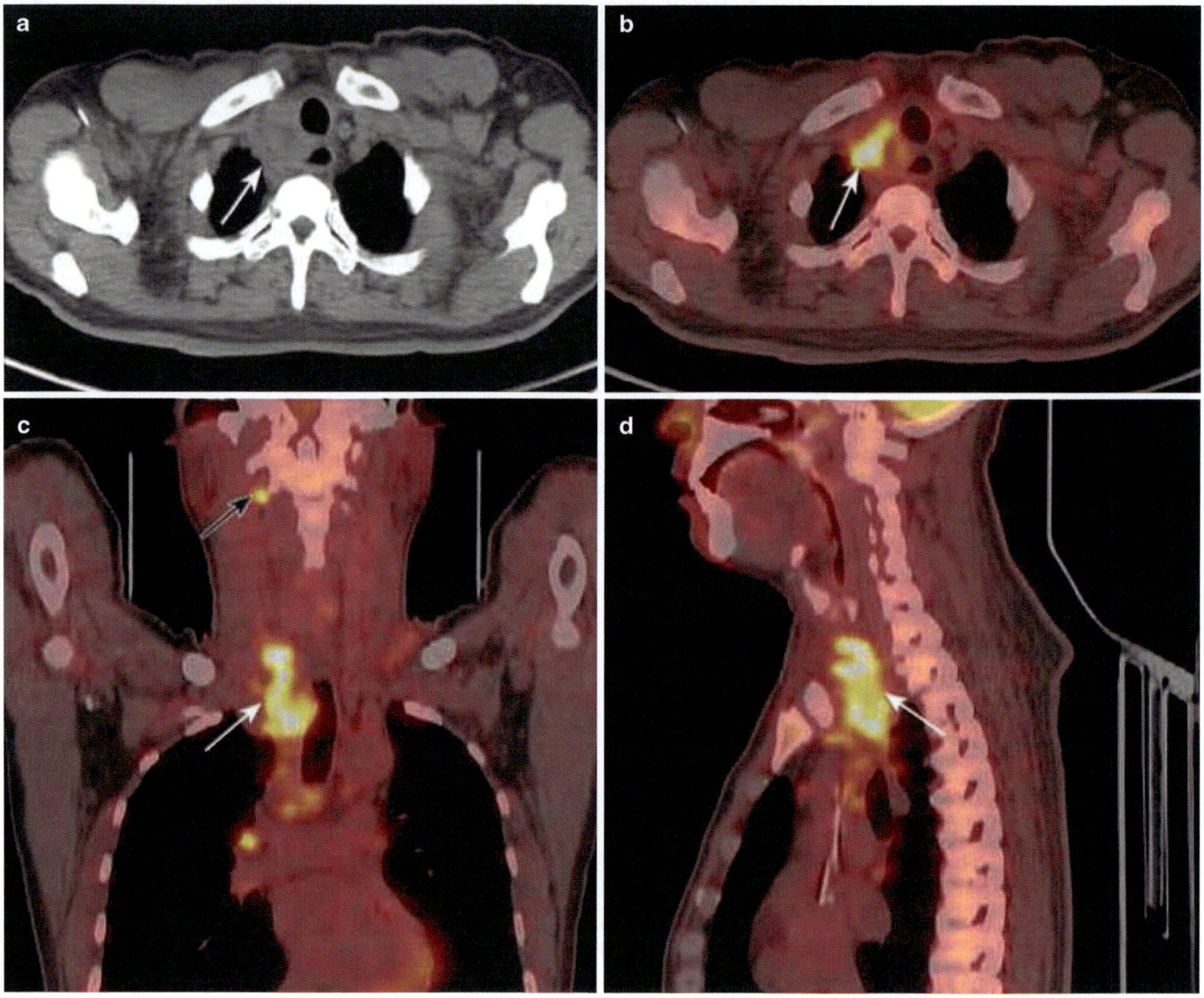

Fig. 18.10 Papillary thyroid carcinoma in the right side and papillary thyroid carcinoma with moderately to poorly differentiated squamous cell carcinoma in the superior mediastinum. (**a**) Irregular and slightly low-density mass in the right lobe of the thyroid, with unclear boundary and lower-density shadow in the center. (**b**) Fusion images showed that the solid part of the mass has an abnormally increased inhomogeneous FDG uptake, SUVmax was about 13.2, and the low-density area in the center was radioactive sparse. (**c** and **d**) The lower pole of the mass reached the superior mediastinum (white arrow), and the right upper cervical enlarged lymph node was seen with abnormal FDG uptake (black arrow)

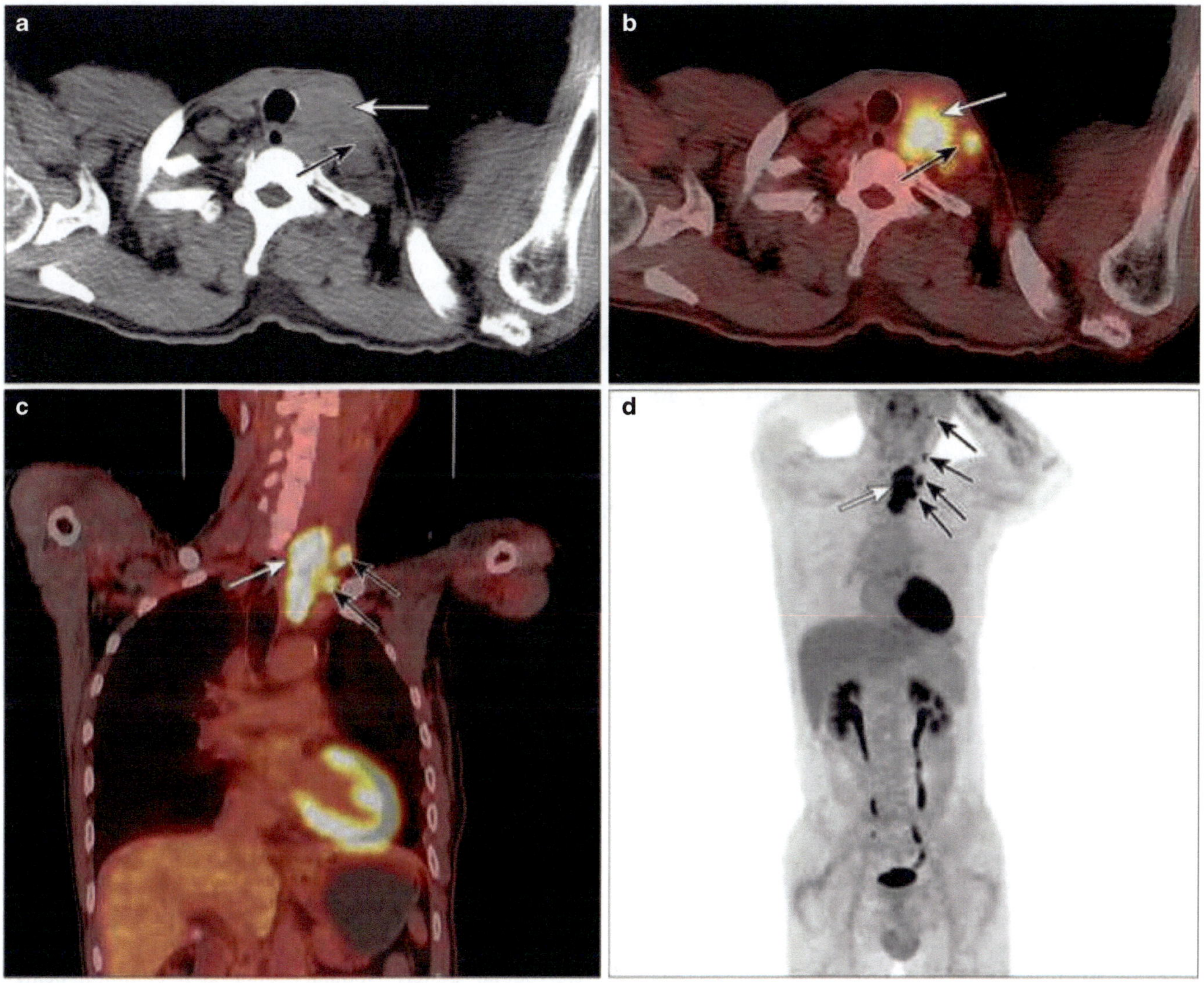

Fig. 18.11 Low-grade B-cell lymphoma of the left thyroid. (**a**) Cross-section of CT scan without contrast: the left thyroid gland was diffusely enlarged, the density was not uniform, there was no obvious low-density shadow, the boundary between the enlarged thyroid and the surrounding blood vessels was not clear, and the trachea and esophagus were not obviously compressed. (**b** and **c**) Cross-section and coronal plane of PET/CT fusion image: the FDG uptake of the left swollen thyroid gland was significantly increased, and the radioactivity distribution was uniform, and its SUVmax was about 21.3 (white arrow); the FDG uptake of multiple enlarged lymph nodes in the left cervical was significantly increased, and SUVmax was 6.5–18.7 (black arrow). (**d**) PET MIP image: No other lesions were found except the left lobe thyroid (white arrow) and left cervical lymph nodes (black arrow) with significantly increased metabolic activity

2.4 Rare Cases

A 53-year-old female with recurrent cervical discomfort for more than 2 years. Postoperative pathology: ① (left carotid artery, superior sternal fossa, left thyroid, and lower part) showing thymus-like differentiated carcinoma (tumor body 3 cm × 2.5 cm × 1.5 cm), invading the striated muscle tissue; ② (left thyroid) thyroid tissue with local nodular hyperplasia; and ③ (around the thyroid) chronic inflammation of two lymph nodes. Immunohistochemical monoclonal antibody and oncogene detection: CK (+), EMA (partial +), LCA (−), CD20 (−), TTF1(−), PAX-8 (+), TG (−), CD5 (+), CD117\c-kit (+), 34βE12 (+), Ki-67 (+, 30%), CD21(−), P40(+), 63(+), and Muc-1(−). Molecular test results: EBER (focus+). Combined with the clinical lesion site, thymic cancer was excluded, and the primary tumor of the thyroid gland was considered (Fig. 18.12).

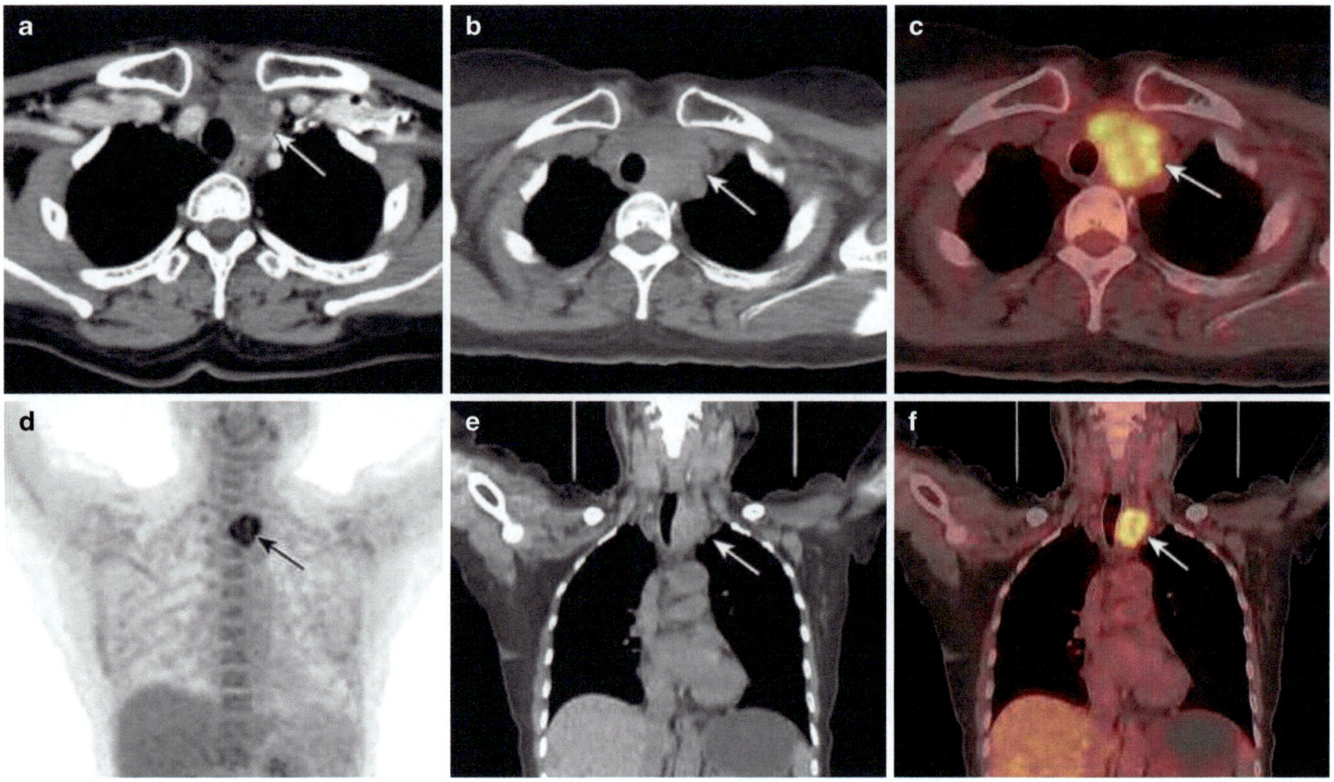

Fig. 18.12 Thymus-like differentiated carcinoma of the left thyroid. (**a**) Cervical enhanced CT: Irregular occupancy of the left lobe of the thyroid gland (arrow), with inhomogeneous density, the lesion surrounding adjacent blood vessels, and inhomogeneous enhancement after enhancement. (**b, c, e, f**) Cross-section and coronal plane of plain CT and fusion image of thyroid PET/CT, respectively: a mass on the lower pole of the thyroid gland (arrow), its density was not uniform, the boundary with the surrounding blood vessels and esophagus was not clear, the lower pole reached the superior sternal fossa, and the FDG uptake of the lesion was abnormally increased annularly and inhomogeneously, and the SUVmax was about 8.5. (**d**) PET MIP image: The left thyroid thymic-like differentiated cancer was shown as a mass with significantly increased metabolic activity on PET MIP image (arrow)

2.5 Summary

Although other malignant tumors of the thyroid have various types and different manifestations, they are relatively rare in clinical practice. When PET/CT finds abnormal FDG uptake in the thyroid with characteristic signs of malignant tumor on CT, the possibility of primary malignant tumors of the thyroid should be considered to avoid missed diagnosis.

3 Benign Thyroid Tumors and Tumor-Like Lesions

3.1 Clinical Overview

Clinically, most thyroid nodules are benign thyroid tumors and tumor-like lesions, and the nodular goiter and thyroid adenoma are the most common.

1. Nodular goiter: Nodular goiter is a common benign space-occupying lesion of the thyroid, which is a proliferative stage of diffuse non-toxic goiter or simple goiter. It is more common in women. The onset may be aggravated during adolescence and pregnancy. There may be a family history of endemic goiter. Clinical manifestations: The goiter is different in size and shape. At the initial stage, the goiter is diffusely enlarged, often symmetrical on both sides. Nodules may form in the later stage, often asymmetrical, with soft texture, which can move up and down with swallowing, and may be accompanied by cystic degeneration. If it is complicated with intrasaccular hemorrhage, the nodules can enlarge rapidly and cause pain in a short time. When the nodules are large, they can compress the trachea, esophagus, nerves, etc. and cause corresponding symptoms, while the thyroid function indicators are basically normal. Pathological manifestations include columnar or papillary hyperpla-

sia of some follicular epithelium, formation of small follicles, degeneration or atrophy of some follicular epithelium, and accumulation of colloid; hyperplasia of interstitial fibrous tissue and formation of nodular lesions with different sizes surrounded by interstitials. In terms of treatment, most of the goiters in adolescence can subside on their own, and some can be supplemented with appropriate amount of thyroid hormone to inhibit excessive endogenous TSH secretion; for those suspected of having malignant transformation in nodular goiter, those with secondary hyperthyroidism, those with huge goiter affecting life and work, those with retrosternal goiter, and those with compression of the trachea, esophagus, and nerves causing clinical symptoms, surgical treatment is required.

2. Thyroid adenoma: Thyroid adenoma is the most common type of benign thyroid tumors. It is divided into follicular and papillary tumors. The former is common, mostly in females, and the age of onset is usually under 40. Most of the patients with thyroid adenomas do not have discomfort and they often accidentally find the cervical mass, which can be single or multiple, round or oval, with smooth surface, no tenderness, and can move up and down with swallowing. The tumor grows slowly; once there is tumor bleeding or cystic degeneration, its volume can suddenly increase, accompanied by pain and tenderness; but it will shrink or disappear after a period of time. When the tumor is large, it will compress the trachea, esophagus, and nerves, causing difficult breathing, difficult swallowing, hoarseness, and so on. Therefore, the most effective treatment for thyroid adenoma is surgical resection, and surgical resection of the affected lobe is generally recommended.

3.2 PET/CT Diagnostic Points

The PET/CT imaging findings of benign thyroid tumors are mostly low or no FDG uptake with uniform radioactivity distribution, and some show focal increased FDG uptake, and most of them are almost round. When it is accompanied by intratumoral hemorrhage, the hemorrhage area lacks FDG uptake.

Normal thyroid tissue has high iodine content and rich blood supply, so the CT value is high, about (70 ± 10) HU. The common feature of plain CT for benign tumors and tumor-like lesions is that the CT value is reduced, which is caused by the decrease of iodine content in the lesion tissue, and it is accompanied by an increase in follicular cells and/or an increase in the proportion of fiber components in the tissue. CT often shows different degrees of enlargement of the thyroid (nodular goiter) or solitary thyroid nodule (thyroid adenoma). The four main signs include regular morphology, dominant cystic degeneration, clear after enhancement, and high enhancement, followed by multiple necrosis, high-density cyst, scattered pleomorphic calcification, varying density, halo sign, massive calcification with artifacts and continuous calcification, etc.

3.3 Typical Cases

A 75-year-old male with a left cervical mass found 3 months ago. Pathology: (left retrosternal) nodular goiter (Fig. 18.13)

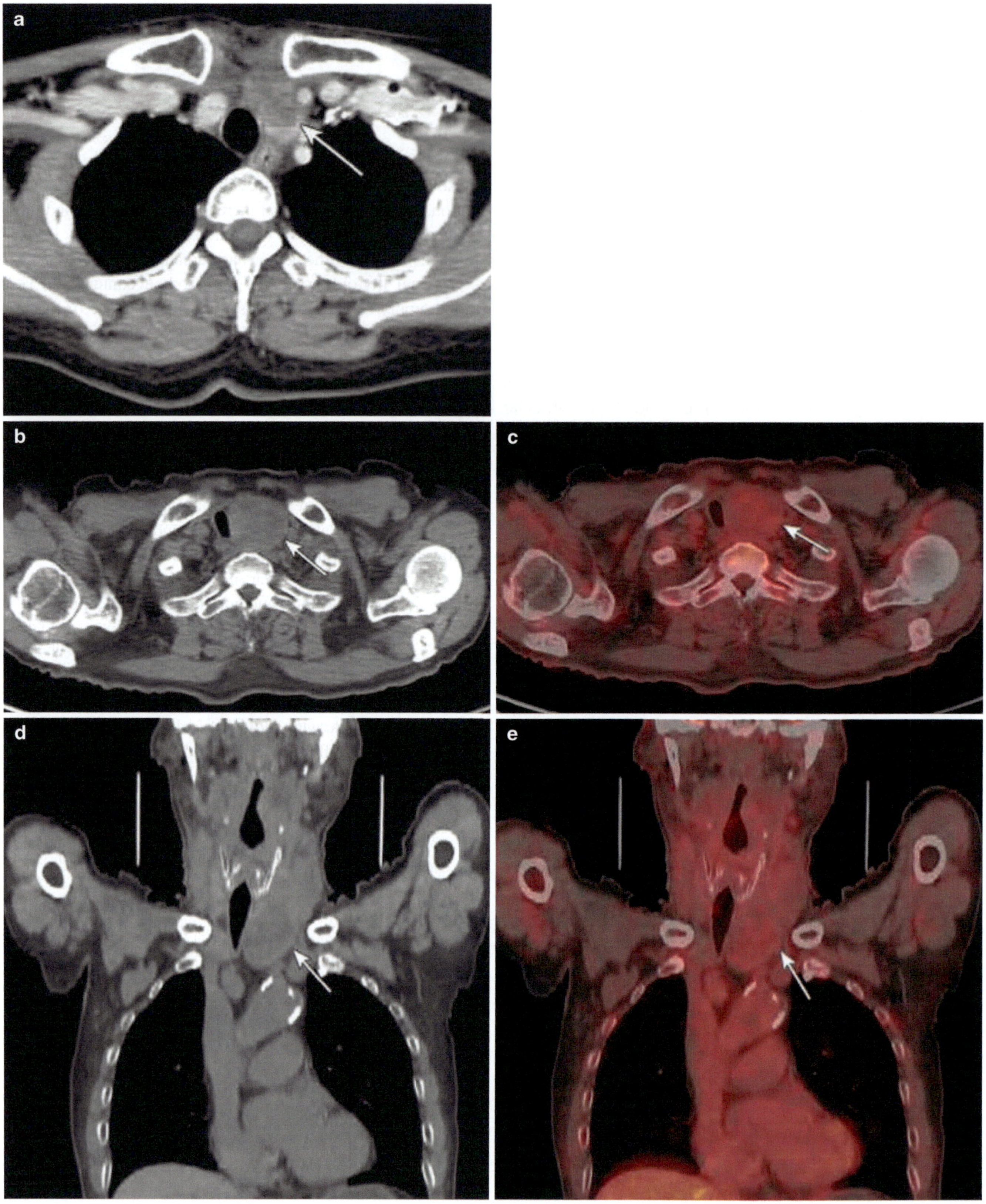

Fig. 18.13 Left retrosternal nodular goiter. (**a**) Cervical enhanced CT: the volume of the left thyroid was significantly increased, and the parenchyma showed an inhomogeneously enhanced mixed density shadow and multiple cystic low-density shadows in the left thyroid, with clear boundary, part of which protruded into the back of the sternum and compressed the trachea to be narrow. (**b, c**) Transverse axial images of the cervical CT and PET/CT fusion images. (**d, e**) Coronal images of the cervical CT and PET/CT fusion images. PET/CT images showed cystic solid mass in the left lobe of the thyroid gland; the trachea was compressed and moved to the right, with clear boundary; the inhomogeneous FDG uptake was slightly increased; and SUVmax was about 2.5

3.4 Summary

Benign thyroid tumors and tumor-like lesions are one of the most common thyroid diseases. Thyroid nodules or goiter is the first clinical manifestation, with or without thyroid function changes. Surgical treatment is still the main clinical treatment. PET/CT images mostly show low uptake or no FDG uptake, and some may show focal high metabolism. When it shows regular morphology, dominant cystic degeneration, clear after enhancement, and high enhancement on CT, the possibility of benign lesions should be considered.

4 Secondary Malignant Tumors of the Thyroid

4.1 Clinical Overview

The thyroid is rich in blood vessels, and malignant tumors in adjacent organs can spread directly or malignant tumors in non-thyroid organs can spread to the thyroid through blood vessels to form secondary thyroid tumors. Squamous cell carcinoma of the larynx is the most common secondary tumor that spreads directly to the thyroid. The most common clinical metastatic carcinoma of the thyroid is clear cell carcinoma of the kidney. Blood metastasis of lung, breast, or colon cancer is also common.

Thyroid metastatic carcinoma has an insidious onset and often has no obvious clinical symptoms. When thyroid metastatic carcinoma is found clinically, attention should be paid to check whether there is metastasis to other parts. Thyroid metastatic carcinoma is generally considered to be the advanced manifestation of malignant tumors, and the prognosis is generally poor, and most patients die in a short time due to widespread systemic metastasis of tumor. In the diagnosis of secondary malignant tumors of the thyroid, it is necessary to pay attention to the key point, that is, the time interval from the diagnosis of the primary tumor to the detection of thyroid metastatic carcinoma in some patients is sometimes quite long, which often misleads the clinical diagnosis. Literature reported that the longest time interval can be up to 26 years, so for patients with previous history of malignant tumor, if a new thyroid tumor is found, the possibility of thyroid metastatic carcinoma needs to be considered. Fine needle aspiration cytology is the first choice for the diagnosis of thyroid metastatic carcinoma.

The pathological diagnosis of thyroid metastatic carcinoma is difficult. In general, thyroid metastatic carcinoma should be considered for multiple nodules. Thyroid metastatic carcinoma has a tendency of interstitial infiltration, which deforms the surrounding follicles, but does not infiltrate and destroy the follicles. This is different from primary thyroid tumors. In addition, thyroid follicular carcinoma often retains cytoplasmic granules, but metastatic carcinoma does not. In recent years, fine needle aspiration biopsy in combination with specific antibodies (such as Napsin A of lung cancer and PAX-8 of thyroid cancer) has been helpful in differentiating primary and secondary thyroid tumors. In addition, fine needle aspiration biopsy of secondary thyroid tumors can provide tissue for the evaluation of molecular changes, which is helpful for the adjuvant treatment of primary tumors. However, it is sometimes unreliable to differentiate primary and secondary thyroid tumors by immunohistochemical staining of immunoglobulin. This mark is usually positive in primary thyroid tumors, while negative in metastatic carcinoma. However, if thyroid follicular cells are embedded in metastatic carcinoma, the result may also be positive. The tumor cells of primary thyroid cancer have hyaloid degeneration, mucinous degeneration, squamous epithelioid degeneration, or columnar epithelial cell carcinoma differentiating into the thymus, which is difficult to distinguish from renal clear cell carcinoma with thyroid metastasis and is often mistaken for metastatic carcinoma.

Although secondary malignant tumors of the thyroid are advanced-stage malignant tumors, if they can be detected early and combined with surgery-based comprehensive treatment, some patients can achieve relatively satisfactory results. The treatment of thyroid metastatic carcinoma should be based on the location of the primary tumor, clinical stage, histological type, systemic condition, and metastasis, and an individualized treatment plan should be formulated. In terms of reducing tumor burden and preventing the further development of tumors from invading the trachea and esophagus, surgical treatment is beneficial. If there is only thyroid metastasis, radical thyroidectomy can be performed, especially in patients whose primary tumor is renal cell carcinoma, and it can be cured.

4.2 PET/CT Diagnostic Points

The PET/CT manifestations of thyroid metastatic carcinoma are diverse, including single nodular type, multiple nodular enlargement type, thick-walled cystic type, etc. The lesions may be accompanied by calcification and cervical lymph node metastasis. Normal thyroid tissue shows diffuse low uptake or no uptake on ^{18}F-FDG PET/CT. If the patient with older age has a history of malignant tumor and has nodules in the thyroid with focal hypermetabolism, especially multiple increased localized metabolism, metastasis should be considered.

4.3 Typical Cases

A 55-year-old male patient had a mass in the upper lobe of the right lung found on CT due to a physical examination of "thyroid mass." Pathology: (upper right) pulmonary nodular type (tumor body 2.8 cm × 2.2 cm × 1.5 cm) infiltrating adenocarcinoma (mainly papillary type, partially solid growth), metastasized to the (right) thyroid tissue, and involved the thyroid envelope (Fig. 18.14)

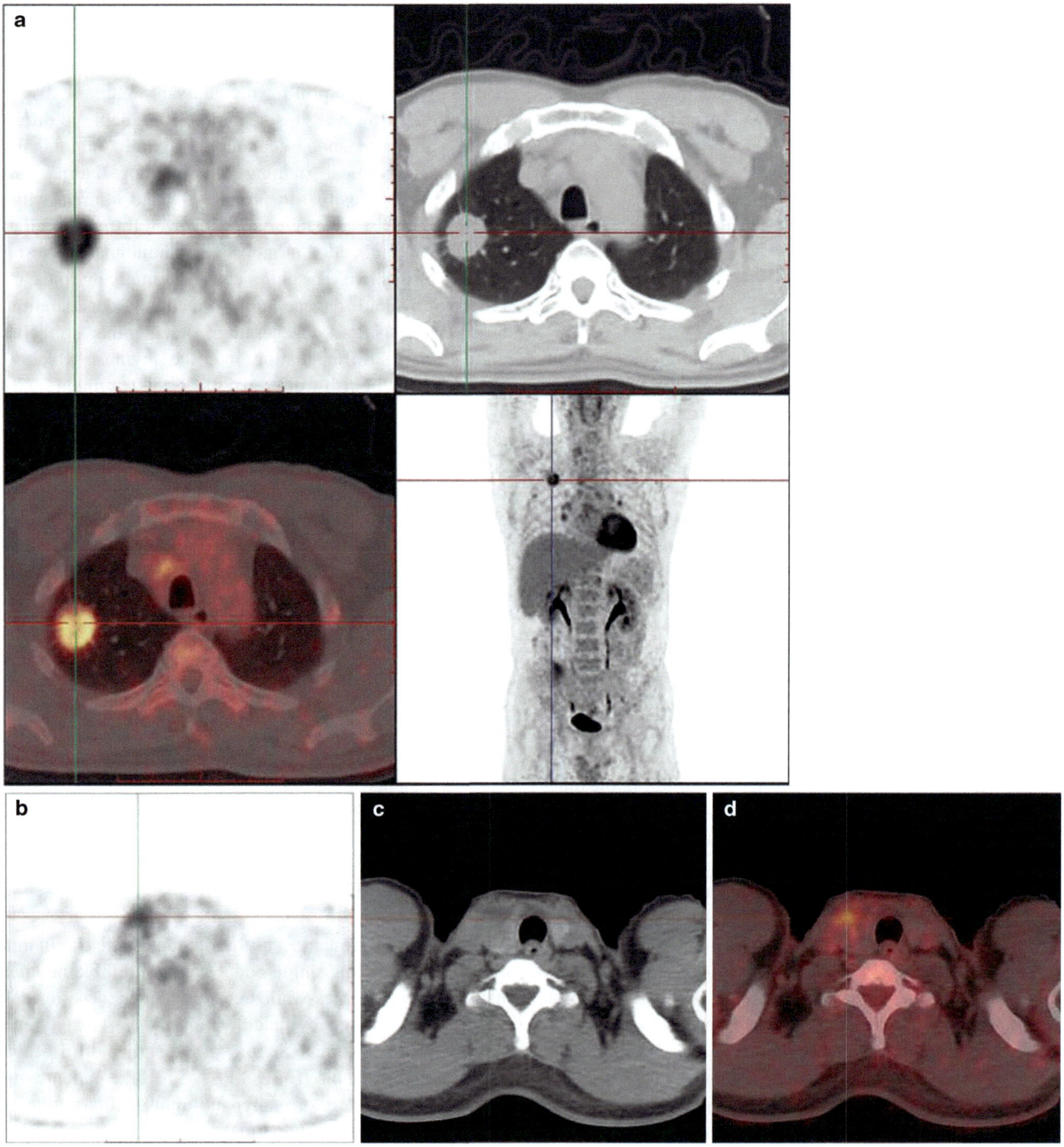

Fig. 18.14 Thyroid metastasis of right lung cancer. (**a**) Soft tissue density mass shadow can be seen in the upper lobe of the right lung, short burrs and pleural traction can be seen in the mass, the size was about 3.2 cm × 2.6 cm, the FDG uptake was abnormally increased, and SUVmax was about 8.4. (**b–d**) Low-density nodule shadow was seen in the right lobe of the thyroid, the density was inhomogeneous, the size was about 2.3 cm × 2.2 cm, the FDG uptake was inhomogeneous and slightly increased, and the SUVmax was about 4.4

4.4 Summary

Secondary malignant tumors of the thyroid are clinically rare, accounting for about 1% of thyroid malignant tumors. Most of patients have a history of malignant tumor. The clinical thyroid metastatic carcinoma is mainly from renal cell carcinoma, and the others are breast cancer, lung cancer, melanoma, and colorectal cancer. The clinical manifestations are mostly insidious, and surgical resection is one of the important means of individualized treatment. PET/CT features are diverse, without characteristic images, and mostly characterized by focal increased FDG uptake which can be single or multiple. Systemic evaluation of primary tumor metastasis and invasion is one of the greatest values of PET/CT.

PET/CT of Salivary Gland Tumors

19

Linfa Li, Weiqiang Pang, Shui Jin, and Yun Wang

1 Common Malignant Tumors of the Salivary Gland

Salivary glands are exocrine glands that produce and secrete saliva. They include three paired major glands (parotid gland, submandibular gland, and sublingual gland) and minor salivary glands that widely exist in the entire respiratory and digestive tract. Many minor salivary gland tumors are located on the hard palate. The global annual incidence of salivary gland tumors is 0.4/100,000–13.5/100,000, and that of malignant tumors is 0.4/100,000–2.6/100,000, accounting for 0.7%–1.6% of all malignant tumors and 2.3%–10.4% of head and neck malignant tumors. Most of the salivary gland tumors are benign, but about 20% of parotid gland tumors are malignant; the incidence of submandibular gland and minor salivary gland malignant tumors is about 50% and 80%, respectively. Nearly 80% of salivary gland tumors occur in the parotid gland, most commonly in the superficial lobe, less than 1% in the sublingual gland, and 9%–23% in the minor salivary glands. The proportion of malignant tumors is different in different parts: 20%–30%, 45%–60%, and 70%–85% in the parotid gland, submandibular gland, and sublingual gland, respectively; 80%–90% of salivary gland tumors in the tongue, floor of the mouth, and retromolar area are malignant. Salivary gland tumors are slightly more common in women, with the peak age of onset ranging from 50 to 70 years, but the peak age of pleomorphic adenoma, mucoepidermoid carcinoma, and acinus cell carcinoma is 20–40 years. Among all salivary gland tumors, pleomorphic adenoma is the most common, accounting for about 50%, usually occurring in young adults aged 30–50 years without significant gender difference. The second most common is Warthin tumor (adenolymphoma), which is common in men over 50 years old; it is usually multiplex or bilateral, mostly located in the inferior superficial lobe of the parotid gland; almost all of Warthin tumors come from the parotid gland or peripheral lymph nodes. Others such as hemangioma, lymphangioma, and lipoma are rare. The most common malignant tumor is mucoepidermoid carcinoma.

The cause of salivary gland tumors is currently unclear. Many studies have shown that ionizing radiation is one of the main risk factors for salivary gland tumors. Radiation from radiotherapy, especially head and neck radiation, significantly increases the risk of salivary gland cancer. When ^{131}I is used to treat thyroid disease, radioiodine is also concentrated in the salivary gland, which may increase the risk of salivary gland tumor. It has been recognized that smoking is closely related to Warthin tumor. Clinically, it is suggested that all current smokers should quit smoking and those who have ever smoked should continue to quit smoking. Furthermore, it may also be related to vitamin A deficiency and exposure to smoke, dust, and chemicals.

The persistent pain in patients clinically diagnosed with salivary gland cancer often indicates a poor prognosis. Compared with patients without pain, their 5-year survival rate drops from 68% to 35%. The overall 10-year survival rate of patients with salivary gland malignant tumors is close to 50%.

1.1 Mucoepidermoid Carcinoma

1.1.1 Clinical Overview

Mucoepidermoid carcinoma of the parotid gland is the most common malignant salivary gland tumor. It is mainly composed of mucous cells, epidermoid cells, and intermediate cells. Based on the ratio and differentiation of the three kinds of cells, they can be divided into three types: well differentiated, moderately differentiated, and poorly differentiated. The parotid gland is the most common site (about 45%), followed by the submandibular gland (about 7%). The minor salivary glands are more common in the palate and buccal mucosa. The disease can occur at any age, mostly in people

L. Li (✉)
Cancer Hospital of the University of Chinese Academy of Sciences, Hangzhou, Zhejiang, China

W. Pang · S. Jin · Y. Wang
Zhejiang Cancer Hospital, Hangzhou, Zhejiang, China

Z. Yao, S. Li (eds.), *Atlas of PET/CT in Oncology - Volume 1*, https://doi.org/10.1007/978-981-99-1172-1_19

aged 30–50 years old, with more females than males, while malignant tumors of the parotid gland in children are usually of this type. Clinically, the well-differentiated type is usually a slow-growing painless mass with medium texture and clear edge; the poorly differentiated type is characterized by fast growth, hard texture, unclear boundary, poor mobility, and adhesion or even fixation with surrounding tissues, it may invade the facial nerve to cause facial paralysis, and it is easy to relapse and metastasize, and the prognosis is poor.

1.1.2 PET/CT Diagnostic Points

Well-differentiated mucoepidermoid carcinoma has the characteristics of general benign tumor, which is similar to pleomorphic adenoma, while poorly differentiated mucoepidermoid carcinoma has the characteristics of general malignant tumor, which is difficult to differentiate from other salivary gland malignant tumors. PET/CT plain scan shows soft tissue density masses. The well-differentiated type often has clear edge and may have cystic degeneration or bleeding. The poorly differentiated type often has unclear edge, is prone to cystic degeneration and bleeding, and is often accompanied by peripheral lymph node metastasis; ^{18}F-FDG uptake shows mild to moderate increase, and it may significantly increase and it is uniform or inhomogeneous.

1.1.3 Typical Cases

A 60-year-old female patient with right facial paralysis gradually aggravated for 1 year and right hemifacial pain for 2 months. She was a case of mucoepidermoid carcinoma of the right parotid gland involving the peripheral nerve wall of V, VI, and VII cranial nerves (Fig. 19.1).

1.1.4 Differential Diagnosis

1. Pleomorphic adenoma: Patients often have a long history of salivary gland masses. The mass develops slowly, with no obvious symptoms or only mild pain. Generally, it is a round or quasi-round mass with clear edge, uniform density, and clear boundary. When the tumor is large, it can push the surrounding tissues.
2. Warthin tumor of the parotid gland: It is more common in middle-aged and elderly men. The lesions are mostly located in the posterior lower pole of the parotid gland, bilateral or multifocal. A history of tumor growth is one of the prominent clinical features of Warthin tumor. A cold or upper respiratory tract infection may induce tumor enlargement.
3. Lymphoma: It is mostly characterized by abnormally high metabolism of ^{18}F-FDG, with soft texture, relatively uniform density, and usually systemic involvement (Fig. 19.2).

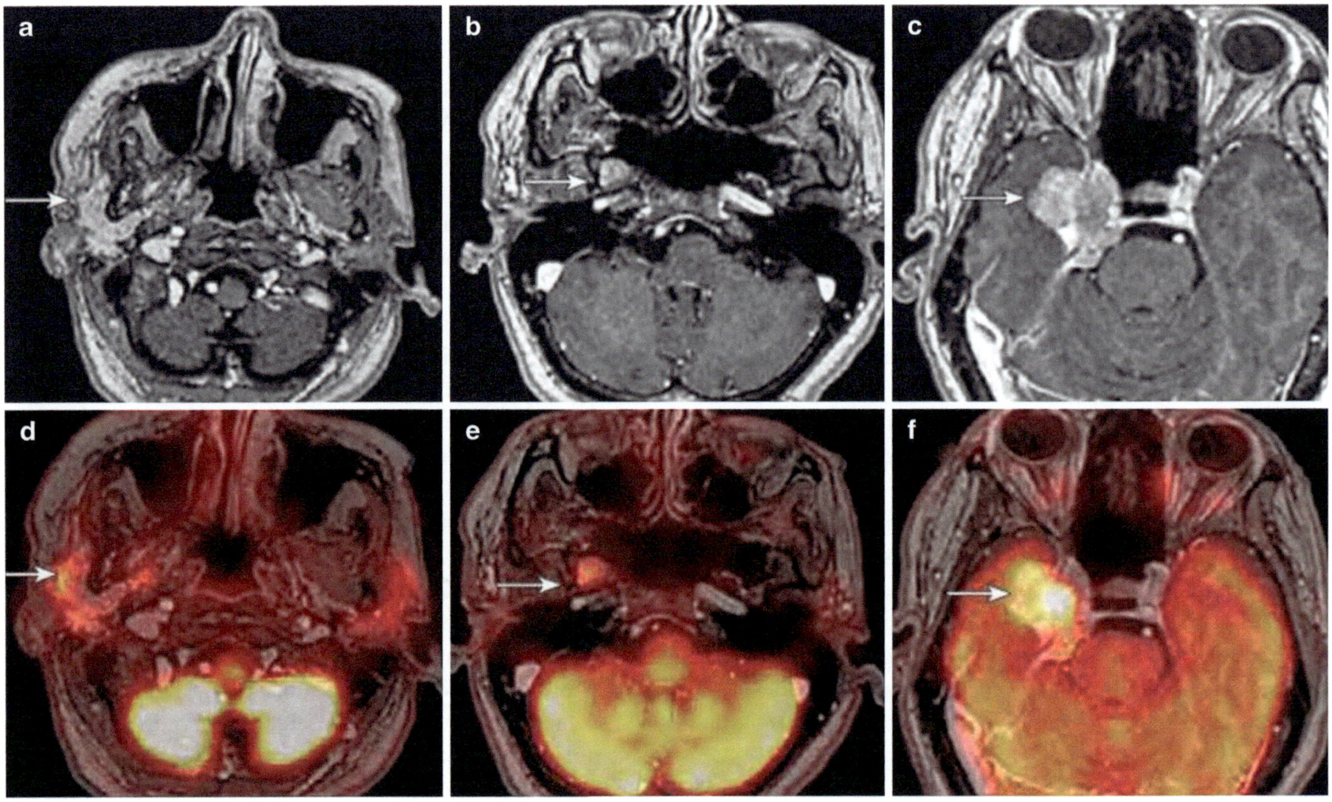

Fig. 19.1 ^{18}F-FDG PET/MR images of mucoepidermoid carcinoma. (**a–c**) Continuous transaxial MR images showed the lesion (arrow) was diffuse and has uniform enhancement, extending from the right parotid gland along the thickened mandibular nerve upward to the right middle cranial fossa (MCF) and anterior cistern. (**d–f**) Continuous transaxial fusion PET/MR images showed that FDG uptake increased in the nodular lesion with clear boundary of the right parotid gland, and continuous curvilinear FDG uptake was seen along the thickened mandibular nerve and extended upward to the mass lesion of MCF

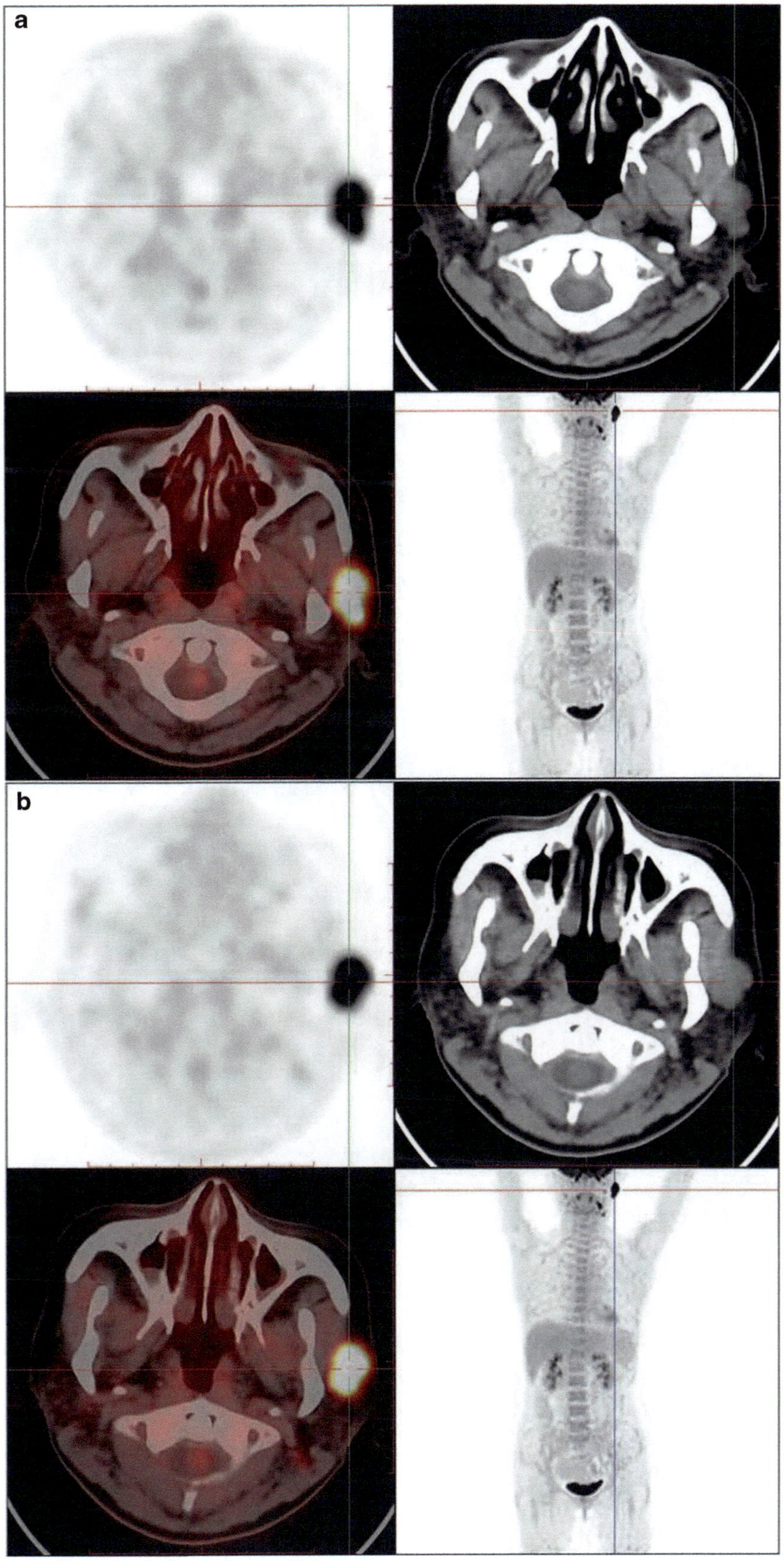

Fig. 19.2 ^{18}F-FDG PET/CT images of left parotid lymphoma. A 55-year-old female patient went to a doctor because a left preauricular mass was found 1 month ago. (**a**) PET/CT image of hypermetabolic nodule in the left parotid gland. (**b**) PET/CT image of hypermetabolic nodule in the left parotid gland. (**c**) PET/CT image of hypermetabolic nodule in the left parotid gland. PET/CT showed that there was a soft tissue mass in the left parotid gland area, which was not clearly separated from the surrounding tissues. Its size was 1.9 cm × 2.5 cm, density was relatively uniform, and shape was irregular, and the FDG uptake was intense (SUVmax 25.8). There were multiple enlarged lymph nodes in bilateral cervical Ib area and II area and left cervical III area. The larger one was about 0.8 cm in short diameter, and the radioactive distribution was concentrated in different degrees, and the SUVmax was about 23.4. Postoperative pathology: (left parotid gland) invasive B-cell lymphoma

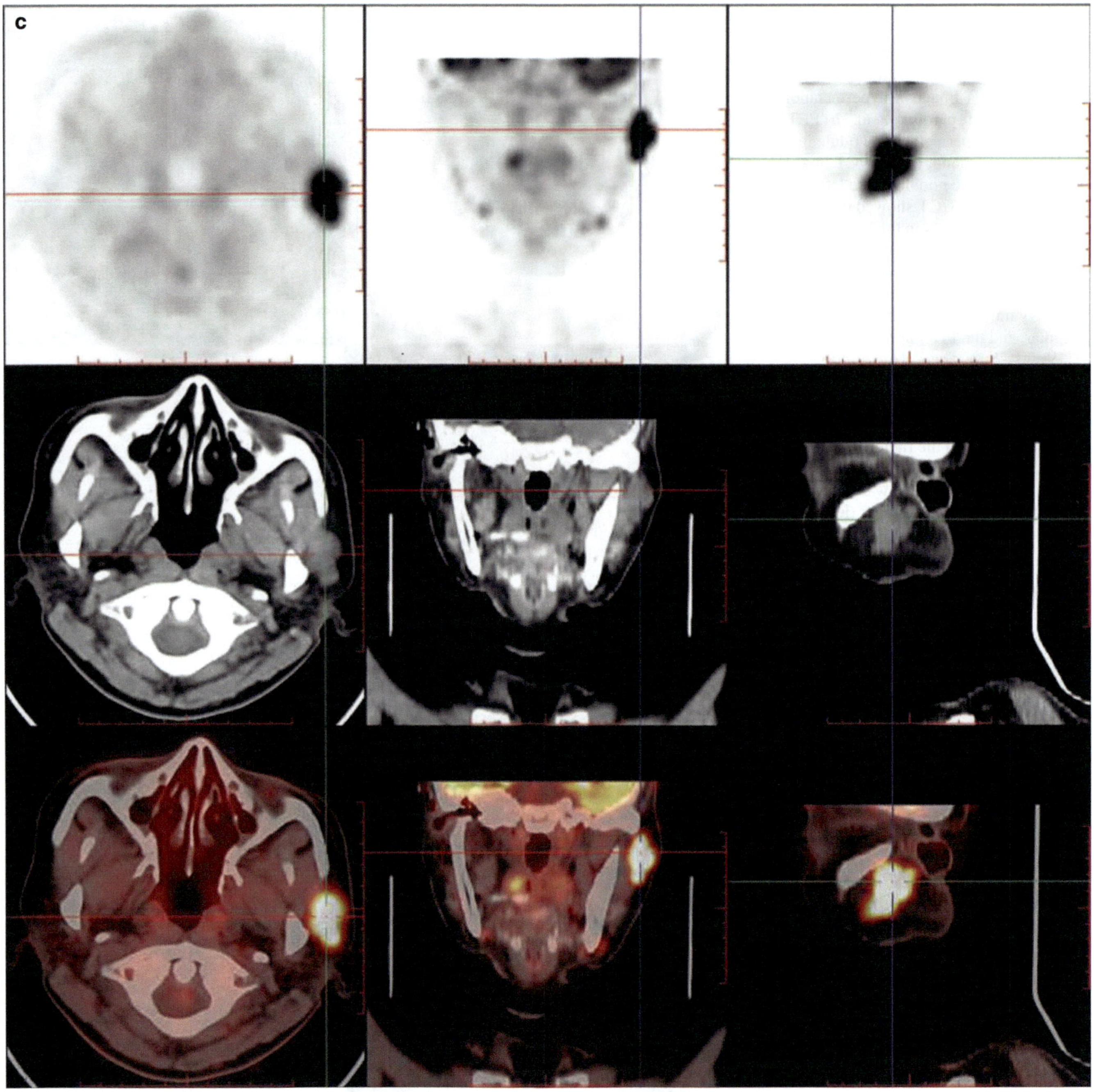

Fig. 19.2 (continued)

4. Adenoid cystic carcinoma: It is more common in the elderly. The tumor grows rapidly, which is fixed, is hard, and often has pain and facial paralysis.
5. Acinar cell carcinoma: Low-grade malignant tumor, similar to benign tumor.

1.1.5 Summary

Salivary gland mucoepidermoid carcinoma is more likely to occur in women or infants aged 30 to 50. FDG PET/CT images are characterized by salivary gland space-occupying lesions with signs of malignant tumor and increased FDG uptake.

1.2 Adenoid Cystic Carcinoma

1.2.1 Clinical Overview

Adenoid cystic carcinoma is a common malignant tumor of the salivary gland epithelium, which accounts for more than one-third of the malignant salivary gland tumors. It mainly occurs in middle-aged people (aged 35–45 years old). It may occur in the parotid gland, especially in the deep part or isthmus of the parotid gland, but it is more common in the submandibular gland, sublingual gland, and other minor salivary glands. The cause is unknown. It is believed that it is related to environmental factors such as chronic injury, inflammatory stimulation, and radiation exposure, as well as internal spirit, immunity, and heredity.

The tumor does not have a complete envelope and originates from the epithelial cells of the salivary gland duct. There are often multiple fluid areas of different sizes within the tumor, and there may be fibrous septum. In the late stage, the tumor grows rapidly in various forms, and they are usually hard, fixed, and with invasive growth. It is low-grade malignancy in early stage, the tumor grows slowly, and it is not easy to differentiate from benign tumors surrounding tissues. It has the characteristics of infiltration and diffusion along the nerve. When the nerve is involved, the pain is obvious. The degree of pain is not directly proportional to the size and growth rate of the tumor. It is more common in middle-aged and elderly people. The early-stage patients have pain or numbness, which is often ignored and delayed in diagnosis, or there are masses in minor salivary gland, which are not taken seriously because of slower early growth. When the tumor is large, the local skin bulges, the mass is fixed, the texture is hard, and the surrounding and cervical lymph nodes may be enlarged. Adenoid cystic carcinoma of the parotid gland often invades the facial nerve, resulting in facial paralysis.

1.2.2 PET/CT Diagnostic Points

When the tumor is small, PET/CT scan shows enlarged salivary gland on the affected side, with the internal localized masses mostly in the size of 2–4 cm. Some masses could completely occupy the whole salivary gland and the shape is irregular, but a few of them could be quasi-circular, with unclear edge and inhomogeneous density. Most are patchy or large patchy low-density areas without incomplete shape in the masses. When the tumor is large, the cystic necrosis area may appear, the cyst wall has irregular shape, the thickness is different, and the edge is lobulated. It often invades superficial and deep lobes. ^{18}F-FDG uptake is often significantly increased, but it may be inhomogeneously increased. In addition, enhanced CT of the salivary glands, or CTS examination, can show signs of compression and displacement to the main duct and branch duct, interruption of erosion, and overflow of contrast medium, which can assist in the differentiation of benign and malignant tumors. Enlarged lymph nodes can be seen around the tumor, and necrotic low-density areas can also be seen in them. ^{18}F-FDG uptake shows a circular increase. Some tumors can destroy the ascending ramus of the mandible, resulting in the destruction and defect of the mandibular bone. Deep tumors can spread to the parapharynx, bulge the pharyngeal wall, and narrow the pharyngeal cavity; sometimes, it is the first symptom of patients, and it is easy to be mistaken for other tumors. At this time, we should pay attention to the position of the carotid sheath. Salivary gland tumors tend to push the carotid sheath backward, while neurogenic tumors in the carotid sheath usually compress the large blood vessels in the neck to move forward and medially.

1.2.3 Typical Cases

A 42-year-old male patient presented with swelling and pain in the right maxillofacial region for more than 2 months. Pathology: (right parotid gland) adenoid cystic carcinoma (Fig. 19.3)

1.2.4 Differential Diagnosis

The differential diagnosis of benign and malignant tumors of the parotid gland is mainly considered from three aspects: the edge, the density of the mass, and the presence or absence of enlarged lymph nodes. Whether the tumor boundary is clear is the key to differentiate between benign and malignant tumors. If the tumor is irregular and shows infiltrative growth and it is significantly enhanced after enhancement and multiple enlarged lymph nodes can be seen at the same time, it is the typical sign of malignant tumor. However, low-grade malignant tumors can also have a clear boundary, and some benign pleomorphic adenomas can also be lobulated or nodular, which should be paid attention to in the differentiation and should be comprehensively analyzed in combination with other clinical manifestations. Facial nerve involvement is also an important clinical symptom in differential diagnosis. Facial nerve paralysis can occur in 12%–14% of malignant tumors of the parotid gland, while facial nerve involvement in benign tumors is rare.

According to the image morphology, the masses in the parotid gland can be divided into three types: ① round or oval tumors, with clear boundary and envelope, more common in benign tumors and inflammatory lesions; ② lobulated tumors with clear boundary and envelope, mainly seen in benign tumors with local erosion and low-grade malignant tumors with slow growth; and ③ invasive tumors, with irregular shape, unclear boundary, and diffuse growth, mostly malignant.

Adenoid cystic carcinoma is a common epithelial malignant tumor of the salivary glands. It is more common in the elderly. The mass grows rapidly, which is fixed and hard, often with pain and facial paralysis. When the tumor is large, the signs are obviously easier to diagnose. When the tumor is small, it should be differentiated from the benign tumor of the salivary gland. It should be observed from the mass location, shape, density, adjacent bones, blood vessels, and peripheral lymph nodes. Benign tumors are characterized by regular shape, uniform density, clear boundary, vascular migration, and no lymph node enlargement, while adenoid cystic carcinoma is characterized by irregular shape, inhomogeneous density, blurry boundary, wrapping or eroding blood vessels, and lymph node enlargement.

1.2.5 Summary

The imaging findings of adenoid cystic carcinoma are diverse, and FDG uptake is increased obviously in the tumor. The important clinical features are neurotropic growth and early hematogenous metastasis.

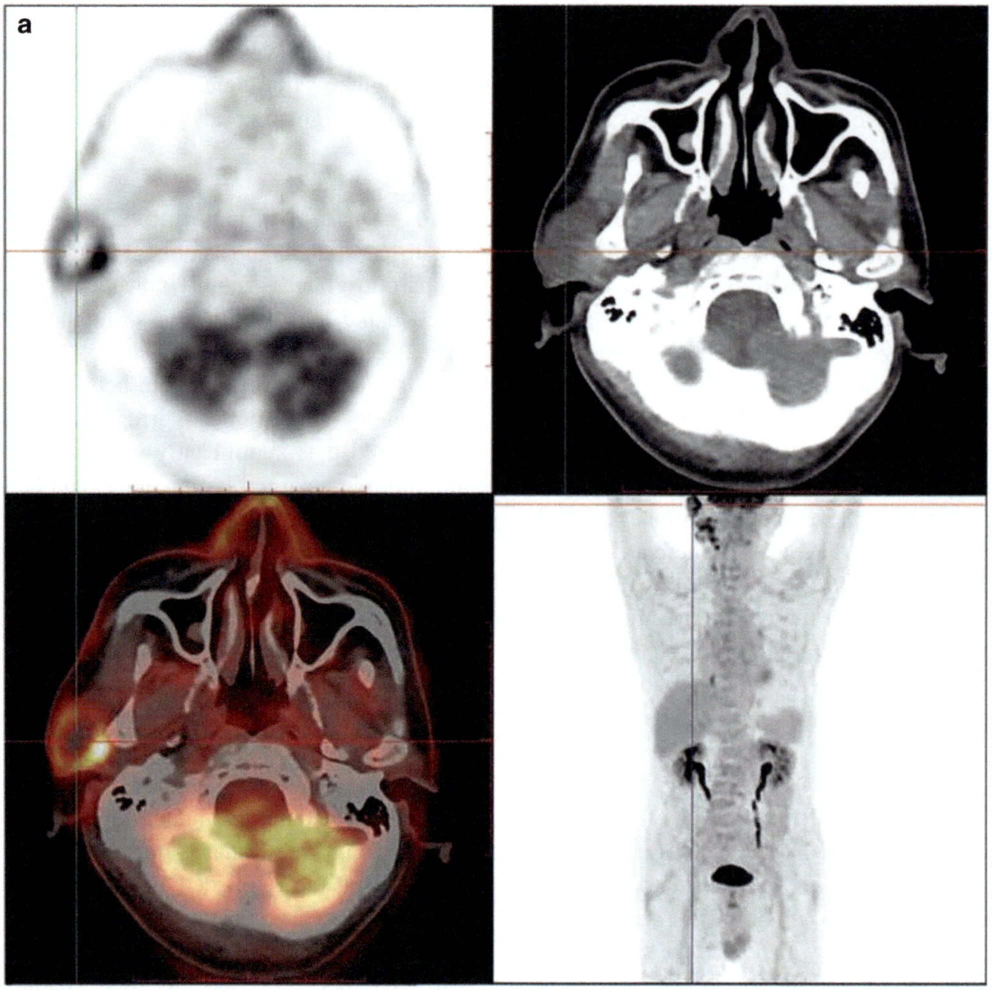

Fig. 19.3 ^{18}F-FDG PET/CT images of adenoid cystic carcinoma of the right parotid gland. (**a**) PET/CT image of hypermetabolic nodules in the right parotid gland; (**b**) PET/CT image of hypermetabolic nodules in the right parotid gland. PET/CT showed that the right parotid gland was enlarged with a cystic and solid nodule (about 3.5 cm × 1.9 cm in size). The nodule was slightly lobulated, irregular in shape with unclear margin, and inhomogeneous density, and it showed intense FDG uptake (SUVmax 14.7). There was necrosis area in the center of the nodule without FDG uptake. Multiple enlarged lymph nodes were found on the right side of the neck, the larger one was about 0.8 cm in short diameter, and there was increased FDG uptake (SUVmax 5.1)

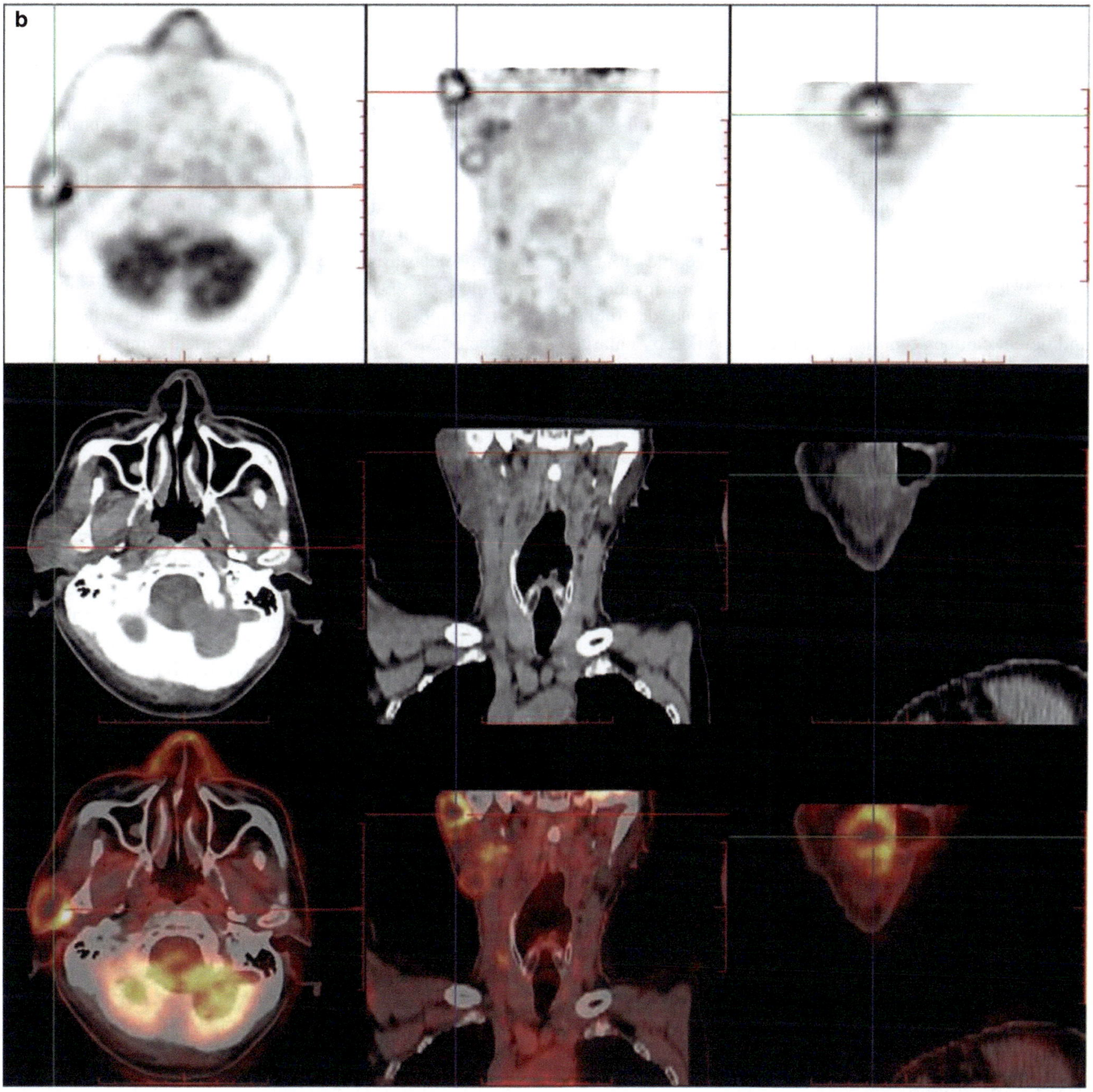

Fig. 19.3 (continued)

1.3 Malignant Mixed Tumor

1.3.1 Clinical Overview

Malignant mixed tumors account for 2%–5% of mixed tumors. Most of them originate from benign transformation, and a few are primary. Patients often have a history of mass in the salivary glands for many years. The patient will go to a doctor due to the mass growing rapidly or pain or facial paralysis. If the tumor occurs in the deep lobe of the parotid gland, the mass tends to protrude into the pharynx and soft palate, causing neck and ear pain, hearing loss, dysphagia, or dyspnea. When the tumor invades the masticatory muscles, the mandible, and the temporomandibular joint, it is difficult to open the mouth. The salivary gland is enlarged, and its internal mass has unclear boundary, with poor activity, tenderness, and hard texture, and some enlarged lymph nodes are palpable.

1.3.2 PET/CT Diagnostic Points

PET/CT scan shows soft tissue mass shadows with unclear boundary, irregular contour, and inhomogeneous density in the salivary gland area. The mass is generally large in size and can involve the deep and superficial parotid gland. Necrosis and liquefaction area can be seen in some tumors with low density. ^{18}F-FDG uptake increases inhomogeneously or increases in a circular shape. When the tumor invades the adjacent muscle, the fat space between the tumor and muscle disappears, the muscle edge becomes blurred, and the density may increase. When the tumor invades the mandible and temporomandibular joint, bone destruction and defect can be seen. It is often accompanied by enlarged lymph nodes around the parotid gland or neck.

1.3.3 Differential Diagnosis

Malignant mixed tumors are mostly caused by malignant transformation of benign mixed tumors. The tumor grows rapidly with pain and adjacent enlarged lymph nodes. Imaging findings show masses in the salivary glands, mostly irregular in shape and inhomogeneous in density, and the boundary between them and the normal salivary glands is not clear. It should be differentiated from benign mixed tumor and chronic abscess of the salivary gland.

1. Benign mixed tumor: Patients with benign mixed tumor often have a long history of mass in the salivary gland area. The mass of benign mixed tumor develops slowly, and the symptoms are not obvious or there is only slight pain; on PET/CT scan, it shows a round or quasi-round mass with clear edge, uniform density, and clear boundary; and large tumor can push and press the surrounding tissues. The mass of malignant mixed tumor grows fast, with obvious pain; the imaging findings show a mass with inhomogeneous density and irregular edge; and sometimes large patchy low-density necrosis in the mass often invades surrounding tissues, with lymph node enlargement.
2. Salivary gland abscess: It is caused by inflammation of the salivary gland. The patients often have a history of painful swelling of the salivary gland in the affected area. The local skin is red with high skin temperature and tenderness. Imaging findings show that the salivary gland is enlarged and there is hypodensity and there is irregular or circular necrotic area in the gland. ^{18}F-FDG uptake is annularly increased in the lesion, with extensive edema surrounding.

1.4 Salivary Duct Carcinoma

1.4.1 Clinical Overview

Salivary duct carcinoma (SDC) is a rare, highly malignant tumor that occurs from the epithelium of the salivary duct. It is classified as an independent tumor in the new WHO classification of salivary gland tumors. This tumor is highly malignant, with significantly more males than females, with a male-to-female ratio of 3:1, and the onset peak age is between 51 and 70 years old. The parotid gland is the most common site, followed by the submandibular gland, and minor salivary glands are rare. The clinical manifestations include that it has strong infiltration; it has invaded the surrounding tissues during early stage, with symptoms of neural paralysis; it is easy to metastasize through lymph and blood circulation; it has a high rate of cervical lymph node metastasis; it often involves in each group of deep cervical lymph nodes; it is prone to distant metastasis; and lung metastasis is the most common, followed by liver and bone metastasis. The tumor grows rapidly, the disease period is short, and most of them are in the advanced stage when they go to a doctor. Most patients have neurological symptoms. Patients with parotid gland tumor mostly have facial paralysis of varying degrees. Patients with submandibular gland tumor may have tongue numbness or tongue dyskinesia and often have local pain.

Its histopathological features are similar to those of breast ductal carcinoma, and the tissue is derived from the reserve cells of the excretory duct. Under the light microscope, the cancer cells are cubic or polygonal, with acidophilic cytoplasm, and may be accompanied by apocrine, with obvious cell atypia; the characteristic structures including papillary, cribriform, solid, and comedo exist alone or in combination, and tumor masses commonly infiltrate extensively around. Some scholars performed immunohistochemical analysis on it and found that S-100 antibody staining is negative and keratin and epithelial membrane antigen reaction is positive; in addition, other studies have confirmed that the tissue source of salivary duct carcinoma is the reserve cells of the salivary gland excretory duct through other special examinations. The treatment of salivary duct carcinoma is mainly surgery. Because of its strong invasion and easy metastasis through lymph and blood, extensive local resection is necessary. Facial nerve is not generally retained for tumors located in the parotid gland. Even if lymph node metastasis is not suspected clinically, cervical lymphatic dissection should be performed, which is supplemented by radiotherapy and chemotherapy to prevent distant metastasis.

1.4.2 PET/CT Diagnostic Points

Salivary duct carcinoma can occur in the gland or outside the gland. The tumors outside the gland are almost enlarged lymph nodes around the gland. Most of the tumors are characterized by diffuse growth of irregular masses with blurred edge and unclear contour and small adjacent fat or fascia space and mostly accompanied by abnormal hypermetabolism of ^{18}F-FDG. The rate of cervical lymph node metastasis is high, and it often involves the deep cervical lymph nodes in each group, with abnormal high metabolism of ^{18}F-FDG.

1.4.3 Typical Cases

Case 1: Male patient, 68 years old. Pathology: poorly differentiated carcinoma of the right parotid gland, which was consistent with salivary duct carcinoma (Fig. 19.4)

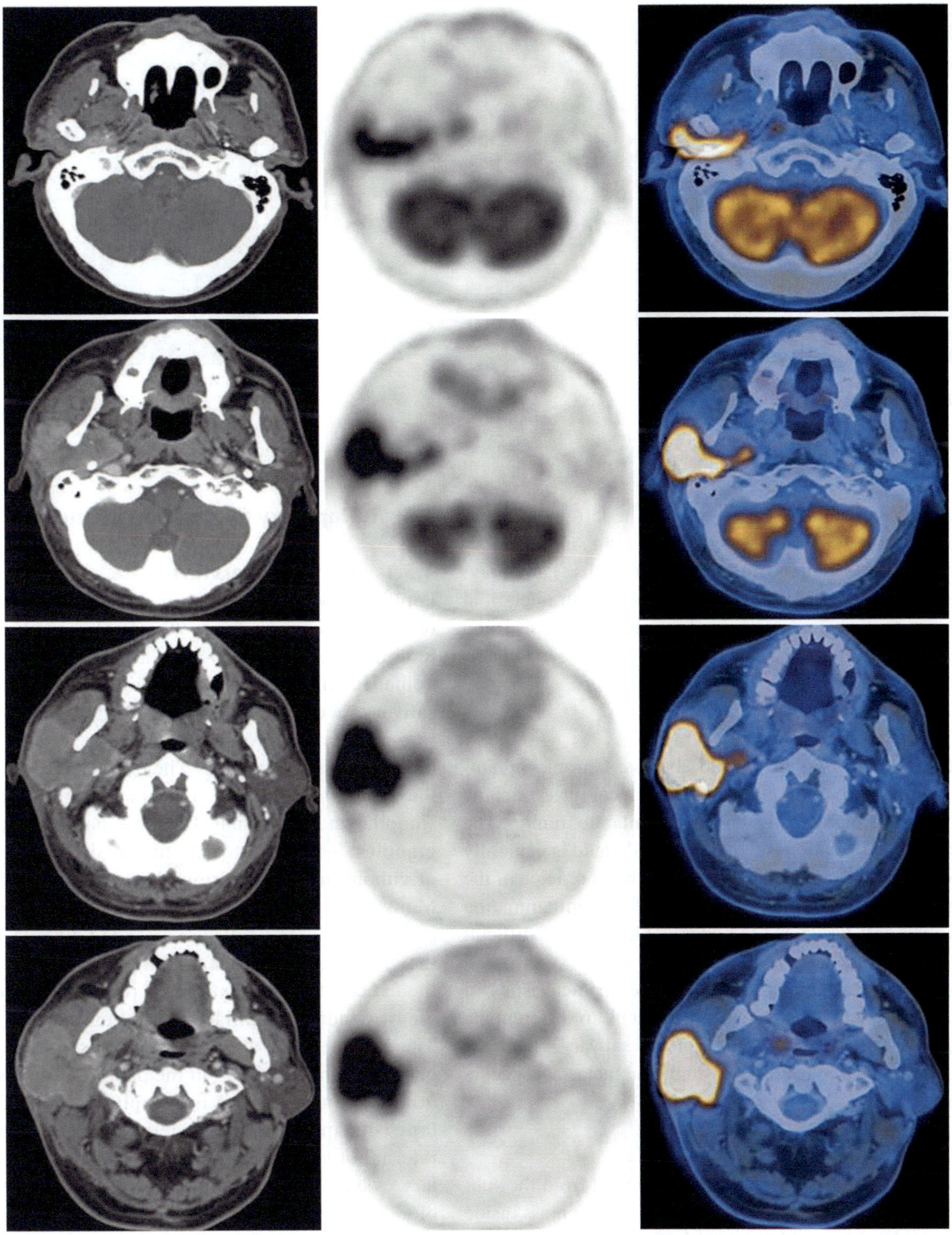

Fig. 19.4 ^{18}F-FDG PET/CT image of right salivary duct carcinoma. The lobulated soft tissue density mass of the right parotid gland showed intense FDG uptake. The SUV was about 17.7, and the largest layer was about 4.6 cm × 5.4 cm. There were low-density necrosis areas and small punctate calcifications with sparse radioactive distribution, and the enhanced scan showed obvious inhomogeneous enhancement. The lesions invaded the right parapharyngeal fat space, and the boundaries with the right masseter muscle, the right medial pterygoid muscle, and the right sternocleidomastoid muscle were not clear. It wrapped the right mandibular ramus and styloid process and pushed the blood vessels in the right carotid sheath area (This case was provided by Lin Xiaoping and Fan Wei from Sun Yat-sen University Cancer Center)

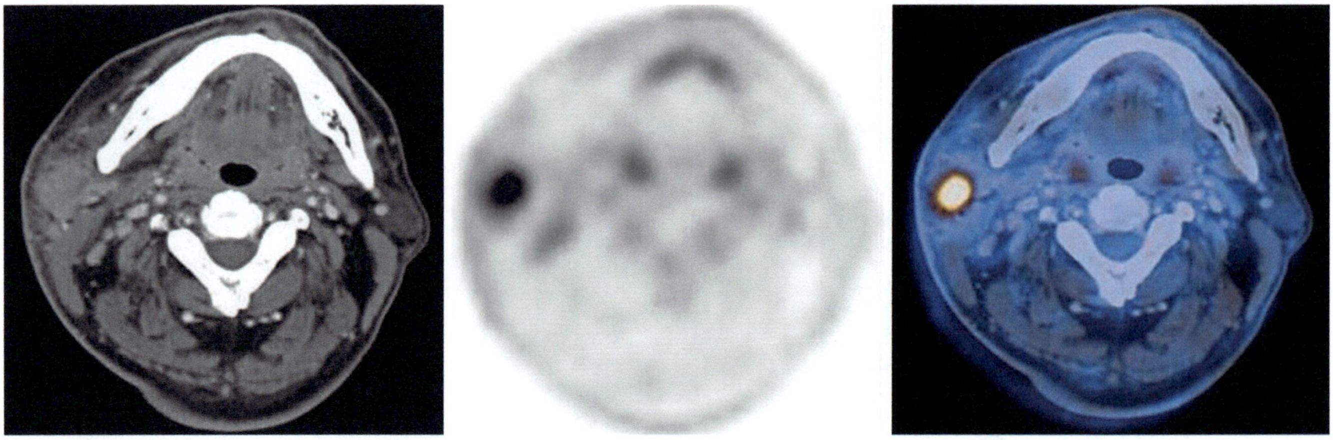

Fig. 19.4 (continued)

Case 2: Male patient, 65 years old. The left preauricular nodule has been found for more than 60 years, and the nodule has increased rapidly in the past 6 months. Pathology: (left parotid gland) salivary duct carcinoma with interstitial collagenization, calcification and massive necrosis, and metastasis or infiltration into the (left cervical) fiber and adipose tissue (Fig. 19.5)

1.4.4 Differential Diagnosis

1. Inflammatory mass or parotid abscess: Chronic inflammation of the parotid gland can form local mass or show inhomogeneous density change, similar to tumor. The typical manifestation is that the parotid gland is generally enlarged and the density is increased, but the shape of the parotid gland is still maintained. If the inflammation involves soft tissue and the edge is blurred, it is difficult to differentiate (Fig. 19.6).
2. Salivary ductal carcinoma: It has the characteristics of most malignant tumors, and it is difficult to differentiate from other malignant tumors of the salivary gland. Its malignant degree is relatively high and metastasis occurs early.

1.4.5 Summary

It should be clear, firstly, whether it is derived from the submandibular gland and, secondly, whether it is the mass inside or outside the submandibular gland. If the plain scan shows there are masses in the submandibular gland and enlarged lymph nodes outside the gland and the FDG uptake is abnormally increased, it mostly is the malignant tumor.

1.5 Papillary Cystadenocarcinoma

1.5.1 Clinical Overview

Papillary cystadenocarcinoma is rare in salivary gland tumors, accounting for 5–7% of salivary gland epithelial tumors. It is often considered as a subtype of adenocarcinoma. Papillary cystadenocarcinoma originates from the salivary duct epithelium. Its pathological morphology resembles mixed tumors, which is round or nodular, mostly without envelope. The cystic cavity is common in the tumor section. The inner wall of the cavity is not smooth, and there may be some papillary processes or granules. The tumor cells vary in size and are columnar or cuboid and form various irregular adenoid structures. Many of the glandular cavities are significantly enlarged to form cysts. The cells are arranged disorderly, although they are arranged in a single layer or multiple layers, and the cancer cells are extremely proliferated, forming single or dendritic papillae, protruding into the cyst cavity. There is a small amount of fibrous tissue interstitium between cancer cells or in the papilla, often infiltrated by inflammatory cells, but no lymphoid tissue. Tumor envelope is incomplete, and sometimes tumor cells invade the internal or surrounding tissues. The growth rate of papillary cystadenocarcinoma varies. It can metastasize along blood and lymphatic channels and also invade nerves, but it is relatively rare.

Papillary cystadenocarcinoma is the most common in the parotid glands, followed by the minor salivary glands in the palate and submandibular glands. It may also occur in the minor salivary glands in the buccal mucosa, floor of the mouth, tongue, and upper lip. The age of onset is 12–72 years old, most common in 30–50 years old, and the ratio of male to female is about 2:1.

The tumors resemble malignant mixed tumors. The common symptom is local painless masses, some of which are larger and nodular. The gland cavity is significantly enlarged to form a cystic shape, and hemorrhage and necrosis can occur, so cystic degeneration often occurs. The palpation part is soft, and bloody secretion can be drawn out by puncture. Generally, there is no obvious adhesion in the early stage and it can be moved.

1.5.2 PET/CT Diagnostic Points

On PET/CT scan without contrast agents, papillary cystadenocarcinoma can be seen as cystic and solid nodules with blurred edge and unclear outline, and the adjacent fat or fascia space is narrowed. ^{18}F-FDG shows a circular metabolic increase, and the circular shape is not obvious or metabolism is not high when the lesion is small.

1.5.3 Differential Diagnosis and Summary

How to differentiate papillary cystadenoma from papillary cystadenocarcinoma is the biggest challenge in histopathological diagnosis. It is often difficult to confirm whether it is

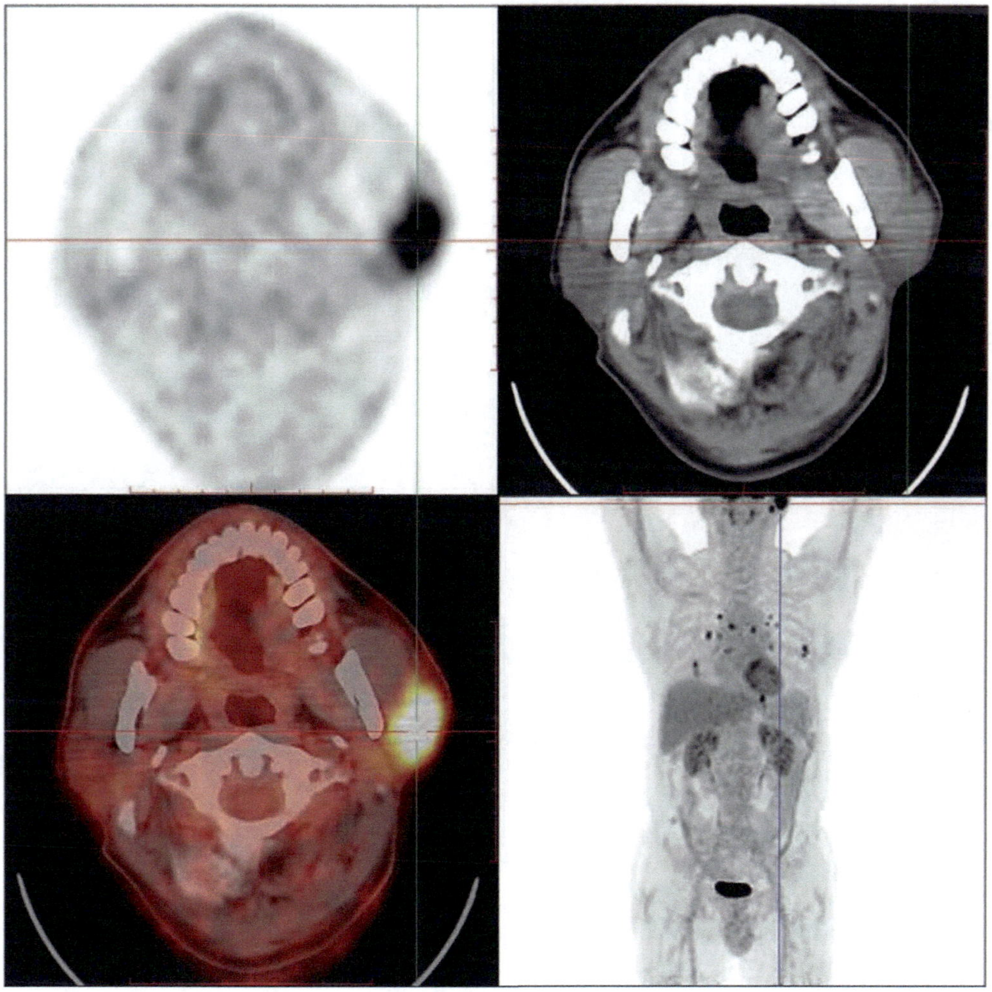

Fig. 19.5 ^{18}F-FDG PET/CT images of left salivary duct carcinoma. A round soft tissue mass was found in the left parotid gland area. Its internal density was inhomogeneous and the boundary was not clear. The size was about 3.8 cm × 2.5 cm. The radioactive distribution was abnormally concentrated, and the SUVmax was about 15.2

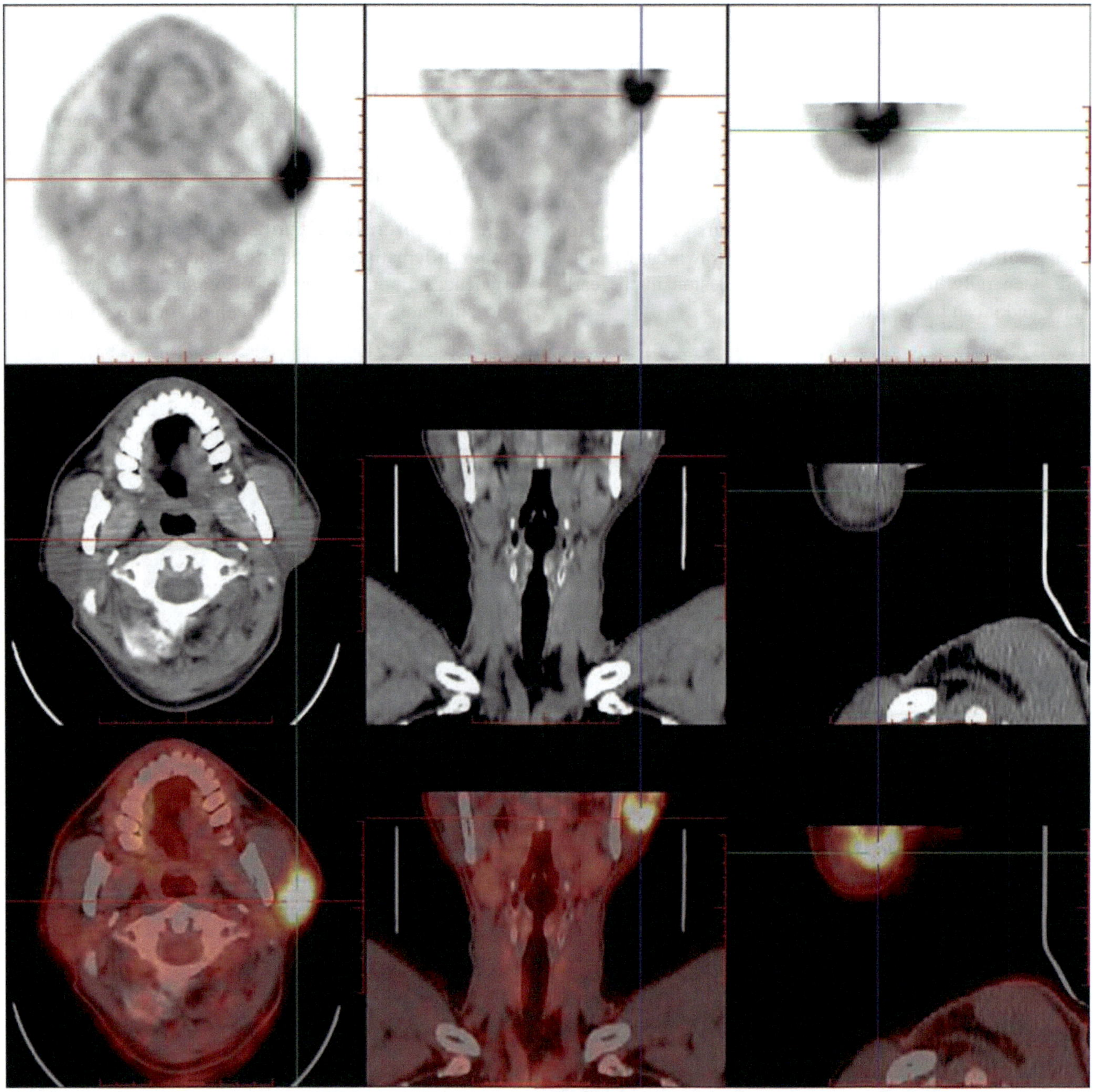

Fig. 19.5 (continued)

benign or malignant due to the similarity between the two in histopathology and cell morphology, especially in some cases of papillary cystadenoma with tumor cells invading the envelope and adjacent glands. However, the main determinant of malignancy is its extensive invasive growth and pleomorphism of cells and nuclei. Clinical symptoms should also be considered. If there are signs of spontaneous pain, recent growth acceleration, facial nerve palsy, etc., malignancy should be considered.

Papillary cystadenocarcinoma of the salivary gland has the characteristics of common malignant salivary gland tumors, so it is difficult to differentiate each other from imaging examination alone.

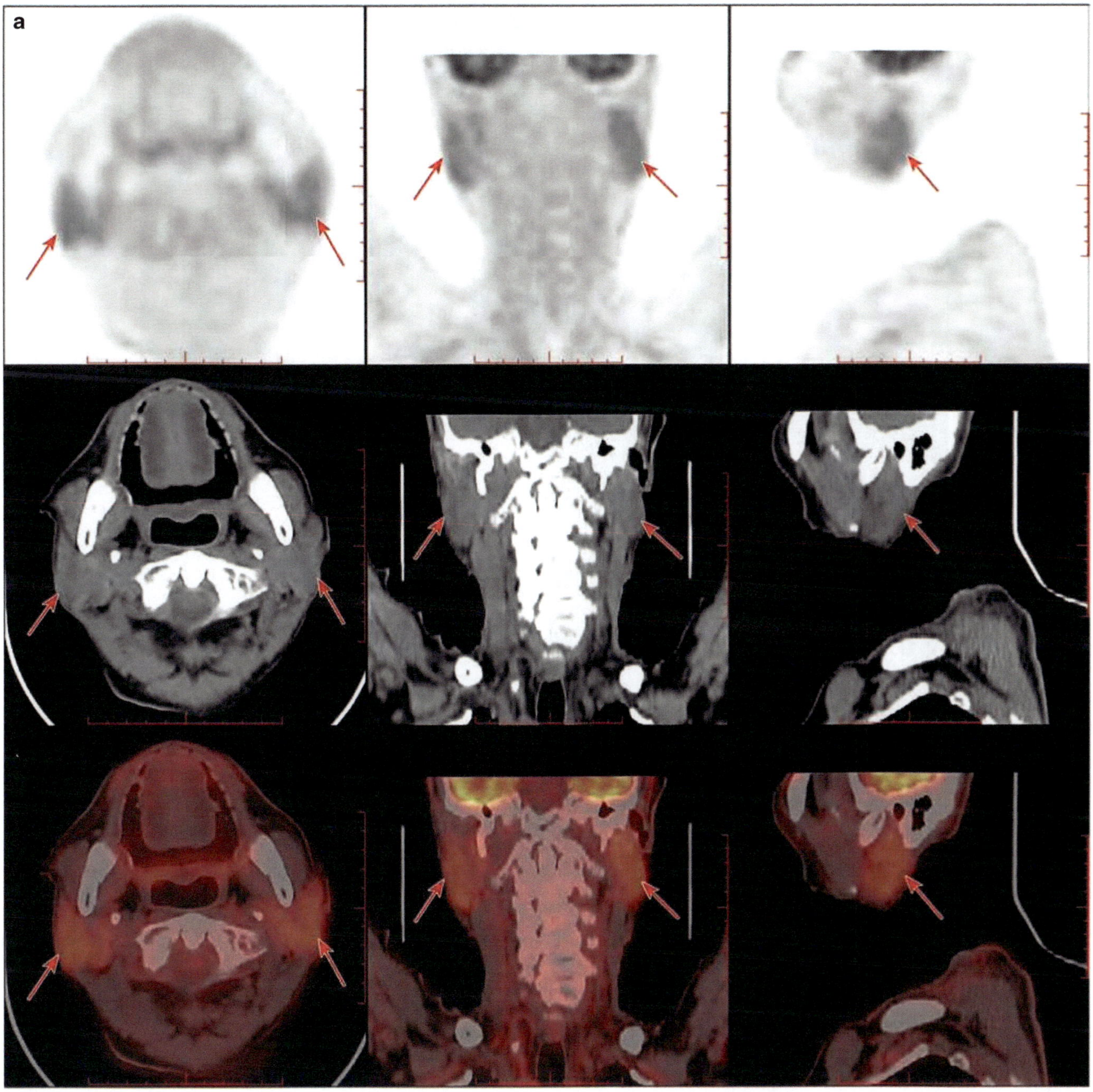

Fig. 19.6 ^{18}F-FDG PET/CT images of bilateral parotid gland inflammation. A 73-year-old male patient with gastric cancer was reexamined in the hospital after operation: (**a**) PET/CT image of diffuse elevated metabolism of bilateral parotid glands; (**b**) PET/CT image of diffuse elevated metabolism of bilateral parotid glands. PET/CT showed bilateral parotid gland enlargement with inhomogeneous increases density, and radioactive distribution increased diffusely. SUVmax was about 5.2

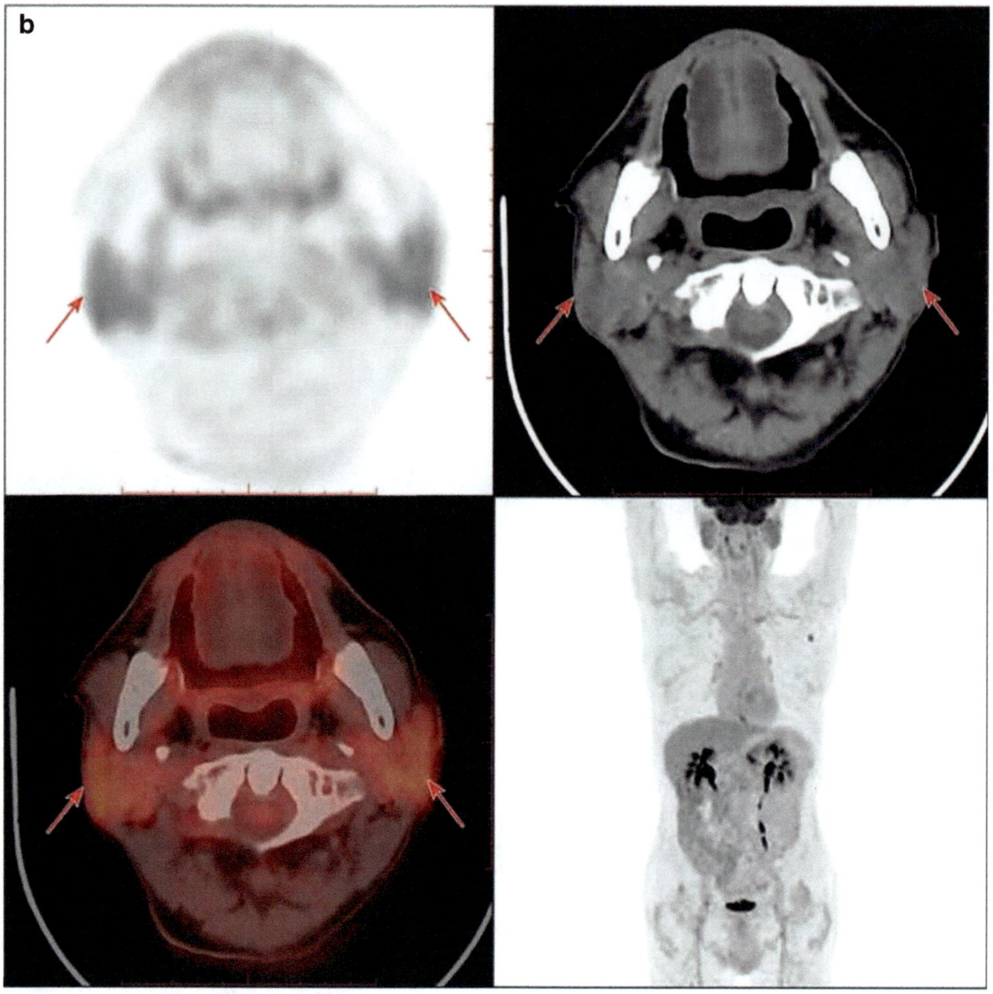

Fig. 19.6 (continued)

2 Common Benign Tumors of the Salivary Gland

2.1 Pleomorphic Adenoma

2.1.1 Clinical Overview

Pleomorphic adenomas of the salivary gland, including pleomorphic adenoma of the parotid gland (also known as mixed tumor of parotid gland), pleomorphic adenoma of the submandibular gland, and pleomorphic adenoma of the minor salivary gland. There are different opinions on histology: Some studies believe that the tumor originates from two germinal layers, so it is named mixed tumor. Later, most scholars believe that the so-called mixed tumor actually originates from the epithelium, including the myoepithelium, glandular epithelium, and tumor matrix, so the name pleomorphic adenoma is more suitable, but most are still used to call it mixed tumor.

Pleomorphic adenoma of the parotid gland is the most common benign tumor of the parotid gland. Pathologically, pleomorphic adenoma of the parotid gland is round or oval with complete envelope. The cross-section of the tumor is solid, off-white, or light yellow. Its main components are light blue cartilage-like tissue and translucent jelly-like mucinous tissue, occasionally bleeding or cystic necrosis, that is, the tumorous epithelial tissue is mixed with mucinous tissue, cartilage-like tissue, and collagen fibers. Under the microscope, the cells are arranged in a cord or sheet shape, which can form cysts of varying sizes, including fibrous tissue, mucinous tissue, and cartilage-like tissue. The mucous-like tissue is the most prominent, and sometimes calcification can be seen. About 25% can be associated with cancer. If the tumor suddenly grows faster and some signs of malignant tumor appear, the possibility of malignant transformation should be considered.

The histopathological characteristics of pleomorphic adenoma of the submandibular gland and minor salivary gland in the oral cavity are similar to that of the parotid gland. Pleomorphic adenoma of the submandibular gland often presents as a painless mass in one side of the submandibular

dibular region with clear boundary and slow growth. Pleomorphic adenoma of the minor salivary gland in the oral cavity usually starts from the oral submucous or vagal minor salivary gland and can occur in any part of the oral mucosa, most commonly in the posterior part of the hard palate, followed by the junction of the posterior hard palate and the soft hard palate on one side, and rarely in the midline and anterior part of the hard palate. Clinically, pleomorphic adenoma of the palate usually presents as a semicircular, oval, or nodular painless mass with smooth mucosal surface, which is often found by accident. Pathologically, pleomorphic adenomas of the submandibular gland and minor salivary gland in the oral cavity with a diameter of less than 3 cm have a smooth surface, and the larger ones may be lobulated, with fibrous tissue envelopes of varying thickness, which are easy to separate from the surrounding tissues. Most of the sections are solid, and cystic degeneration areas can be seen in larger sections. Under the light microscope, it shows the pleomorphism of the tissue structure rather than the cell itself. It is often mixed with mucus-like or cartilage-like tissue between the epithelial and mutated myoepithelial cell components.

2.1.2 PET/CT Diagnostic Points

Pleomorphic adenoma of the parotid gland usually occurs in the superficial lobe of the parotid gland and often involves the parapharyngeal space in the deep lobe. Most of the lesions are round or oval with clear edge. PET/CT scan without contrast agents shows equal or slightly high density, and sometimes low-density cystic necrosis or punctate calcification can be seen. The FDG uptake of the solid part of the tumor is increased or slightly higher, which may be inhomogeneous. Salivary gland angiography shows that the salivary duct is compressed and bent, presenting a "ball-holding sign," which was a characteristic manifestation.

Polymorphic adenomas of the submandibular gland are mostly masses with uniform density on PET/CT scan without contrast agents, which can be lobulated, and the density can be higher than that of the surrounding glandular tissues. The boundary is clear. The larger ones have inhomogeneous density. Sometimes, punctate calcification can be seen. The FDG uptake of the solid part of the tumor is increased or slightly higher, which may be inhomogeneous. The FDG uptake of the small ones may not be increased.

The PET/CT scan without contrast agents shows polymorphic adenoma of the minor salivary gland in the oral cavity is round, oval, or lobulated soft tissue mass similar to or slightly less than the adjacent muscles in density, with clear boundary and uniform density. Some of them show cystic degeneration, necrosis, compression, and absorption of adjacent bone, and they may penetrate the hard palate and invade the nasal cavity or completely locate in the maxilla. Sclerotic margin is often seen in adjacent bone. FDG uptake is increased or slightly higher, which may be inhomogeneous, or there may be no significant increase in metabolism.

2.1.3 Typical Cases

A 70-year-old male patient with PET/CT reexamination after lung cancer surgery. Pathology: (right parotid gland) pleomorphic adenoma (Fig. 19.7)

2.1.4 Differential Diagnosis

This disease mainly needs to be differentiated from adenolymphoma (also known as lymphopapillary cystadenoma, Warthin tumor), parapharyngeal space tumor, parotid lymphadenitis, eosinophilic granuloma, retromandibular mandibular vein, parotid malignant tumor, etc. The smaller pleomorphic adenomas are not characteristic and cannot be differentiated from other benign salivary gland tumors or low-grade malignant salivary gland tumors. If a large lobulated soft tissue mass in the parotid or submandibular gland area is found, pleomorphic adenoma should be considered first.

Adenocarcinoma is a common benign parotid tumor in the second position, which is often multiple. It can involve bilateral parotid glands or there are multiple lesions in one side of the gland. There are often cystic areas of varying sizes, and ^{18}F-FDG uptake is increased. The differential diagnosis between small single adenolymphoma and pleomorphic adenoma is difficult, and the diagnosis mainly depends on the incidence. Adenolymphoma is more common in male, but it can be multiple and small in size. The mass is soft and often has a history of growth and decline. Usually, there is cyst in the mass, which can be as a sign for identification.

Parotid gland lymphadenitis and small mixed tumor of eosinophilic granuloma are not easy to differentiate from parotid gland lymphadenitis and eosinophilic granuloma, which should be analyzed in combination with medical history.

Parapharyngeal space tumors often cause the fat in the parapharyngeal space to move outward, while tumors in the deep lobe of the parotid gland often cause the fat tissue in the parapharyngeal space to move inward. Parapharyngeal space tumors can be neuronal tumors or ectopic minor salivary gland tumors. Neurolemmoma usually occurs in the space of the carotid sheath and is prone to cystic degeneration, and the edge of the cystic lesion area is clear. The malignant tumors of the parotid gland have mixed density, irregular edge, unclear boundary, and blurred fat space, the metabolism of ^{18}F-FDG is abnormally increased, and sometimes the destruction of mastoidale or styloid process bone or cervical enlarged lymph nodes can be seen.

Pleomorphic adenoma of the oral small salivary gland should be differentiated from other benign tumors in the palate, including myoepithelioma, papilloma, and fibroma. The abovementioned tumors are difficult to differentiate from pleomorphic

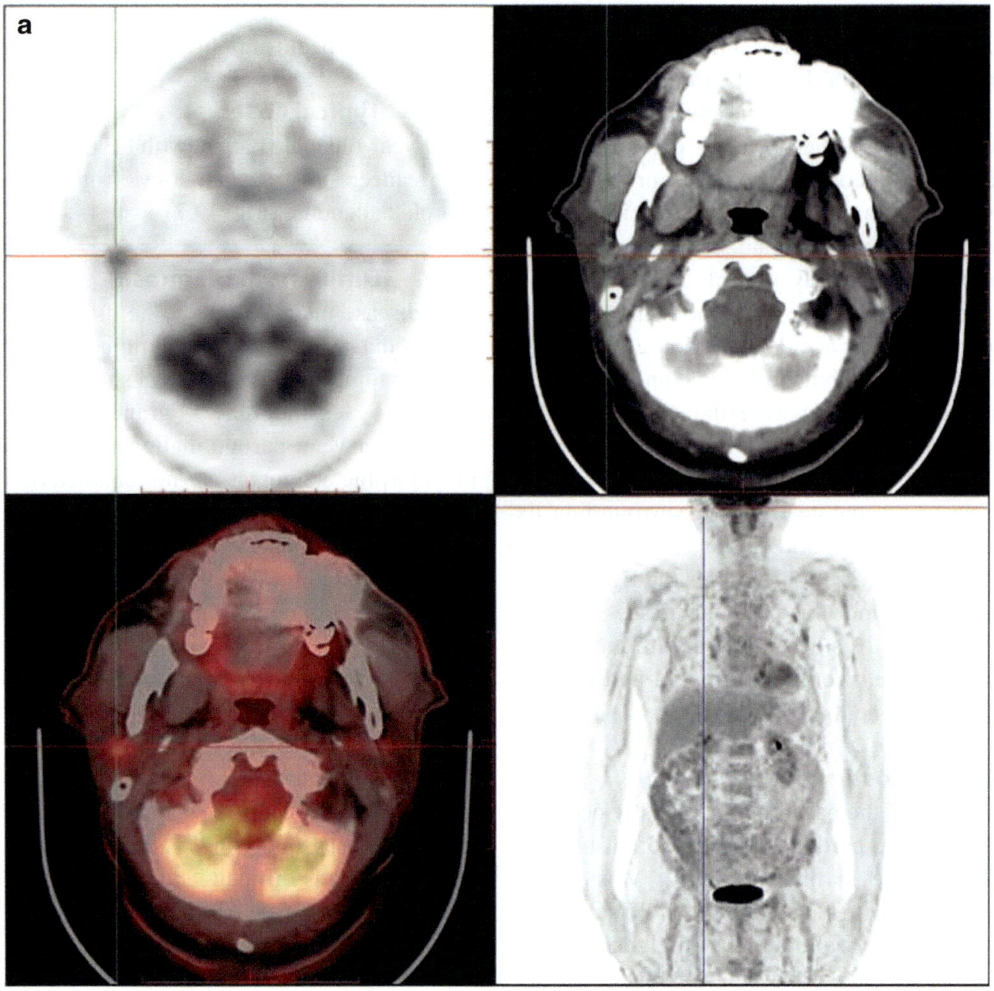

Fig. 19.7 ^{18}F-FDG PET/CT images of pleomorphic adenoma of the right parotid gland. (**a**) PET/CT image of hypermetabolic nodules of the right parotid gland; (**b**) PET/CT image of hypermetabolic nodules of the right parotid gland. PET/CT showed a round slightly high-density nodule shadow in the superficial lobe of the right parotid gland, with clear edge and a diameter of about 0.9 cm, the radioactivity distribution increased, and the SUVmax was about 5.7. Pathology: (right parotid gland) pleomorphic adenoma

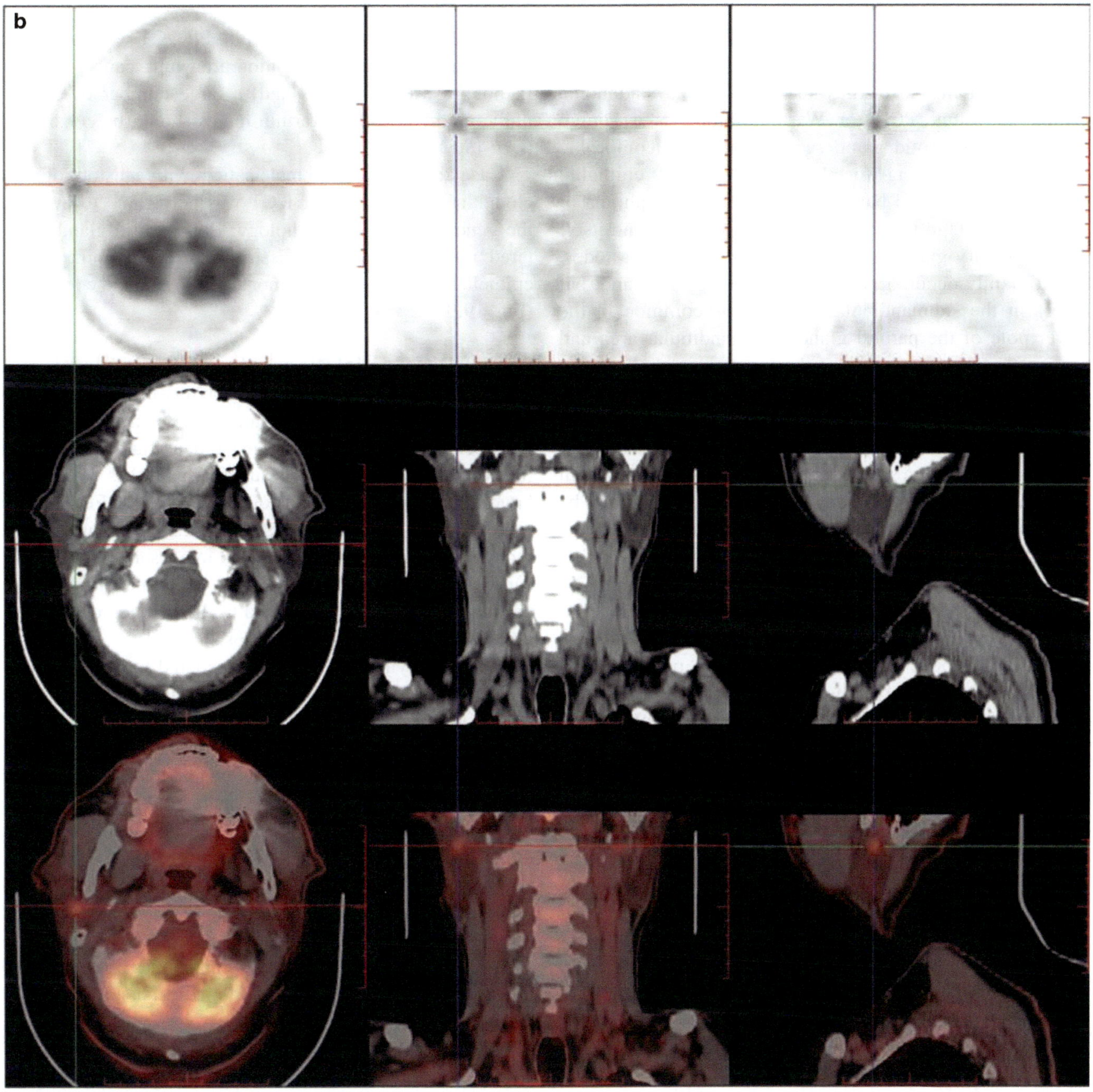

Fig. 19.7 (continued)

adenomas by imaging examination alone, but their incidence is significantly lower than that of pleomorphic adenoma. Malignant tumors are often accompanied by local pain, the surface of the lesion is not smooth, and there may be ulcers. Most of the lesions show infiltrative growth, with unclear boundary; cystic degeneration, necrosis, and hemorrhage are common; and metastatic enlarged cervical lymph nodes can be seen.

2.1.5 Summary

Most pleomorphic adenomas have high ^{18}F-FDG uptake, but this is not specific. The occasional high uptake of ^{18}F-FDG in the parotid gland is common in metastases, physiological uptake, and infectious diseases. In the reports on the application of ^{18}F-FDG PET/CT in the differential diagnosis of parotid benign and malignant lesions, most studies believe that SUV cannot effectively differentiate between benign and malignant parotid lesions. Pleomorphic adenomas, Warthin tumors, large eosinophilic tumors, and other benign tumors can also show high uptake of ^{18}F-FDG. Therefore, differential diagnosis is difficult at times, and the differential diagnosis from other parotid benign tumors mainly depends on the incidence.

2.2 Adenolymphoma

2.2.1 Clinical Overview

Adenolymphoma, also known as papillary cystadenoma lymphomatosum (PCL) or Warthin tumor, is a benign tumor of the parotid gland second only to pleomorphic adenoma, accounting for 15.3% of parotid epithelial tumors and 20.6% of benign tumors. Adenolymphoma of the salivary gland is derived from the salivary gland itself or the salivary gland tissue enclosed in the lymph nodes, and it mainly occurs in one side of the parotid gland, but rarely in the submandibular gland. It is common in the lower pole of the parotid gland and mandibular area and rare in the preauricular area; the location is shallow, the growth is slow, the tumor is generally small, and the diameter is rarely more than 3 cm, with soft, smooth texture and mild activity; after anti-infection treatment, there is no obvious reduction in size, which can be distinguished from inflammation. The occurrence of adenolymphoma may be the result of multiple factors such as gender, region, heredity, age, tobacco, infection, and immunity. Smoking is closely related to the occurrence of adenolymphoma. The disease is a kind of ectopic adenoma and benign epithelial tumor which mainly occurs in the parotid gland, so it is considered to be a disease specific to the parotid gland area. Although adenolymphoma has a benign histological morphology, it has the characteristics of multicentric growth and is accompanied by other types of tumors, which can occur simultaneously on both sides. Clinically, for elderly patients with long-term smoking history, when a soft mass with a diameter of about 3 cm is found in the parotid gland, the possibility of Warthin tumor of the parotid gland should be highly suspected. The history of mass growth and decline is one of the prominent clinical features of Warthin tumor. A cold or upper respiratory tract infection can induce tumor enlargement. The disease rarely has malignant transformation, and the epithelial component can become squamous cell carcinoma or mucoepidermoid carcinoma; the interstitial component mostly becomes mucosal-associated lymphoma.

2.2.2 PET/CT Diagnostic Points

Adenolymphoma usually occurs in the superficial lobe of the parotid gland. It can be multiple in one side or concurrently involves bilateral parotid glands. It is the most common tumor of bilateral glands. PET/CT scan without contrast agents shows round or oval shape with clear edge, mostly less than 2 cm in diameter, and the density can be uniform, comparable to the muscle density at the same level. The low-density area of tumor-associated cyst can be seen. The metabolism of ^{18}F-FDG is slightly or moderately increased.

2.2.3 Typical Cases

Case 1: Male patient, 66 years old. PET/CT was performed to evaluate the general condition after lung cancer surgery. Pathology: (left parotid gland) a large number of eosinophilic epithelial cells; Warthin tumor should be considered (Fig. 19.8).

Case 2: A 66-year-old male patient with a history of non-Hodgkin's lymphoma. PET/CT was performed to evaluate the general condition. Pathology: (left parotid gland) scattered inflammatory cells, tissue cells, eosinophilic ductal epithelial cells; Warthin tumor should be first considered (Fig. 19.9).

2.2.4 Differential Diagnosis

Pleomorphic adenoma: a small unilateral single Warthin tumor is difficult to differentiate from it on imaging. The diagnosis mainly depends on the incidence and pathological results. Large single Warthin tumor usually has a relatively large glandular cavity or bad void cavity, and ^{18}F-FDG uptake can be slightly increased. MRI shows that it is characterized by hyperintensity nodules on T1WI images and T_2WI signal can be hypointensity, isointensity, or hyperintensity. The signal intensity was closely related to the histological components, which can assist the diagnosis.

Sjogren's syndrome (SS) is considered to be an autoimmune disease, which is more common in middle-aged and elderly women. It is characterized by diffuse enlargement of unilateral or bilateral parotid glands, and the submandibular or sublingual glands can also be enlarged at the same time. Clinically, dry eyes, dry mouth, rheumatoid arthritis history, and bilateral lacrimal gland enlargement contribute to the diagnosis of the disease.

Malignant lymphoma may involve bilateral parotid glands, mostly extranodal type. Nodules in parotid gland lymphoma often complicate with enlarged lymph nodes in the neck space, and the enlarged lymph nodes often fuse into blocks, grow fast, and have a short medical history.

2.2.5 Summary

Adenolymphoma of the salivary gland has no specific clinical manifestations. Adenolymphoma is often found accidentally in the PET/CT diagnosis of other diseases. Patients with cystic solid mass are easily misdiagnosed as mixed tumor of the salivary gland, lymphadenitis, or cyst. Therefore, imaging examinations cannot be used as the only basis for diagnosis, and the diagnosis must be made in combination with medical history and clinical manifestations. When the middle-aged and elderly male patients with long-term smoking history have a round soft tissue mass in the posterior lower pole of the parotid gland, with clear edge; solid or cystic solid, bilateral or multifocal; and increased ^{18}F-FDG uptake, Warthin tumor of the parotid gland is suggested.

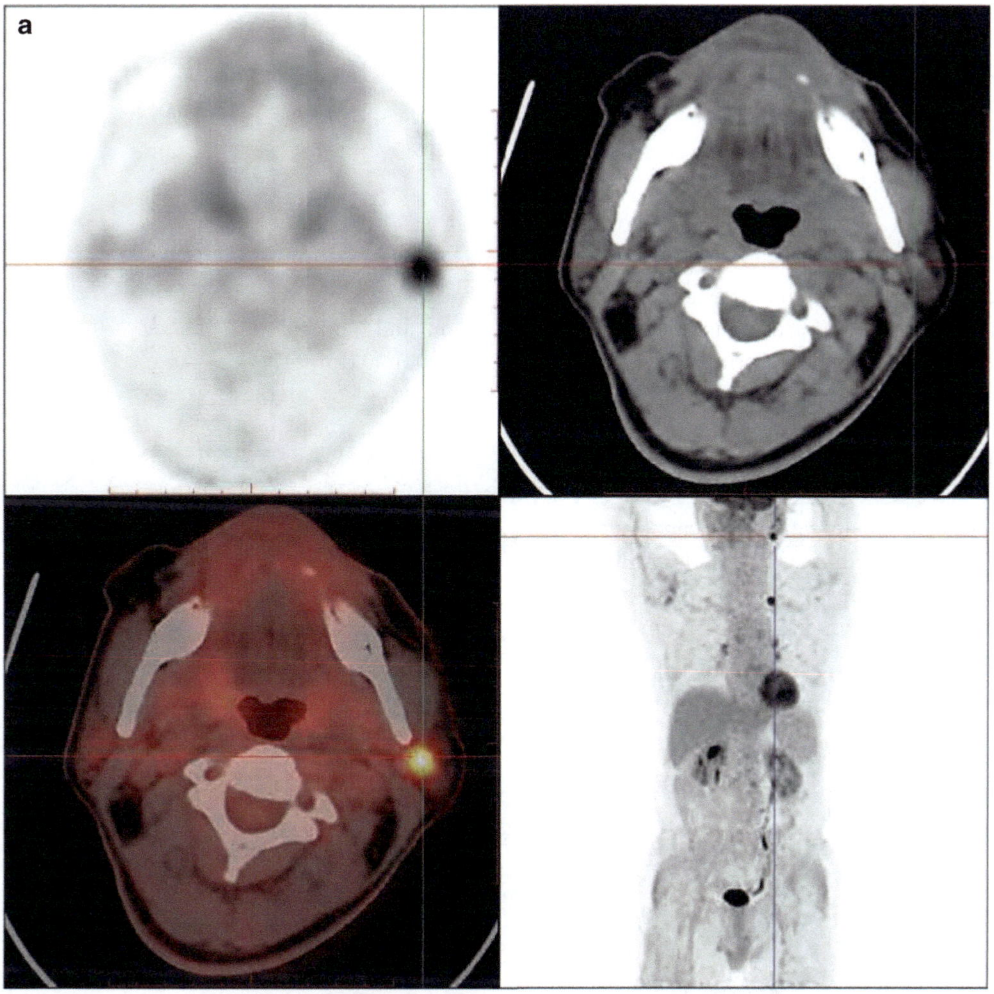

Fig. 19.8 ^{18}F-FDG PET/CT images of Warthin tumor of the left parotid gland. (**a–c**) PET/CT images of hypermetabolic nodules in the left parotid gland. PET/CT showed that there was a round, slightly high-density, small nodule shadow in the lower pole of the left parotid gland, with clear edges and a size of about 1.0 cm × 0.9 cm. The density was uniform, comparable to the muscle density at the same level. The radioactive distribution was abnormally concentrated, and the SUVmax was about 15.6

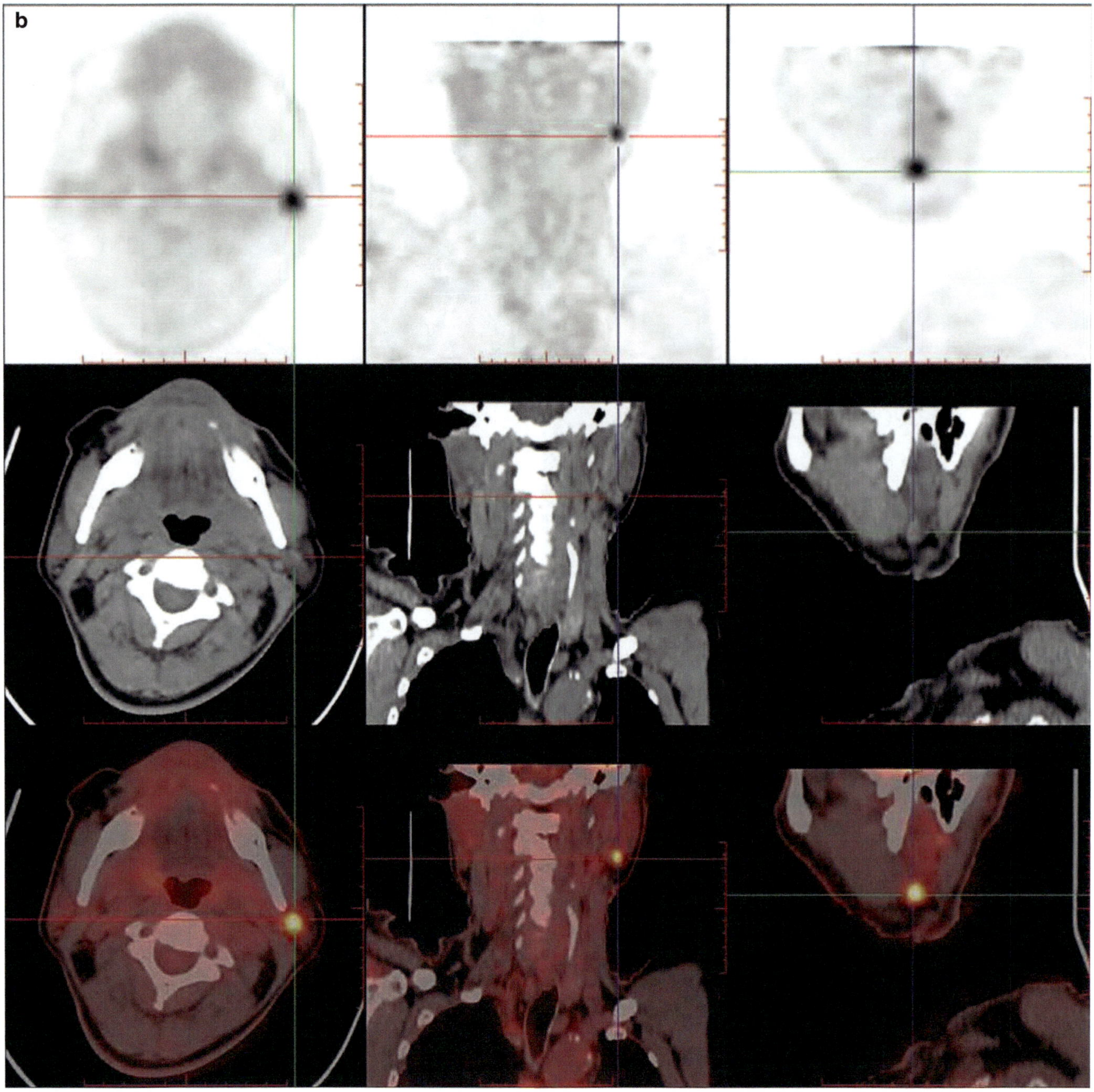

Fig. 19.8 (continued)

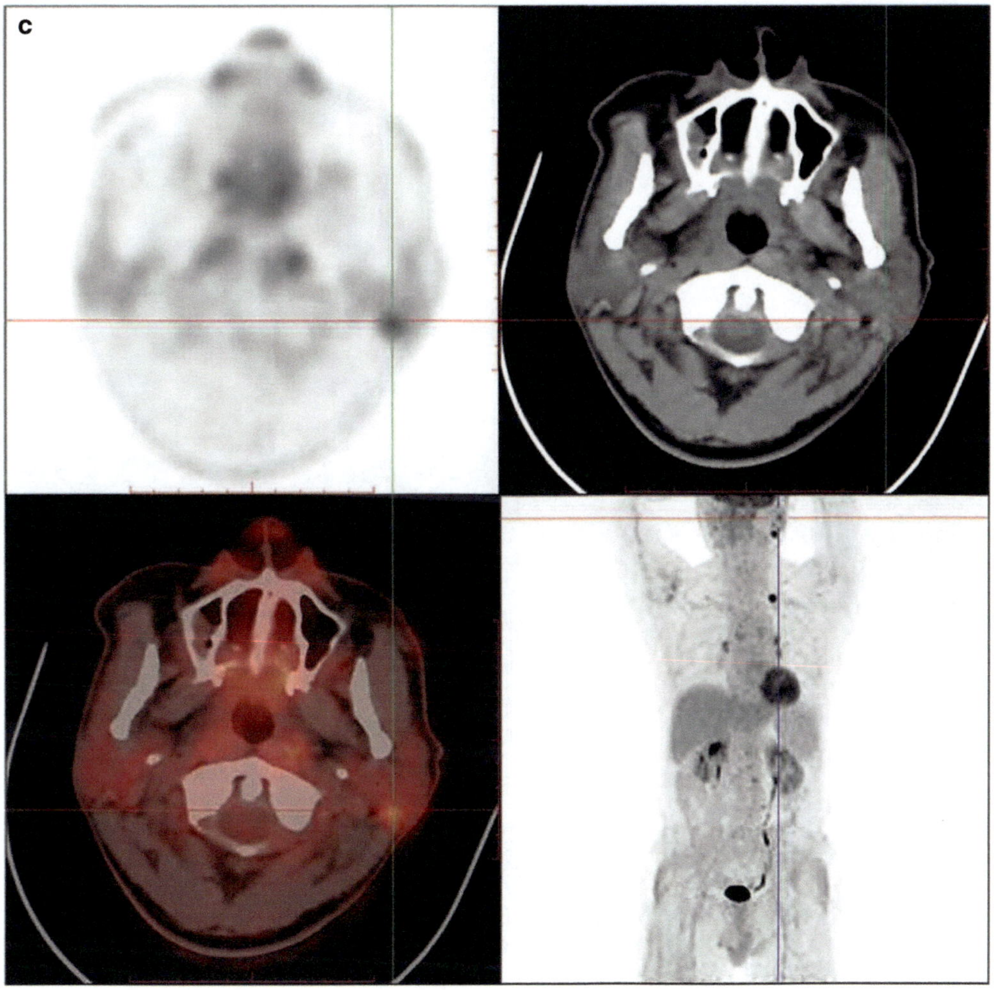

Fig. 19.8 (continued)

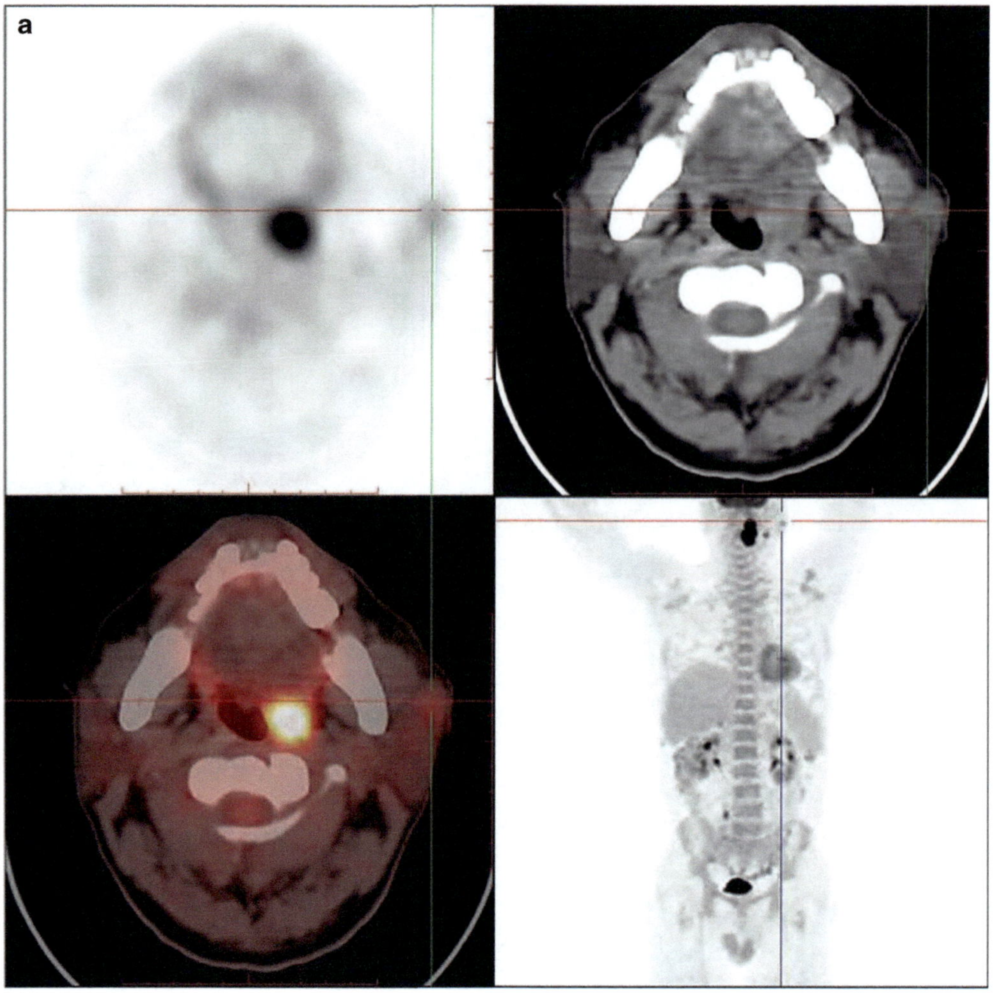

Fig. 19.9 ^{18}F-FDG PET/CT images of non-Hodgkin's lymphoma with Warthin tumor. (**a**) PET/CT image of a slightly hypermetabolic nodule on the anterior outer edge of the left parotid gland (before treatment), with clear edge, about 1.0 cm in diameter, with uniform density and slightly increased FDG uptake (SUVmax 2.3). (**b**) PET/CT image of a slightly hypermetabolic nodule in the left parotid gland (after treatment). The patient underwent PET/CT reexamination after 4 months of treatment. The nodule size did not change significantly. The radioactivity distribution was slightly higher than before, and SUVmax was about 2.5

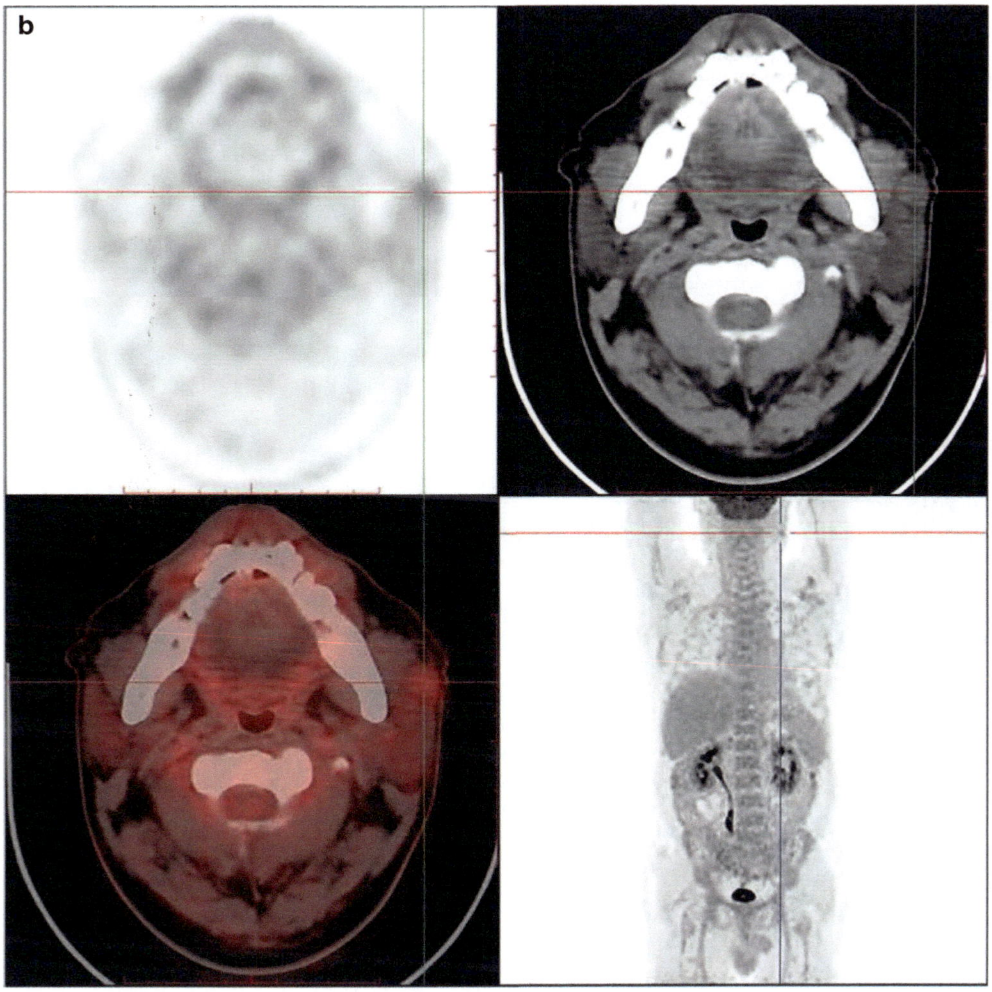

Fig. 19.9 (continued)

Further Reading

Hsieh C E, Ho K C, Hsieh C H, et al. Pretreatment primary tumor SUVmax on ^{18}F-FDG PET/CT images predicts outcomes in patients with salivary gland carcinoma treated with definitive intensity-modulated radiation therapy. Clin Nucl Med 2017; 42(9):655-662.

Jeong H S, Chung M K, Son Y I, et al. Role of ^{18}F-FDG PET/CT in management of high-grade salivary gland malignancies. J Nucl Med, 2007; 48(8):1237-1244.

Kim M J, Kim J S, Roh J L, et al. Utility of ^{18}F-FDG PET/CT for detecting neck metastasis in patients with salivary gland carcinomas: preoperative planning for necessity and extent of neck dissection. Ann Surg Oncol 2013; 20(3):899-905.

Nguyen B D, Roarke M C. Salivary duct carcinoma with perineural spread to facial canal ^{18}F-FDG PET/CT detection. Clin Nucl Med 2008; 33(12):925-928.

Park M J, Oh J S, Roh J L, et al. ^{18}F-FDG PET/CT versus contrast-enhanced CT for staging and prognostic prediction in patients with salivary gland carcinomas. Clin Nucl Med, 2017; 42(3):e149-e156.

Ryu I S, Kim J S, Roh J L, et al. Prognostic value of preoperative metabolic tumor volume and total lesion glycolysis measured by ^{18}F-FDG PET/CT in salivary gland carcinomas. J Nucl Med, 2013; 54(7):1032-1038.

Sharma P, Jain T K, Singh H, et al. Utility of ^{18}F-FDG PET/CT in staging and restaging of patients with malignant salivary gland tumours: a single-institutional experience. Nucl Med Commun, 2013; 34 (3):211-219.

Toriihara A, Nakamura S, Kubota K, et al. Can dual-time-point ^{18}F-FDG PET/CT differentiate malignant salivary gland tumors from benign tumors?. AJR Am J Roentgenol, 2013; 201(3):639-644.

PET/CT of Cervical Lymphatic Metastases

20

Yuetao Wang, Chun Qiu, and Rong Niu

Among the neck malignant tumors, 20% are primary tumors and 80% are metastatic. Among them, 85% are primary tumors of the head and neck, 20% are metastatic tumors of the chest and abdomen, and the remaining 3–9% have unknown primary tumors. The pathological types of metastatic lymph nodes in the neck are mostly squamous cell carcinoma, mainly from the mouth, sinuses, throat, and pharynx, while some are adenocarcinoma, mostly from the thyroid, salivary gland, nasal cavity, lung, breast, gastrointestinal tract, etc.

1 Clinical Overview

The probability and location of cervical lymphatic metastasis of various primary tumors may vary. The incidence of cervical lymphatic metastasis is 86–90%, tonsil cancer 58–76%, hypopharyngeal cancer 52–72%, tongue bottom cancer 50–83%, and oropharyngeal cancer 50–71%. Due to the abundance of pharyngeal lymph nodes, there are often overlapping lymphatic networks on both sides, and the probability of bilateral cervical lymphatic metastasis is also high, among which nasopharyngeal cancer is the most common occurrence of bilateral metastasis (32.8%), followed by soft palate cancer, supraglottic throat cancer, tongue bottom cancer, and oropharyngeal cancer.

Metastatic lymph nodes in different areas of the neck also have different primary lesions. Metastatic lymph nodes in region I are most frequently found in prelingual carcinoma, bottom of mouth carcinoma, gingival carcinoma (posterior triangle of molar), and carcinoma of the tonsil anterior column. Any squamous cell carcinoma of the head and neck may metastasize to lymph nodes in the region II, while metastatic lymph nodes in the region III are mostly from the carcinoma of the tongue, nasopharyngeal carcinoma, oropharyngeal carcinoma, hypopharyngeal carcinoma, gingival carcinoma, and supraglottic laryngocarcinoma, while metastatic lymph nodes in the region IV are mostly from the nasopharyngeal carcinoma, thyroid carcinoma, tonsil carcinoma, tongue bottom carcinoma, and hypopharyngeal carcinoma. Metastatic lymph nodes in region V are rare and can come from nasopharyngeal carcinoma, among which supraclavicular (VB) metastasis is more common in lung cancer, followed by thyroid cancer and gastrointestinal tumor. Metastatic lymph nodes in region VI and superior mediastinum (region VII) are mostly from thyroid carcinoma (Table 20.1).

The regions where metastatic lymph nodes are most common in primary tumors are also different. Oral cancer, submaxillary adenocarcinoma, and sublingual adenocarcinoma usually metastasize to regions I and II first. Laryngeal cancer and hypopharyngeal cancer are successively in regions III, IV, and V. Parotid cancer is seen in the anterior ear and around the parotid gland and lymph nodes in the parotid gland. If there is no lymphatic metastasis at the initial site, the probability of lymphatic metastasis at other sites is very small. The site of lymphatic metastasis of thyroid carcinoma is different from that of squamous cell carcinoma, and the most common metastasis is to regions IV, VI, and VII.

The accuracy of palpation, CT, MRI, and B-mode ultrasound-guided fine needle biopsy in detecting metastatic lymph nodes in the neck is 56%, 66%, 75%, and 86%, respectively. Compared with puncture biopsy, various non-invasive imaging methods to determine the nature of cervical lymph nodes are still the first choice in clinical practice. In addition to the above conventional examination methods, the diagnostic value of PET/CT has gradually gained clinical recognition, especially for the clinical staging and treatment decision-making of nasopharyngeal carcinoma.

According to the difference of primary tumor and clinical stage, the treatment of cervical lymphatic metastasis also

Y. Wang (✉)
Changzhou Key Laboratory of Molecular Imaging, The First People's Hospital of Changzhou, The Third Affiliated Hospital of Soochow University, Changzhou, Jiangsu, China

C. Qiu · R. Niu
The First People's Hospital of Changzhou, Changzhou, Jiangsu, China

Z. Yao, S. Li (eds.), *Atlas of PET/CT in Oncology - Volume 1*, https://doi.org/10.1007/978-981-99-1172-1_20

Table 20.1 Common primary lesion of metastatic lymph nodes in different neck regions

Metastatic lymph node area in the neck	Primary lesion
Region I	Anterior tongue cancer, bottom of mouth cancer, gingival cancer (posterior triangle of molar), tonsil anterior column cancer
Region II	Any squamous cell carcinoma of the head and neck
Region III	Cancer of the tongue bottom, nasopharynx, oropharynx, hypopharynx, gingiva, and supraglottic larynx
Region IV	Nasopharyngeal cancer, thyroid cancer, tonsil cancer, tongue bottom cancer, hypopharyngeal cancer
Region V	Nasopharyngeal cancer, thyroid cancer, lung cancer, gastrointestinal tumor
Regions VI and VII	Thyroid cancer, esophageal cancer

varies. Radiotherapy is the main treatment for nasopharyngeal carcinoma, synchronous chemoradiotherapy is the preferred choice for local advanced stage, and surgical treatment is the alternative for survival or recurrence of metastatic lymph nodes in the neck after radiotherapy. Surgical treatment is mainly used for the newly diagnosed thyroid cancer, and lymph nodes in the central region are routinely dissected. When lymphatic metastasis in other regions is suspected prior to surgery, or serum globulin/calcitonin is significantly increased, selective lymph node dissection shall be performed at the same time. Cervical lymphatic metastasis occurs after the operation of differentiated thyroid carcinoma. If ^{131}I fails, surgical resection needs to be taken. Radical dissection of cervical lymph nodes should be performed for salivary gland tumors with cervical lymphatic metastasis; selective dissection of cervical lymph nodes should be performed for patients with facial nerve palsy; postoperative adjuvant radiotherapy is feasible for parotid carcinoma with cervical lymphatic metastasis. In principle, chemotherapy mainly applies to cervical metastatic lymph nodes from thoracic or abdominal tumors.

Patients with ipsilateral lymphatic metastasis have a 50% lower survival rate than those without lymphatic metastasis. For those with contralateral or bilateral lymphatic metastasis, the survival rate decreased to 25% of those without metastasis. With bilateral lymphatic metastasis accompanied by lymph node capsular invasion, the survival rate is only 12.5% of those without metastasis. Additionally, the incidence of distant metastases is increased in patients with lymphatic metastases, and death from cervical lymphatic metastases can occur even if the primary tumor is locally controlled. Detecting lymphatic metastasis before treatment in patients with head and neck tumors is of great clinical significance for therapeutic strategies and prognosis assessment.

2 PET/CT Diagnostic Points

The sensitivity and specificity of ^{18}F-FDG PET/CT in detecting metastatic lymph nodes in the neck are 90% and 94%, which has more advantages over CT and MRI, and have important guiding significance for whether cervical lymph node dissection should be performed in patients with head and neck squamous cell carcinoma. It is crucial to the prognosis of patients whether there is regional lymphatic metastasis or not, so the detection of cervical lymphatic metastasis by PET/CT is of great value in determining clinical staging, making therapy decisions, and evaluating prognosis. However, FDG can be ingested in both inflammatory and metastatic lymph nodes, which makes differential diagnosis difficult. Using methionine or tyrosine as imaging agents can improve the specificity of differential diagnosis.

The main criteria for imaging used for the diagnosis of metastatic lymph nodes by ^{18}F-FDG PET/CT are the size of lymph nodes, whether there is central necrosis, and FDG uptake. Moreover, lymph node morphology, number, and whether there is a junction of the invasion also have a certain diagnostic value. In general, the uptake of ^{18}F-FDG in metastatic lymph nodes is significantly increased, especially in lymph nodes with enlargement and necrosis or fusion. However, it is still possible that there is only slight uptake or no significant uptake in some metastatic lymph nodes. A meta-analysis found that CT, MRI, PET/CT, and ultrasound showed no significant difference in the detection accuracy of cervical lymphatic metastasis in head and neck tumors. Therefore, the level of uptake of ^{18}F-FDG cannot be used as a basis for the identification of metastatic lymph nodes.

The PET/CT imaging features of metastatic lymph nodes in the neck are as follows:

1. Size of lymph node: It is generally believed to be measured by the smallest (shortest) diameter. For cervical lymph nodes, some scholars proposed that different diagnostic thresholds should be set in different regions. It is believed that the lymph nodes at the top of area II ≥11 mm and the other areas ≥10 mm were more reliable as diagnostic thresholds. The minimum diameter ≥8 mm was used as the CT diagnostic threshold for II–IV regions, with a sensitivity of 91.67% and specificity of 98.61%, and that the smallest diameter ≥5 mm was used as the threshold value of metastatic lymph nodes in the tracheoesophageal groove, with a sensitivity of 69.23% and a specificity of 100%. Metastatic lymph nodes of thyroid carcinoma are smaller than those of squamous cell carcinoma, and the smallest lymph nodes with a diameter of 5 mm should also be taken into account. The presence of lymph nodes of any size in the tracheoesophageal groove should be a matter of high vigilance against the possibility of metastatic lymph nodes. It

should be noted that lymph node size alone should not be used as a diagnostic criterion for metastatic lymph nodes.

2. Lymph node density and internal structure: The CT findings of metastatic lymph nodes can be classified into four types: (1) uniform density and degree of enhancement similar to muscle; (2) the density is significantly higher than that of muscle, with uniform or non-uniform enhancement; (3) edge enhancement and low density in the center; and (4) thin ring enhancement and uniform density in the central area (similar to muscle). Of them, type 3 is the most typical metastatic manifestation of squamous cell carcinoma. The pathological basis is that tumor cells first invade the marginal sinus of the cortex and then infiltrate into the medulla, resulting in the obstruction of lymphoid reflux and subsequent necrosis of the medulla. The low density of the center shown on CT is tumor necrosis, keratin, fibrous tissue, interstitial effusion or edema, and viable cancer cells. Calcification in cervical lymph nodes is most common in papillary thyroid cancer and medullary cancer, followed by prostate cancer, testicular cancer, colon cancer, ovarian cancer, breast cancer, lung adenocarcinoma, osteosarcoma, etc. In addition, it is necessary to exclude calcification following radiotherapy for lymphoma. Cystic degeneration may also occur in some metastatic lymph nodes of papillary thyroid carcinoma.
3. Morphology and number of lymph nodes: The lymph nodes with normal or reactive hyperplasia are generally in renal shape, with a ratio of approximately 2:1 in length to short diameter. Metastatic lymph nodes are mostly spherical with similar length and short diameter. In patients with head and neck malignant tumors, there are three or more lymph nodes distributed in clusters in the lymph drainage area, and the possibility of metastatic lymph nodes should be warned even if the smallest diameter is 5–8 mm.
4. Extracapsular lymph node invasion: It is manifested as irregular enhancement of lymph node margin, varying thickness, infiltration of adjacent fat, unclear boundary from surrounding structures, and invasion of the carotid artery, pair IX–XII cranial nerves, skull base, etc. The larger the metastatic lymph node is, the greater the possibility of invasion is. For those with a maximum diameter of >3 cm, 3/4 of them have extracapsular invasion, while for those with a maximum diameter of 1 cm, 1/4 of them can still have extracapsular invasion.
5. MRI signal features of metastatic lymph nodes: T_1-weighted signals are mostly medium and low, and T_2-weighted signals are mostly medium and high, and the signals can be uniform or non-uniform. The necrotic area of tumor in lymph nodes often presents T_1- and T_2-weighted heterogeneous signals. The T_2-weighting for metastatic lymph nodes usually presents medium and high signals, which is significantly different from surrounding muscles, indicating that lymph nodes in the retropharyngeal group are more advantageous than those in CT. With cystic degeneration in metastatic lymph nodes of papillary thyroid carcinoma, those with high content of internal globulin present high T_1- and T_2-weighted signals, while those with low content are similar to cyst signals.
6. FDG uptake characteristics of metastatic lymph nodes: There are limitations in judging properties of lymph node solely based on morphological basis. ^{18}F-FDG PET/CT mainly takes metabolic changes of lymph nodes as the diagnostic basis, which can help to detect involvement of unenlarged lymph nodes. Metastatic lymph nodes in the neck usually show high uptake of FDG. Due to differences in pathological types of the primary tumor, some metastatic lymph nodes show low uptake or no uptake. For those with necrotic lymph nodes, the necrotic area presents relatively low uptake or no uptake. Metabolic changes in metastatic lymph nodes after treatment may be used to indicate therapeutic efficacy, which is often earlier than morphological changes. However, cervical lymph nodes often present different degrees of physiological uptake. High uptake of FDG also shows in benign lymph node hyperplasia and lymphadenitis, while the distribution is usually symmetrical. However, when lymph nodes show with asymmetric increased uptake, with or without abnormal anatomical changes, it needs to be alert for metastatic lymph nodes.

3 Typical Cases

Case 1: A 60-year-old female patient had low-differentiated squamous cell carcinoma of the right maxillary gingiva. No other treatment was performed 5 months after the operation. A right neck mass was found half a month ago, gradually increasing. PET/CT images showed that a 2.0 cm short lymph node with FDG increased metabolic uniformity (SUVmax was 28.0) in region II of the right neck, which was considered as metastatic lymph node. After "lymph node dissection on the right omohyoid," 2.5 cm lymph nodes behind the right mandibular angle were found during the operation, and pathological findings showed squamous cell carcinoma metastasis in lymph nodes (Fig. 20.1).

Case 2: A 60-year-old male patient presented with a left mandibular mass for 3 weeks. Biopsy of the mass on the left mandibular oral floor showed highly atypical hyperplasia of squamous epithelial mucosa and partial cancerism. PET/CT evaluation was conducted before treatment (Figs. 20.2 and 20.3).

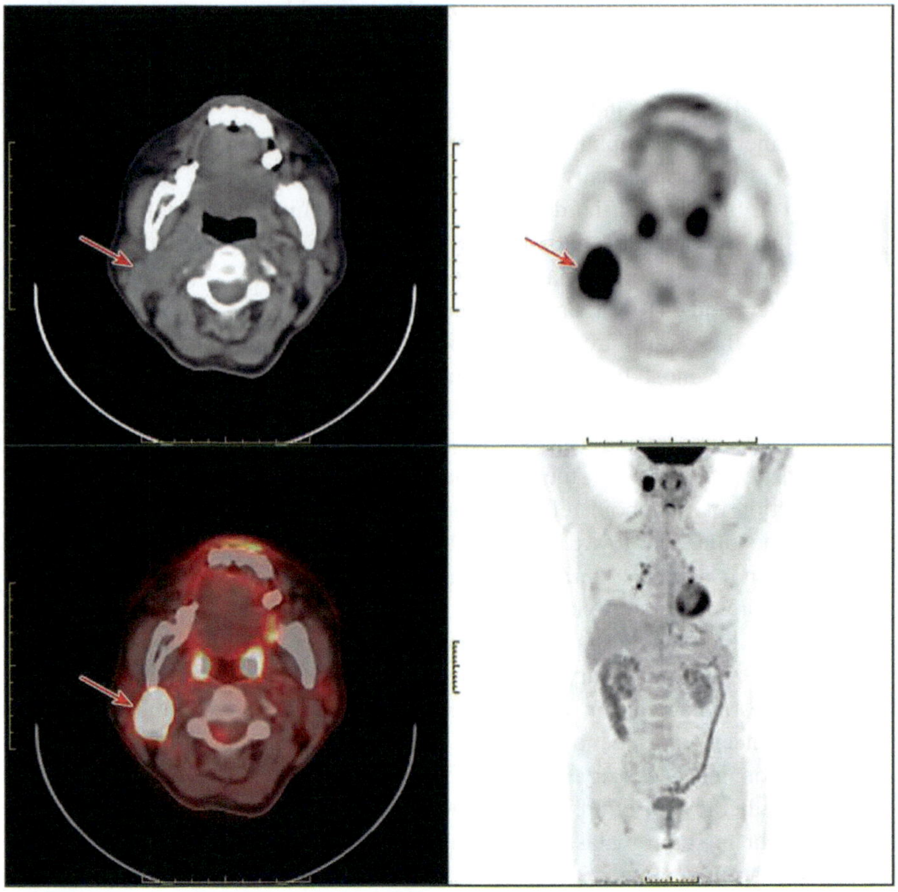

Fig. 20.1 Lymphatic metastasis in the right neck after surgery for gingival squamous cell carcinoma

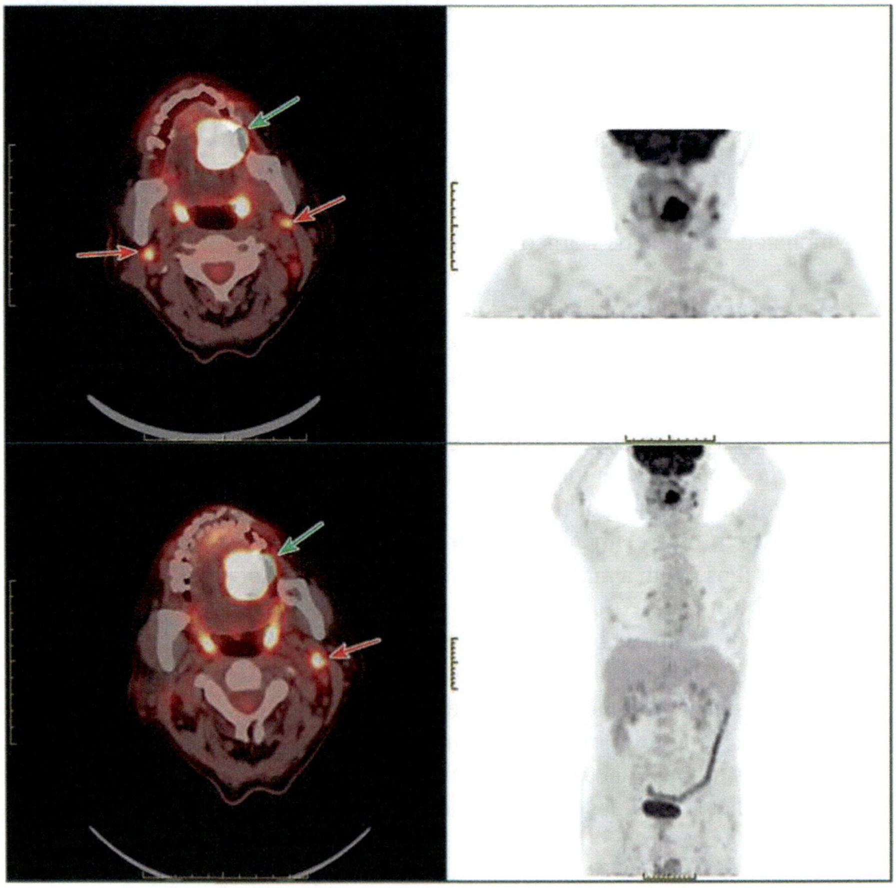

Fig. 20.2 Oral bottom squamous cell carcinoma with bilateral cervical lymphatic metastasis. PET/CT images showed a mass at the bottom of the mouth (left side of the lower margin of the tongue) with abnormal increased FDG uptake, which was considered as malignant lesion (green arrow). Multiple lymph nodes in region I of both sides of the neck indicated increased FDG uptake (larger ones with a short diameter of 0.8 cm with SUVmax of 11.1), which were considered as multiple metastatic lymph nodes (red arrow)

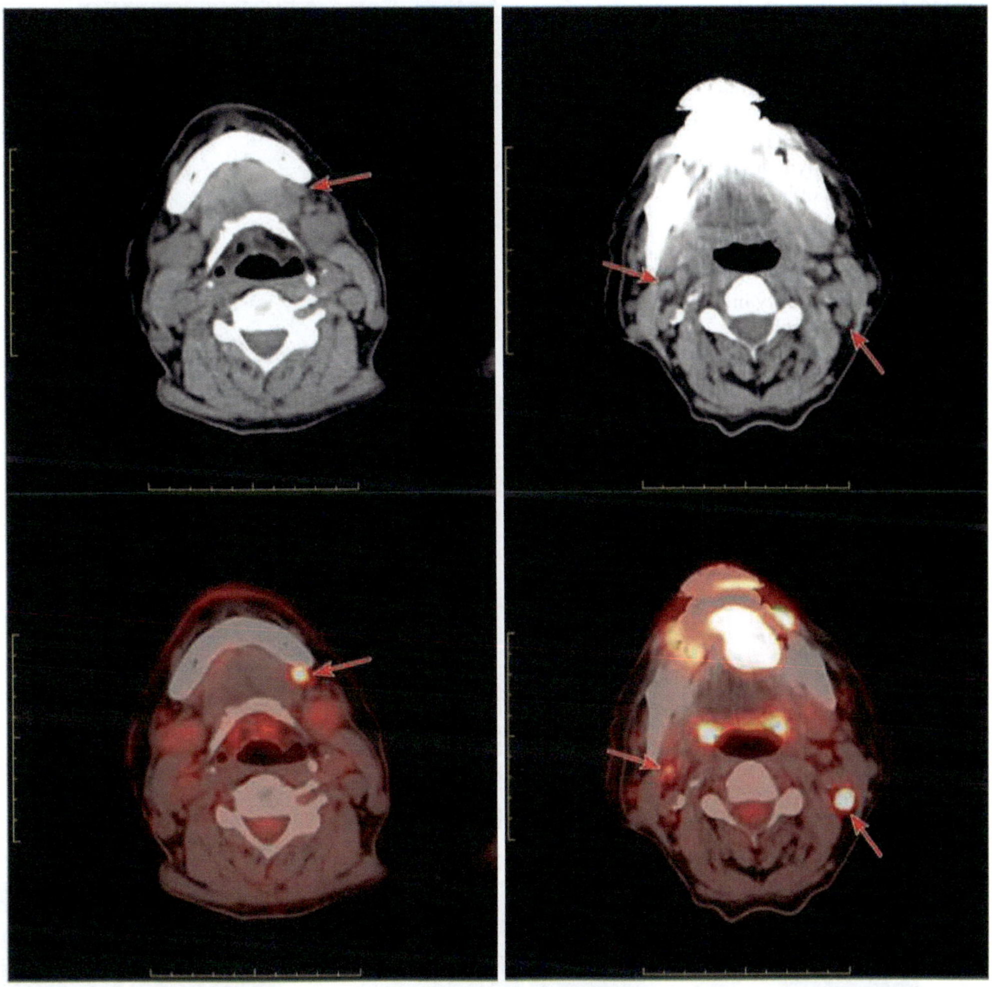

Fig. 20.3 Squamous cell carcinoma at the oral bottom with bilateral cervical lymphatic metastasis. PET/CT images showed increased FDG uptake in multiple lymph nodes in region I of the left neck and region II of both sides of the neck (with short diameter of 0.8 cm and SUVmax of 11.1 in the larger group), which was considered as multiple metastatic lymph nodes. The clinical stage was $T_2N_2M_0$ and IVa stage. After one course of induced chemotherapy was given first, the mass at the bottom of the mouth was significantly reduced, followed by radical radiotherapy

Case 3: A 63-year-old male patient was diagnosed with non-keratinized low-differentiated carcinoma of the nasopharynx with pharyngorhinoscopy and was evaluated by PET/CT images before treatment (Figs. 20.4 and 20.5).

Case 4: A 32-year-old female presented with poorly differentiated squamous cell carcinoma of the nasopharynx (Figs. 20.6 and 20.7).

Case 5: A 73-year-old male patient presented, 1 month after laryngeal cancer surgery (total laryngectomy), with the images showing moderately to poorly differentiated squamous cell carcinoma which invaded the outer membrane, and abnormal cell masses were observed in the lamella propria of the upper resection margin. The pathological stage was $pT_2N_0M_0$, stage II. PET/CT evaluation was performed before radiotherapy (Figs. 20.8 and 20.9).

Case 6: A 55-year-old male presented with laryngoscopy showing two new organisms in the right arytenoid region and the right pyriform pit, and the pathology showed squamous cell carcinoma. PET/CT evaluation was performed prior to the treatment (Fig. 20.10).

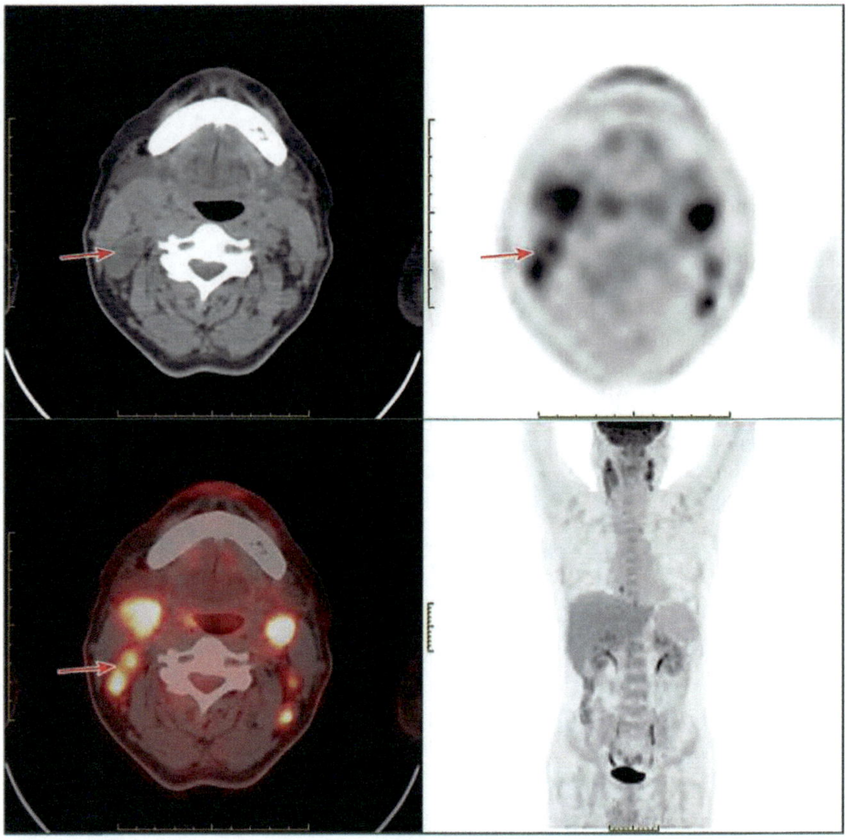

Fig. 20.4 Nasopharyngeal carcinoma with multiple lymphatic metastases on both sides of the neck, with partial necrosis PET/CT images showing increased FDG uptake in multiple lymph nodes in region II of both sides of the neck, which was considered as multiple metastatic lymph nodes. Among them, the density in the center of one lymph node in the right neck (as shown in the arrow) was reduced (necrosis), and FDG uptake in the necrotic area was lower than that in the surrounding area (short diameter of 1.3 cm with SUVmax of 6.4)

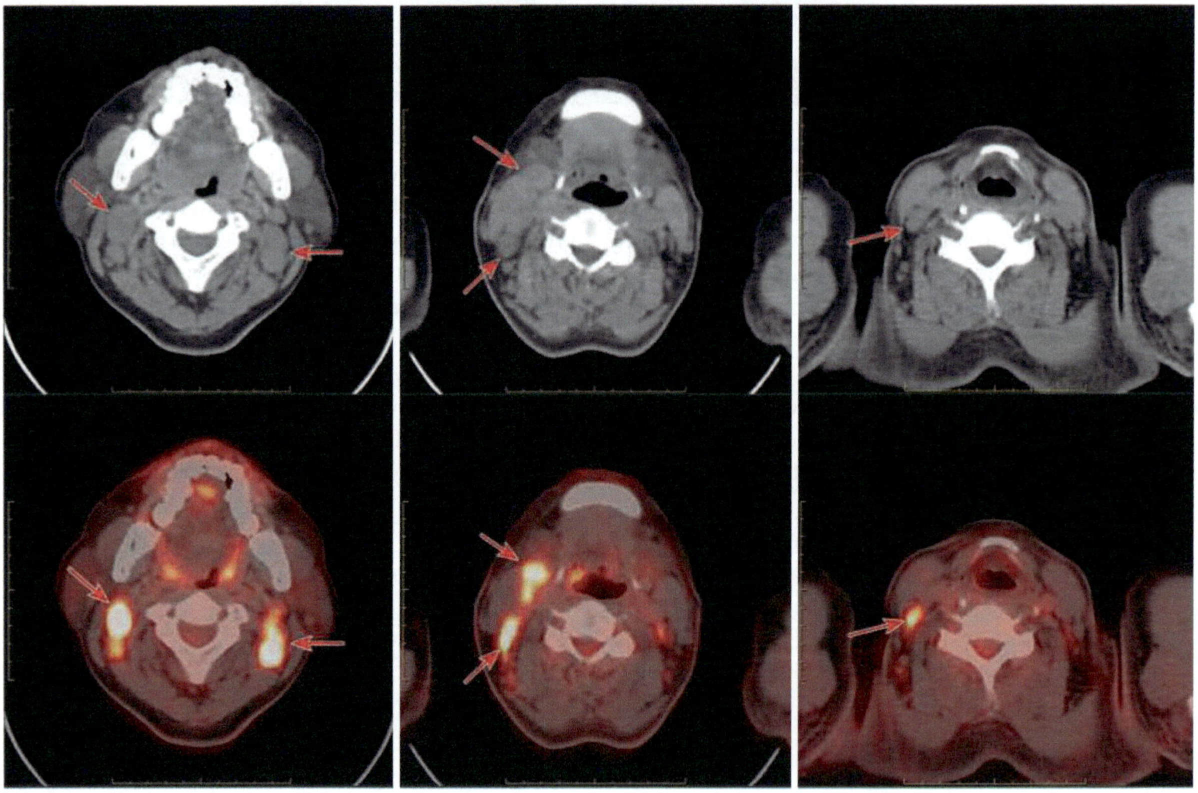

Fig. 20.5 Nasopharyngeal carcinoma with multiple lymphatic metastases on both sides of the neck. PET/CT images showed increased FDG uptake in multiple lymph nodes in II–V regions on both sides of the neck (the larger one with short diameter of 2.4 cm and SUVmax of 10.9), and the lymph node density was equal to or slightly lower than the surrounding muscles, which was considered as multiple metastatic lymph nodes

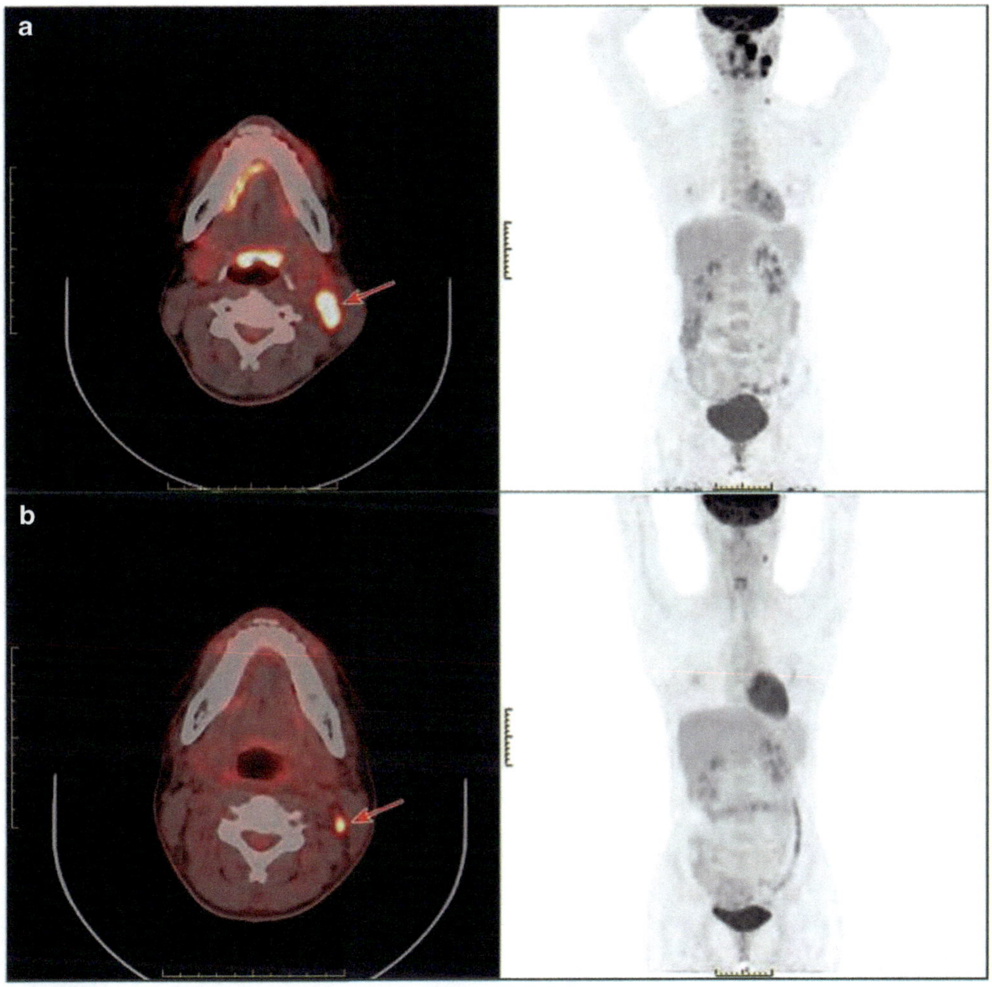

Fig. 20.6 Nasopharyngeal carcinoma with lymphatic metastasis in the left neck (PET/CT evaluation before and after treatment). (**a**) PET/CT evaluation before treatment showed increased FDG uptake (short diameter, 1.3 cm; SUVmax, 13.1) of enlarged lymph nodes in region III of the left neck, with the clinical stage of $cT_2N_3M_0$, IVa stage. The patient underwent two courses of induced chemotherapy, one course of radical radiotherapy, and synchronous molecular targeted therapy. (**b**) PET/CT performed 4 months after the end of treatment showed reduced lymph nodes in region III of the left neck and decreased FDG uptake (short diameter, 0.6 cm; SUVmax, 5.6)

Case 7: A 53-year-old male presented with a mass in the right neck, and puncture biopsy showed metastasis with unknown primary lesion. PET/CT images (Fig. 20.11) revealed a malignant lesion in the right aryepiglottic fold with bilateral cervical lymphatic metastasis. Total laryngectomy and cervical lymph node dissection were performed. Postoperative pathology showed poorly differentiated squamous cell carcinoma in the right lower laryngeal epiglottis invading the muscularis propria. Metastasis was seen in 4/11 lymph nodes in the right neck and 2/20 lymph nodes in the left neck.

Case 8: A 73-year-old female patient was found with a right subauricular mass. Postoperative pathology showed adenoid cystic carcinoma of the right salivary gland (parotid) (11 cm × 6 cm × 4 cm), and 1/2 of the suprahyoid lymph node (1.5–2 cm) was seen with carcinoma metastasis (Fig. 20.12).

Case 9: A 36-year-old male patient presented with left parotid carcinoma after surgery, after chemoradiotherapy, and after local recurrence and metastasis (Figs. 20.13, 20.14, and 20.15).

Case 10: A 65-year-old male presented with 1 month after the operation of squamous cell carcinoma of the right submandibular gland (pathology showed nodules of right submandibular squamous cell carcinoma, involving peripheral nerve fibers and rhabdomyo tissue, and that lymphatic metastasis was seen on 10/10 of lymph node). PET/CT image evaluation was performed before radiotherapy (Fig. 20.16).

Case 11: A 56-year-old female presented with a mass resection of the right neck, and pathology showed metastatic

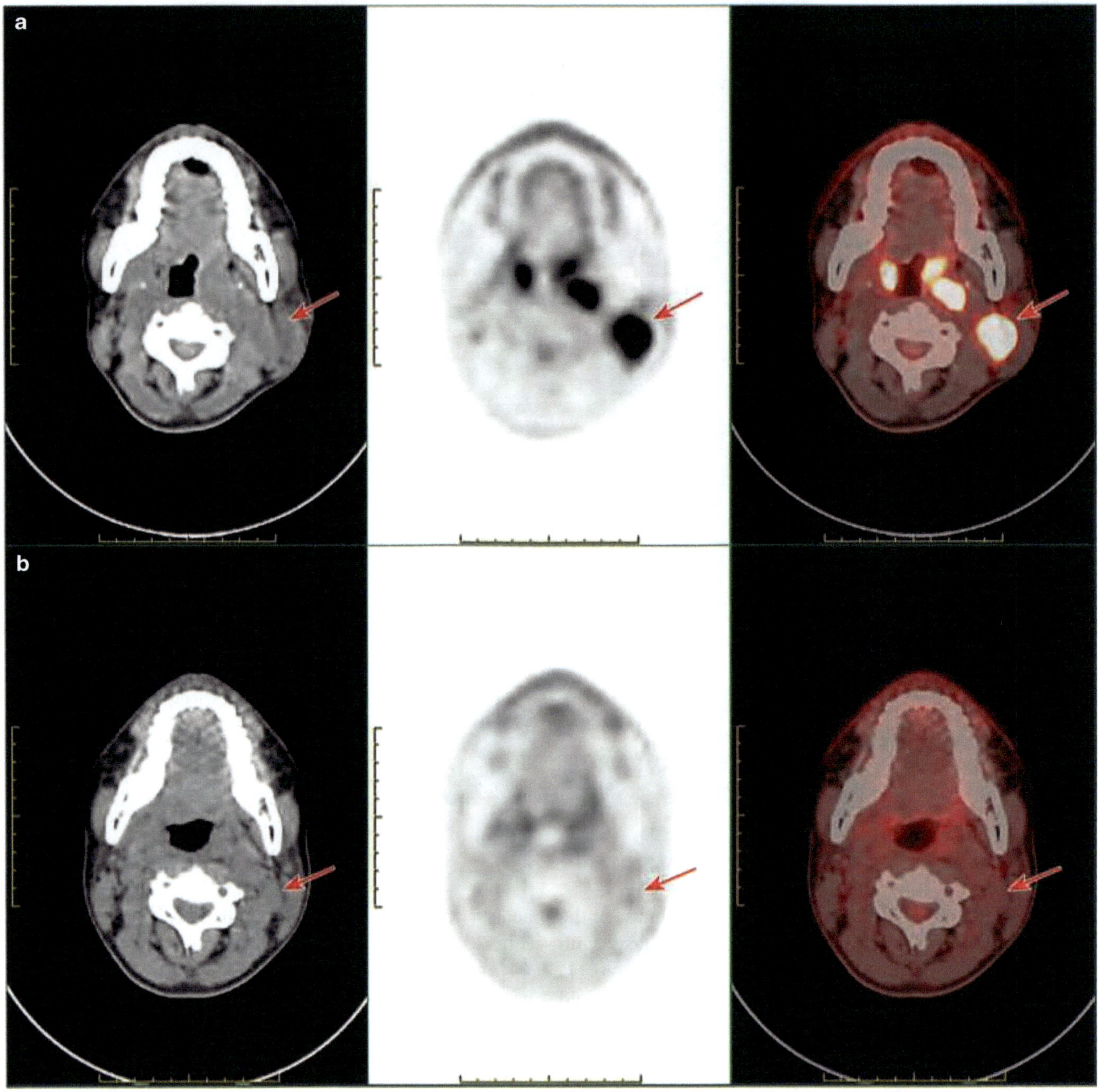

Fig. 20.7 Nasopharyngeal carcinoma with lymphatic metastasis in the left neck (PET/CT evaluation before and after treatment). (**a**) PET/CT before treatment showed increased FDG uptake in the left parapharyngeal space and lymph nodes in region II of the left neck (2.3 cm in short diameter and 22.6 in SUVmax for the larger one), with slightly lower density than the muscle and unclear boundary; (**b**) PET/CT images 4 months after the end of treatment showed that the left parapharyngeal space and lymph nodes in region II of the left neck significantly shrunk (among which, lymph nodes in region II of the left neck were 1.0 cm in short diameter), and FDG uptake decreased to be similar to that of surrounding muscles (no uptake)

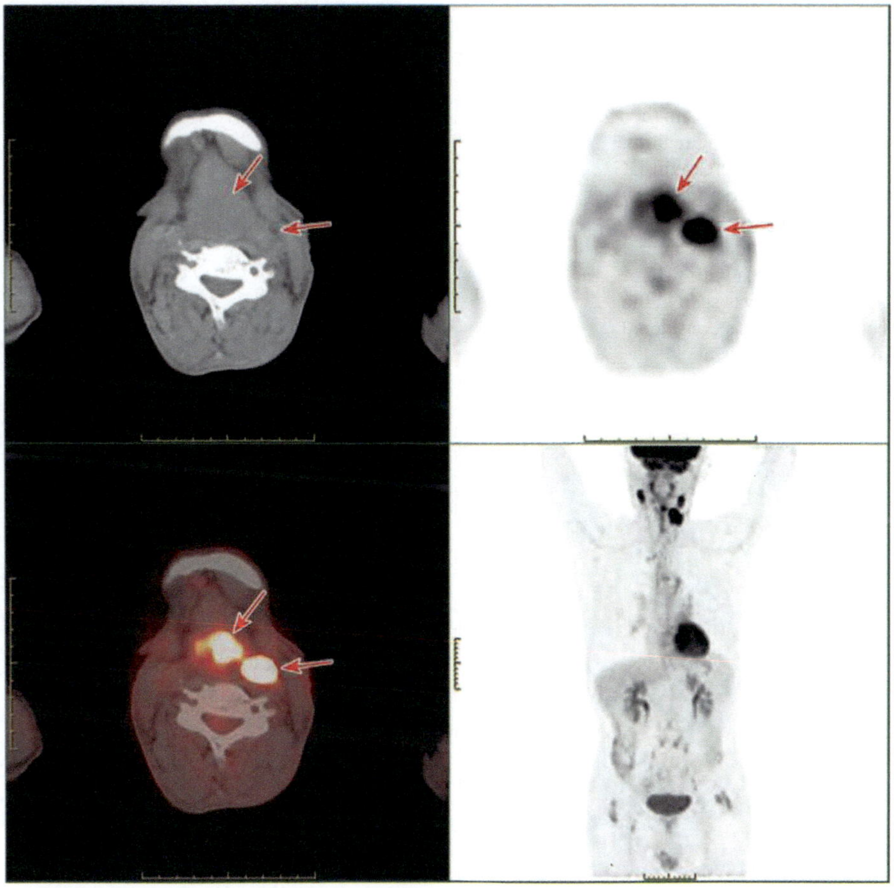

Fig. 20.8 Residual laryngeal carcinoma with lymphatic metastasis in both sides of the neck. PET/CT images showed swelling of the soft tissue in the operative area of the larynx accompanied by increased metabolism of irregular mass and patchy FDG (SUVmax was 16.6), which was considered as residual tumor tissue. Enlarged lymph nodes in region III area of the left neck showed increased FDG uptake (1.7 cm in short diameter, 37.5 in SUVmax), with similar density to surrounding soft tissues, and with unclear boundary with the lesion in the operative area of the larynx, which was considered as metastatic lymph nodes

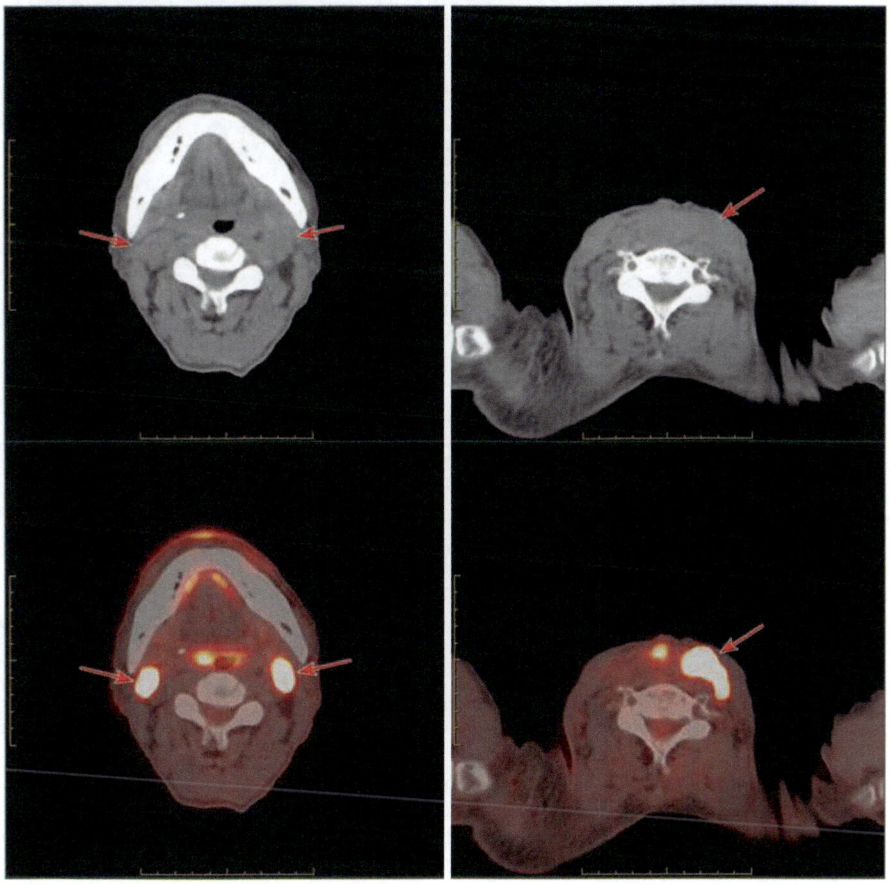

Fig. 20.9 Bilateral cervical lymphatic metastasis after laryngeal cancer surgery. PET/CT images showed multiple enlarged lymph nodes in region II of the neck and region IV of the left neck on both sides with increased FDG uptake, which had similar density with the surrounding soft tissues, whose boundary was unclear, with mutual fusion (the larger one with a short diameter of 1.3 cm and SUVmax of 24.6), so that they were considered as multiple metastatic lymph nodes. Both lungs were also found to be metastatic by PET/CT, so the clinical stage was changed to $cT_2N_2M_1$ and palliative radiotherapy was given

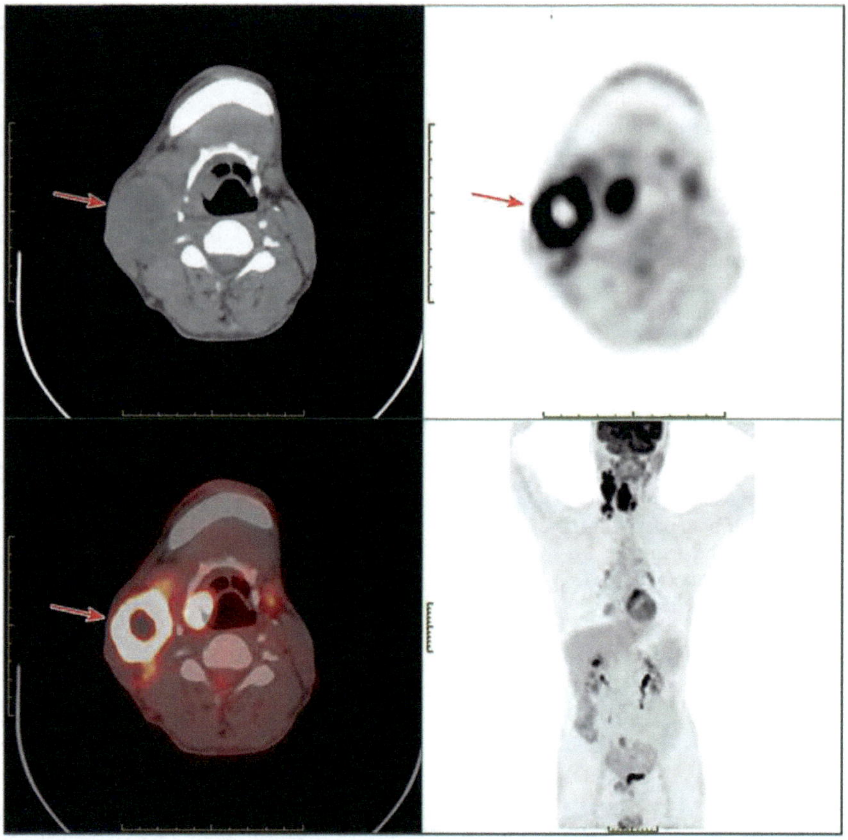

Fig. 20.10 Laryngeal carcinoma with lymphatic metastasis in the right neck. In PET/CT images (arrow), enlarged lymph nodes in the right neck (involving regions II–IV) showed increased FDG uptake ring (3.5 cm in short diameter, 26.5 of SUVmax), with clear boundary. Circular low-density area with FDG uptake defect was seen in the center, which was considered as central necrosis of metastatic lymph nodes

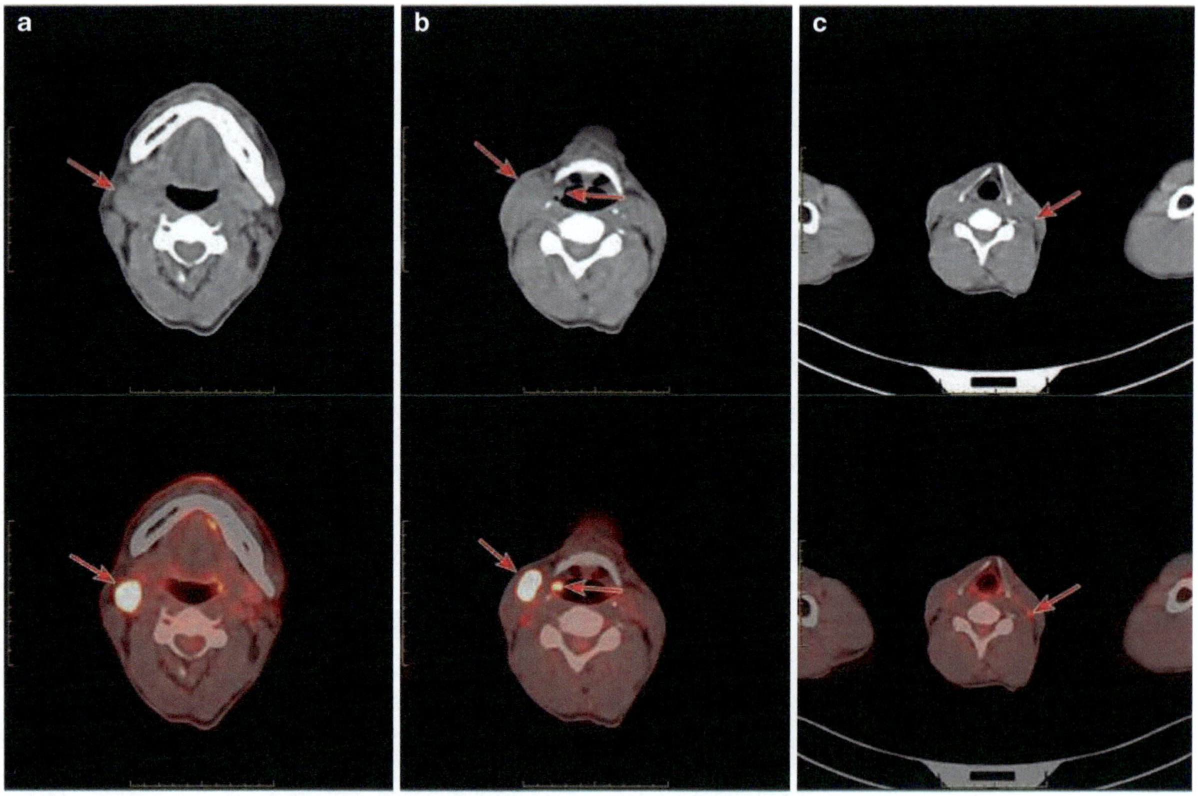

Fig. 20.11 Squamous cell carcinoma in the throat epiglottis with bilateral cervical lymphatic metastasis. (**a**) Increased FDG uptake in the lymph nodes in region II of the right neck (short diameter, 1.8 cm; SUVmax, 17.3). (**b**) Focal FDG uptake of the right aryepiglottic fold increased (diameter, 1.1 cm; SUVmax, 12.9), and FDG uptake of region III in lymph nodes increased (short diameter, 2.0 cm; SUVmax, 24.7). (**c**) FDG uptake in region IV in lymph nodes in the left neck increased (short diameter, 0.8 cm; SUVmax, 3.8)

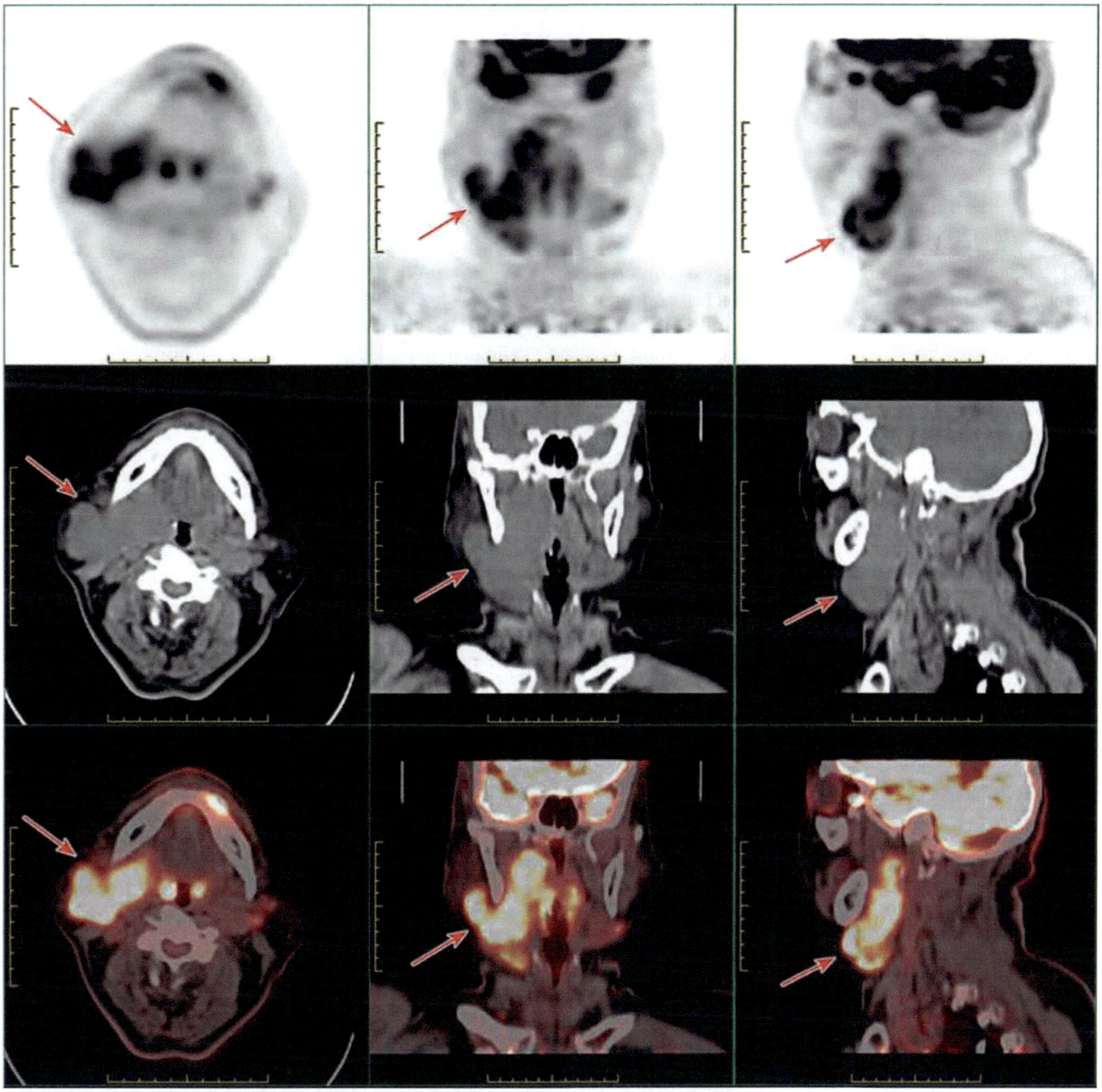

Fig. 20.12 Adenoid cystic carcinoma in the right parotid gland with right suprahyoid lymphatic metastasis on the right hyoid. Parotid origin tumor was considered in CT image. PET/CT images showed increased FDG uptake in the shadow of irregular soft tissue of the right parotid gland region—submandibular gland region (SUVmax was 8.6). Multiple enlarged lymph nodes from the right parapharyngeal space to the right submaxillary region showed increased FDG uptake, which were fused with unclear boundary with the above shadow of the soft tissue (the larger one had a short diameter of 2.9 cm, and SUVmax was 7.4), which was considered as parotid malignant tumor with lymph node metastasis in the right neck

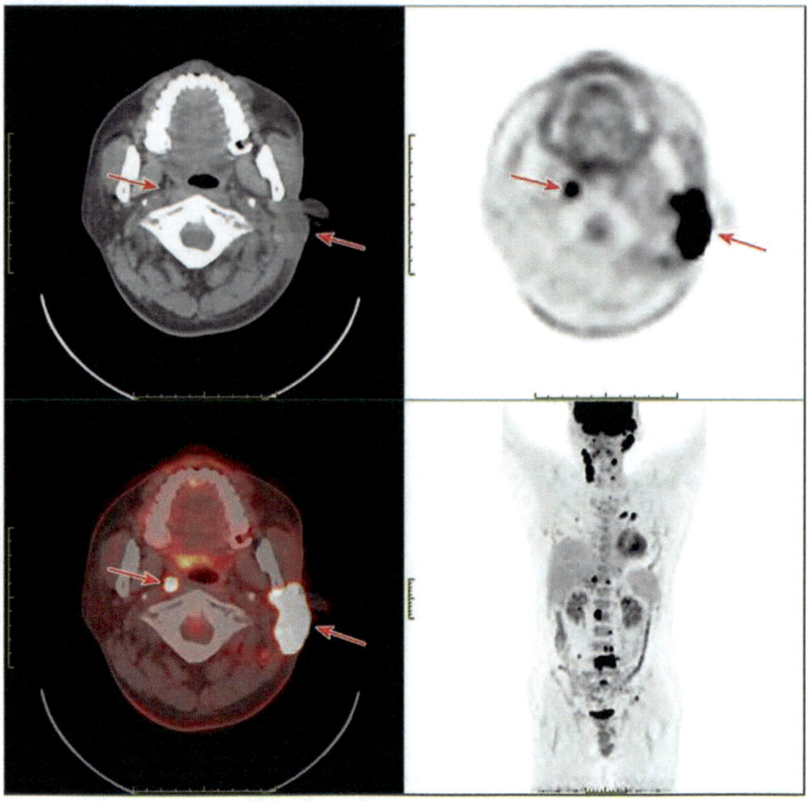

Fig. 20.13 Left parotid carcinoma recurred after treatment with cervical lymphatic metastasis. PET/CT images showed increased FDG uptake (larger cross-section, 4.8 cm × 2.1 cm; SUVmax, 50.8) in soft tissue mass of the left parotid gland, which was considered to be recurrence. Increased FDG uptake in lymph nodes in the right parapharyngeal space (0.5 cm in short diameter and 19.0 in SUVmax) was considered as metastatic lymph nodes. MIP map shows extensive systemic metastases (not shown on the fault map)

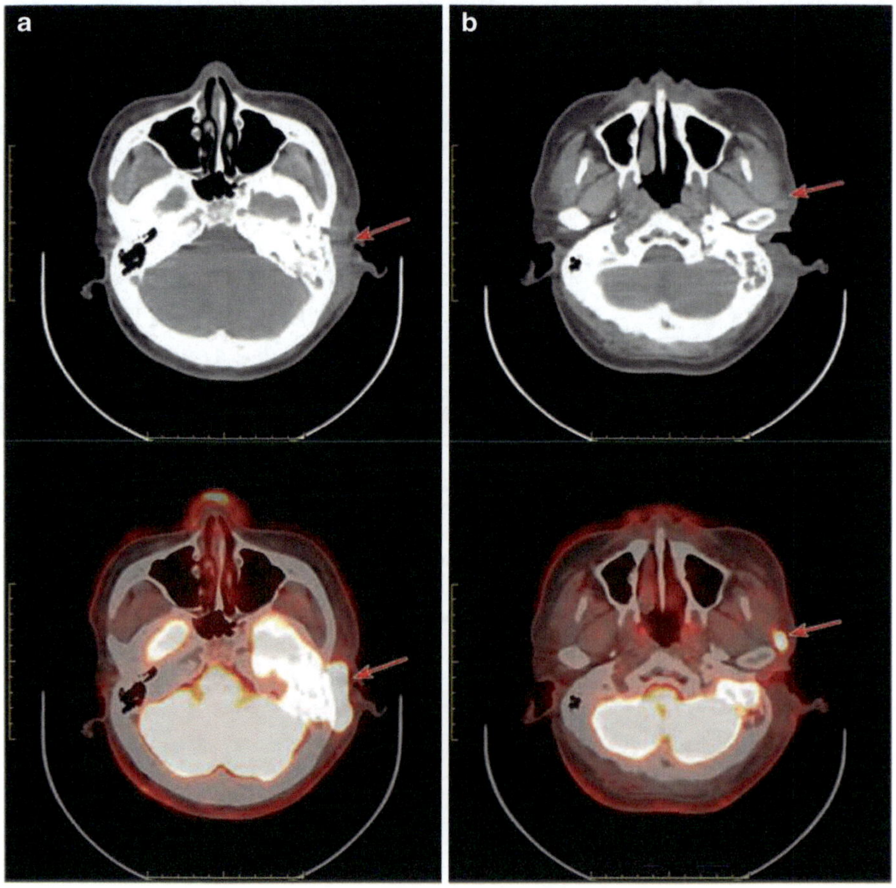

Fig. 20.14 Recurrence of left parotid carcinoma and metastasis of the left external auditory canal and cervical lymph nodes. (**a**) Increased FDG uptake (SUVmax was 42.7) in the left external auditory canal—mastoid soft tissue mass, which was considered as local metastasis. (**b**) Increased FDG uptake in the left preauricular lymph nodes (0.8 cm in diameter and 12.0 in SUVmax) was considered as metastatic lymph nodes

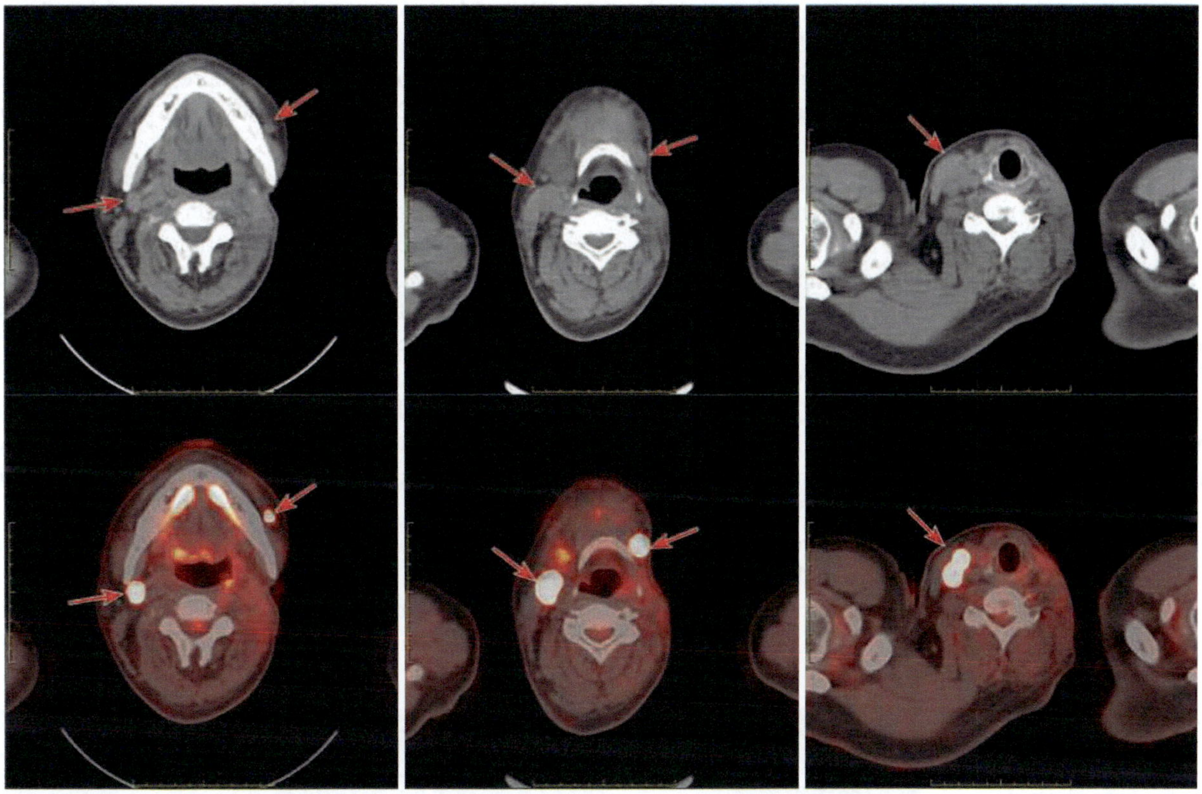

Fig. 20.15 Recurrence of left parotid carcinoma with bilateral cervical lymphatic metastasis. PET/CT images showed increased FDG uptake in multiple lymph nodes in regions II–IV of the right neck and region I of the left neck (the larger one with short diameter of 1.5 cm and SUVmax of 52.0), which was considered as multiple lymphatic metastasis

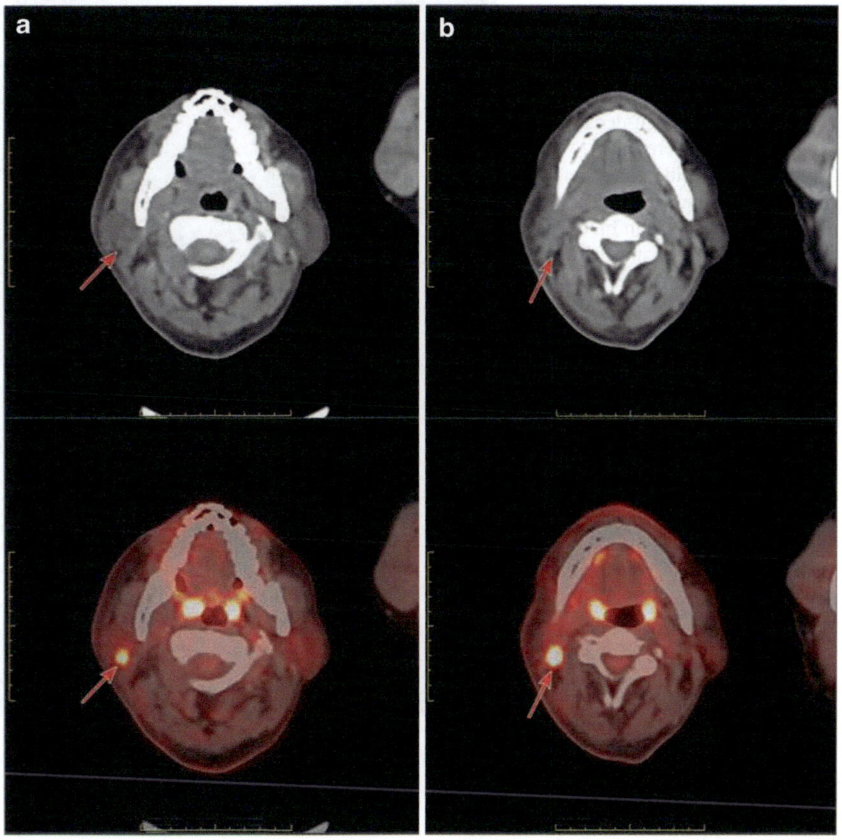

Fig. 20.16 Squamous cell carcinoma of the right submandibular gland with lymphatic metastasis. (**a**) FDG uptake in the right parotid lymph node increased (short diameter, 0.7 cm; SUVmax, 5.9). (**b**) FDG uptake of lymph nodes in region II in the right neck (short diameter, 0.8 cm; SUVmax, 13.0). The above lesions were considered as multiple metastatic lymph nodes in the right neck

squamous cell carcinoma with unknown primary lesion. After PET/CT imaging (Fig. 20.17), lymph node dissection in the right neck (radical resection) and right oropharyngeal malignant tumor enlargement were performed. The pathology showed poorly differentiated squamous cell carcinoma of the tonsils at the root of the right tongue, and reactive hyperplasia of lymph nodes showed in regions I–V of the right neck (0/31).

Case 12: A 54-year-old male patient presented with squamous cell carcinoma of the bilateral maxillary sinus and squamous cell carcinoma of the left upper lip, and submental lymph node metastasis, with left nostril and right suborbital mass (Figs. 20.18 and 20.19).

Case 13: A 57-year-old male patient with elevated CEA (5.4 ng/mL) was found in physical examination. B-mode ultrasonography showed nodules in two lobes of the thyroid, and two nodules in the right lobe of the thyroid were detected by biopsy to reveal atypia cells and papillary cancer cells. Preoperative PET/CT evaluation was performed (Figs. 20.20, 20.21, and 20.22).

Case 14: A 65-year-old female presented with progressive increased calcitonin 4 months after surgery for bilateral medullary thyroid carcinoma. The result in the final examination was 3522 pg/mL and CEA was 16.62 ng/mL (Figs. 20.23 and 20.24).

Case 15: A 68-year-old female presented with ovarian cancer more than 1 year after surgery and multiple postoperative chemotherapy. Reexamination results showed a significant increase in CA125 (868.3 U/mL). PET/CT images showed FDG uptake increased in lymph nodes in region IV of the right neck (0.5 cm in short diameter and 7.2 in SUVmax), which was considered as metastatic lymph nodes. MIP showed multiple lymphatic metastases in the mediastinum, right hilum, and retroperitoneum, with extensive peritoneal metastasis and left lung metastasis (not shown in CT) (Fig. 20.25).

Case 16: A 64-year-old female patient with a left neck mass was found. Pathology of puncture biopsy showed the tendency of metastatic lymph nodes, and PET/CT was performed to find out the primary lesion (Figs. 20.26 and 20.27).

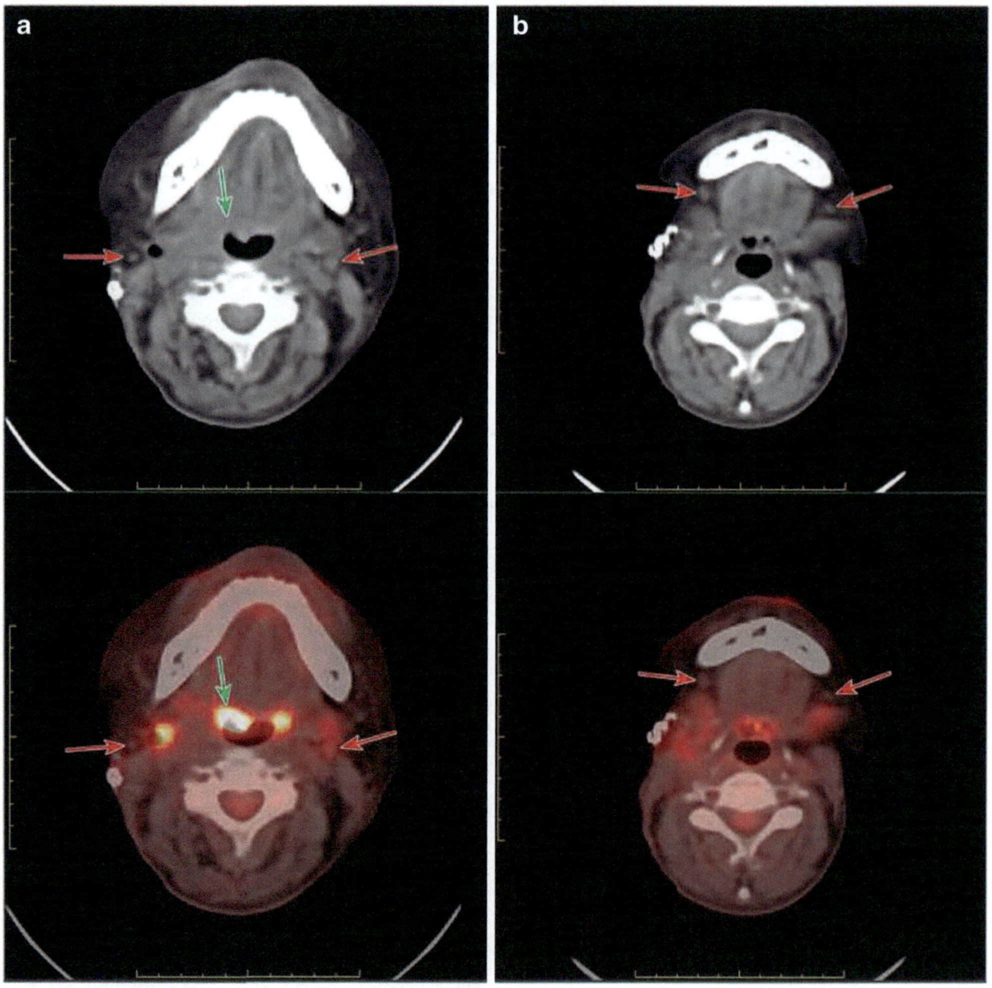

Fig. 20.17 Tonsillar squamous cell carcinoma of the base of the right tongue with reactive hyperplasia of lymph nodes in the right neck. (**a**) FDG uptake (longer diameter, 1.7 cm; SUVmax, 11.1) in the right soft tissue elevation of the oropharynx increased, which is considered as malignant lesion (green arrow); FDG uptake increased in the right cervical area (SUVmax was 5.5), and gas and high-density suture shadows were seen, which were considered as postoperative changes. There was a slight increase in FDG uptake in the lymph nodes in region IIA of the left neck (short diameter, 0.6 cm; SUVmax, 2.3). (**b**) No increase in FDG uptake was observed in small lymph nodes of both sides in region IB (short diameter: 0.5 cm). These lymph nodes were considered inflammatory lymph nodes (red arrows)

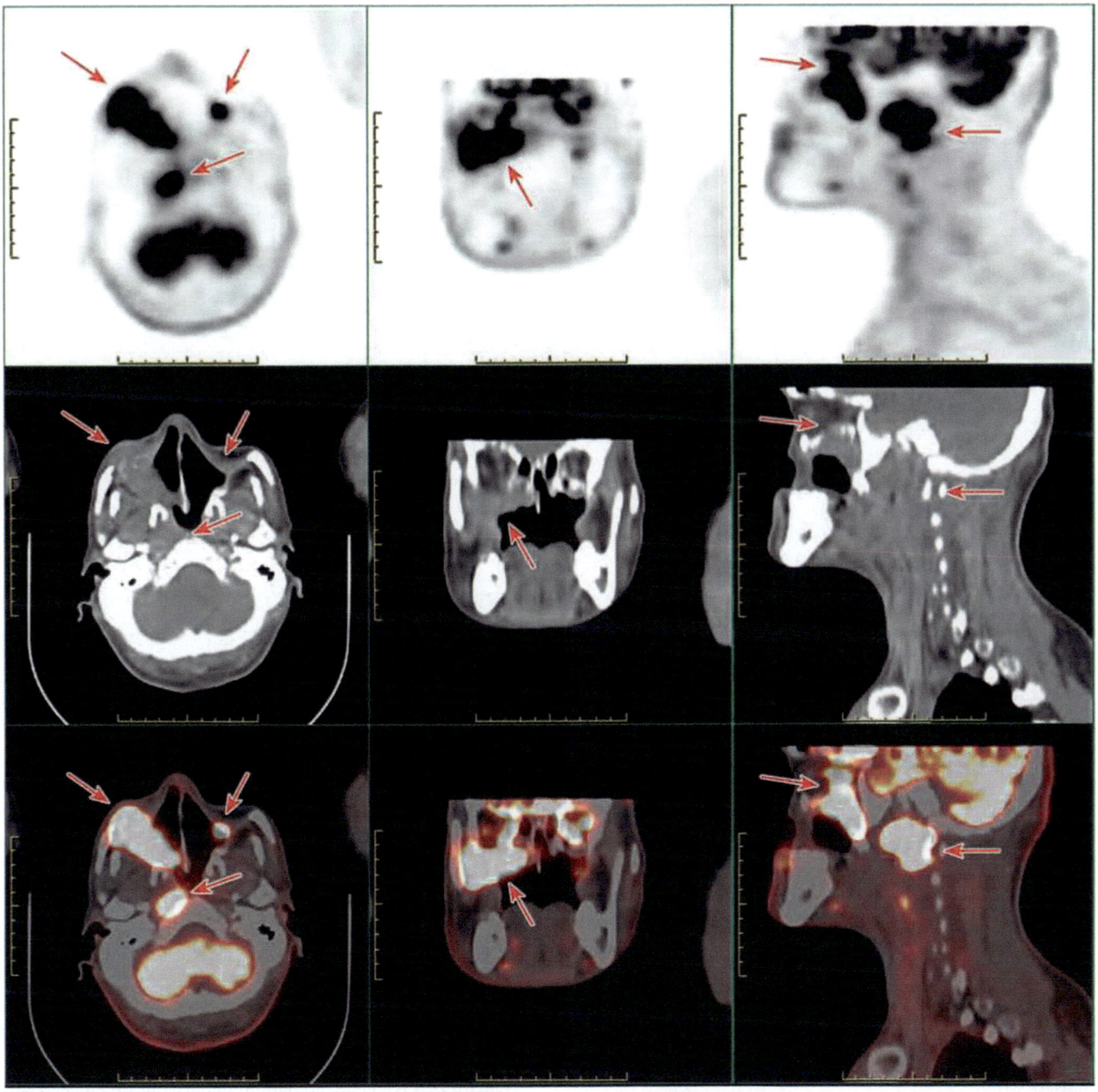

Fig. 20.18 Postoperative recurrence of squamous cell carcinoma in the bilateral maxillary sinus and left upper lip with bilateral cervical lymphatic metastasis. PET/CT images showed increased FDG uptake (SUVmax: 28.6) in both sides of the primary maxillary sinus (right side is more prominent), right maxillofacial area, and part of the ethmoid sinus, and right nasopharyngeal soft tissue mass invaded the skull and surrounding soft tissues, which were considered as recurrence of tumor accompanied by skull invasion

Case 17: A 77-year-old male patient presented with a mass in the left neck. Needle aspiration pathology revealed metastatic carcinoma with unknown primary lesion. PET/CT images showed FDG uptake increased in multiple lymph nodes in region V of the left neck (1.3 cm in diameter, 26.2 in SUVmax), which was considered as metastatic lymph nodes. MIP showed multiple abnormal increased FDG uptake in the left lung, left hilum, mediastinum, and left neck, which was considered to be malignant lesion of the left lung with multiple lymphatic metastasis (not shown on the tomography). A biopsy of the posterior upper left lung showed poorly differentiated squamous cell carcinoma (Fig. 20.28).

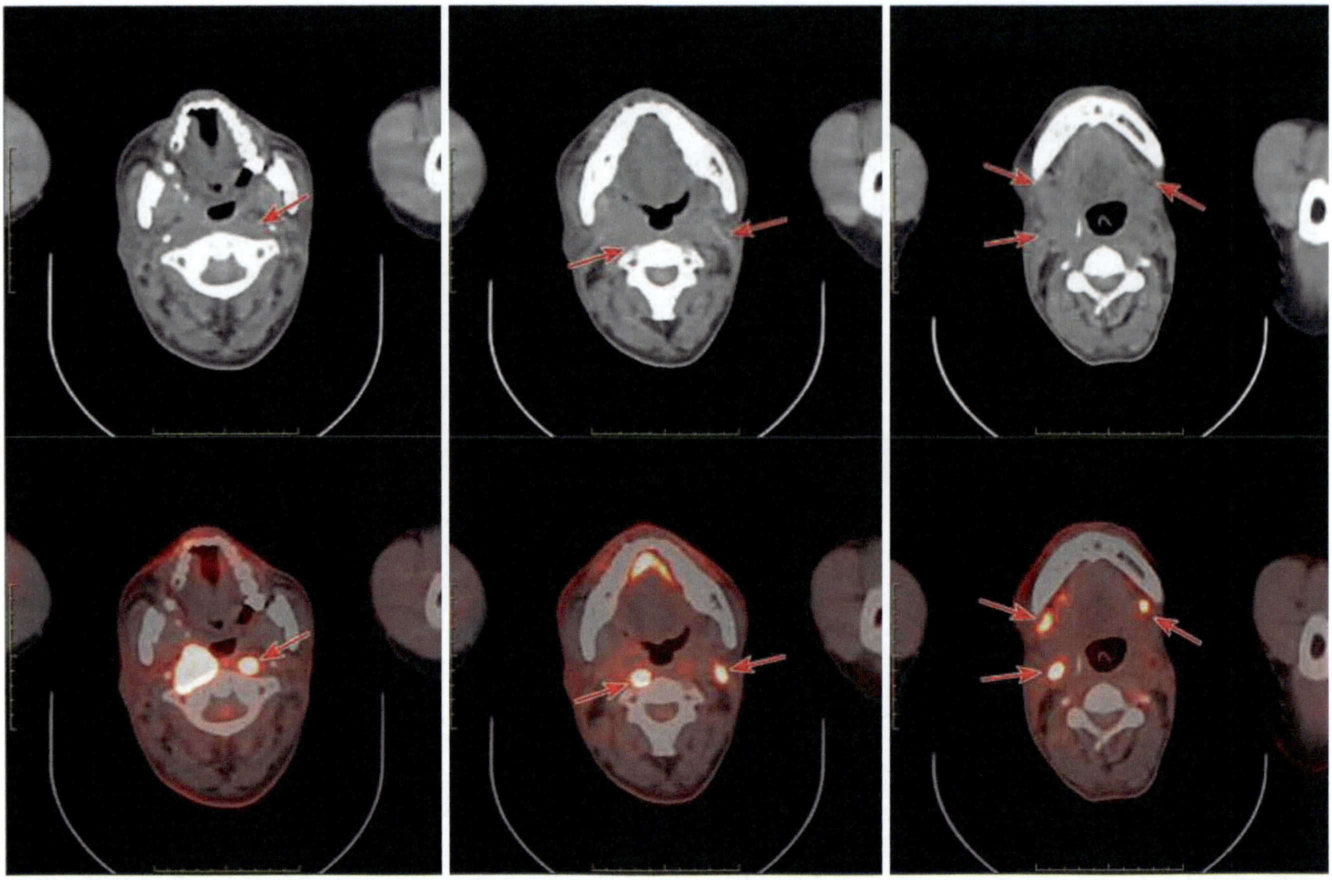

Fig. 20.19 Postoperative recurrence of squamous cell carcinoma of the bilateral maxillary sinus and left upper lip with bilateral cervical lymphatic metastasis. PET/CT images showed FDG uptake increased in multiple lymph nodes in regions IB and IIA in the bilateral retropharyngeal lymph nodes and bilateral neck (the larger one had a short diameter of 1.1 cm and SUVmax of 14.9), and the boundary between bilateral retropharyngeal lymph nodes and surrounding soft tissues was unclear, which was considered as multiple lymphatic metastasis in both sides of the neck. Adjuvant chemotherapy was followed by radiotherapy (the target region of the lymph nodes: left and right posterior pharynx, regions IB and IIA in both sides of the neck)

Case 18: A 69-year-old male patient presented with gastroscope indicating esophageal squamous cell carcinoma 20–25 cm from incisors. Biopsy of enlarged lymph nodes in the clavicle showed metastatic carcinoma, and PET/CT assessment was performed before radiotherapy (Figs. 20.29 and 20.30).

Case 19: A 65-year-old male patient underwent total gastrectomy with pathology showing ulcerative adenocarcinoma of the cardia glands, with medium-low differentiation. PET/CT evaluation was performed after the third course of chemotherapy (Fig. 20.31).

Case 20: A 70-year-old female patient presented 13 years after surgery for left breast cancer, who underwent PET/CT examination for neck mass due to hoarseness (Fig. 20.32).

Case 21: A 61-year-old patient underwent PET/CT examination due to "left shoulder mass" (Fig. 20.33). Pathology of mass puncture in the left shoulder showed thyroid carcinoma metastasis; thyroid surgery was pathologically confirmed as left lobe follicular carcinoma.

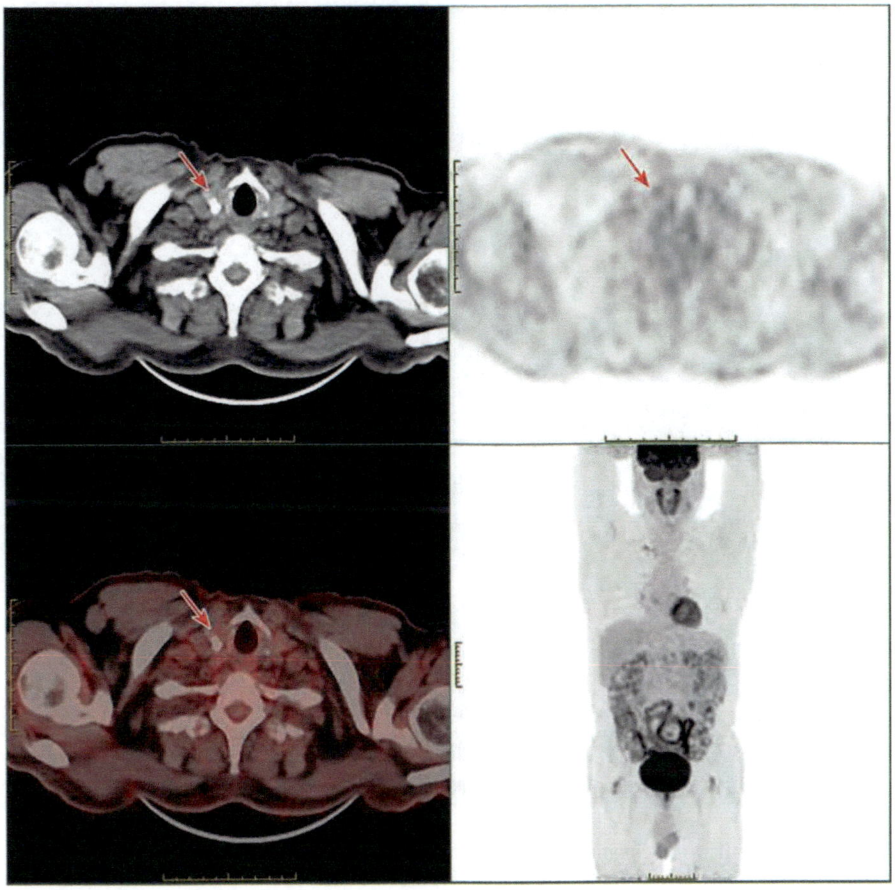

Fig. 20.20 Papillary carcinoma of both thyroid lobes accompanied with lymphatic metastasis in the right neck. No abnormal rise in FDG uptake was seen in the thyroid, and multiple thick calcifications were observed in the right lobe (arrow). Postoperative pathology confirmed bilateral papillary thyroid carcinoma

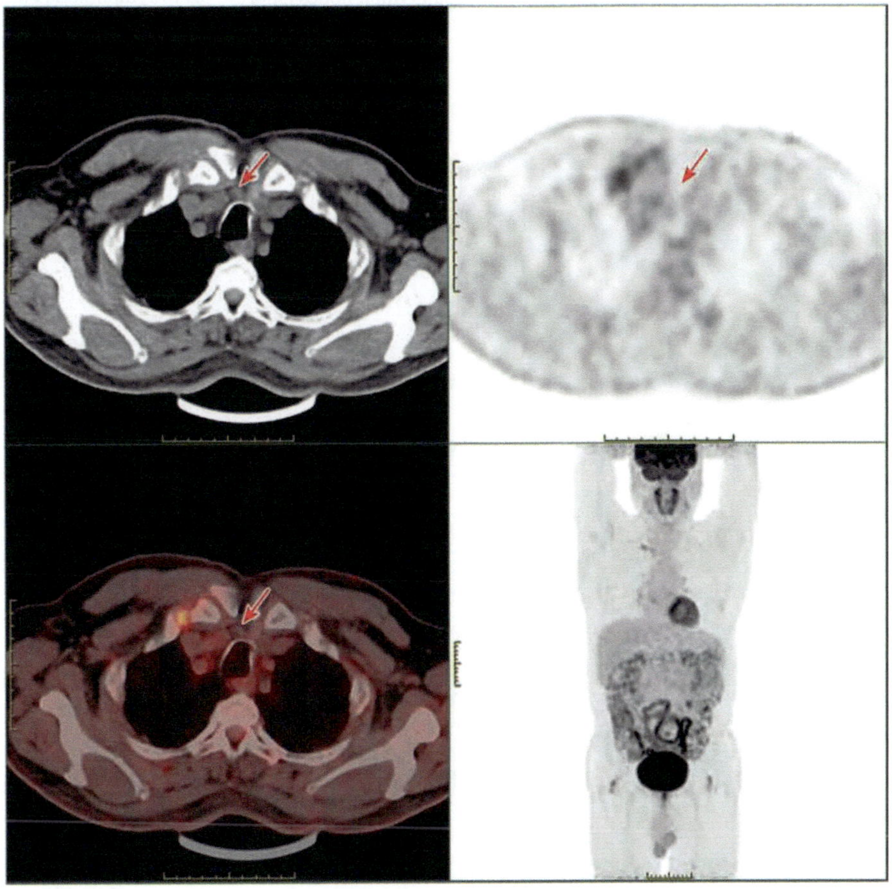

Fig. 20.21 Papillary carcinoma of both thyroid lobes accompanied with lymphatic metastasis in the right neck. Preoperative PET/CT assessment: No rise in FDG uptake was seen in the right anterior tracheal lymph nodes (region VI) (short diameter: 0.8 cm). Cervical lymph node dissection was performed later (right regions II–VI, left VI area), and pathology showed carcinoma metastasis in the right central lymph node (9/10)

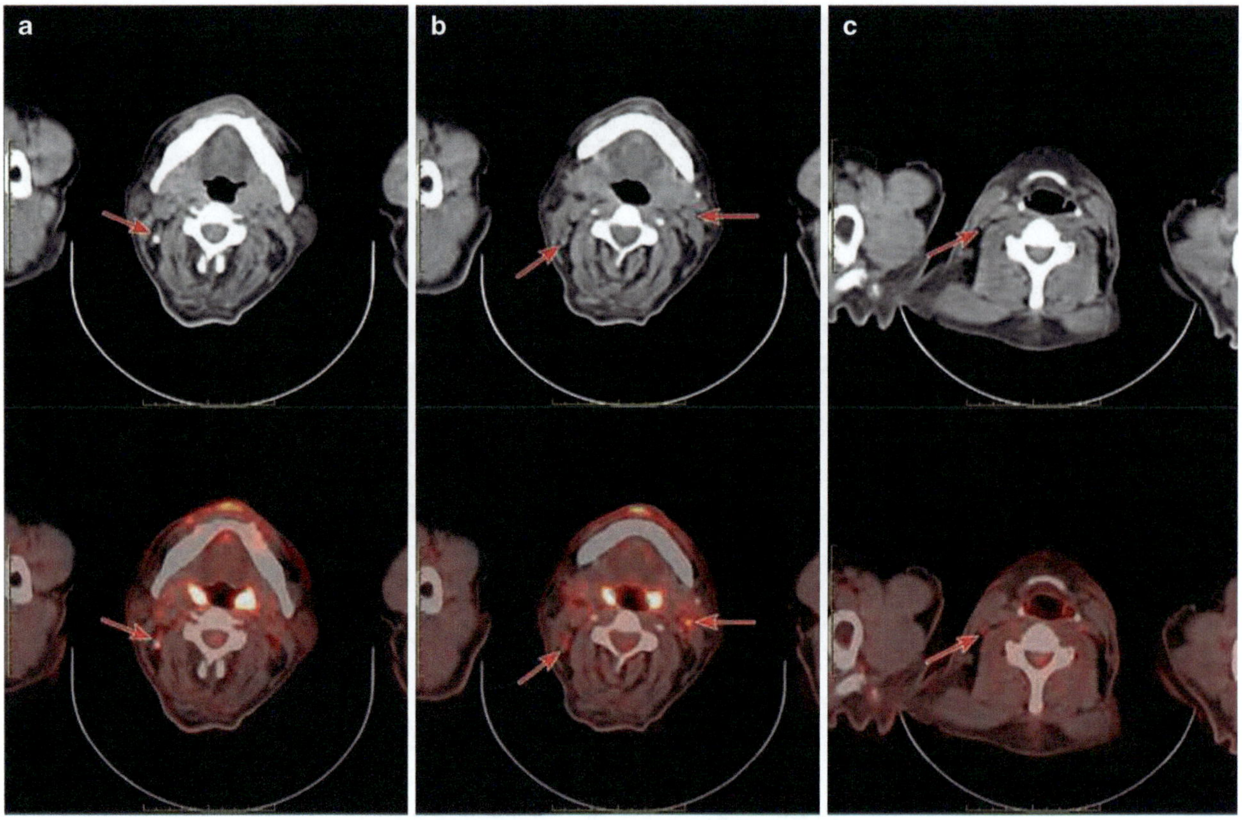

Fig. 20.22 Papillary carcinoma of both thyroid lobes accompanied with lymphatic metastasis from the right neck. Figure **a–c** showed that there was a slight increase in FDG uptake in regions II–III in the right neck and region II in the left neck scattered in small lymph nodes (short diameter, 0.3–0.6 cm; SUVmax, 2.1), in which there was a lymph node with calcification in region II of the right neck (as shown in Figure **a**). Cervical lymph node dissection was performed later (right regions II–VI and region VI on the left). Postoperative pathology showed metastasis to lymph nodes in 9/10 of the right central region, 5/11 of the right neck (II–V regions), and 0/7 of the left central region

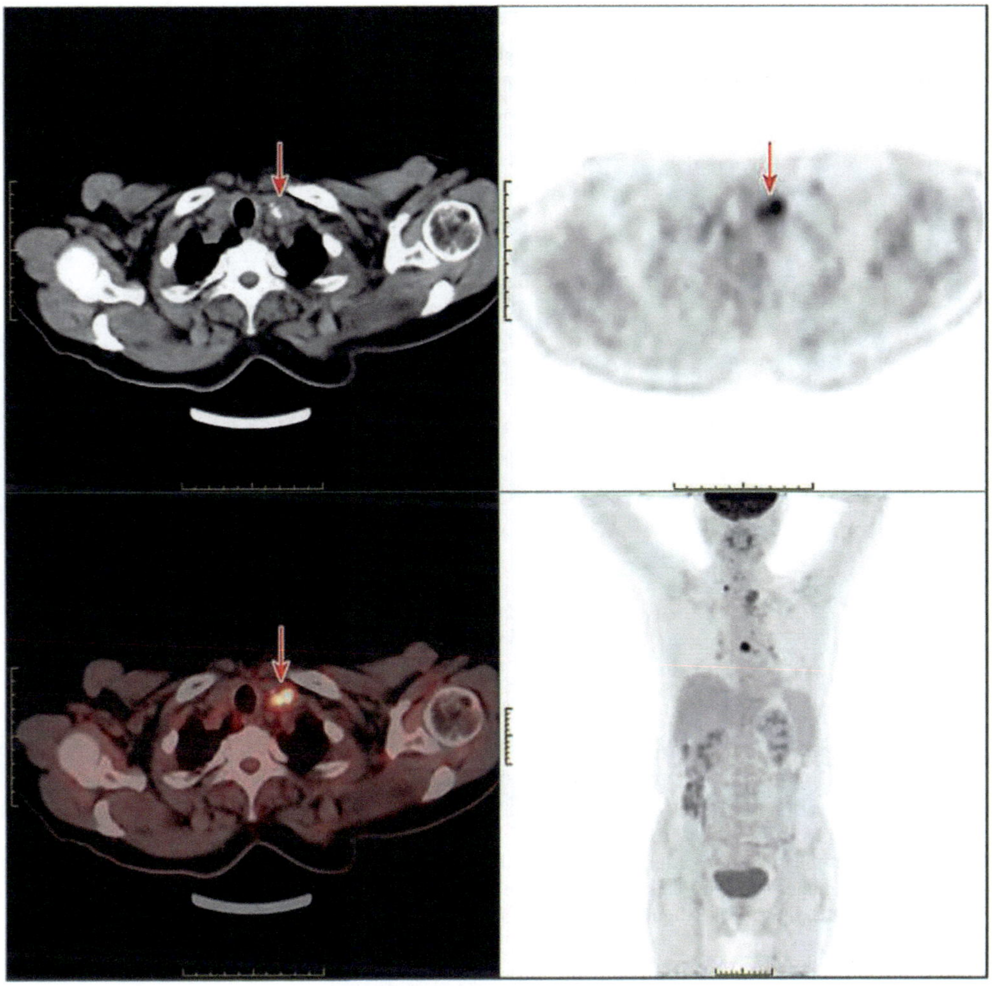

Fig. 20.23 Lymphatic metastasis in the left clavicle area after surgery for bilateral medullary thyroid carcinoma. PET/CT images showed FDG uptake increased in enlarged lymph nodes in the left clavicle (short diameter, 1.5 cm; SUVmax, 10.7), accompanied with irregular calcification, which was considered as lymphatic metastasis

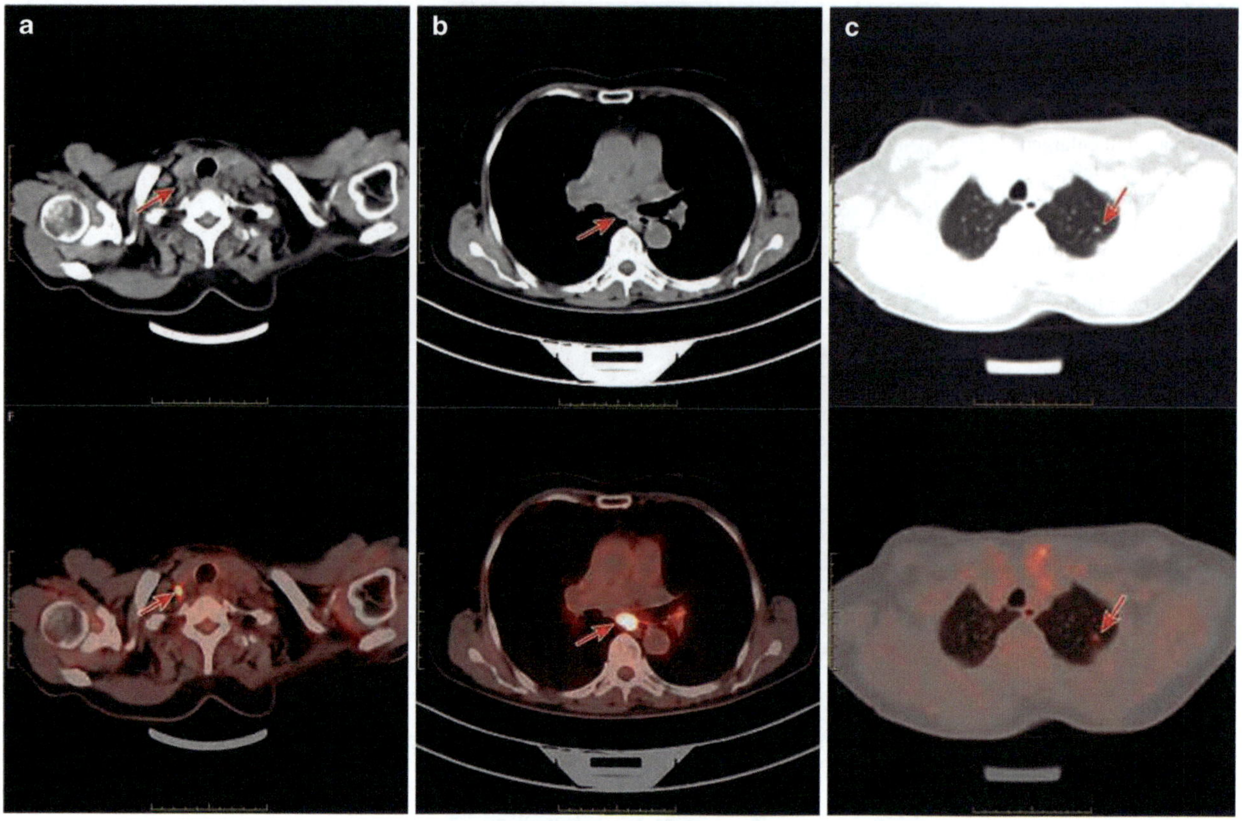

Fig. 20.24 Multiple metastases after bilateral medullary thyroid carcinoma. PET/CT images showed FDG uptake increased in lymph nodes in region IV in the right neck (Figure **a**), the lymph nodes under the mediastinal carina (Figure **b**), and the small nodules in the left lung (Figure **c**), which were considered as multiple metastasis

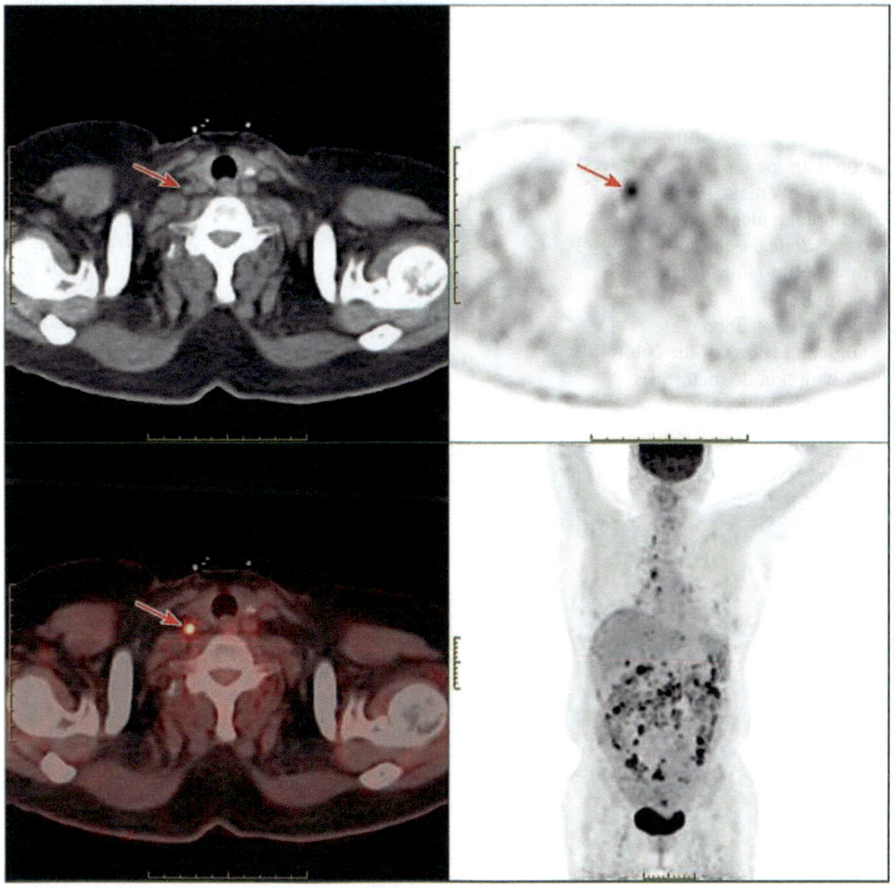

Fig. 20.25 Right cervical lymphatic metastasis after surgery and chemotherapy for ovarian cancer

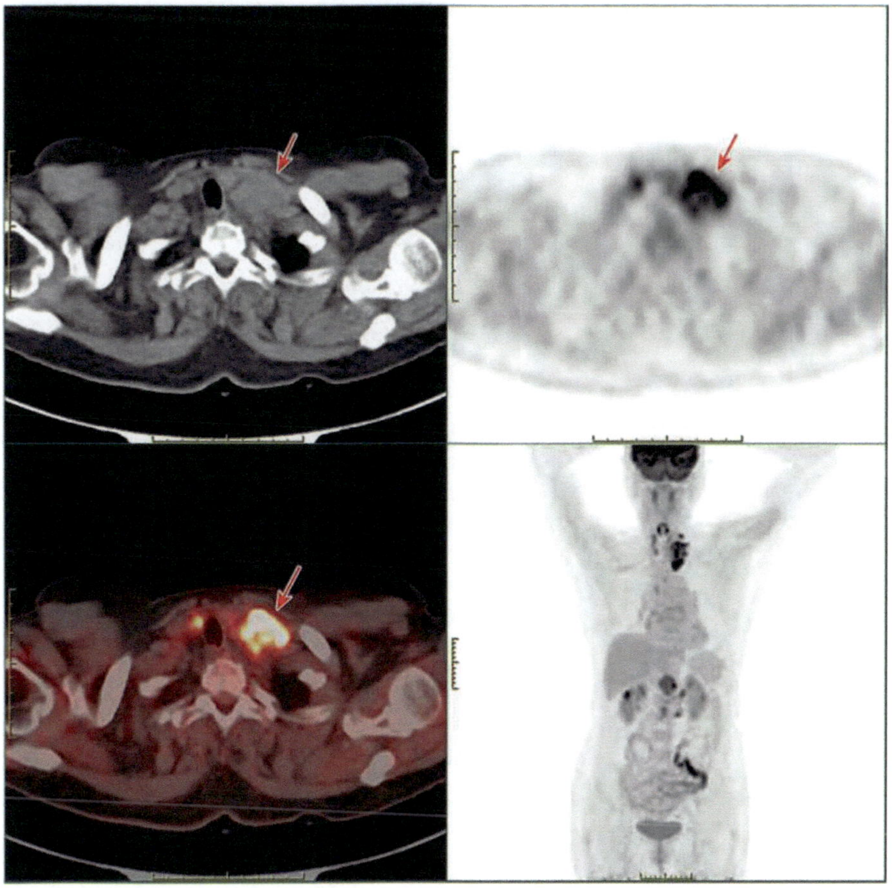

Fig. 20.26 Transverse colon cancer with lymphatic metastasis in the left clavicle area. PET/CT images (arrow) showed multiple lymph nodes in the left clavicle with increased FDG uptake characterized with inhomogeneous increase and partial fusion (the larger one with a short diameter of 3.3 cm, and SUVmax was 20.0), and the trachea was slightly shifted to the right due to slight pressure, which was considered as metastatic lymph nodes

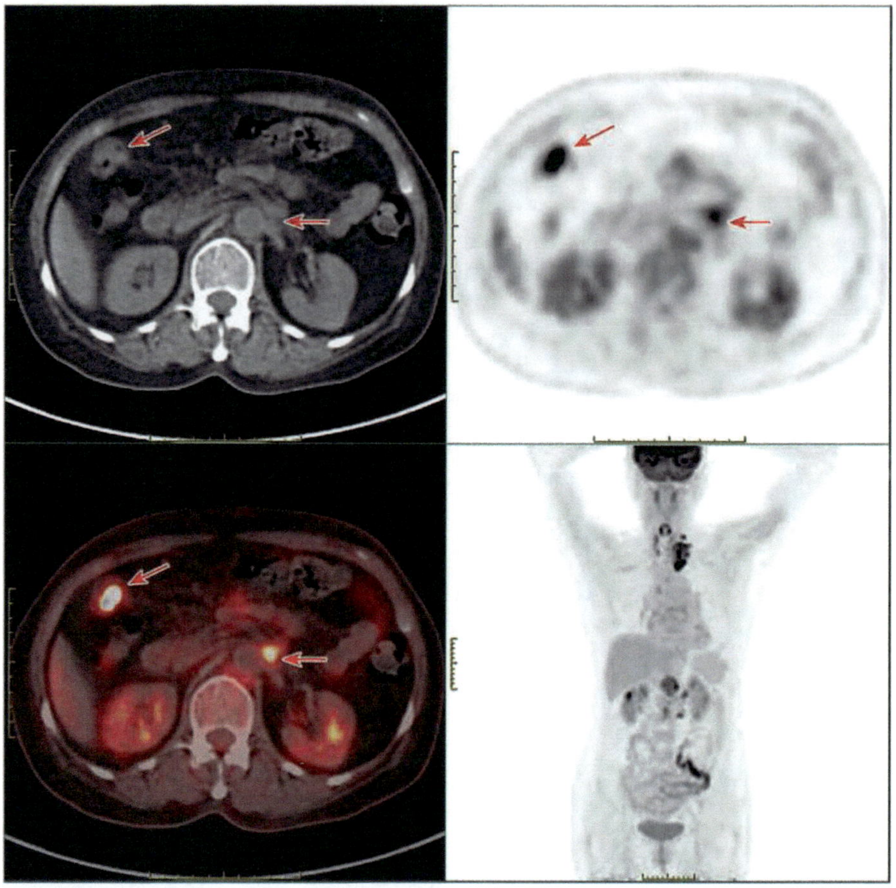

Fig. 20.27 Transverse colon cancer accompanied with retroperitoneal lymphatic metastasis. PET/CT images showed the thickening wall of the hepatic flexure of the colon with increased FDG uptake (SUVmax: 19.6), and FDG uptake increased in retroperitoneal enlarged lymph nodes (short diameter, 1.6 cm; SUVmax, 15.1) which was considered as malignant lesions of the colon with lymph node metastasis. Posterior colonoscopy confirmed transverse colon cancer

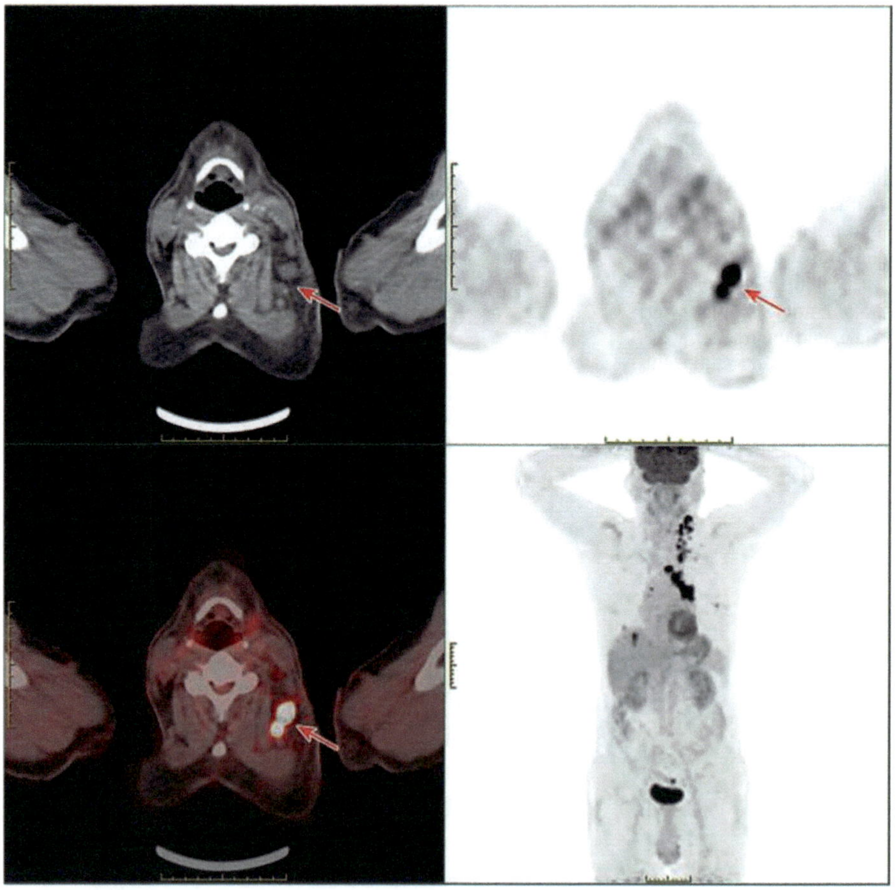

Fig. 20.28 Left lung cancer accompanied with lymph node metastasis in the left neck

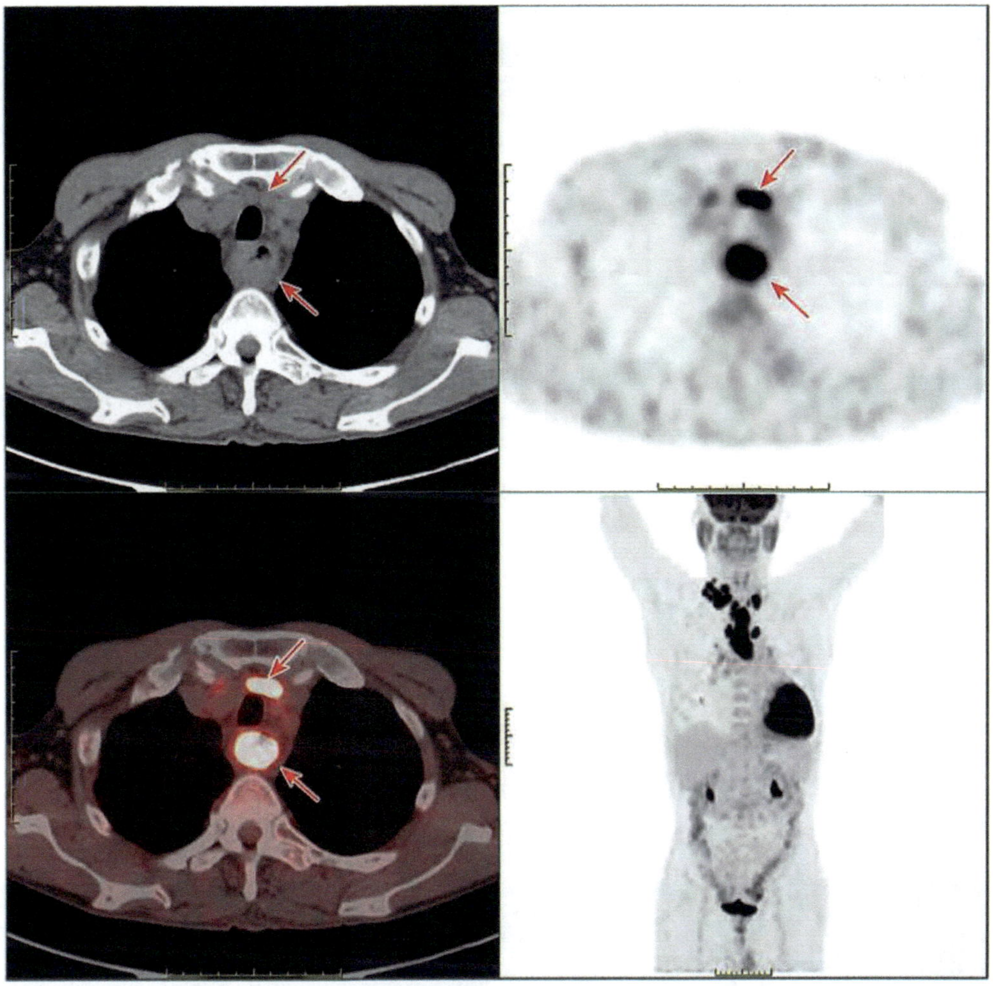

Fig. 20.29 Esophageal carcinoma accompanied with bilateral cervical lymphatic metastasis. PET/CT images showed thickening of the middle and upper esophageal wall with increased FDG uptake (the long diameter, 9.4 cm; SUVmax, 29.4) and increased FDG uptake in multiple lymph nodes in the upper mediastinum (region VII) (short diameter, 0.9 cm; SUVmax, 17.4), which were considered as malignant esophageal lesions accompanied with multiple lymphatic metastasis

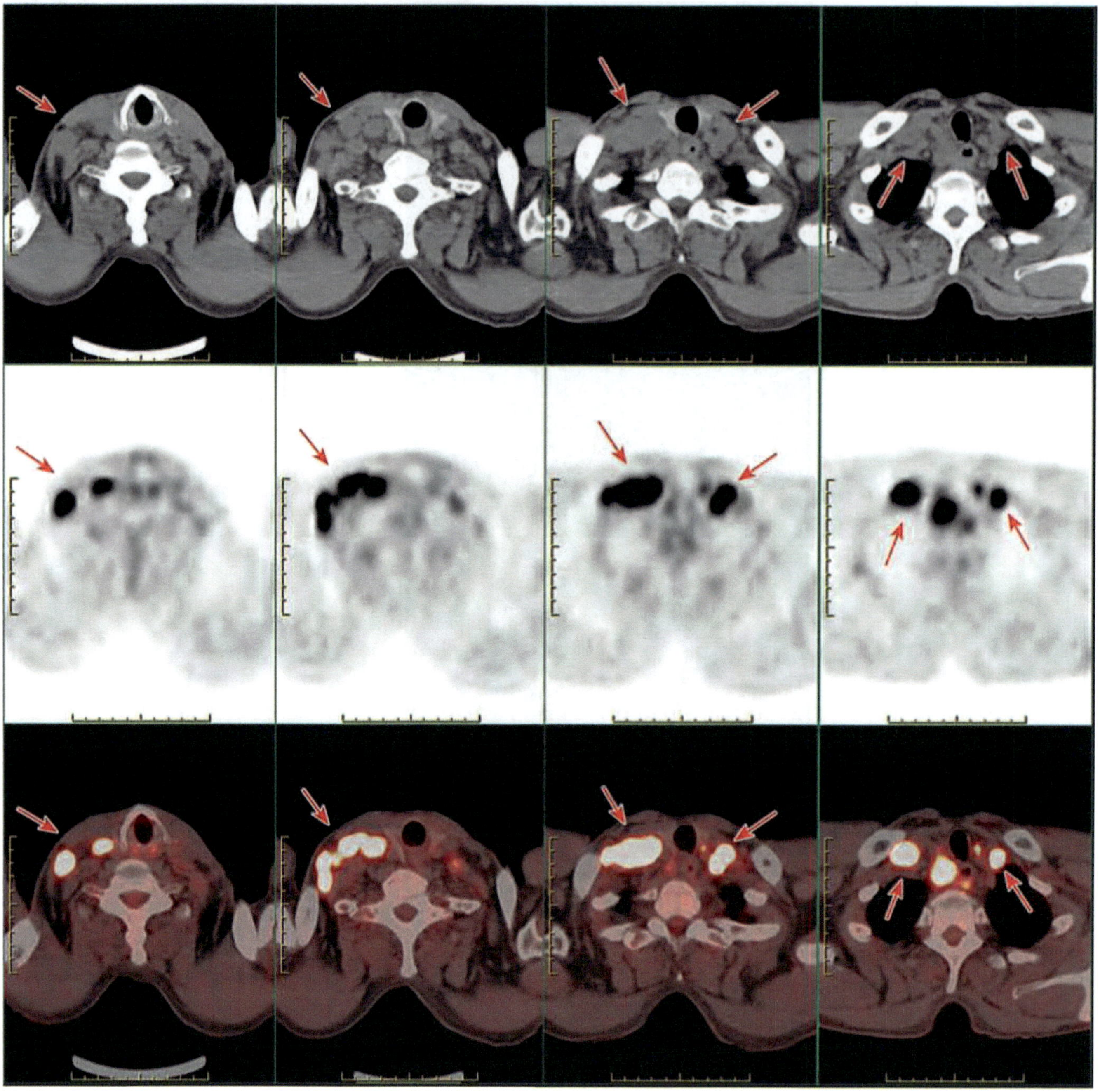

Fig. 20.30 Esophageal carcinoma accompanied with bilateral cervical lymphatic metastasis. PET/CT images showed increased FDG uptake, partial fusion, and absence of obvious necrosis in regions V–VI in both sides and clavicular region (2.3 cm in short diameter and 23.2 in SUVmax for the larger ones), which were considered as multiple metastatic lymph nodes

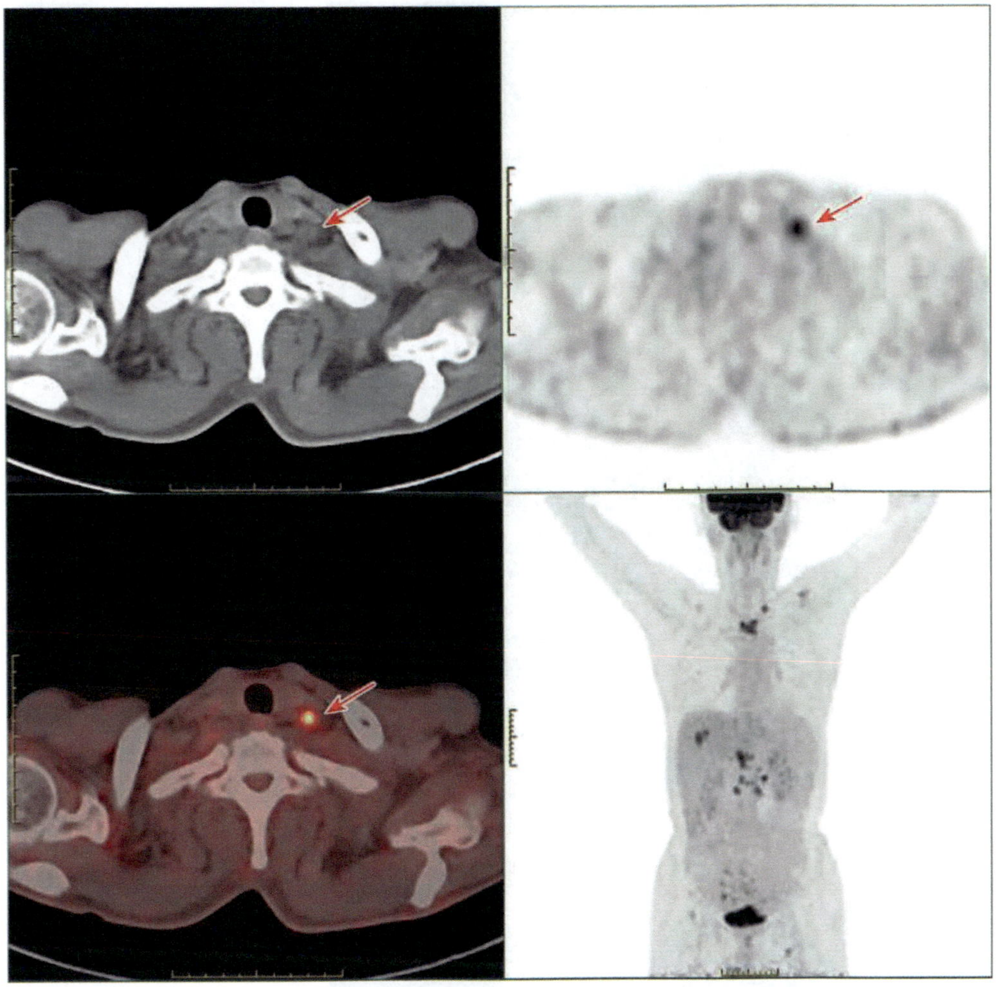

Fig. 20.31 Lymphatic metastasis in the left clavicle area after postoperative chemotherapy for gastric cancer. PET/CT images showed FDG uptake increased in lymph nodes in the left clavicle area (short diameter, 1.1 cm, and SUVmax, 7.4), which was considered as metastatic lymph nodes. MIP revealed multiple metastases to the retroperitoneal lymph nodes, liver, and bone (not shown on the sectional view)

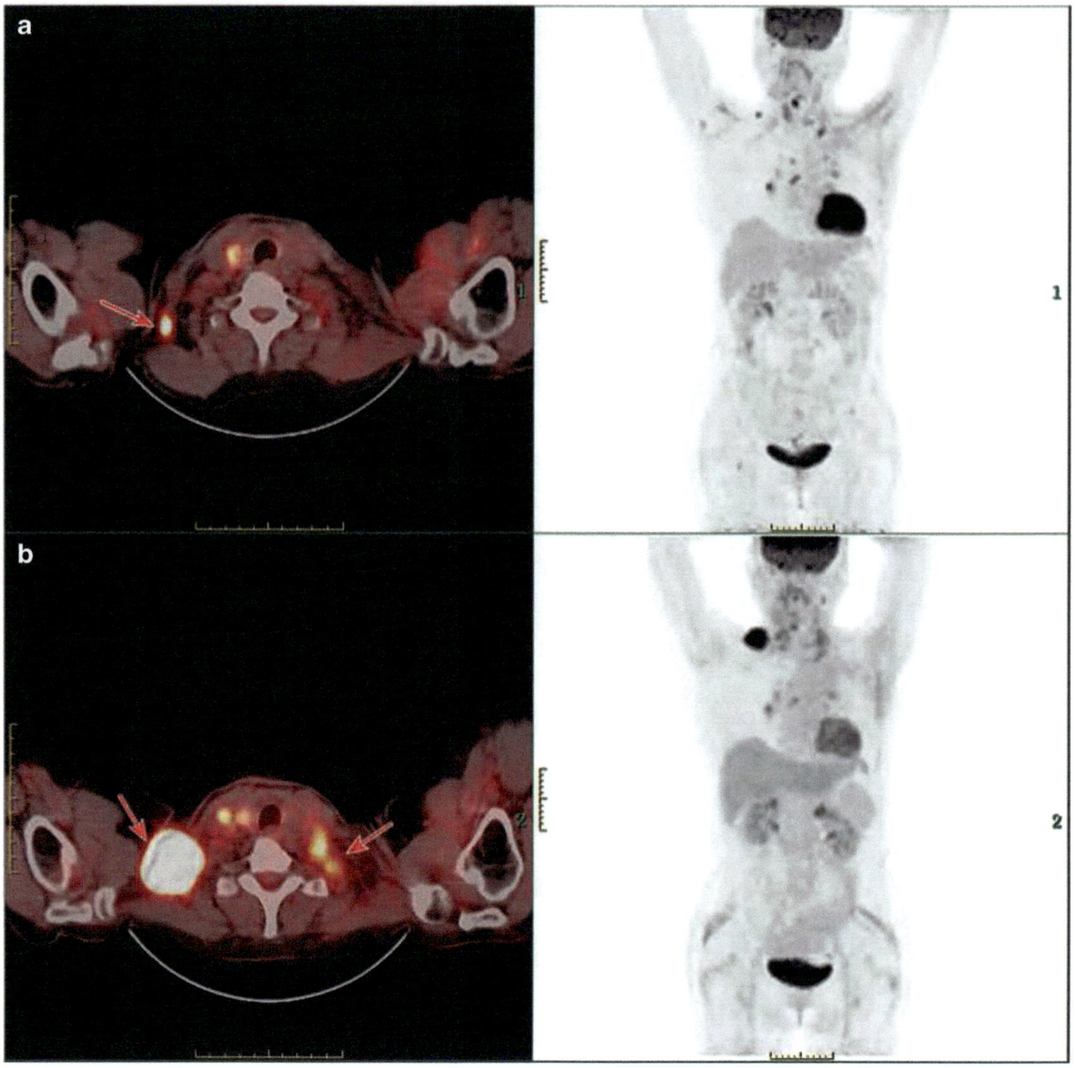

Fig. 20.32 Bilateral cervical lymphatic metastasis after surgery for left breast cancer. (**a**) PET/CT images showed FDG uptake (1.8 cm in short diameter and 7.2 in SUVmax) increased in lymph nodes in region V of the right neck, which was considered as metastatic lymph nodes, and chemotherapy combined with endocrine therapy was performed for the patient. (**b**) PET/CT reexamination after treatment showed that cervical lymph nodes were enlarged and the number increased compared with that before treatment. FDG uptake increased with partial fusion. The short diameter of lymph nodes in the right supraclavicular VB region was 3.2 cm, and SUVmax was 19.6, indicating the disease progression

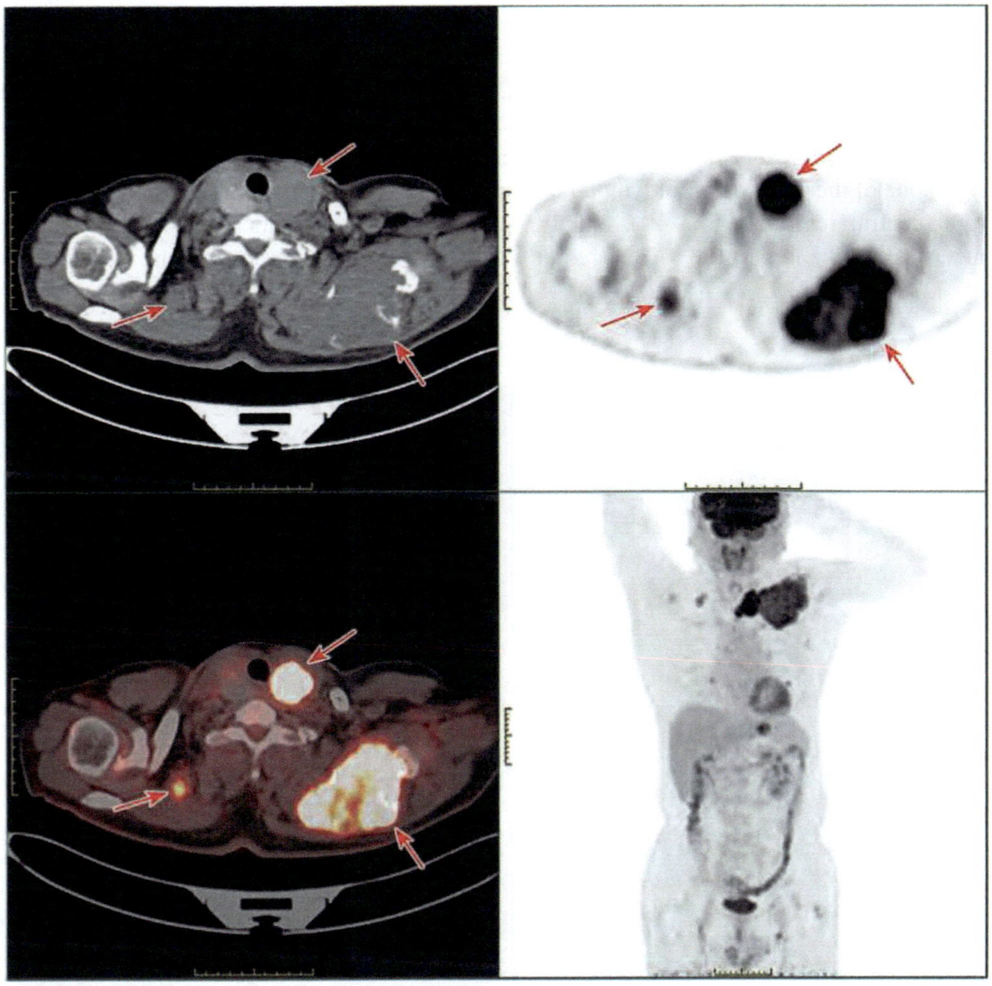

Fig. 20.33 Thyroid follicular carcinoma with extensive systemic metastases. PET/CT images showed low-density nodules in the left lobe of the thyroid with increased FDG uptake, longer diameter of 4.0 cm, and SUVmax of 16.1, which were considered as malignant lesions. FDG uptake (short diameter, 2.7 cm; SUVmax, 5.1) increased in enlarged lymph nodes in region V of the right neck, which was considered as metastatic lymph nodes. Bone destruction in the left scapula accompanied with increased FDG uptake in soft tissue mass (SUVmax was 10.0) was considered as bone metastasis

4 Rare Cases

The patient, a 51-year-old male, underwent PET/CT examination due to elevated CEA found in physical examination (Fig. 20.34). Surgical pathology: medullary carcinoma of the right lobe of the thyroid, 1/3 of lymph node metastasis in the right central region (region VI), and 0/5 of lymph node metastasis in the left central region (region VI).

5 Differential Diagnosis

The diseases that need to be differentiated from metastatic lymph nodes in the neck can be divided into two categories: (1) non-metastatic lymph node lesions, lymphoma, lymphatic tuberculosis, sarcoidosis, etc., and (2) non-lymphatic tumor in the neck, schwannoma, thyroglossal duct cyst, lymphangioma, etc.:

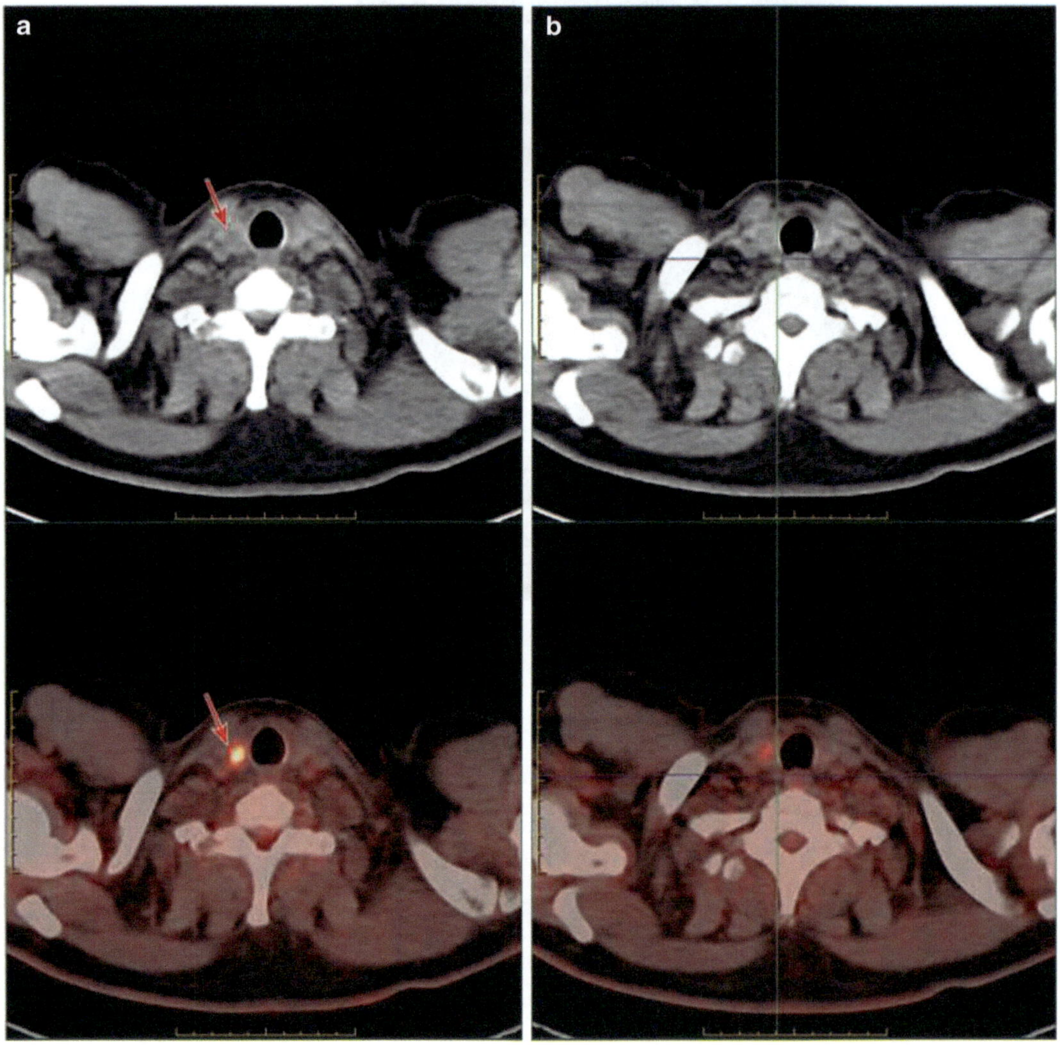

Fig. 20.34 Medullary thyroid carcinoma accompanied with lymphatic metastasis in the right central region. (**a**) A round low-density lesion in the right lobe of the thyroid (longer diameter, 1.0 cm; SUVmax, 5.4) was considered as malignant lesion. (**b**) No increase in FDG uptake was observed in lymph nodes in region VI of the right neck, with a short diameter of about 0.5 cm

1. Lymphoma: Lymphomas often involve cervical lymph nodes, which are typically manifested as multiple enlarged lymph nodes on both sides, with a diameter of 1–10 cm, characterized with uniform density, and slightly uniform enhancement on enhanced scan. In addition to inert lymphoma and some low-degree malignant lymphoma, most pathological types of lymphoma showed evident high uptake of ^{18}F-FDG. If the treatment is effective, the lesions can shrink and disappear, with possible decrease in central density (necrosis), decrease in uptake, or no uptake at all. It is also possible, but less common, for lymphomas to infiltrate beyond the capsule. According to histological studies, when lymphatic vessels are unobstructed and only blood supply is impaired, central necrosis of lymph nodes involved with lymphoma does not necessarily result. However, extensive central necrosis of lymph nodes can occur when the tumor invades the lymphatic sinuses, resulting in obstructed lymphatic reflux, which, at the same time, results in the compression or invasion of blood vessels of the lymphatic hilum. Patients may have irregular fever, emaciation, and other symptoms, and they may also present with enlargement of other lymph nodes, hepatosplenomegaly, and other manifestations. Diagnosis is mainly based on the pathology of lymph node biopsy. The imaging findings of neck lymphoma and metastatic tumor are similar, and it cannot be differentiated by PET/CT alone. Medical history and other clinical data should be combined (Figs. 20.35 and 20.36).
2. Lymph node tuberculosis: The global incidence of tuberculosis has increased in recent years, and TB infection among people with immunodeficiency is very common. Cervical lymph node is the most common site of extrapulmonary tuberculosis. Cervical lymph node tuberculosis is more common in adolescents and females. The pathological process of tuberculous lymphadenitis can be divided into four stages: (1) proliferative granuloma; (2) cheesy or liquefactive necrosis in lymph nodes with intact capsule; (3) destruction of lymph node envelope and mutual fusion, accompanied with perilymph node inflammation; and (4) cheesy material penetrates the surrounding soft tissue to form cold abscesses or sinus tract. The

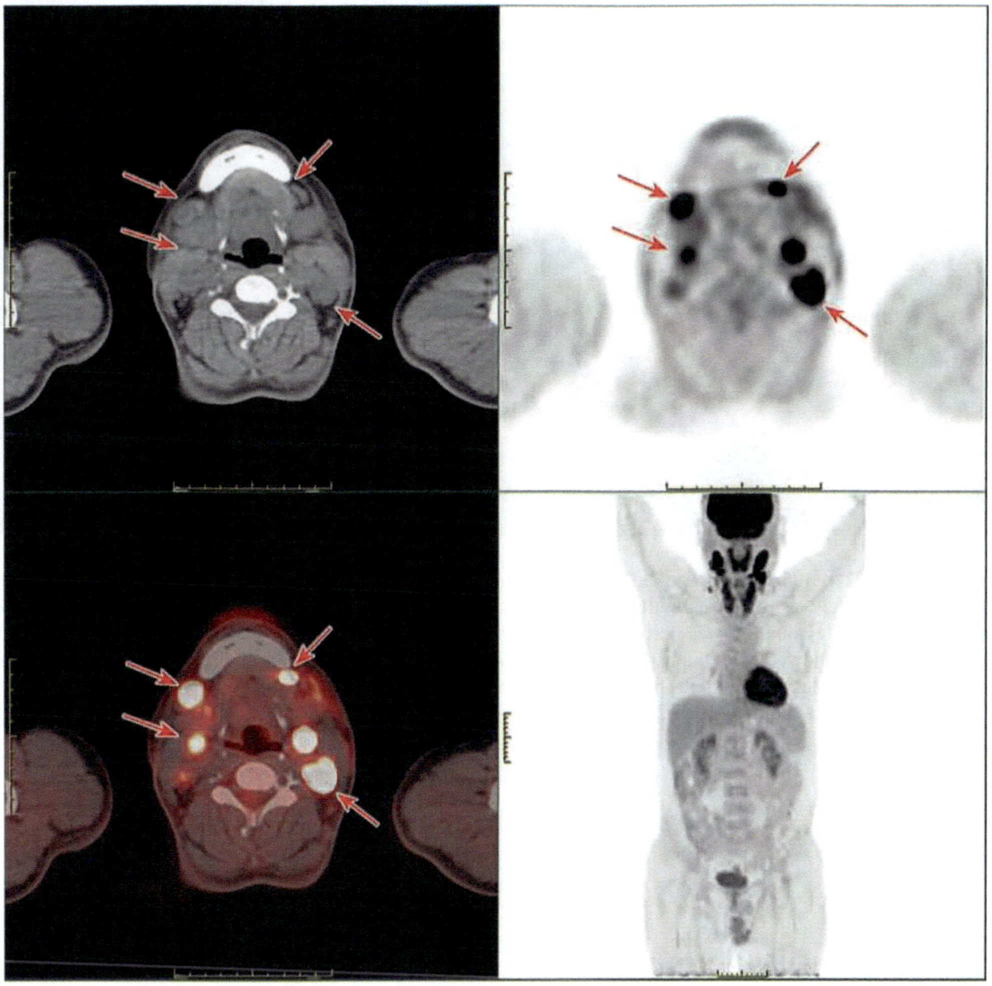

Fig. 20.35 Diffuse large B-cell lymphoma accompanied with cervical lymph node infiltration. The patient was a 49-year-old male with lymph node biopsy of the left submaxillary node showing diffuse large B-cell lymphoma. PET/CT evaluation was performed for the patient before chemotherapy. PET/CT images showed FDG uptake (short diameter, 2.4 cm; SUVmax, 29.7) increased in multiple enlarged lymph nodes in regions I–III of both sides of the neck, which was considered as lymphoma infiltration

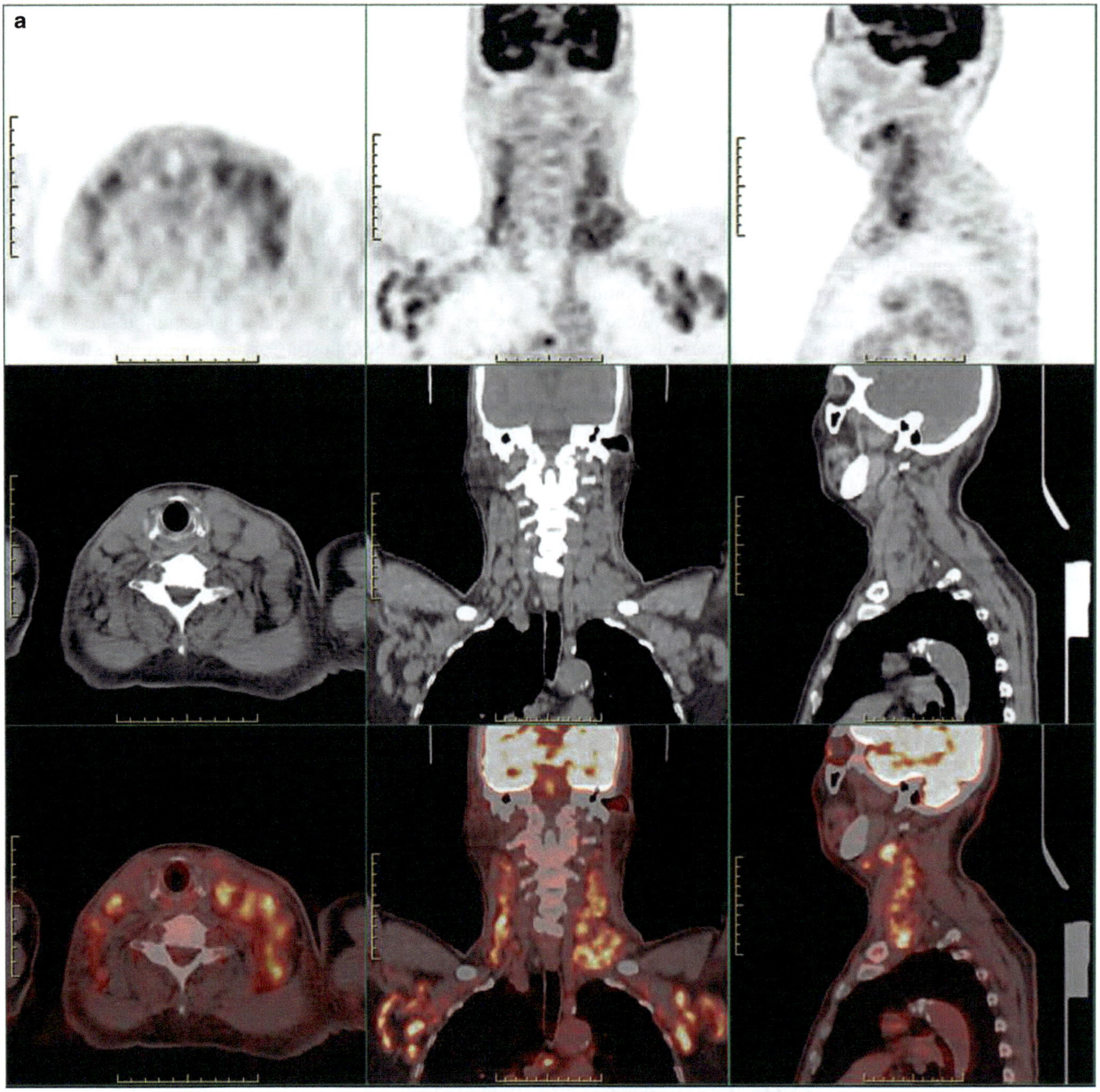

Fig. 20.36 T lymphoblastic leukemia/lymphoma. The patient, a 77-year-old male, was diagnosed with T lymphoblastic leukemia/lymphoma. PET/CT evaluation was performed before chemotherapy: (**a**) PET/CT images showed that regions I–V in both sides of the neck were full of lymph nodes of different sizes, accompanied with increased FDG uptake (short diameter, 0.3–2.2 cm; SUVmax, 2.6–6.9), which was considered as lymphoma infiltration. (**b**) PET/CT images showed that regions I–V on both sides were full of lymph nodes of different sizes accompanied with FDG uptake increasing in different degrees (short diameter of 0.3–2.2 cm, SUVmax of 2.6–6.9), which was considered as lymphoma infiltration

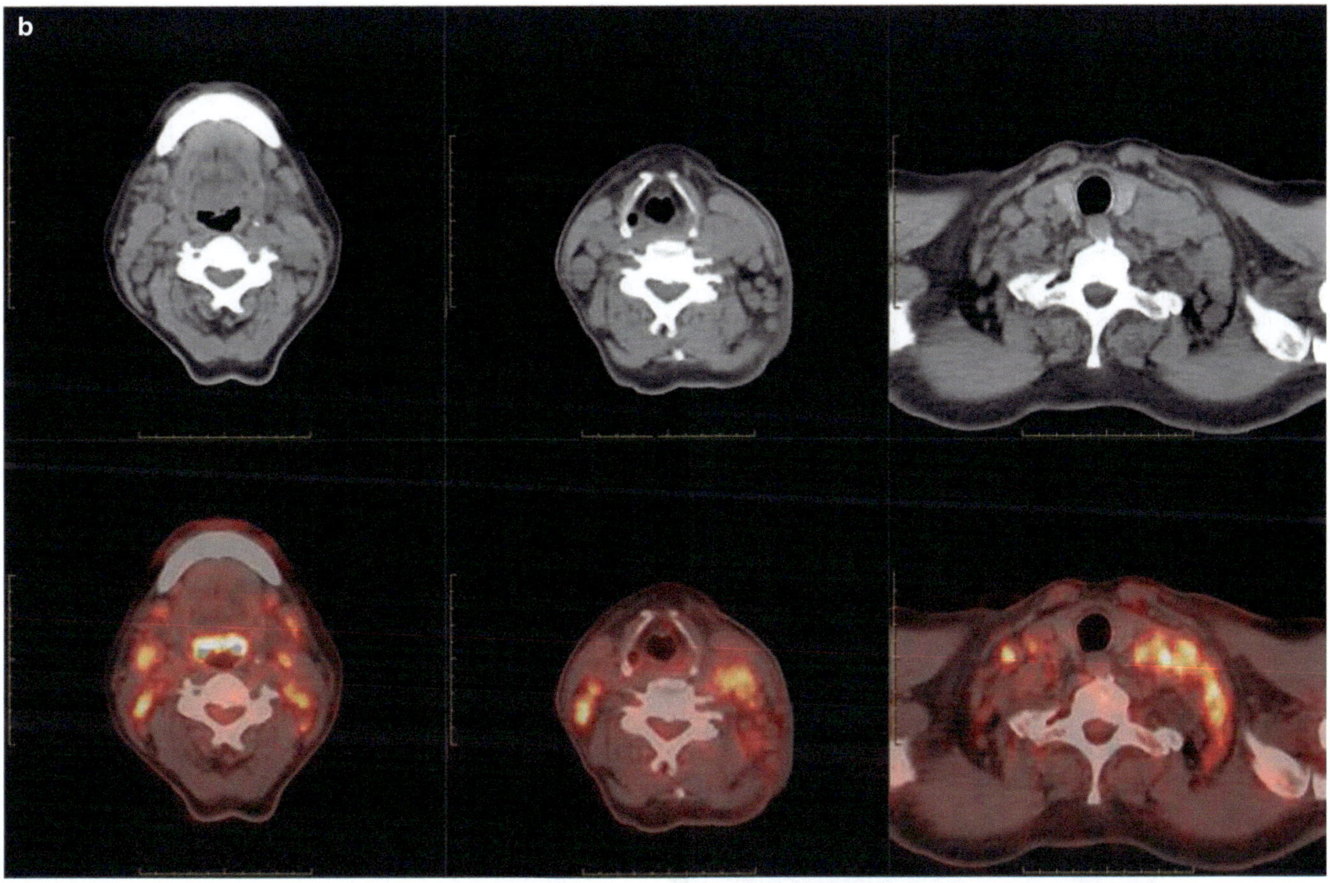

Fig. 20.36 (continued)

tuberculosis of the cervical lymph node in the second to fourth stages is common clinically, and the lesions in each stage often exist simultaneously.

Tuberculosis of the cervical lymph nodes is more likely to occur in lymph nodes of region IV, followed by region II and region V, often involving more than one region.

The typical imaging findings of tuberculosis of the cervical lymph nodes are basically consistent with the pathological changes, and the pathological changes at all stages are also common:

(a) Proliferative type, single or multiple lymph node enlargement with uniform density.
(b) Peripheral granulation tissue showed increased annular uptake and central cheesy or liquefactive necrosis, presenting a low-density area with decreased uptake or without uptake, where lesions can be fused to form flower ring.
(c) The surrounding area is grid-like when accompanied with inflammation, with unclear boundaries, and when it is surrounded by fibrous tissue, the boundaries are clear.
(d) Calcification is occasionally observed.

The metastatic sites of cervical lymph nodes of non-head and neck squamous cell carcinoma (lung cancer, gastric cancer, esophageal cancer, breast cancer, etc.) are similar to those of tuberculosis, but there are few peripheral inflammatory reactions. Metastatic lymph nodes of head and neck squamous cell carcinoma rarely occur in region IV or region V, but central necrosis and invasion of surrounding tissues can also occur, but fusion is rare (Figs. 20.37 and 20.38).

3. Sarcoidosis: Sarcoidosis is a multi-system non-caseous granulomatous lesion of unknown origin, which generally shows a benign process with self-limiting involvement in the lymph nodes, lungs, pleura, skin, bones, eyes, liver, spleen, parotid gland, tonsils, and other organs. Sarcoidosis is more common in women aged 20–40 years. It is a chronic disease with mild clinical symptoms.

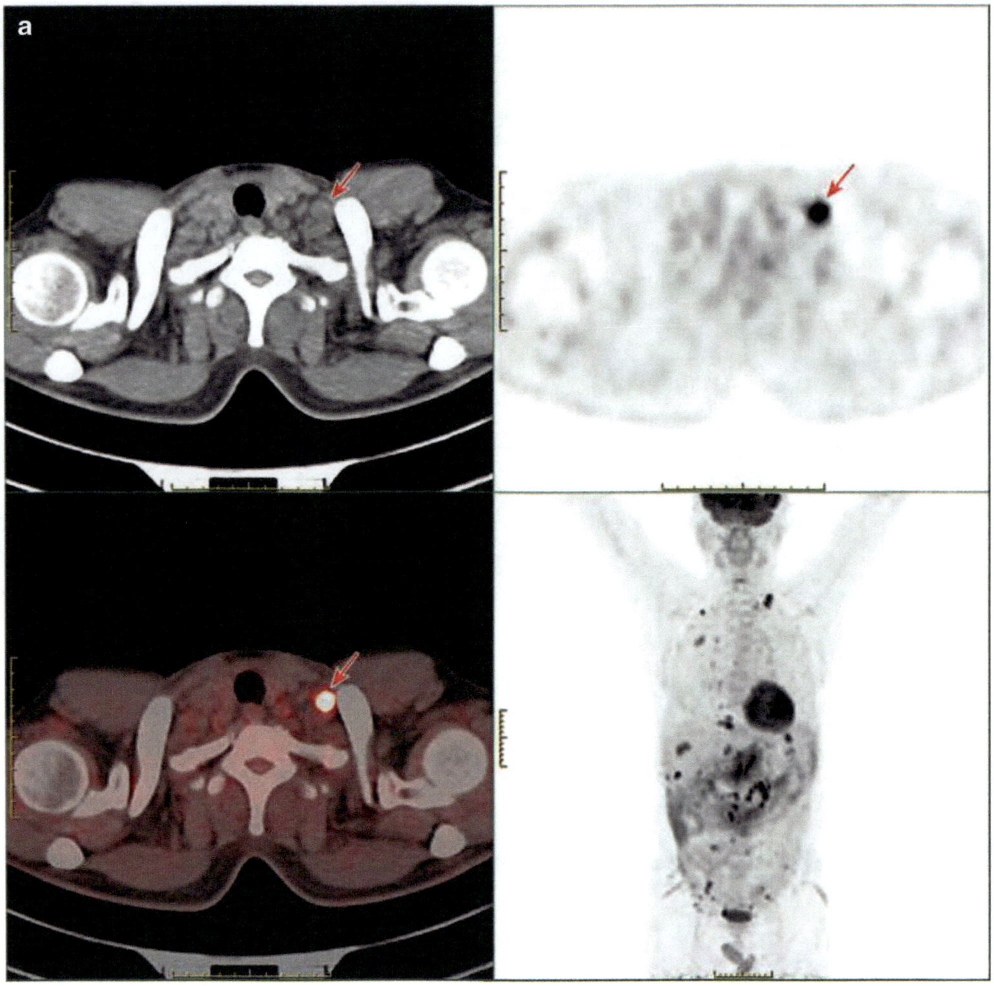

Fig. 20.37 Tuberculous involvement of cervical lymph nodes. The patient was a 61-year-old male with repeated abdominal distension. CT showed pleural and abdominal pelvic effusion and abdominal lymph node enlargement: (**a**) PET/CT images showed FDG uptake increased in enlarged lymph nodes in region V of the left neck (short diameter, 1.2 cm; SUVmax, 12.8). MIP showed FDG uptake increased in multiple abdominal and pelvic lymph nodes (not displayed). (**b**) PET/CT images showed FDG uptake increased in multiple lymph nodes in the regions IV–VI of the left neck and the right clavicle area (the short diameter was 1.2 cm and the SUVmax 12.8 in the larger group). A biopsy of a lymph node in the left neck indicated granulomatous inflammation (tuberculosis)

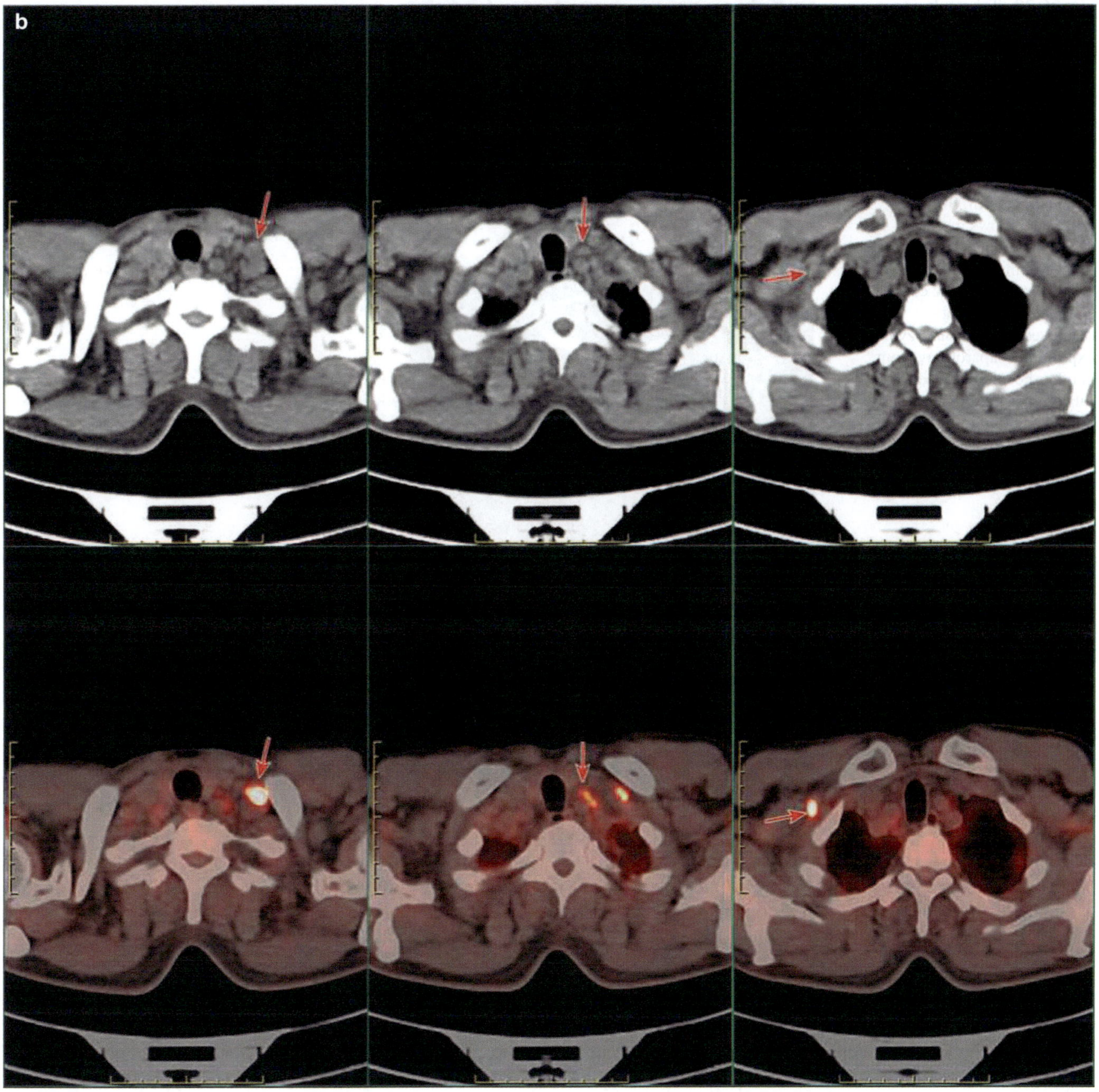

Fig. 20.37 (continued)

Bilateral cervical lymph nodes are enlarged after involvement, most of which are symmetrical in distribution, uniform in density, rarely fused with each other, and rare in central necrosis (Fig. 20.39).

4. Suppurative lymphadenitis: It usually has typical clinical symptoms of infection, namely, "redness, swelling, fever, and pain," accompanied by changes in inflammatory indicators; images are characterized with low density in the central abscess cavity with reduced or no uptake, increased annular uptake at the margin, and surrounding inflammatory edema, some of which resembles tuberculosis (Figs. 20.40 and 20.41).
5. Schwannoma: Schwannoma is a benign tumor originating from the nerve sheath cells. It is commonly found in the carotid artery space and comes from the vagus, hypoglossal nerve trunk, and cervical sympathetic plexus. It is more likely to occur among population of 30–40 years old, and the disease course is longer. CT images show isolated soft tissue mass in the carotid space, usually round and well-defined. Small tumors present uniform

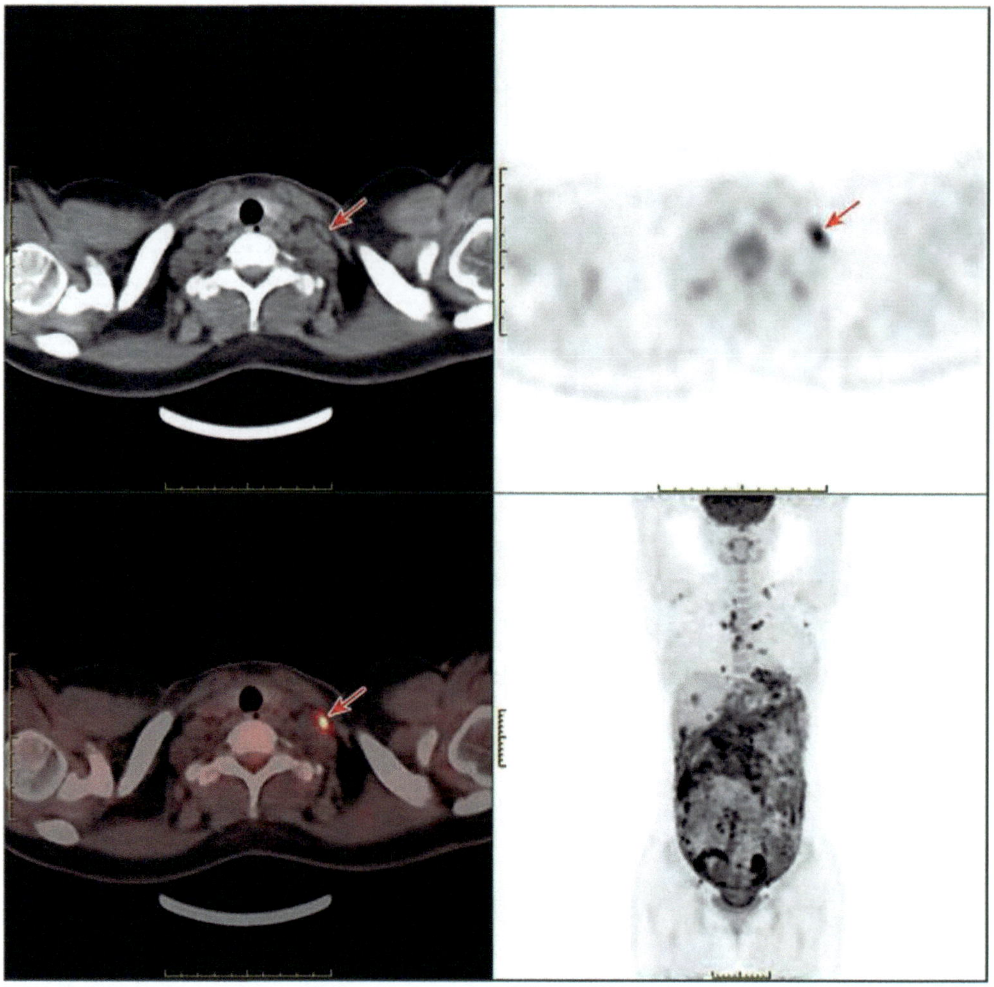

Fig. 20.38 Tuberculosis involving cervical lymph nodes. The female patient, 26 years old, presented with abdominal effusion 4 months after delivery. PET/CT images showed FDG uptake increased in the lymph nodes in region V of the left neck (short diameter, 0.4 cm; SUVmax, 6.9). MIP shows multiple lesions with increased FDG uptake in the mediastinum, abdominal and pelvic cavity, and peritoneum (not displayed). The pathology of exploratory laparotomy from another hospital proved to be tuberculosis, which was improved after anti-tuberculosis treatment

density, while large tumors can show central necrosis and cystic degeneration, and can push the internal and external carotid artery forward (Figs. 20.42 and 20.43).

6. Lymphangioma: Lymphangioma belongs to congenital lymphatic malformation, which is more common in children. It is painless, grows slowly, and is easy to be complicated with bleeding and infection. It occurs most often in the posterior cervical triangle and can occur in adults in the sublingual, submaxillary, parotid, and parapharyngeal spaces and can also extend to the mediastinum. Lymphangioma can be divided into three pathological subtypes: simple, capillary, and spongy. Simple lymphangioma is a single chamber and can be completely resected. The remaining two types can be infiltrated growth, which are not easy to be completely resected. Imaging findings are single or multi-locular thin-walled cystic masses with watery density inside, but with increased density and a liquid-liquid plane if bleeding occurs.
7. Others:
   (a) HIV infection: It is characterized with extensive lymph node enlargement on both sides of the neck, some of which are lymph node reactive hyperplasia with relatively uniform density; some of them are caused by HIV infection combined with Kaposi's sarcoma and lymphoma, among which the enlarged lymph nodes of Kaposi's sarcoma show characteristic high density.

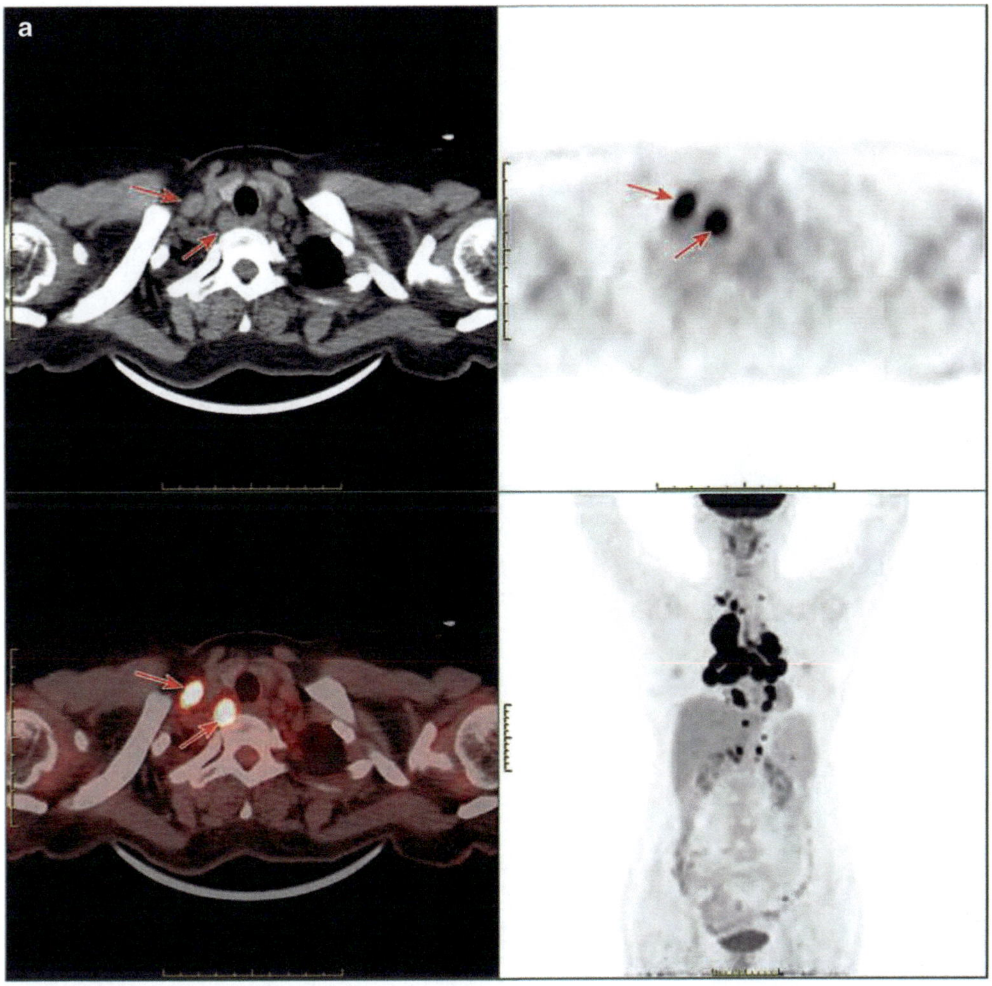

Fig. 20.39 Sarcoidosis involving cervical lymph nodes. PET/CT examination was performed on a 57-year-old female patient due to multiple enlarged lymph nodes in the mediastinum: (**a**) PET/CT images showed FDG uptake increased in region IV and region VI of the right neck (1.1 cm in short diameter and 14.1 in SUVmax for larger ones); MIP showed multiple lesions with increased FDG uptake in the mediastinum and in the hilum of both lungs and retroperitoneum (not shown on the CT images). (**b**) PET/CT images showed FDG uptake increased in regions V–VI of the right neck and region V of the left neck with multiple enlarged lymph nodes (1.1 cm in short diameter and 14.1 in SUVmax). Mediastinoscopy biopsy showed multiple focal granulomatous lesions (sarcoidosis) in the right subclavicular, right superior mediastinal, and inferior mediastinal lymph nodes

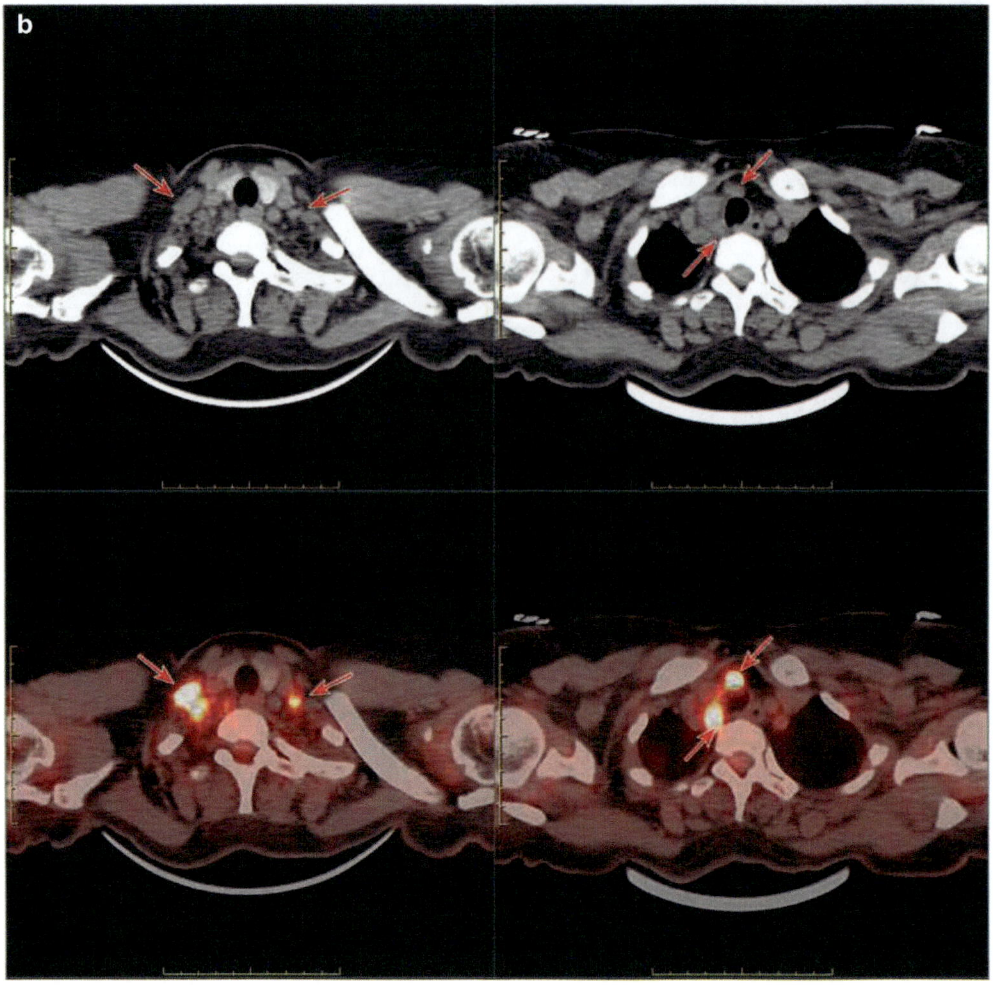

Fig. 20.39 (continued)

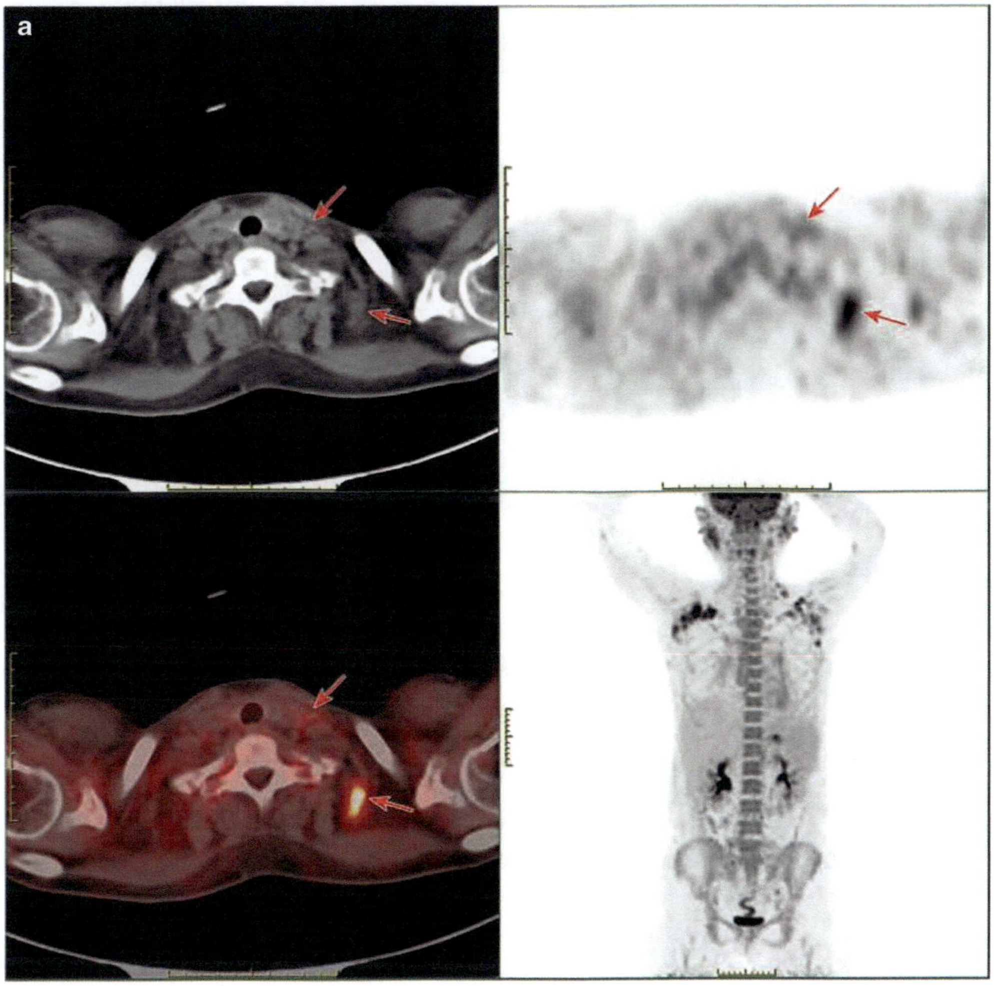

Fig. 20.40 Necrotizing lymphadenitis of the neck. The patient was a 27-year-old female with fever to be determined: (**a**) PET/CT images showed multiple lymph nodes in regions IV and V of the left neck with increased FDG uptake (short diameter, 0.4–0.8 cm; SUVmax, 2.6–8.3). There were many lymph nodes with different sizes and different FDG uptakes. MIP images showed FDG uptake increased in multiple lymph nodes in the bilateral parotid region, axilla, and abdomen and pelvis (not shown on the CT image). (**b**) PET/CT images showed FDG uptake increased in multiple lymph nodes in regions I–V of the right parotid gland and both sides of the neck (short diameter, 0.4–0.8 cm; SUVmax, 2.6–8.3). There were many lymph nodes with different sizes and different FDG uptakes. Necrotizing lymphadenitis was pathologically diagnosed by two biopsies of cervical lymph nodes, which was improved after anti-inflammatory treatment

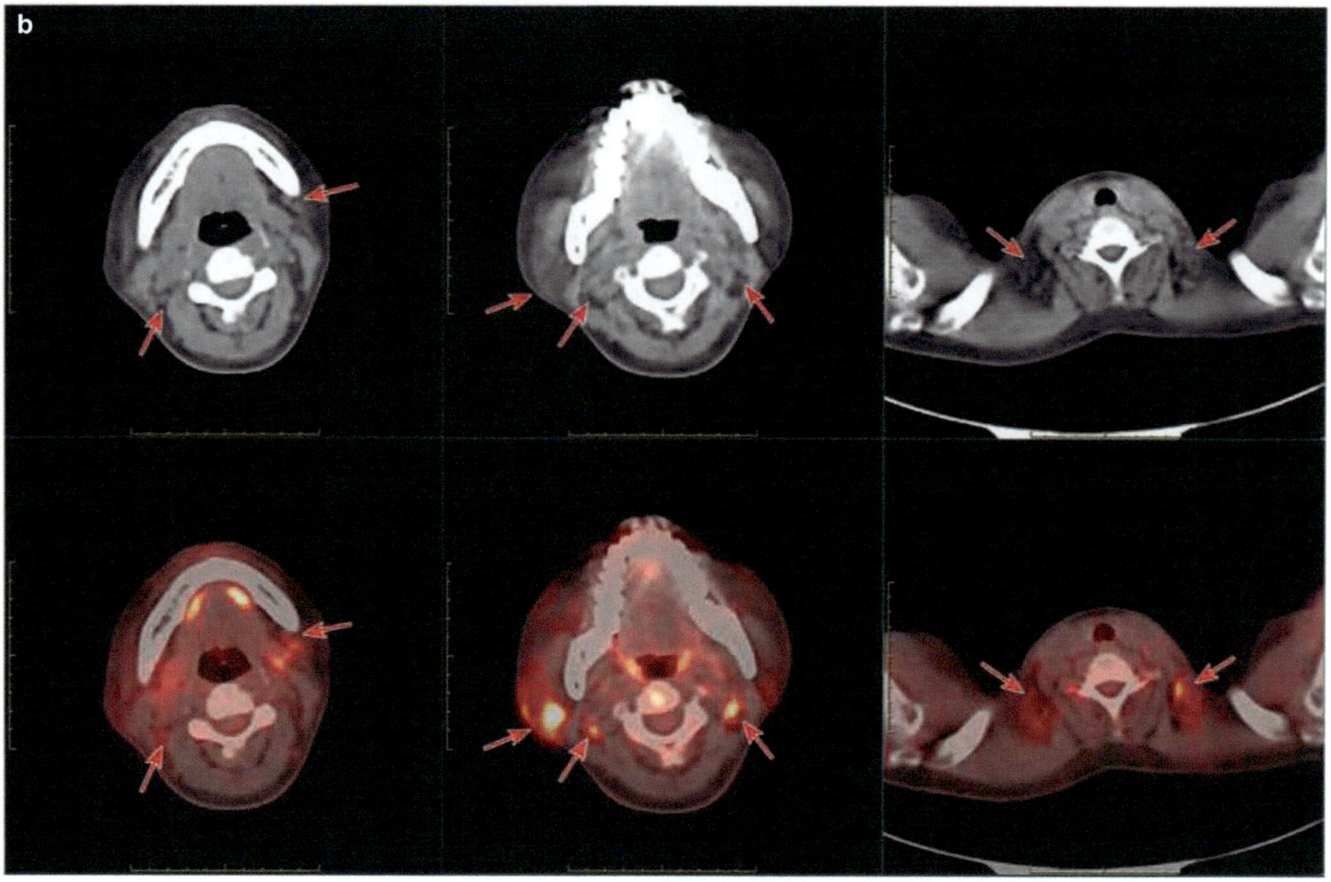

Fig. 20.40 (continued)

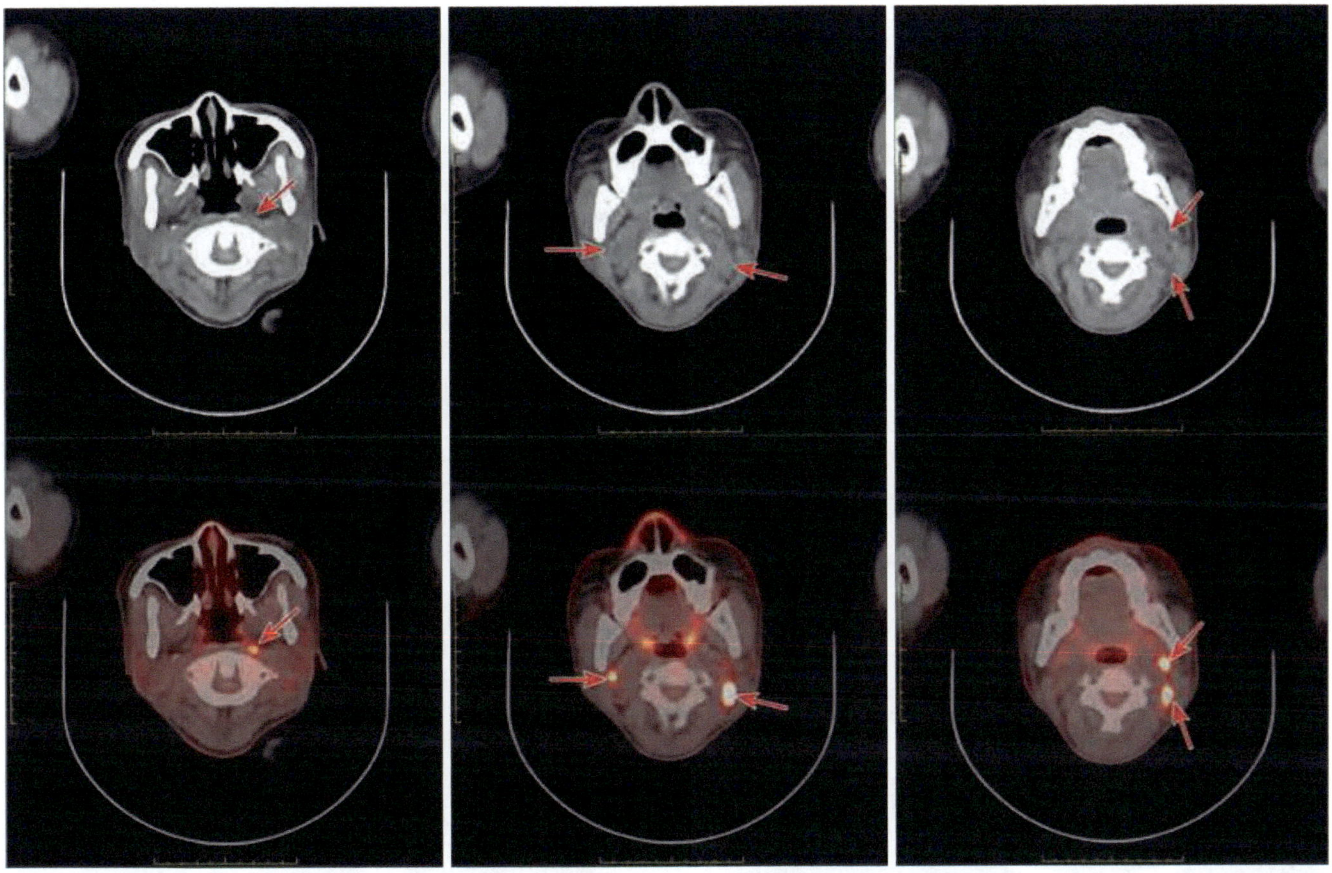

Fig. 20.41 Inflammatory hyperplasia of cervical lymph nodes. The patient, a 22-year-old female, presented with fever to be examined. PET/CT images showed FDG uptake (short diameter 0.4–1.0 cm, SUVmax 2.6–21.8) increased in multiple lymph nodes in the left parapharyngeal space and bilateral neck mouth area, and the lymph nodes were different in sizes and levels of FDG uptake. The biopsy pathology of cervical lymph nodes indicated proliferative lesion of lymph nodes, which was improved after anti-inflammatory treatment

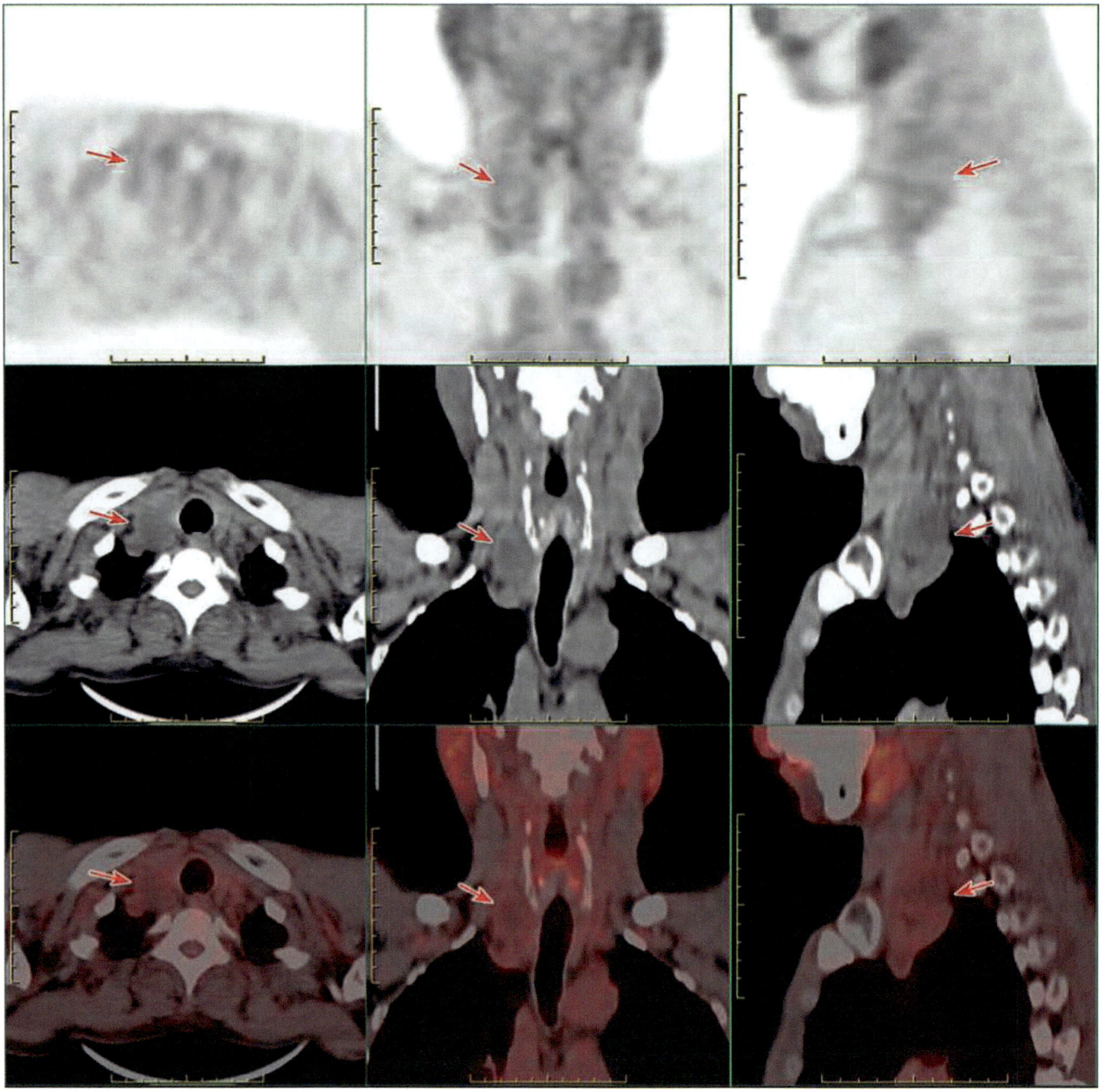

Fig. 20.42 Schwannoma of the neck. The patient, a 59-year-old male, developed a mass in his right neck. PET/CT images showed a rounded low-density shadow in the right clavicle (behind the right lobe of the thyroid), with a clear boundary and a size of about 3.4 cm × 2.3 cm. The CT value was 24 HU. FDG uptake was close to the background of the surrounding muscle tissues (SUVmax was 2.1), and the FDG uptake in the central area was slightly lower than that in the background (SUVmax was 1.5). Surgery confirmed it was a right cervical vagus schwannoma

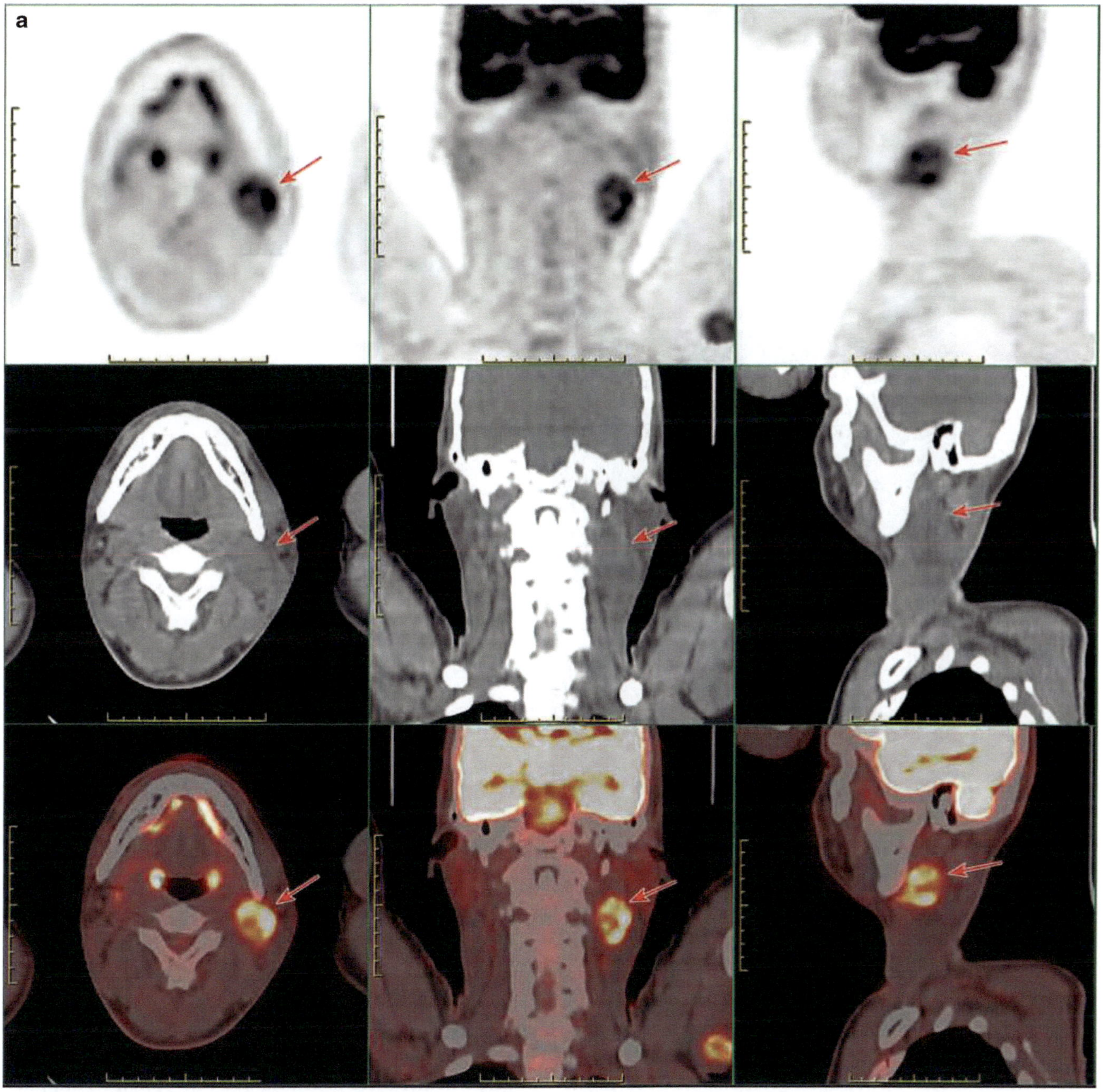

Fig. 20.43 Cervical schwannoma (multiple). The patient, a 25-year-old male, was found with a painless mass in the left neck: (**a**) PET/CT images showed increased metabolism inhomogeneity of the left neck with circular low-density shadow (about 3.9 cm × 2.5 cm in size, with CT value of 27HU and SUVmax of 7.8); the pathology of left cervical mass resection showed schwannoma with hemorrhage and cystic changes. (**b**) PET/CT images showed FDG uptake increased (size, 2.4 cm × 2.3 cm; CT value, 36HU; SUVmax, 5.8) in the right clavicle. MIP images showed multiple abnormal increased FDG uptake in the left neck, left armpit, double upper arm, chest, and abdomen basin. The pathology of mass resection of the left neck showed schwannoma

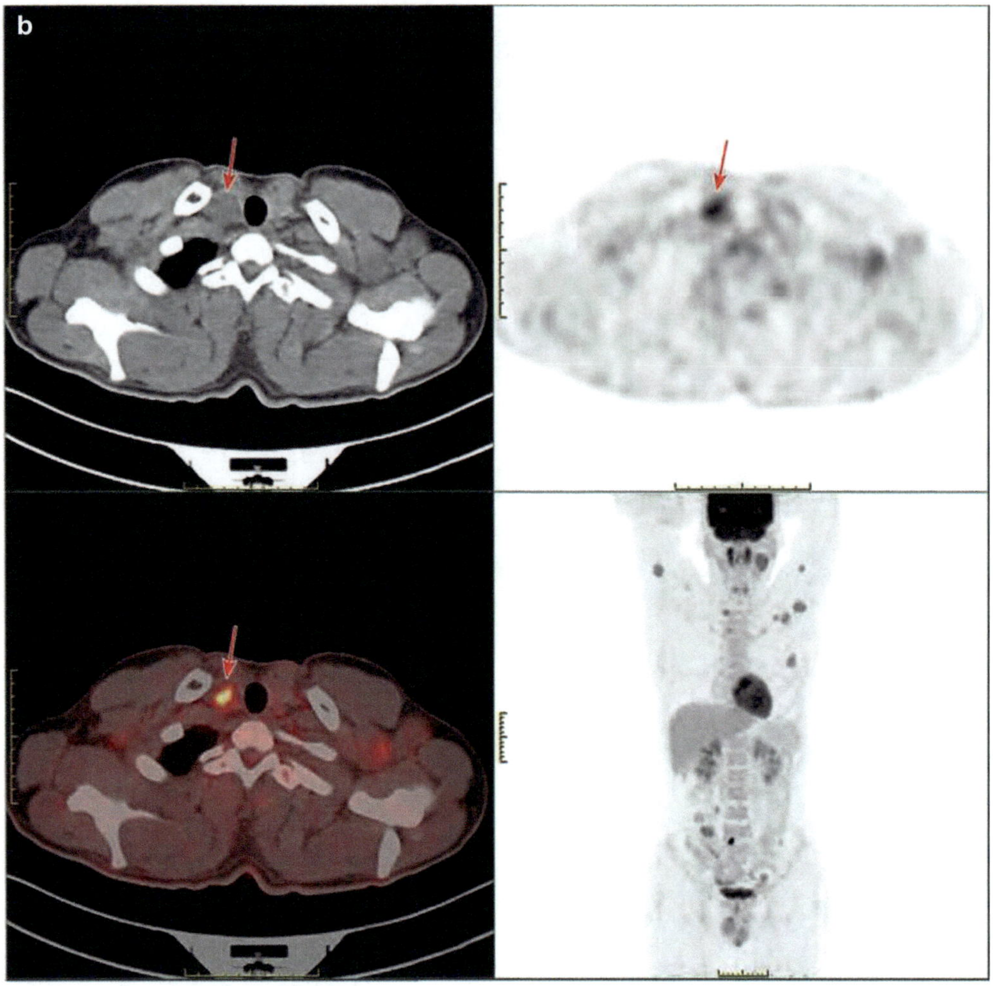

Fig. 20.43 (continued)

(b) Cat-scratch fever: It is self-limiting due to infection by gram-negative bartonella. It is characterized with enlargement of lymph nodes, extensive surrounding edema, and non-uniformed enhancement of lymph nodes, and there may be central necrosis.
(c) Hyperplasia of giant lymph node: It is more common in the mediastinum, and it can also be seen in the neck, with enlarged lymph nodes characterized with mean changes in density.
(d) Thyrolingual cyst: A non-degenerated cyst forms at the base of the tongue at the upper end of a thyroglossal canal in the embryonic stage, usually located near the hyoid bone, and completely or partially opens to form a leaky canal. Imaging findings show a round cystic mass in the anterior cervical middle, with clear boundaries, smooth edges, thin walls, and uniform fluid density, whose posterior edge is seen with handle-like protuberance, extending into the glossoepigolttic ligaments and the posterior thyroid cartilage.

6 Summary

The detection of metastatic lymph nodes in the neck by PET/CT is of great clinical significance for clinical staging, decision-making in treatment, and prognosis assessment. Based on the characteristics such as the size of the lymph nodes; whether there is central necrosis or not; its morphology, quantity, presence, and absence of external invasion; and whether there is a high ^{18}F-FDG uptake, it is possible to undertake the diagnosis of metastasis lymph nodes. However, there are also some of the metastasis lymph nodes only with mild intake or without intake. Therefore, the level of uptake of ^{18}F-FDG cannot be used as a basis for the identification of metastatic lymph nodes, and it needs to be determined in close combination with other clinical information. In practice, it is necessary to make differential diagnosis among inflammatory lymph node, lymphoma, tuberculosis, and other lymph node lesions.

GPSR Compliance

The European Union's (EU) General Product Safety Regulation (GPSR) is a set of rules that requires consumer products to be safe and our obligations to ensure this.

If you have any concerns about our products, you can contact us on ProductSafety@springernature.com

In case Publisher is established outside the EU, the EU authorized representative is:

Springer Nature Customer Service Center GmbH
Europaplatz 3
69115 Heidelberg, Germany

Batch number: 10731524

Printed by Printforce, the Netherlands